Human Enterovirus Infections

Human Enterovirus Infections

Edited by

Harley A. Rotbart

Departments of Pediatrics and Microbiology
Infectious Diseases and Epidemiology Sections
University of Colorado Health Sciences Center
Denver, Colorado

ASM Press • Washington, D.C.

Copyright © 1995 American Society for Microbiology
1325 Massachusetts Ave., N.W.
Washington, DC 20005

Library of Congress Cataloging-in-Publication Data

Human enterovirus infections/edited by Harley A. Rotbart.
   p. cm.
   Includes index.
   ISBN 1-55581-092-6
   1. Enterovirus diseases. I. Rotbart, Harley A.
   [DNLM: 1. Enterovirus Infections. WC 500 H9185 1995]
RC114.55.H85   1995
616'.0194—dc20
DNLM/DLC   94-39792
for Library of Congress   CIP

All Rights Reserved
Printed in the United States of America

Cover photos: (Top left) Egyptian stele (c. 1500 B.C.) depicting the priest Ruma, afflicted with paralytic poliomyelitis. Note the withered leg, high arched foot, and cane. Photo courtesy of the NY Carlsberg Glyptotek, Copenhagen. (Bottom) Ribbon diagram showing the binding of a candidate anti-enteroviral compound to the VP1 pocket of a human picornavirus (for details, see chapter 18). Photo courtesy of Dr. Edward Arnold, Center for Advanced Biotechnology and Medicine, Rutgers University.

*To my wife, Sara,
and our kids,
Matthew, Emily, and Samuel,
who fill our lives with infectious smiles, contagious laughter,
and pandemic love*

*And to my mom,
who has her own germ theory but never published it*

CONTENTS

Contributors ix
Preface xiii
Acknowledgments xvi

I   SCIENTIFIC PRINCIPLES

1. Epidemiology
David M. Morens and Mark A. Pallansch
3

2. Enterovirus Genetics
Christopher U. T. Hellen and Eckard Wimmer
25

3. Early Events in Infection: Receptor Binding and Cell Entry
Vincent R. Racaniello
73

4. Viral RNA Synthesis
Kyle L. Johnson and Peter Sarnow
95

5. Translation and Host Cell Shutoff
Aurelia A. Haller and Bert L. Semler
113

6. Cell Biology of Enterovirus Infection
Andreas Schlegel and Karla Kirkegaard
135

7. Enterovirus Structure and Assembly
Christopher U. T. Hellen and Eckard Wimmer
155

8. Host Immune Responses to Enterovirus Infections
Steven Tracy, Nora M. Chapman, Ronald J. Rubocki, and Melinda A. Beck
175

II CLINICAL MANIFESTATIONS

9. Poliomyelitis and Poliovirus Immunization
John F. Modlin
195

10. Perinatal Enterovirus Infections
Mark J. Abzug
221

11. Nonpolio Enteroviruses and the Febrile Infant
Ron Dagan and Marilyn A. Menegus
239

12. Respiratory Infections
Tasnee Chonmaitree and Linda Mann
255

13. Meningitis and Encephalitis
Harley A. Rotbart
271

14. Enteroviral Myocarditis and Dilated Cardiomyopathy: a Review of Clinical and Experimental Studies
Tamara A. Martino, Peter Liu, Martin Petric, and Michael J. Sole
291

15. The Possible Role of Enteroviruses in Diabetes Mellitus
Marian Rewers and Mark Atkinson
353

16. Enteroviruses and Human Neuromuscular Diseases
Marinos C. Dalakas
387

III DIAGNOSIS AND TREATMENT

17. Laboratory Diagnosis of Enteroviral Infections
Harley A. Rotbart and José R. Romero
401

18. Development of Antiviral Agents for Picornavirus Infections
John O'Connell, Randi Albin, Deborah Blum, Paul Grint, and Jerome Schwartz
419

Index
435

CONTRIBUTORS

Mark J. Abzug
Department of Pediatrics, Section of Infectious Diseases, University of Colorado School of Medicine, and The Children's Hospital, Denver, Colorado 80218

Randi Albin
Department of Antiviral Chemotherapy, Schering-Plough Research Institute, Kenilworth, New Jersey 07033

Mark Atkinson
Department of Pathology, University of Florida, Gainesville, Florida 32610

Melinda A. Beck
FPG Child Development Center, Department of Pediatrics, University of North Carolina at Chapel Hill, Chapel Hill, North Carolina 27599-8180

Deborah Blum
Anti-Infectives Clinical Research, Schering-Plough Research Institute, Kenilworth, New Jersey 07033

Nora M. Chapman
Department of Pathology and Microbiology, University of Nebraska Medical Center, Omaha, Nebraska 68198-6495

Tasnee Chonmaitree
Pediatric Infectious Diseases Division, University of Texas Medical Branch, The Children's Hospital, Galveston, Texas 77555-0371

Ron Dagan
Pediatric Infectious Disease Unit, Soroka University Medical Center, and Faculty of Health Sciences, Ben-Gurion University of the Negev, Beer-Sheva, Israel

Marinos C. Dalakas
Neuromuscular Diseases Section, Medical Neurology Branch, National Institute of Neurological Disorders and Stroke, National Institutes of Health, Bethesda, Maryland 20892-1428

Paul Grint
Anti-Infectives Clinical Research, Schering-Plough Research Institute,
Kenilworth, New Jersey 07033

Aurelia A. Haller
Department of Microbiology and Molecular Genetics, College of Medicine,
University of California, Irvine, California 97217

Christopher U. T. Hellen
Department of Microbiology and Immunology, State University of New York Health
Sciences Center at Brooklyn, Brooklyn, New York 11203-2098

Kyle L. Johnson
Department of Biochemistry and Molecular Genetics, The University of Alabama at
Birmingham, Birmingham, Alabama 35294-0005

Karla Kirkegaard
Department of Molecular, Cellular, and Developmental Biology, Howard Hughes
Medical Institute, University of Colorado, Boulder, Colorado 80309

Peter Liu
The Center for Cardiovascular Research, The Toronto Hospital,
Toronto, Ontario M5G 2C4, Canada

Linda Mann
Department of Pathology, Clinical Microbiology Division, University of Texas
Medical Branch, Galveston, Texas 77555-0743

Tamara A. Martino
The Center for Cardiovascular Research, The Toronto Hospital,
Toronto, Ontario M5G 2C4, Canada

Marilyn A. Menegus
Department of Microbiology and Immunology, University of Rochester
Medical Center, Rochester, New York 14642

John F. Modlin
Departments of Pediatrics and Medicine, Dartmouth Medical School,
Dartmouth-Hitchcock Medical Center, Lebanon, New Hampshire 03756

David M. Morens
Epidemiology Section, School of Public Health, and Department of Tropical
Medicine, School of Medicine, University of Hawaii, Honolulu Hawaii 96822

John O'Connell
Department of Antiviral Chemotherapy, Schering-Plough Research Institute,
Kenilworth, New Jersey 07033

Mark A. Pallansch
Enterovirus Section, Respiratory and Enteric Viruses Branch, Division of Viral and
Rickettsial Diseases, National Center for Infectious Diseases, Centers for Disease
Control and Prevention, Atlanta, Georgia 30333

Martin Petric
The Virology Laboratory, Department of Microbiology, The Hospital for Sick
Children, Toronto, Ontario M5G 1X8, Canada

Vincent R. Racaniello
Department of Microbiology, College of Physicians and Surgeons, Columbia University, New York, New York 10032

Marian Rewers
Departments of Preventive Medicine and Biometrics and Pediatrics, School of Medicine, University of Colorado, Denver, Colorado 80262

José R. Romero
Combined Division of Pediatric Infectious Diseases, Creighton University/University of Nebraska Medical Center, Omaha, Nebraska 68178

Harley A. Rotbart
Departments of Pediatrics and Microbiology, Infectious Diseases and Epidemiology Sections, University of Colorado Health Sciences Center, Denver, Colorado 80262

Ronald J. Rubocki
Department of Pathology and Microbiology, University of Nebraska Medical Center, Omaha, Nebraska 68198-6495

Peter Sarnow
Department of Biochemistry, Biophysics, and Genetics and Department of Microbiology, University of Colorado Health Sciences Center, Denver, Colorado 80262

Andreas Schlegel
Department of Molecular, Cellular, and Developmental Biology, Howard Hughes Medical Institute, University of Colorado, Boulder, Colorado 80309

Jerome Schwartz
Department of Antiviral Chemotherapy, Schering-Plough Research Institute, Kenilworth, New Jersey 07033

Bert L. Semler
Department of Microbiology and Molecular Genetics, College of Medicine, University of California, Irvine, California 97217

Michael Sole
The Center for Cardiovascular Research, The Toronto Hospital, Toronto, Ontario M5G 2C4, Canada

Steven Tracy
Department of Pathology and Microbiology, University of Nebraska Medical Center, Omaha, Nebraska 68198-6495

Eckard Wimmer
Department of Microbiology, State University of New York at Stony Brook, Stony Brook, New York 11794-8621

PREFACE

In August of 1982 I had just completed my residency training in Pediatrics and was beginning my subspecialty fellowship in Infectious Diseases. I was called to the newborn intensive care unit at Children's Hospital of Denver to see an ill one-week-old baby with a rash. The prenatal course was unremarkable until 38 weeks gestation when the baby's mother developed abdominal and back pain, uterine tenderness, fever, and an elevated leukocyte count; she and several family members also had upper respiratory infections. The obstetrician induced labor for fear that the mother's symptoms heralded bacterial chorioamnionitis, an infection treated by prompt delivery of the infant and administration of antibiotics.

The first 4 days of little "Briana's" life were entirely normal. On day 5, at home, she developed poor feeding and lethargy. By the time she was readmitted the next day, she was hypothermic, minimally responsive to external stimuli, and bleeding from both upper and lower gastrointestinal tracts. Laboratory studies confirmed disseminated intravascular coagulation, hepatitis, meningitis, pneumonia, and renal impairment. She was treated with broad-spectrum antibiotics and vidarabine (anti-herpesvirus medication) with the presumed diagnosis of overwhelming bacterial or herpesvirus sepsis.

Her pneumonia required assisted ventilation for more than 2 weeks. Her meningitis evolved into meningoencephalitis, with difficult to control seizures, profoundly abnormal brain waves by electroencephalograpy, and coma, but her neurologic condition stabilized and returned to normal by 4 weeks of age. Her renal disease gradually resolved. By 4 weeks of age Briana was breast-feeding, alert, and active. Her hepatitis, however, progressed to full-blown liver failure; she became progressively more jaundiced and edematous, continuing to ooze blood from multiple body sites. Although the jaundice gradually faded, the synthetic capacity of her liver never recovered and she died with massive ascites and pulmonary edema at 3 months of age.

Viral cultures of blood, cerebrospinal fluid, urine, and nasopharyngeal aspirate all grew echovirus 11, the same agent which undoubtedly caused her family's upper respiratory infection symptoms and her mother's lower abdominal pain. Early induction of labor may have precluded maternal antibody from developing in time to cross the placenta and protect the baby from transplacental enterovirus infection. Bacterial and herpesvirus cultures were negative.

It took 6 hospital days before we knew the cause of Briana's overwhelming sepsis, but the slow laboratory diagnosis probably did not harm her, since there was nothing other than supportive care to offer for neonatal enteroviral sepsis. When the culture results were known, we administered plasma obtained from her mother in the hope that by then enough maternal antibody to echovirus 11 had formed to neutralize some of the virus in Briana; there was no sound evidence that such an approach would help, but we had nothing else.

There may be 2,000 or more babies like Briana who die of this infection every year in the United States, but she was the first that I had seen, and the impact on me was enormous. I watched her die from a virus that causes adults to cough and sneeze. Knowledge of the pathogenesis of such infections was rudimentary, diagnostic tools were inadequate, and there was no meaningful treatment. So we watched her die.

Now, 12 years later, understanding and awareness of human enterovirus infections have increased logarithmically. The genomes of these pathogens have been cloned and sequenced, virulence determinants have been mapped, atomic structures have been resolved, cellular receptors have been identified, and immune responses have been characterized. Diagnosis can now be made in a few hours, promising antiviral drugs are in the final stages of development, and the knowledge is in place for the design of new vaccines to protect us from both the polio and nonpolio enteroviruses.

This is a worthy list of achievements in a field already rich in scientific heritage. Indeed, the discoveries which preceded the current molecular era of enterovirus research include no less than the first propagation of animal viruses in continuous cell culture. That Nobel Prize winning accomplishment allowed the development of the vaccines which have now eradicated wild-type poliovirus infections from the Western Hemisphere.

The progress we have seen over the past 12 years in the field of human enterovirus infections is the result of a unique synergy between basic science and clinical medicine, reflected in the subject and spirit of this book. The chapter authors are the preeminent scholars in their fields, which assures the reader that the basic science contributions are written with an eye toward clinical implications and that the clinical chapters are steeped in relevant science. Necessarily, there is some overlap and some controversy between the chapters—both of which I hope will provide the reader with the fullest possible perspective on these important pathogens and the diseases they cause. Our goal in preparation of this monograph was that it be a definitive and current resource for scientists wanting clinical correlates, clinicians seeking explanations, and medical scientists pursuing cures.

Which brings us back to little Briana. Her picture is shown below as a reminder to us all of why we do what we do.

HARLEY A. ROTBART
October 1994

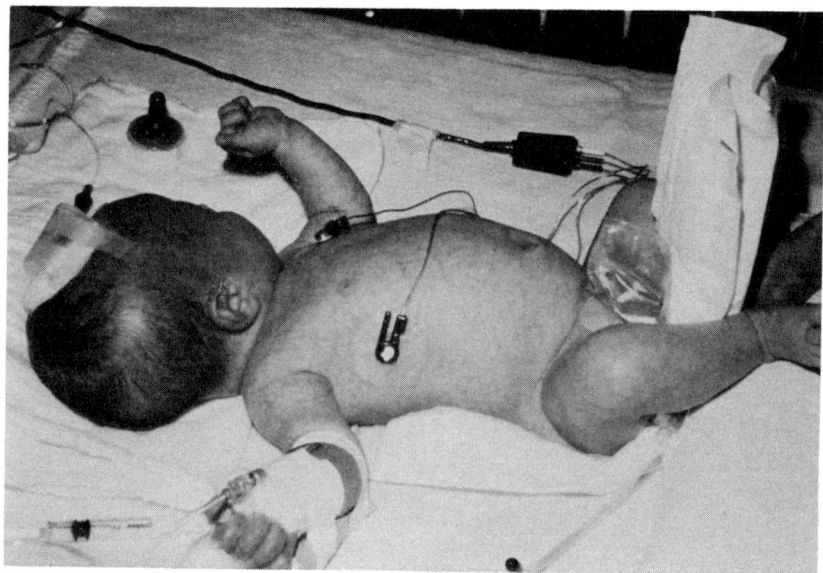

Briana

ACKNOWLEDGMENTS

I am grateful to the contributing authors of this book, not only for their fine chapters but also for their collaboration and friendship over the years. I thank my colleagues and mentors Myron Levin, Lewis Pizer, and John Sninsky for their invaluable, longstanding support. Thanks also go to Patrick Fitzgerald and Pamela Wilks of ASM Press for their encouragement and efficiency.

SCIENTIFIC PRINCIPLES

I

EPIDEMIOLOGY

David M. Morens and Mark A. Pallansch

1

There are 67 distinct human enteroviruses, most of which have been associated with many of over 20 clinically recognized syndromes, including poliomyelitis and polioencephalitis, aseptic meningitis, encephalitis, perinatal enteroviral disease, myocarditis, pericarditis, pleurodynia, respiratory illnesses, febrile illnesses, exanthems, enanthems, nonspecific conjunctivitis and acute hemorrhagic conjunctivitis (AHC), uveitis, gastroenteritis, hepatitis, arthritis, pancreatitis, chronic infections in immunocompromised hosts, and conceivably (in some cases implausibly) diabetes mellitus, urinary tract disorders, orchitis, Reye's syndrome, sudden infant death syndrome, rhabdomyolysis, "glandular fever," and postviral fatigue syndrome (84).

Almost any attempted generalization about this important group of viruses is contradicted by exceptions. The profusion and complexity of the enteroviruses are discouraging to scholars and students who seek to understand human disease. Fortunately, enteroviral epidemiology constitutes a framework for understanding not only the clinical illnesses caused by enteroviruses but also viral genetic variation, pathogenesis, and opportunities for prevention.

Salient organizing principles for understanding the epidemiology of enterovirus infection and disease include evolutionary and adaptational strategies, the interaction of the virus with its human host and the environment, and characteristic modes of transmission.

Since enteroviral genetics is discussed in detail in the following chapter (chapter 2), only general points are made here. Enteroviruses are relatively well adapted to humans (the term "enterovirus" is here taken to mean human enteroviruses and excludes enteric animal picornaviruses). Enteroviruses have no known extrahuman hosts or reservoirs; to survive, they have developed a balanced relationship with their human hosts so that the hosts will continue to replicate them efficiently. Part of the bargain, of course, is that enteroviruses must not often kill or seriously injure their hosts, lest virus and host replications diminish or cease.

At the cellular level, such adaptation is accomplished by a strategy of targeting enteric

---

David M. Morens, Epidemiology Section, School of Public Health, and Department of Tropical Medicine, School of Medicine, University of Hawaii, Biomed D103, 1960 East-West Road, Honolulu, Hawaii 96822. *Mark A. Pallansch*, Enterovirus Section, Respiratory and Enteric Viruses Branch, Division of Viral and Rickettsial Diseases, National Center for Infectious Diseases, Centers for Disease Control and Prevention, Atlanta, Georgia 30333.

Human Enterovirus Infections, Edited by Harley A. Rotbart,
© 1995 American Society for Microbiology, Washington, DC 20005

and respiratory tract epithelial cells for infection (see chapter 3). These cells not only replicate virus efficiently, but also facilitate excretion and expulsion of viruses directly into the environment, where they are likely to encounter additional human hosts. Consequently, enteroviruses are primarily adapted to cells of the human gastrointestinal tract, and they face the selection pressures of local secretory and cell-mediated gut immunity.

Unlike many agents of gastroenteritis, enteroviruses are usually excreted for prolonged periods because they do not deplete the virus-replicating host cells or adversely change the ecologic habitat in the gut. It is therefore not an accident that of the many diseases caused by enteroviruses, neither vomiting, diarrhea, cramps, abdominal pain, nor other gastrointestinal complaints are prominent. In addition, it is most likely that almost all of the serious conditions caused by enteroviruses result from spillover viremia leading to secondary infection of nongastrointestinal cells that do not contribute to the survival of the virus. Infections of these tissues, e.g., poliomyelitis (caused by destruction of cells of the spinal cord), pleurodynia (involving pleural cells), and carditis (involving myocardial cells), probably do not exert significant selection pressures on the viruses that are transmitted.

Teleologically, such human diseases can be considered accidents in which the eager virus, trying to achieve maximum replication, instead strays too far in the direction of harming the virus-replicating host. While such an imbalance might at first suggest incomplete adaptation, this is far from certain. Enteroviruses rarely kill their hosts, a fact consistent with adaptation. Furthermore, serious enteroviral illnesses are, in general, less common in very young children than in older children and adults. Since enteroviruses must have evolved for millennia in undeveloped populations with high birth rates (i.e., populations in which highly infectious agents are typically encountered early in life), it should not be surprising to find that they are best adapted to their typical host. In fact, poliomyelitis is relatively uncommon today in the poorest countries with the poorest hygiene, where infection occurs early in life. It is only when nations begin to develop and to improve sanitation and hygiene that poliomyelitis rates begin to rise. This is so because social development leads to delay in the age at which polioviruses are first encountered. In young children, paralysis is rare. In older children and adults, paralysis is a more common outcome of infection.

An additional aspect of enterovirus evolution and adaptation, reflected in molecular epidemiologic observations discussed below, is the capacity for mutational and genetic drift (see also chapter 2). Long before the era of molecular genetics, it was suspected because of the large number of antigenically distinct serotypes that enteroviruses were capable of rapid genetic and antigenic drift. This strategy presumably developed as a way to escape the selective pressures of human immunity. As is true for certain other RNA viruses (e.g., bunyaviruses and togaviruses), the existence of multiple serotypes, variants, and strains that differ widely in degree of interrelatedness has been considered implicit evidence for evolutionary capacity, and perhaps evidence for a specific survival strategy as well. Most human enterovirus infections of a single serotype contain a heterogeneous population of viruses that constitutes a quasispecies. This genetic variability provides, in a single infected host, the raw material for selecting distinct new genetic strains. Over multiple viral generations, accumulated genomic changes in conjunction with possible recombination events may lead to the observed diversity of the enterovirus genus. Thus, rather than being a confusing accident, the existence of so many different enteroviruses causing so many different diseases may actively reflect a basic and possibly stable adaptational relationship between virus and host.

Enterovirus diseases can also be considered from the vantage point of the interaction of the virus with its human host and the environment. That enteroviruses must survive a gastric pH of 2.5 to reach the enteric tract implies viral adaptation of specific properties of structural stability under adverse conditions. Such necessary adaptation may also have resulted in environmental survival advantages. Indeed, enteroviruses are relatively hardy, surviving for long periods on hands and fomites, in water, and even on crops fertilized with night soil. While there is little evidence that environmental persistence is a principal means of enterovirus transmission, viral stability must enhance the capacity for fecal-oral transmission by maximizing viability between generations of hosts.

A second important selection pressure may be the human immune response (see chapter 8). After natural enterovirus infection, humoral, secretory, and cell-mediated immunities are elicited; the last two of these may prevent productive reinfection with the same serotype. There is little doubt that population immunity acts to select new influenza A strains (producing shifts and drifts of both the hemagglutinin and the neuraminidase). Does the same phenomenon operate to select new enteroviruses, but at a slower pace? Although perhaps the answer to this question will be inferred from current and future molecular studies (see below), the birth of new virus serotypes from existing parent viruses has not been demonstrated since the advent of molecular virology. The pandemic spread of enterovirus 70 (EV70) that began in the 1960s may represent the most recent example of this process among the enteroviruses.

Enteroviral disease thus not only may result from virulence properties of the agents themselves, but also may reflect a shaping role by human hosts and environmental factors. Nowhere is the standard epidemiologic maxim more true than with the enteroviruses: disease is the outcome of interactions between the agent, the host, and the environment.

Finally, there can be no singular enterovirus epidemiology but, rather, multiple enterovirus epidemiologies. The epidemiology of a particular agent, or of a disease associated with a particular agent, reflects not only the properties of the agent, host, and environment but also the mode of transmission. Enteroviruses are transmitted by six different routes: (i) fecal-oral (i.e., fecal transmission with oral acquisition), (ii) water, (iii) food, (iv) respiratory, (v) inoculation (general and venereal), and (vi) blood (including vertical transmission from mothers to fetuses). Each of these routes will be discussed in greater detail below. It is important to note that the mode of transmission or acquisition may not only reflect properties of the agent but may also determine the epidemiologic and clinical picture.

In summary, the spectrum of enteroviral infection and disease can be better understood and categorized according to epidemiologic features that include modes of transmission as well as evolutionary-adaptational aspects of the relationships between the viral agents, their human hosts, and the environment.

EPIDEMIOLOGIC SURVEILLANCE DATA

Information about enterovirus epidemiology and about epidemics is published widely in the scientific literature and can easily be accessed through computer searches or examination of the *Index Medicus*. Descriptions of cases, clusters, outbreaks, and enterovirus surveillance information are also found in epidemiologic reports such as the World Health Organization's (WHO) *Weekly Epidemiologic Record,* the Centers for Disease Control and Prevention's *Morbidity and Mortality Weekly Report,* supplemented by periodic *Poliomyelitis Surveillance Reports* and *Enterovirus Surveillance Reports*; the *Canada Diseases Weekly Report/Rapport hebdomadaire des maladies au Canada,* published by the Canadian Department of National Health and Welfare; the United Kingdom Public Health Laboratory Service's *Communicable Disease Report*; and many other national and local publications (84).

Interpretation of enterovirus surveillance data requires an appreciation of the high degree of selection of most surveillance systems, which emphasize unusual and severe occurrences. Surveillance systems usually depend on passive case finding of enteroviral disease. Such surveillance systems are likely to hear about a case if it is easily recognizable and diagnosed by someone who decides to report it. Not surprisingly, such surveillance systems overestimate the true proportion of serious complications, particularly those of the central nervous system. In the United States, for example, the only notifiable enteroviral diseases (i.e., those for which the physician making the diagnosis is required to notify the local health department) are poliomyelitis, aseptic meningitis, and encephalitis; the last two are reportable only by diagnostic category (i.e., encephalitis and meningitis) rather than by etiology (e.g., echovirus meningitis). An example of passive surveillance follows. In 1963, the WHO established a surveillance system for viral neurologic diseases not caused by arboviruses. The first 10-year surveillance report, covering 1967 to 1976, summarized 59,281 reports from over 30 countries on five continents (6). As of 1975, 119 WHO Virus Reference Centers and other national laboratories in 47 countries were participating in diagnosis and reporting to the WHO Virus Unit in Geneva. Such complication-based surveillance provides the most accessible but least representative of all surveillance data.

Active surveillance is exemplified by prospective studies such as the Virus Watch studies conducted in various U. S. cities in the early 1960s (16, 63, 101). These studies depended on regular follow-up visits and virologic sampling of subjects in selected households over long periods. While difficult and extremely expensive, such prospective cohort studies avoid many of the pitfalls of passive surveillance and allow interpretations of both infection and disease incidence.

A second point important for interpretation of surveillance data is that enterovirus excretion (or carriage) does not necessarily imply association with disease, since enteroviruses are common and most such excretion is asymptomatic. This word of caution applies particularly to developing countries, where enteroviruses are ubiquitous and childhood infections are commonplace and characteristically silent.

Epidemiologic studies are often designed to supply information about either the incidence of infection or the prevalence of disease or infection. To determine prevalence, the number of cases of the infection (or disease) at a single point in time is established, with laboratory documentation improving the overall quality of the data. An important type of prevalence study is the serosurvey, in which the proportion of persons with antibody titers at or above some predetermined minimum level is sought. For example, the prevalence of detectable poliovirus antibodies in a population of clinic attendees during the 1979 U.S. poliomyelitis outbreak was between 78 and 89% for each of the three poliovirus types (11). Serologic prevalence studies do not distinguish between vaccine-elicited and natural infection-elicited antibodies.

To determine incidence, the number of new cases of infection (or, in some cases, of disease) in a population over a specified time interval is established. For example, the incidence of poliomyelitis in the United States in 1979 (as determined by passive surveillance) was 0.01/100,000 persons per year, or 0.01/100,000 person-years (11). This type of study is also greatly improved by laboratory confirmation of cases. Incidence studies generally rely on virus isolation or documentation of a rise or fall in specific serum antibodies (seroconversion).

Finally, enterovirus activity in populations may be either sporadic or epidemic. Certain enterovirus types are associated with both sporadic and epidemic disease occurrence, although they may typically be limited to one or the other (76). The reported occurrence of a given enteroviral disease may be actually or artifactually increased in an outbreak situation, when there is a sudden focus of attention that improves diagnosis and reporting of cases, but this may also increase reporting of noncases. The clinician should ideally maintain a high index of suspicion for sporadic cases as well as outbreak-associated cases of enteroviral diseases, especially during summer months. Suspicion should be reinforced by local surveillance information, typically provided by the city, county, or state health department, or by virology laboratories in referral medical centers.

DESCRIPTIVE EPIDEMIOLOGY

Descriptive epidemiologic characterization of disease emphasizes the classic triad of person, place, and time. "Person" alludes to the host's typical age, gender, health, socioeconomic status, ethnicity, and susceptibility status. "Place" refers to certain environmental aspects of disease occurrence including geographic limitations, latitude and longitude, climate, elevation, rainfall, rural-urban occurrence, crowding index, environmental persistence, and others. "Time" refers not only to seasonality but also to endemicity and epidemicity and to secular trends in epidemic occurrence, including potential for epidemic cyclicity.

Person

AGE

Age is one of the most important determinants of enteroviral infection outcome. Different age groups have different susceptibilities to infection, different clinical manifestations and degrees of severity, and different prognoses following enteroviral infection. Nevertheless, certain generalizations are possible. Young children are probably the most important transmitters of enteroviruses: in one study, echovirus 9 disease attack rates were 50 to 70% in children but only 17 to 33% in adults (68), a fact that probably reflects the increased exposure of children. Age-specific attack rates of echovirus 30 per 1,000 persons, computed during an outbreak in the United Kingdom in 1966, ranged from 19.70 for children 0 to 9 years old to 7.11, 4.85, 4.73, 1.50, and 0.00 for each succeeding 10-year age cohort (45).

Severity of disease in infected persons may also be strikingly age related. Coxsackie B virus infections may be more severe in newborns than in older children and adults, often causing fulminant viral "sepsis" with myocarditis, encephalitis, hepatitis, and sometimes death. Although the precise route of infection in newborns cannot usually be determined, the apparent increased risk of disease may well be due to large viral inocula associated with transplacental transmission or fecal exposure at birth. With poliovirus infection, on the other hand, adults are more likely than children to be severely affected, with the former tending to acquire paralytic poliomyelitis rather than nonparalytic poliomyelitis (poliovirus aseptic meningitis), abortive illness, or asymptomatic infection (34, 39). Adults appear also to be more susceptible to other complications such as myocarditis and pleurodynia. For the most part, diseases associated with coxsackie A viruses and echoviruses are also milder in children than in adults. Exceptions include coxsackievirus A16, which tends to be more often symptomatic and sometimes more severe in younger persons (95). In a 10-year surveillance summary from the United States (83), adults tended to be overrepresented among cases of severe disease (paralysis, encephalitis, meningitis, carditis) compared to the age distribution of the enterovirus-infected population as a whole.

Childhood poliomyelitis appears to be more common in developing nonindustrialized countries, in which control through vaccination has not yet been achieved, than in wealthier industrialized countries. The reasons for this are discussed below. Encephalitis and aseptic meningitis due to nonpolio enteroviruses appear to be most frequent among children 5 to 14 years old.

In mice, susceptibility to disease is related to such factors as age at infection, virus and strain type, and principal target organ (60). There are marked differences in the abundance of sedimentable murine receptor site material at different ages and in different tissues (65). Human cell receptors are discussed elsewhere (chapter 3). In humans, the different age susceptibilities and different tissue tropisms have been thought to result from differences in the relative abundance of cell receptor sites (65,

71), as well as from epidemiologic factors such as inoculum and route of viral acquisition.

GENDER DISTRIBUTION

A large body of data supports the observation that enteroviral diseases, and possibly also enteroviral infections, occur more frequently in males than in females (84). The male-female ratio for apparent disease appears to range generally between about 1.5:1 and 2.5:1, meaning that approximately 60 to 70% of such diseases occur in males. Male predominance tends to be greater for the more severe diseases (e.g., central nervous system disease or carditis) than for the less severe diseases (e.g., pleurodynia, hand-foot-and-mouth disease, respiratory disease, rash, or undifferentiated febrile illness). The reasons for the apparent predominance of enteroviral infections in males is obscure. On the basis of a study of healthy children (24), several possibilities have been suggested: (i) longer duration of virus excretion in males than in females (leading to more complete ascertainment of infected males than of infected females), (ii) higher virus titers in the feces of males (with similar improvement in infection ascertainment), or (iii) more frequent infections in males owing to greater exposure (parental treatment and play habits of little boys and, later, greater activity among older boys). That human myopericarditis is more common in adolescent and adult males than in females, except pregnant and postpartum females (111), could reflect endocrine effects.

HEALTH STATUS

Enteroviral infections typically occur in otherwise healthy persons. Although severe disease is occasionally observed in immunocompromised hosts (see chapter 13), enteroviral infections are not prominent among those conditions seen frequently in persons with cancer or AIDS or in persons receiving steroids or anticancer chemotherapy. Chronic severe enteroviral infections are sometimes diagnosed in persons with congenital deficiency of cell-mediated immunity (e.g., severe combined immunodeficiency disorder, Nezelof syndrome) or with certain collagen-vascular disorders, but even in persons with these disorders, severe enteroviral diseases seem to be uncommon. Strenuous physical exertion before onset of poliomyelitis, coxsackie B myocarditis, and occasionally other severe enteroviral diseases has frequently been noted in adults. Muscle damage, increased blood flow, and other mechanisms have been postulated, but the true role of exertion in influencing enteroviral pathogenesis is unknown (84).

SOCIOECONOMIC STATUS

Enteroviruses are more prevalent among persons of lower socioeconomic status living in urban areas. In a 1951 to 1953 West Virginia study utilizing active surveillance of healthy children, the rate of isolations among children in a lower socioeconomic setting was two to seven times higher than that among children in a higher socioeconomic setting (33); these results may have been confounded by the greater number of persons per household and per room in the lower socioeconomic groups. A similar study in Ghana during 1971 to 1973 further indicated that isolations were significantly more frequent from children in areas with poorer sanitation and in urban areas during both the rainy and the dry seasons (88). Other data from a prospective cohort study of newborns in Rochester, N.Y., suggest that socioeconomic status is also a predictor of neonatal infection (49). Presumably, socioeconomic status is a marker for other, more direct risk factors such as crowding and sanitation.

Paradoxically, poliomyelitis and perhaps some nonpolio enteroviral diseases tend to be diseases of development (76). In the case of poliomyelitis, improvement in a country's hygienic and socioeconomic conditions leads to a transition phase in disease experience characterized by a delay in age at first infection and a temporary increase in the paralysis-to-infection ratio until vaccination programs successfully reduce the incidence of paralysis to its ultimate low level. Before the introduction of poliovirus vaccine in the United States and other developed countries, paralytic poliomyelitis was disproportionately a disease of the middle and upper socioeconomic classes, a reflection of delay of infection to an older age, when paralysis was a more frequent complication—a delay occasioned, ironically, by improved hygiene. The infant mortality rate, a general indicator of a country's level of health development, may thus be inversely correlated with the incidence of poliomyelitis in the absence of good immunization programs (76, 90).

ETHNIC IDENTITY

Enteroviral infection rates in the United States appear to be greater for nonwhites than for whites, probably reflecting socioeconomic and other confounding variables rather than strictly racial or ethnic characteristics (24).

SUSCEPTIBILITY STATUS

Enteroviral infection usually elicits long-lasting type-specific immunity. Live and inactivated polio vaccines also elicit long-lasting humoral immunity, although inactivated vaccines, especially earlier formulations, may not induce substantial gut immunity. For all enterovirus infections, including vaccination, gut immunity wanes with time after exposure, allowing for reinfection with virus. The anamnestic immune response, however, limits systemic spread within the sequentially infected host and curtails the amount and duration of virus excretion.

Place

GEOGRAPHIC PARAMETERS, CLIMATE, ELEVATION, AND RAINFALL

Enteroviruses circulate worldwide in all geographic areas of human habitation and are not known to be affected by elevation above sea level. It is well known that enteroviral seasonality (see below) is markedly affected by latitude (84). In tropical climates, enteroviral circulation tends to be less seasonal, whereas in temperate climates, summer-fall seasonality is universal. Curiously, in tropical climates, enteroviral circulation may increase during the rainy season, a period that is usually cooler than the dry season.

RURAL-URBAN OCCURRENCE

In developed countries, enteroviruses tend to circulate more widely in urban areas, presumably because of greater crowding (84). The difference may be slight, however, and nonpolio enteroviral infections are quite common even in rural areas of the United States.

CROWDING

As is true of almost all infectious agents transmitted from person to person, enteroviral circulation is facilitated by crowding. This is especially true for crowded locales with many young children. Enterovirus outbreaks in families may frequently follow index cases, and intrafamily transmission is well known for both wild and vaccine polioviruses. In fact, a major benefit of live polio vaccines is said to be the degree to which they spread (secondarily infect others) in the family and in the community. The two agents of AHC are both associated with crowding and low socioeconomic status, which are probably markers for imperfect hygiene leading to hand- and fomite-associated viral spread. In the 1981 Miami epidemic of EV70, for example, disease was confined largely to the poorer, more crowded sections of the city (89). This and other epidemics of EV70 have demonstrated that community epidemics may be seeded by transmission within schools, particularly where young children are taught in crowded classrooms (87).

ENVIRONMENTAL PERSISTENCE

Although human enteroviruses have been isolated from various environmental sources, humans are thought to be the only important natural reservoir (22, 76). No extrahuman reservoir or focus of overwintering is known; in small, closed populations, transmission may be explosive but quickly dies out, and the viruses disappear completely (84). Long-term carriage of enteroviruses (beyond a few weeks) does not normally occur. Since viruses cannot replicate outside of living cells, infectious enteroviral particles can only decrease in number in the environment. However, enteroviruses are so hardy that they can survive for months in favorable environmental conditions such as neutral pH, moisture, and low temperatures, especially in the presence of organic matter that protects them against inactivation (22). However, at elevated temperatures or upon drying, the virus is rapidly inactivated.

Although there is little evidence that enteroviruses found in the environment are of public health importance (22), concern has been expressed about the possible dangers of contaminated water sources and contaminated shellfish intended for consumption. Recreational swimming water has been investigated in several studies: enteroviruses have been isolated from swimming and wading pools in the absence of fecal coliforms and in the presence of recommended levels of free residual chlorine. Although outbreaks of adenovirus pharyngoconjunctival fever and Norwalk-like viral gastroenteritis have been attributed to swimming pool transmission, no such outbreaks have been documented for enteroviruses. However, in one study, the relative risk of enterovirus infection among Wisconsin children was significantly higher for beach swimmers, especially for those less than 4 years old (18). In a 1972 outbreak at a boys' camp in Vermont, coxsackievirus B5 was isolated from the unchlorinated lake swimming area, but the outbreak itself was explained by person-to-person transmission (30).

Enteroviruses have been found in surface and groundwaters throughout the world (22). In the tropics, virus survival is prolonged in groundwater because groundwater is cooler than surface water. As in water from swimming pools, these viruses are often found, even after chlorination, in the absence of fecal coliforms. In industrialized countries, enterovirus transmission from potable water is apparently uncommon but is a constant source of concern for public health investigators, since the usual conditions under which city drinking water is chlorinated (residual chlorine concentrations of 0.2 to 0.4 ppm in water of pH 7.0 for 10 min) may be insufficient to completely inactivate enteroviruses.

Enteroviruses have been isolated from raw or partly cooked mollusks and crustacea and their overlying waters (19, 22, 28). Shellfish rapidly concentrate many viruses, including enteroviruses, which may survive in oysters for 3 weeks at temperatures of 1 to 21°C (22). Depuration in clean, warm, flowing water removes 99.9% of viruses in 24 h (22). Such cleansing is important, as some enteroviruses can survive in shellfish that have been stewed, fried, baked, or steamed (22), and in any case, hepatitis A and Norwalk-like gastroenteritis have both been acquired by ingestion of contaminated shellfish. To date, no outbreak of enteroviral disease has been attributed to consumption of shellfish. However, food-borne transmission has been documented on at least one occasion (see below).

The poliomyelitis literature is replete with investigation of polioviruses in sewage. In industrialized countries in the prevaccine era, these studies demonstrated distinct seasonality, but an absence of seasonality is apparent today in countries widely using live attenuated poliovirus vaccine. Today, enteroviruses are still more prevalent in sewage from areas with low socioeconomic conditions or with large proportions of young children (22). Sewage workers have a higher prevalence of serum antibodies to enteroviruses than highway maintenance workers (14), a fact consistent with occupational risk. Enteroviruses can be inactivated by proper sewage treatment, and there appears to be no risk from discharge of primary-treated sewage into clean water.

Soil and crops also provide conditions favorable to enteroviruses, which survive well in sludge and remain on the surface of sludge-treated soil and even on crops (22). Because of this survival, it is recommended that when night soil or sludge is used agriculturally, drying periods of 3 to 5 days be allowed between applications (22). Air samples from aerosolized spray irrigants using contaminated effluents have also been found to contain enteroviruses (22, 82). Protective face wear may be desirable for workers involved in or downwind of such irrigation.

To prevent transmission from potential fomite sources, as in hospitals or day-care centers, it is recommended that articles be cleaned first and then disinfected (21). Cleaning can be accomplished with soap and water, and disinfection can be done with any high- or intermediate-level germicide, such as 5% sodium hypochlorite disinfectant solution, for 30 s (20).

Time

SEASONALITY

In temperate climates, enteroviruses are characteristically summer viruses. When compared with the live attenuated polioviruses of the oral poliomyelitis vaccine, the naturally occurring (wild) enteroviruses have a distinct seasonal pattern of circulation that varies by geographic area. In tropical and semitropical areas, circulation tends to be year-round (76) or associated with the rainy season, whereas in temperate climates, circulation in summer and early fall is increased. In 10 years of surveillance in the United States, 82% of enterovirus isolations were made during the five summer and fall months of June to October (83). In a 6-year study of viral diseases of the central nervous system, 85% of enteroviral diseases but only 12 to 26% of diseases due to other viral agents occurred between June and November (78). The 10-year surveillance summary from the United States also indicated that polioviruses (mostly vaccine strains) were isolated year-round, reflecting the routine administration of poliomyelitis vaccine to children. Knowledge of the seasonal pattern of enteroviral activity, especially in temperate climates, is an extremely important diagnostic clue. All clinicians should be aware of the seasonal pattern of enteroviral circulation in their own locales and should maintain a high index of suspicion during times of enterovirus prevalence.

ENDEMICITY-EPIDEMICITY

Various studies have suggested that certain enteroviruses occur predominantly in epidemic form, whereas others are identified only in sporadic cases (76). When a particular strain is predominant in a community, there may be a tendency for other strains to be excluded (8, 75), although large communities with summer enteroviral disease typically support cocirculation of several different types simultaneously and in no particular discernible pattern. In many urban centers, enterovirus-associated cases of aseptic meningitis and other syndromes appear regularly at about the same time each summer.

SECULAR TRENDS IN OCCURRENCE AND EPIDEMIC CYCLICITY

For many of the less prevalent enteroviruses, secular trends in occurrence have not been detected, although cyclicity may be noted for some syndromes, e.g., meningitis (2). Even in the modern vaccine era, secular trends in poliovirus circulation may be noted. For example, in southern India, epidemics have been regularly noted every 3 years (73). As was true for measles (every 3 years) and rubella (every 6 or 7 years) in the prevaccine era, epidemic cyclicity typically reflects the relationship between the virus and the susceptibility of the population. Highly transmissible agents that generate high levels of immunity may eventually put themselves out of business until the population has had sufficient time to add susceptible persons through its birth rate; further endemic or epidemic circulation occurs when herd immunity cannot protect an increasing cohort of susceptible persons (infants and young children who have lost placentally acquired maternal antibody).

INCIDENCE AND PREVALENCE

Incidence data about diseases caused by particular enterovirus types are often based on an active or passive case finding and computation of attack rates, using population estimates for a given point in time. For example, the age-specific attack rates of illness during an echovirus 4 aseptic meningitis outbreak in an Iowa community in 1955, determined by house-to-house survey, ranged from 46 to 308/1,000 population during the 6 weeks of the epidemic, with an overall attack rate of 191/1,000 (67).

Better incidence data may be derived from prospective longitudinal surveillance of a defined population or of a sample of the population in which the occurrence of disease or infection can be more reliably determined. This type of study is exemplified by the Virus Watch program in U.S. cities (16, 63, 101), in which specimens from children were obtained every 2 weeks for virologic evaluation. Although these children could have had infections not detected by biweekly sampling, the studies probably came closer than any others to estimation of true attack rates of enteroviral infections.

Less useful is information based on passive case finding. Typically, such data are reported by laboratories testing specimens submitted by clinicians for diagnosis and may include the total number of specimens examined and the number positive for the virus in question. For example, one study reporting data from a 10-year period in Ontario, Canada, showed an overall 11% virus isolation rate among 21,698 specimens tested, with enteroviruses constituting 82% of all positive specimens (52). Another method of passive case finding is surveillance for only positive laboratory specimens. For example, 10 years of data from WHO surveillance for viral neurologic disease revealed that 56% of all reported virus-positive cases were enteroviral infections (6). Since such data frequently indicate neither how many ill persons were not reported nor how many ill persons had negative laboratory tests, the information is mostly of qualitative value, though it may be useful in indicating trends.

In developing countries, lameness surveys may be conducted to determine the prevalence of residual effects of paralytic poliomyelitis by age or the overall burden of cumulative paralytic cases (1, 59).

TRANSMISSION

As noted above, there are six recognized modes of enterovirus transmission. Each of these transmission modes influences the epidemiologic picture associated with infection. The six modes of transmission are (i) fecal-oral, (ii) waterborne, (iii) food borne, (iv) respiratory, (v) inoculation (general and [potentially] venereal), and (vi) blood borne (including vertical transmission from mothers to fetuses).

Fecal-oral transmission-acquisition is the classic mode of enterovirus spread and probably explains patterns of spread in developing countries, where hygiene and sanitation may be imperfect, and in day-care centers in developed countries. Despite the unsavory term "fecal-oral," transmission normally involves an intermediate step in which hands or fomites are contaminated with fecal material. For example, small children in day-care centers might contaminate their fingers by touching their own soiled diapers and then touch other children or toys played with by other children. When the contaminated toys or the fingers of the second child are placed in his or her mouth, fecal-oral transmission is accomplished. Since urine-soaked diapers efficiently diffuse fecal contaminants and since the environment seems to be full of potential fomites, fecal-oral transmission typically occurs in the absence of visible fecal contamination. A recent investigation also established the risk of more severe disease among parents during an outbreak of echovirus 30 among children in a day-care center (31).

Waterborne transmission-acquisition can be thought of as an extension of fecal-oral transmission in which the intermediate vector is water instead of hands or fomites. Hepatitis A virus, a related picornavirus not currently considered an enterovirus, is routinely transmitted by the waterborne route. On theoretical grounds, acquisition of enteroviral infection by drinking contaminated water is possible, yet such occurrences are rarely documented. Enteroviruses have occasionally been associated with suspected swimming pool outbreaks, in which swallowing of contaminated pool water could conceivably account for transmission. However, there is no proof that this type of transmission actually occurs.

Food-borne transmission-acquisition of enteroviruses is rarely documented, and most epidemiologists assume that, at least in developed countries, it rarely occurs. Food-borne acquisition of echovirus type 4, leading in some cases to aseptic meningitis, was nevertheless documented on one occasion in Pennsylvania (84). The implicated food was cole slaw. Survival of enteroviruses on vegetable food crops exposed to contaminated water or fertilizer has not been proved to be associated with transmission of infection.

Respiratory transmission-acquisition might include either aerosol spread (as occurs, for example, with influenza, varicella, and measles) or spread via direct contact with respiratory secretions. While it is believed that almost all enteroviruses (except those causing AHC) can be transmitted by the fecal-oral route, it is not known whether most are also transmitted by the respiratory route. Respiratory spread may result from passage of viruses from the bloodstream into the saliva or from virus replication in upper respiratory tract tissues during the early phase of infection.

Inoculation acquisition is the principal means of spread of the agents of AHC (EV70 and coxsackievirus A24 variant [CA24v]) and probably also accounts for spread of many other enteroviruses. As discussed above, inoculation of fecally contaminated material into the mouth is considered fecal-oral transmission-acquisition. Inoculation acquisition is usually (but not exclusively) taken to mean hand- or fomite-mediated inoculation of contaminated respiratory secretions (for example, in the case of AHC, secretions on towels, washcloths, or pillowcases) into the mouth, nose, or eye. Inoculation of fecally contaminated materials into the nose or eye would also constitute inoculation acquisition, but in practice, this seems to be an uncommon mode of spread. For at least one syndrome, AHC, transmission may be exclusively mediated by direct contact with contaminated hands or fomites (64).

A related mode of spread is venereal inoculation (most venereal diseases are associated with genital inoculation). There is no evidence that venereal transmission is important in spreading enteroviruses, although certain sexual practices, particularly those of some homosexual men (e.g., anilingus, rectal intercourse, and "fisting"), seem likely to increase transmission. However, enteroviral infections do not appear to be highly prevalent in persons with AIDS or other illnesses associated with the human immunodeficiency virus, suggesting that such infections, if they occur, are transient and either mild or inapparent.

Enteroviruses, especially polioviruses, are regularly found in sewage (36) and have been isolated from flies (76, 77), leading to a suspicion that houseflies (*Musca domestica*) and various filth flies may be vehicles of mechanical transmission, but this has not been proved.

Blood-borne transmission-acquisition may be the chief means of acquisition of the most severe forms of neonatal enteroviral disease; this is suggested by the tendency for neonatal fatalities to occur in babies with onset of illness at or within about 4 days after birth, versus within 4 to 12 days after birth, and by the tendency for secondary nursery-associated cases to be mild (see chapter 10). Presumably, the mild late-onset primary neonatal cases and the mild early- and late-onset secondary neonatal cases represent fecal-oral or respiratory transmission to the infant from an infected infant, parent, or hospital staff member, whereas many of the more severe early-onset cases represent transmission of virus across the placenta before birth. Severe disease may conceivably be related to both a high viral inoculum and viral seeding of multiple target organs before establishment of a preliminary immune response. Blood-borne transmission is also suggested by the occurrence of enterovirus-linked fetal illnesses and death in the third trimester (84).

Direct bloodstream inoculation, usually by laboratory accidents, including needle sticks and shattered glass vials, may result in enteroviral infection, but neither blood transfusion nor mosquito or other insect bites appear to transmit infection. A combination of the inability of insect vectors to biologically transmit enteroviruses and the transience of viremia of modest titer in the relatively few individuals who become viremic at any given time may explain the failure of insect transmission.

Enteroviruses are routinely isolated from both the lower and the upper alimentary tracts and can be transmitted by both the fecal-oral and respiratory routes (35, 76). Fecal-oral transmission may predominate in areas with poor sanitary conditions, while respiratory transmission may be important in more developed areas (35). It is also likely that enteroviruses are transmitted in the same manner as viruses that cause the common cold, that is, by hand contact with secretions (e.g., on the hand of another person) and autoinoculation to the mouth, nose, or eyes (see chapter 12).

Transmission within households has been well studied for both polioviruses and nonpolio enteroviruses. Enteroviruses are generally introduced into the family by small children (5), although in some outbreaks of AHC, young adults make up the majority of index cases. Intrafamily transmission may be rapid (15) and relatively complete, depending on (i) duration of virus excretion, (ii) household size, (iii) number of siblings, (iv), socioeconomic status, (v) immunity status of household members, and (vi) other risk factors (84). Transmission is generally greatest in large families of lower socioeconomic status with more 5- to 9-year-old children and apparent serologic susceptibility to the virus type studied. Not surprisingly, infections in different family members may result in different clinical manifestations and different clinical syndromes (84).

Household secondary attack rates in susceptible members may be greatest for the agents of AHC (EV70 and CA24v) and for the polioviruses and of lesser magnitude for the coxsackieviruses and echoviruses. In some studies, secondary attack rates may be 90% or more, although they are typically lower (25, 63). New York Virus Watch data indicated that enterovirus infections were more frequent among 2- to 9-year-old children (63) and that secondary coxsackievirus infections were more frequent in mothers (78%) than in fathers (47%). In the same study, coxsackieviruses spread to 76% of exposed susceptible persons versus 25% of exposed persons who had detectable antibody to the infecting type; echoviruses infected 43% of susceptible persons and only one person with antibody (63). The greater spread of polioviruses and coxsackieviruses may derive from longer periods of viral excretion (25, 76). Observations of household transmission of various enteroviruses suggest that many infected contacts do not become ill (84) and that the extent of secondary transmission varies with different enteroviruses (84).

Nosocomial transmission, typically in newborn nurseries, has also been well documented for including coxsackieviruses of groups A and B and the echoviruses (84). EV70 is highly transmissible and may cause outbreaks in ophthalmology clinics when instruments (e.g., tonometers) are inadequately cleaned between patients. An apparent outbreak of coxsackievirus A1 in bone marrow transplant recipients, including fatal cases, has also been reported (84). Laboratory-acquired infections are occasionally documented.

Like many other viruses, enteroviruses can be rapidly transmitted within institutions when circumstances—for example, crowding, poor hygiene, or contaminated water—permit. School teams or activity groups and institutionalized ambulatory retarded children or adults may be at special risk (3). Despite crowding, in institutions where good sanitation is usual (e.g., university dormitories or military barracks), enterovirus transmission is not usually accelerated to a noticeable degree.

Of great interest is the existence of poliovirus-susceptible enclaves (usually religious groups) in countries with an otherwise high prevalence of poliovirus immunity. Such enclaves have in recent years become foci for outbreaks in countries such as the United States, Canada, and the Netherlands, which have reasonably effective vaccination programs and high herd immunity (9–12). Apparently, herd immunity may be of only limited value in protecting groups of susceptible persons who have regular contact with each other, raising questions about virus control strategies and the risks that such groups may pose to the community at large.

MOLECULAR EPIDEMIOLOGY

In the past 15 years, the epidemiology of enteroviruses has been greatly clarified by newer techniques that allow characterization of genetic and antigenic differences between isolates. Older techniques, such as serologic tests to distinguish isolates (e.g., cross-neutralization), were cumbersome and imprecise. The newer molecular techniques allow inferences about strain evolution and also have implications for prevention. Some of these implications are discussed in later chapters. In this section, the promise of these molecular techniques is highlighted in the context of enteroviral diseases of particular interest, including poliovirus infections and AHC associated with EV70 and CA24v. Although enteroviral genome detection has been greatly improved by the wide application of PCR techniques, which provide information of epidemiologic importance (32, 50, 98, 99, 105), PCR is discussed more fully in chapter 17, in the context of laboratory diagnosis. The following discussion of molecular epidemiology focuses on three of the most useful techniques: partial genome sequencing, analysis of RNA genome relationships by screening oligonucleotide mapping of the entire genome, and analysis of viral epitope distribution by use of monoclonal antibodies. These methods are considered in the context of important public health problems for which epidemiologic information is sought.

The best-studied example of the relationship between molecular characteristics of enteroviruses and epidemic occurrence was the 1984 to 1985 outbreak of type 3 poliovirus infection in Finland (38), in which 10 cases of poliomyelitis and an estimated 100,000 infections were detected. As Finland had for many years had a high degree of vaccine coverage with inactivated polio vaccine to all three serotypes and had gone for many years without any evidence of virus circulation (through both case investigation and environmental sampling), the outbreak was unexpected. Even before epidemic control was instituted on an emergency basis with oral polio vaccines, isolates from affected persons were gathered and studied. These and subsequent studies (37, 41, 43, 44, 61, 72, 91) that relied on molecular techniques revealed that the epidemic was caused by a widely prevalent strain from the Mediterranean region. However, serologic studies both before and after the outbreak demonstrated that significant segments of the population in Finland had failed to adequately respond to the type 3 component of the inactivated polio vaccine and were therefore unprotected from the wild poliovirus. This finding had important implications for prevention strategies: the problem lay not in exotic or virulent strains, but rather in reduced vaccine-induced immunity.

The basic mutability of the poliovirus was demonstrated during this outbreak through antigenic characterization of isolates by use of panels of monoclonal antibodies. By using first a panel of five monoclonal antibodies directed to a 12-amino-acid VP1 site (37, 44) and subsequently an expanded panel of monoclonal antibodies (61), extremely rapid molecular evolution during the epidemic, including evolution of strains isolated sequentially from infected individuals, was detected (61). It was also discovered that neutralization-resistant outbreak strains appeared to spontaneously mutate to partially resistant strains (strains neutralized by at least one of the five selected monoclonal antibodies). It is possible that the inherent instability of the VP1 epitope array of all polioviruses may contribute to a selective advantage for the virus in epidemic circulation.

The extent of antigenic strain differences detected by monoclonal antibodies directed to surface proteins was confirmed by whole (41) and partial (44, 91, 92) nucleotide sequence analyses. Using the unique viral sequences from the outbreak isolates, workers developed an oligonucleotide hybridization test with a 17-nucleotide probe to screen poliovirus type 3 isolates for outbreak-associated strains. Initial studies revealed that the test identified 100% of 88 outbreak-associated strains but few type 3 strains from other sources. The investigative team next used the same probe to search existing libraries of type 3 isolates for the origin of the 1984 to 1985 epidemic. Study of 80 international type 3 isolates collected over a period of 34 years revealed that only 5 isolates were oligonucleotide hybridization positive (92). Each of these five was partially sequenced in two genomic regions. Sequence comparisons revealed that the Finnish outbreak strains were different from three of the five isolates—obtained from the United States and Europe in the 1950s—but highly similar (80 to 100% identity at each of the two sites) to 1980 and 1981 isolates from the Mediterranean region (92). These last two strains were further related to European strains prevalent as long as 8 years before the epidemic. Thus, the Finnish epidemic was linked to prevalent strains circulating regionally at least 4 years before the epidemic.

In recent years, molecular techniques have been increasingly used to study the epidemiology of other polioviruses. At about the same time that monoclonal antibodies were first being produced, oligonucleotide mapping was first applied to the study of polioviruses. The technique of oligonucleotide mapping produces characteristic patterns for given strains of viruses that have been referred to as "fingerprints."

Fingerprint studies of wild and vaccine polioviruses have revealed many fascinating aspects of poliovirus molecular epidemiology (54, 55, 85). Fingerprints of poliovirus strains that are epidemiologically distinct, that is, those that are isolated sporadically or from persons in different epidemics, are unequivocally different. Poliovirus genomes appear to spontaneously and randomly mutate during replication in humans, resulting in variation in fingerprint types isolated during epidemics, presumably reflecting single and multiple generations of person-to-person transmission. Investigation of one epidemic in which contact tracing was possible revealed that the fingerprint changed during infection of each case or contact, attesting to the remarkable rapidity of poliovirus evolution (85). However, changes do not appear so rapidly that it is impossible to detect related strains. In one instance, an unsuspected epidemiologic link was established when it was discovered that wild poliovirus type 1 isolates from apparently unrelated fatal cases in New York and Ohio had similar fingerprints (85).

Fingerprinting studies have also been performed with vaccine polioviruses (85). Patterns for the live attenuated (Sabin) type 1 poliovirus vaccine, and for the prototype Mahoney strain from which it was derived, are quite similar. However, as is the case with wild viruses, vaccine viruses predictably change during human infection.

All three molecular approaches noted above have been utilized in addressing the classic problem of differentiating wild and vaccine-derived polioviruses (17, 23, 29). Early attempts at differentiation of wild from vaccine polioviruses were insensitive. Typically, poliovirus isolates were grown at low (35.5°C) and high (39.9°C) temperatures with the assumption that temperature-sensitive vaccine polioviruses would not grow at the higher temperature. However, it was eventually learned that roughly 30% of the wild viruses would also not grow at such temperatures, making interpretation problematic. Another test intended to differentiate between wild and vaccine viruses depended on cross-absorbed antibody. Separate aliquots of hyperimmune serotype-specific antisera were reacted with either wild or vaccine virus to absorb cross-reacting antibodies. The two resulting sera could then be used in neutralization tests to determine which serum neutralized an unknown virus better. More recently, investigators have distinguished between wild and vaccine polioviruses by using cross-absorbed rabbit immunoglobulin G in an enzyme-linked immunosorbent assay (26, 27).

Other techniques used to study poliovirus strain differences include restriction fragment length polymorphism (109), genomic sequence analyses (48, 102, 108, 113), and monoclonal antibody characterization of viral epitopes (48) (the last two are described above with respect to the 1984 to 1985 Finish outbreak). Such techniques have supplemented earlier techniques in epidemiologic investigation of the occurrence of vaccine-associated poliomyelitis (48, 57, 58).

A second problem of public health importance investigated by molecular epidemiologic techniques is the appearance and pandemic spread of AHC associated with both EV70 and CA24v. Both viruses appeared suddenly at about the same time (in West Africa and Southeast Asia, respectively), and both have a pronounced tendency for rapid and recurrent epidemic-pandemic spread.

Several studies using oligonucleotide fingerprinting have examined isolates of EV70. Fingerprints of isolates obtained from multiple sites worldwide during the 1981 to 1982 pandemic showed that all of the isolates were very closely related, supporting a single agent as the etiology of the global outbreak (56). Further studies demonstrated that the changes in the EV70 genome were progressive, with increased numbers of changes with time over a 10-year period (103). Quantitative analysis of these fingerprint data suggested a common origin for all EV70 isolates, with an estimated date of origin of 1966 to 1967, likely in West Africa, 2 or 3 years prior to the first known pandemic of this disease (80, 103).

Studies of CA24v also reveal progressive genomic changes linked to outbreak occurrence and pandemic spread. For nearly 15 years (1970 to 1984), the disease appeared to be confined to Southeast Asia and the Indian subcontinent. In 1985, however, it spread to Japan, Taiwan, Oceania, Central America, and Africa. The occurrence of three sequential outbreaks in Taiwan (1985, 1986, 1988) was studied by sequence analysis of a 549-nucleotide part of the $3C^{Pro}$ region of the genome. By this technique, the 1985 and 1986 isolates appeared to be closely related, while the 1988 isolates were genetically distinct (69). Japanese-Okinawan epidemics of 1985, 1986, 1988, and 1989 were also studied by these techniques. The 1985 Japanese strain, shown by oligonucleotide mapping to be markedly different from the 1970 Singapore prototype strain (81), was found to match the 1985 Taiwanese strain; similarly, the 1986 Japanese and Taiwanese strains were indistinguishable (46). However, the 1988 Japanese mainland isolates were different from the 1988 Taiwanese isolate, being similar to isolates from Singapore in 1987 and from China in 1988 (46, 70). The 1988 Taiwanese strain eventually did become established in mainland Japan a year later (1989), by which time the 1988 epidemic virus appeared to have become extinct (46). These three specific strains had evolved as distinct entities prior to the epidemic spread. Standard phylogenetic estimates suggested that the viruses causing the 1985 and 1986 epidemics in Taiwan and Japan-Okinawa had diverged from the viruses causing the 1988 Taiwanese epidemics as early as 1982 (70). The closest relative of another strain was commonly circulating in the region around 1981 (47).

Thus, it appears that the outbreaks of AHC in these Asian countries can be described as three successive waves of genetically distinct CA24v strains. The first strain of CA24v caused an outbreak in 1985 and 1986 in Taiwan, Okinawa, and Japan. The second strain caused the outbreak that spread from Singapore in 1987 to China and Japan in 1988. The third strain then caused the outbreaks that began in 1988 in Taiwan and proceeded to Japan in 1989. The molecular characterization of these isolates provides a much clearer picture of the transmission pathways of the viruses and a more discrete description of the relationship between individual overlapping outbreaks of disease.

As with poliovirus, even within a single outbreak, a large degree of genetic diversity can be observed. Oligonucleotide mapping data from a 1987 outbreak in Accra, Ghana, suggested a surprising degree of genomic diversity (7). The investigators concluded that phylogenetic divergence had occurred 11 to 26 months before the epidemic. Almost certainly, some low-level circulation must have occurred for some time before the epidemic was recognized.

In addition to characterization of polioviruses and the agents of AHC, molecular epidemiology has been used to investigate outbreaks in newborn nurseries (74), and community outbreaks (106, 107), to determine strain identity in community outbreaks (66, 97), to implicate or absolve enteroviral infection in childhood myocarditis (32, 51), to correlate clinical and environmental isolates (40, 41), to follow serial genomic changes (79, 86) or genomic variation within outbreaks (93, 94), to study viral geographic distribution patterns (96), and to characterize viral evolution (104).

In summary, molecular epidemiology promises new insights into the origin, evolution, and prevention of human enteroviruses. The complexities of genetic and antigenic diversification may be matched by those of host and environmental selection pressures. The molecular epidemiologic data generated from investigation of the 1984 to 1985 polio type 3 epidemic in Finland suggest that worldwide eradication is likely to be a better control strategy than even the best vaccine delivery programs.

POLIOVIRUS ERADICATION

With little fanfare and much humility at the daunting task that lies ahead, an aggressive program of poliovirus control in the Americas led in 1985 to a plan for regional eradication (4) and in 1988 to a goal of global eradication by the year 2000 (13, 42, 100, 110, 112). Despite the profound epidemiologic differences between smallpox and enteroviruses, the eradication home stretch is likely to be dominated by some of the same operational difficulties in impoverished nations experiencing famines, wars, population displacements, and national disasters.

In other respects, poliovirus eradication is more complicated than smallpox eradication. There are three viruses instead of one. Furthermore, eradication efforts may be confronted by discouraging importations into previously controlled areas (as occurred in Canada in 1993 [12]) and by difficulties in proving local eradication. Unlike smallpox, neither infection nor vaccination with poliovirus leaves a visible record to facilitate control. In addition, poliomyelitis may affect only about 1 in 200 infected persons, so surveillance for paralytic disease might well be unproductive even in the face of continued poliovirus circulation. Proof of eradication thus depends on laboratory and epidemiologic efforts (53), which may be greatly complicated by the persistence of enteroviruses in environmental sources, the use of live poliovirus vaccines that enter the environment, and the absence of simple and rapid field techniques to distinguish wild from vaccine strains.

Even so, the goal of worldwide eradication is achievable with existing knowledge and prevention expertise. Only the existence of the international political will and commitment necessary to achieve eradication is in doubt. Epidemiology will continue to play the leading role in poliovirus eradication, but it is deeply wished by all involved in the creation of this book—epidemiologists, virologists, cell and molecular biologists, and clinicians alike—that a second edition will feature a discussion of polioviruses in a new chapter entitled "History."

ACKNOWLEDGMENTS

We thank Virginia Tanji, Jo-Anne Nakamoto, and Ratna Soetjahja Morens for help in manuscript research and preparation. We also thank Melinda Moore and other colleagues from the Centers for

Disease Control and Prevention who over the years have shared many valuable thoughts about enteroviral epidemiology.

REFERENCES

1. **Acharya, D., and B. K. Chakladar.** 1989. The epidemiological study of paralytic poliomyelitis cases in Kasturba Hospital, Manipal. *J. Commun. Dis.* **21:**183–189.
2. **Aleraj, B., V. Kruzic, and B. Borcic.** 1990. [Epidemiology of enteroviral meningitis in Croatia 1958–1988 with special emphasis on the great epidemic of 1988.] *Lijec-Vjesn* **112:**305–309.
3. **Alexander, J. P., L. E. Chapman, M. A. Pallansch, W. T. Stephenson, T. J. Torok, and L. J. Anderson.** 1993. Coxsackievirus B2 infection and aseptic meningitis: a focal outbreak among members of a high school football team. *J. Infect. Dis.* **167:**1201–1205.
4. **Andrus, J. K., C. A. de Quadros, and J. M. Olive.** 1992. The surveillance challenge: final stages of eradication of poliomyelitis in the Americas. *Morbid. Mortal. Weekly Rep.* **41:**21-26.
5. **Artenstein, M. S., F. C. Cadigan, and E. L. Beuscher.** 1964. Epidemic coxsackie virus infection with mixed clinical manifestations. *Ann. Intern. Med.* **60:**196–203.
6. **Assaad, F., R. Gispen, M. Kleemola, L. Syrucek, and K. Esteves.** 1980. Neurological diseases associated with viral and *Mycoplasma pneumoniae* infections. *Bull. W.H.O.* **58:**297–311.
7. **Brandful, J. A. M., N. Takeda, T. Yoshii, et al.** 1991. A study of the evolution of coxsackievirus A24 variant in Ghana by viral RNA fingerprinting analysis. *Res. Virol.* **142:**57–65.
8. **Brown, E. H.** 1972. Enterovirus infections. *Br. Med. J.* **2:**169–171.
9. **Center for Disease Control.** 1978. Poliomyelitis—Netherlands. *Morbid. Mortal. Weekly Rep.* **27:**222.
10. **Center for Disease Control.** 1979. Poliomyelitis—Pennsylvania, Maryland. *Morbid. Mortal. Weekly Rep.* **28:**49–50.
11. **Centers for Disease Control.** 1981. *Poliomyelitis Surveillance Summary 1979.* U.S. Department of Health and Human Services, Atlanta.
12. **Centers for Disease Control and Prevention.** 1993. Isolation of wild poliovirus type 3 among members of a religious community objecting to vaccination—Alberta, Canada, 1993. *Morbid. Mortal. Weekly Rep.* **42:**337–339.
13. **Centers for Disease Control and Prevention.** 1993. Progress toward global eradication of poliomyelitis, 1988–1991. *Morbid. Mortal. Weekly Rep.* **42:**486–487, 493–495.
14. **Clark, C. S., A. B. Bjornson, G. M. Schiff, et al.** 1977. Sewage worker's syndrome. *Lancet* **i:**1009.
15. **Clemmer, D. I., F. Li, D. R. Le Blanc, and J. P. Fox.** 1966. An outbreak of subclinical infection with coxsackievirus B3 in southern Louisiana. *Am. J. Epidemiol.* **83:**123–129.
16. **Cooney, M. L., C. E. Hall, and J. P. Fox.** 1972. The Seattle Virus Watch. III. Evaluation of isolation methods and summary of infections detected by virus isolation. *Am. J. Epidemiol.* **96:**286–305.
17. **Crainic, R., P. Couillin, B. Blondel, et al.** 1983. Natural variation of poliovirus neutralization epitopes. *Infect. Immun.* **41:**1217–1225.
18. **D'Alessio, D. J., T. E. Minor, C. I. Allen, A. A. Tsiatis, and D. B. Nelson.** 1981. A study of the proportions of swimmers among well controls and children with enterovirus-like illness shedding or not shedding an enterovirus. *Am. J. Epidemiol.* **113:**533–541.
19. **Denis, F. A.** 1973. Coxsackie group A in oysters and mussels. *Lancet* **i:**1262.
20. **Drulak, M., A. M. Wallbank, I. Lebtag, L. Werboski, and L. Poffenroth.** 1978. The relative effectiveness of commonly used disinfectants in inactivation of coxsackievirus B5. *J. Hyg. Camb.* **81:**389–397.
21. **Favero, M. S.** 1980. Sterilization, disinfection, and antisepsis in the hospital, p. 952–959. *In* E. H. Lennette, A. Balows, W. J. Hausler, Jr., and J. P. Truant (ed.), *Manual of Clinical Microbiology,* 3rd ed. American Society for Microbiology, Washington, D.C.
22. **Feachem, R., H. Garelick, and J. Slade.** 1981. Enteroviruses in the environment. *Trop. Dis. Bull.* **78:**185–230.
23. **Ferguson, M., D. I. Magrath, P. D. Minor, and G. T. Schild.** 1986. WHO collaborative study on the use of monoclonal antibodies for the intratypic differentiation of poliovirus strains. *Bull. W.H.O.* **64:**239–246.
24. **Gelfand, H. M., A. H. Holguin, G. E. Marchetti, and P. M. Feorino.** 1963. A continuing surveillance of enterovirus infections in healthy children in six United States cities. I. Viruses isolated during 1960 and 1961. *Am. J. Hyg.* **78:**358–375.
25. **Gelfand, H. M., D. R. LeBlanc, J. P. Fox, and D. P. Conwell.** 1957. Studies on the development of natural immunity to poliomyelitis in Louisiana. II. Description and analysis of episodes of infection observed in study group households. *Am. J. Hyg.* **65:**367–385.
26. **Glikmann, G., M. Moynihan, I. Petersen,**

and B. F. Vestergaard. 1983. Intratypic differentiation of poliovirus strains by enzyme-linked immunosorbent assay (ELISA): poliovirus type 1. *Dev. Biol. Stand.* **55:**199–208.
27. **Glikmann, G., M. Pedersen, and I. Petersen.** 1987. Intratypic differentiation of poliovirus strains by enzyme-linked immunosorbent assay (ELISA): poliovirus type 2 and poliovirus type 3. *J. Virol. Methods* **18:**25–36.
28. **Goyal, S. M., C. P. Gerba, and J. L. Melnick.** 1979. Human enteroviruses in oysters and their overlying waters. *Appl. Environ. Microbiol.* **37:**572–581.
29. **Guo, R., E. H. Tang, H. Wang, et al.** 1987. Preliminary studies on antigenic variation of poliovirus using neutralizing monoclonal antibodies. *J. Gen. Virol.* **68:**989–994.
30. **Hawley, H. B., D. P. Morin, M. E. Geraghty, J. Tomkow, and A. Phillips.** 1973. Coxsackievirus B epidemic at a boy's summer camp. Isolation of virus from swimming water. *JAMA* **226:**33–36.
31. **Helfand, R. F., A. S. Khan, M. A. Pallansch, J. P. Alexander, H. B. Meyers, R. A. DeSantis, L. S. Schonberger, and L. J. Anderson.** 1994. Echovirus 30 infection and aseptic meningitis in parents of children attending a day care center. *J. Infect. Dis.* **169:**1133–1138.
32. **Hilton, D. A., S. Variend, and J. H. Pringle.** 1993. Demonstration of coxsackie virus RNA in formalin-fixed tissue sections from childhood myocarditis cases by *in situ* hybridization and the polymerase chain reaction. *J. Pathol.* **170:**45–51.
33. **Honig, E. I., J. L. Melnick, P. Isacson, et al.** 1956. An endemiological study of enteric virus infections. Poliomyelitis, Coxsackie, and orphan (ECHO) viruses isolated from normal children in 2 socio-economic groups. *J. Exp. Med.* **103:**247–262.
34. **Horstmann, D. M.** 1955. Poliomyelitis: severity and type of disease in different age groups. *Ann. N.Y. Acad. Sci.* **61:**956–967.
35. **Horstmann, D. M.** 1967. Enterovirus infection of the central nervous system. The present and future of poliomyelitis. *Med. Clin. N. Am.* **61:**681–693.
36. **Horstmann, D. M., J. Emmons, L. Gimpel, T. Subrahmanyan, and J. T. Riordan.** 1973. Enterovirus surveillance following a community-wide oral poliovirus vaccination program: a 7-year study. *Am. J. Epidemiol.* **97:**173–186.
37. **Hovi, T.** 1989. The outbreak of poliomyelitis in Finland in 1984–1985: significance of antigenic variation of type 3 polioviruses and site specificity of antibody responses in antipolio immunization. *Adv. Virus. Res.* **37:**243–275.
38. **Hovi, T., K. Cantell, A. Huovilainen, E. Kinnunen, et al.** 1986. Outbreak of paralytic poliomyelitis in Finland: widespread circulation of antigenically altered poliovirus type 3 in a vaccinated population. *Lancet* **i:**1427–1432.
39. **Howe, H. A.** 1953. Poliomyelitis, p. 300–337. *In* T. M. Rivers (ed.), *Viral and Rickettsial Infections of Man.* J. B. Lippincott, Philadelphia.
40. **Hughes, M. S., E. M. Hoey, and P. V. Coyle.** 1993. A nucleotide sequence comparison of coxsackievirus B4 isolates from aquatic samples and clinical specimens. *Epidemiol. Infect.* **110:**389–398.
41. **Hughes, P. J., D. M. A. Evans, P. D. Minor, et al.** 1986. The nucleotide sequence of a type 3 poliovirus isolated during a recent outbreak of poliomyelitis in Finland. *J. Gen. Virol.* **67:**2093–2102.
42. **Hull, H. F., and N. A. Ward.** 1992. Progress towards the global eradication of poliomyelitis. *World Health Stat. Q.* **45:**280–284.
43. **Huovilainen, A., T. Hovi, L. Kinnunen, et al.** 1987. Evolution of poliovirus during an outbreak: sequential type 3 poliovirus isolates from several persons show shifts of neutralization determinants. *J. Gen. Virol.* **68:**1373–1378.
44. **Huovilainen, A., L. Kinnunen, M. Ferguson, and T. Hovi.** 1988. Antigenic variation among 173 strains of type 3 poliovirus isolated in Finland during the 1984 to 1985 outbreak. *J. Gen. Virol.* **69:**1941–1948.
45. **Irvine, D. H., A. B. H. Irvine, and P. S. Gardner.** 1967. Outbreak of ECHO virus type 30 in a general practice. *Br. Med. J.* **4:**774–776.
46. **Ishiko, H., N. Takeda, K. Miyamura, et al.** 1992. Phylogenetically different strains of a variant of coxsackievirus A24 were repeatedly introduced but discontinued circulating in Japan. *Arch. Virol.* **126:**179–193.
47. **Ishiko, H., N. Takeda, K. Miyamura, et al.** 1992. Phylogenetic analysis of a coxsackievirus A24 variant: the most recent worldwide pandemic was caused by progenies of a virus prevalent around 1981. *Virology* **187:**748–759.
48. **Jarzabek, Z., J. Zabicka, A. John, et al.** 1992. Application of monoclonal antibody panels in the virological and epidemiological review of poliomyelitis in Poland, 1981–1990. *Bull. W.H.O.* **70:**327–333.
49. **Jenista, J. A., K. R. Powell, and M. A. Menegus.** 1984. Epidemiology of neonatal enterovirus infection. *J. Pediatr.* **104:**685–690.
50. **Johnston, S. L., G. Sanderson, P. K. Pattemore, et al.** 1993. Use of polymerase chain reaction for diagnosis of picornavirus in-

fection in subjects with and without respiratory symptoms. *J. Clin. Microbiol.* **31:**111–117.
51. **Keeling, P. J., S. Jeffrey, A. L. Caforio, et al.** 1992. Similar prevalence of enteroviral genome within the myocardium from patients with idiopathic dilated cardiomyopathy and controls by the polymerase chain reaction. *Br. Heart J.* **68:**554–559.
52. **Kelen, A. E., and N. A. Labzoffsky.** 1967. Variations in the prevalence of enterovirus infections in Ontario, 1956–1965. *Can. Med. Assoc. J.* **97:**797–801.
53. **Kew, O., L. De, C.-F. Yang, B. Nottay, E. da Silva, and M. Pallansch.** 1993. The role of virological surveillance in the global initiative to eradicate poliomyelitis, p. 215–246. *In* E. Kurstak (ed.), *Control of Virus Diseases.* Marcel Dekker, Inc., New York.
54. **Kew, O. M., and B. K. Nottay.** 1984. Molecular epidemiology of polioviruses. *Rev. Infect. Dis.* **6**(Suppl. 2)**:**S499–S504.
55. **Kew, O. M., B. K. Nottay, M. H. Hatch, J. H. Nakano, and J. F. Obijeski.** 1981. Multiple genetic changes can occur in the oral poliovaccines upon replication in humans. *J. Gen. Virol.* **56:**337–347.
56. **Kew, O. M., B. K. Nottay, M. H. Hatch, J. C. Hierholzer, and J. F. Obijeski.** 1983. Oligonucleotide fingerprint analysis of enterovirus 70 isolates from the 1980 to 1981 pandemic of acute hemorrhagic conjunctivitis: evidence for a close genetic relationship among Asian and American strains. *Infect. Immun.* **41:**631–635.
57. **Kew, O. M., B. K. Nottay, R. Rico-Hesse, and M. A. Pallansch.** 1990. Molecular epidemiology of wild poliovirus transmission, p. 199–221. *In* E. Kurstak, R. G. Marusyk, F. A. Murphy, and M. H. V. van Regenmortel (ed.), *Applied Virology Research,* vol. 2. Plenum Publishing, New York.
58. **Kew, O. M., M. A. Pallansch, B. K. Nottay, R. Rico-Hesse, L. De, and C.-F. Yang.** 1990. Genotypic relationships among wild polioviruses from different regions of the world, p. 357–365. *In* M. A. Brinton and F. X. Heinz (ed.), *New Aspects of Positive-Strand RNA Viruses.* American Society for Microbiology, Washington, D.C.
59. **Khajura, R., N. Datta, R. Kumar, T. Kaur, M. K. Kaushal, S. Singhi, and V. Kumar.** 1989. Impact of annual immunization programme with oral polio vaccine on the prevalence of paralytic poliomyelitis. *Indian J. Pediatr.* **56:**343–347.
60. **Khatib, R., J. L. Chason, B. K. Silberberg, and A. M. Lerner.** 1980. Age-dependent pathogenicity of group B coxsackieviruses in Swiss-Webster mice: infectivity for myocardium and pancreas. *J. Infect. Dis.* **141:**394–403.
61. **Kinnunen, L., A. Huovilainen, T. Pöyry, and T. Hovi.** 1990. Rapid molecular evolution of wild type 3 poliovirus during infection in individual hosts. *J. Gen. Virol.* **71:**317–324.
62. **Kinnunen, L., T. Pöyry, and T. Hovi.** 1991. Generation of virus genetic lineages during an outbreak of poliomyelitis. *J. Gen. Virol.* **72:**2483–2489.
63. **Kogon, A., I. Spigland, T. E. Frothingham, et al.** 1969. The Virus Watch program: a continuing surveillance of viral infections in metropolitan New York families. VII. Observations on viral excretion, seroimmunity, intrafamilial spread and illness association in coxsackie and echovirus infections. *Am. J. Epidemiol.* **89:**51–61.
64. **Kono, R.** 1975. Apollo 11 disease or acute hemorrhagic conjunctivitis: a pandemic of a new enterovirus infection of the eyes. *Am. J. Epidemiol.* **101:**383–390.
65. **Kunin, C. M.** 1962. Virus-tissue union and the pathogenesis of enterovirus infections. *J. Immunol.* **8:**556–569.
66. **Kutitova, O. K., G. I. Lipskaia, and S. V. Maslova.** 1990. [The molecular epidemiology of poliomyelitis: the characteristics of the strains isolated from patients in Moscow in 1973–1986.] *Zh. Mikrobiol. Epidemiol. Immunobiol.* **1990:**43–49.
67. **Lehan, P. H., E. W. Chick, I. L. Doto, et al.** 1957. An epidemic illness associated with a recently recognized enteric virus (Echo virus type 4). I. Epidemiologic and clinical features. *Am. J. Hyg.* **66:**63–75.
68. **Lerner, A. M., J. O. Klein, J. D. Cherry, and M. Finland.** 1963. New viral exanthems. *N. Engl. J. Med.* **269:**678–685.
69. **Lin, K. H., N. Takeda, K. Miyamura, S. Yamazaki, and C. W. Chen.** 1991. The nucleotide sequence of 3C proteinase region of the coxsackievirus A24 variant: comparison of the isolates in Taiwan in 1985–1988. *Virus Genes* **5:**121–131.
70. **Lin, K. H., H. L. Wang, M. M. Sheu, et al.** 1993. Molecular epidemiology of a variant of coxsackievirus A24 in Taiwan: two epidemics caused by phylogenetically distinct viruses from 1985 to 1989. *J. Clin. Microbiol.* **31:**1160–1166.
71. **Loria, R. M., N. Shadoff, S., Kibrick, and S. Breitman.** 1976. Maturation of intestinal defenses against peroral infection with group B coxsackievirus in mice. *Infect. Immun.* **13:**1397–1401.

72. **Magrath, D. I., D. M. A. Evans, M. Ferguson, et al.** 1986. Antigenic and molecular properties of type 3 poliovirus responsible for an outbreak of poliomyelitis in a vaccinated population. *J. Gen. Virol.* **67**:899–905.
73. **Mahadevan, S., S. Ananthakrishnan, S. Srinavasan, P. Nalini, and R. K. Puri.** 1989. Poliomyelitis: the Pondicherry experience. *J. Trop. Med. Hyg.* **92**:416–421.
74. **Matsumoto, K., T. Kobayashi, and Y. Kimura.** 1990. Isolation and preliminary characterization of antigenic variant of echovirus type 11. *J. Med. Virol.* **31**:253–258.
75. **McLean, D. M., M. A. Coleman, and R. P. B. Larke.** 1966. Viral infections of Toronto children during 1965. I. Enteroviral disease. *Can. Med. Assoc. J.* **94**:839–843.
76. **Melnick, J. L.** 1989. Enteroviruses, p. 191–263. *In* A. S. Evans (ed.), *Viral Infections of Humans, Epidemiology and Control*, 3rd ed. Plenum, New York.
77. **Melnick, J. L., E. W. Shaw, and E. C. Curnen.** 1949. A virus isolated from patients diagnosed as nonparalytic poliomyelitis or aseptic meningitis. *Proc. Soc. Exp. Biol. Med.* **71**:344–349.
78. **Meyer, H. M., R. T. Johnson, I. P. Crawford, H. E. Dascomb, and N. G. Rogers.** 1960. Central nervous system syndromes of "viral" etiology. A study of 713 cases. *Am. J. Med.* **29**:334–347.
79. **Minor, P. D., A. John, M. Ferguson, and J. P. Icenogle.** 1986. Antigenic and molecular evolution of the vaccine strain of type 3 poliovirus during the period of excretion by a primary vaccinee. *J. Gen. Virol.* **67**:693–706.
80. **Miyamura, K., M. Tanimura, N. Takeda, R. Kono, and S. Yamazaki.** 1986. Evolution of enterovirus 70 in nature: all isolates were recently derived from a common ancestor. *Arch. Virol.* **89**:1–14.
81. **Miyamura, K., K. Yamashita, N. Takeda, et al.** 1988. The first epidemic of acute hemorrhagic conjunctivitis due to a coxsackievirus A24 variant in Okinawa, Japan, in 1985–1986. *Jpn. J. Med. Sci. Biol.* **41**:159–174.
82. **Moore, B. E., B. P. Sagik, and C. A. Sorber.** 1979. Procedure for the recovery of airborne human enteric viruses during spray irrigation of treated waste water. *Appl. Environ. Microbiol.* **38**:688–693.
83. **Moore, M.** 1982. Enteroviral disease in the United States, 1970–1979. *J. Infect. Dis.* **146**:103–108.
84. **Morens, D. M, M. A. Pallansch, and M. Moore.** 1991. Polioviruses and other enteroviruses, p. 427–497. *In* R. B. Belshe (ed.), *Textbook of Human Virology*, 2nd ed. Mosby Yearbook, St. Louis.
85. **Nottay, B. K., O. M. Kew, M. H. Hatch, J. T. Heyward, and J. F. Obijeski.** 1981. Molecular variation of type 1 vaccine-related and wild polioviruses during replication in humans. *Virology* **108**:405–423.
86. **O'Neil, K. M., M. A. Pallansch, J. A. Winkelstein, T. M. Lock, and J. F. Modlin.** 1986. Chronic group A Coxsackievirus infection in agammaglobulinemia: demonstration of genomic variation of serotypically identical isolates persistently excreted by the same patient. *J. Infect. Dis.* **157**:183–186.
87. **Onorato, I. M., D. M. Morens, L. B. Schonberger, M. H. Hatch, R. M. Kaminski, and J. P. Turner.** 1985. Acute hemorrhagic conjunctivitis caused by enterovirus type 70: an epidemic in American Samoa. *Am. J. Trop. Med. Hyg.* **34**:984–991.
88. **Otatume, S., and P. A.-K. Addy.** 1975. Ecology of enteroviruses in tropics. I. Circulation of enteroviruses in healthy infants in tropical urban areas. *Jpn. J. Microbiol.* **19**:201–209.
89. **Patriarca, P. A., I. M. Onorato, V. Sklar, et al.** 1983. Acute hemorrhagic conjunctivitis: investigation of a large-scale community outbreak in Dade County, Florida. *JAMA* **249**:1283–1289.
90. **Payne, A. M.-M.** 1955. Poliomyelitis as a world problem, p. 393–400. *In* M. Fishbein (ed.), *Poliomyelitis Papers and Discussions Presented at the Third International Poliomyelitis Conference*. J. B. Lippincott, Philadelphia.
91. **Pöyry, T., L. Kinnunen, and T. Hovi.** 1989. Restricted variability of a 17 nucleotide stretch within the 5'-noncoding region of poliovirus genome. *Epidemiol. Infect.* **103**:671–683.
92. **Pöyry, T., L. Kinnunen, J. Kapsenberg, O. Kew, and T. Hovi.** 1990. Type 3 poliovirus/Finland/1984 is genetically related to common Mediterranean strains. *J. Gen. Virol.* **71**:2535–2541.
93. **Prabhakar, B. S., M. V. Haspel, P. R. McClintock, and A. L. Notkins.** 1982. High frequency of antigenic variants among naturally occurring human coxsackie B4 virus isolates identified by monoclonal antibodies. *Nature* (London) **300**:374–376.
94. **Prabhakar, B. S., M. A. Menegus, and A. L. Notkins.** 1985. Detection of conserved and nonconserved epitopes on Coxsackievirus B4: frequency of antigenic change. *Virology* **146**:302–306.
95. **Public Health Laboratory Service.** 1976. Hand, foot and mouth disease. *Br. Med. J.* **1**:350.

96. Rico-Hesse, R., M. A. Pallansch, B. K. Nottay, and O. M. Kew. 1987. Geographic distribution of wild poliovirus type 1 genotypes. *Virology* **160**:311–322.
97. Rossouw, E., C. W. A. Tsilimigras, and B. D. Schoub. 1991. Molecular epidemiology of a coxsackievirus B3 outbreak. *J. Med. Virol.* **34**:165–171.
98. Rotbart, H. A. 1990. Diagnosis of enteroviral meningitis with the polymerase chain reaction. *J. Pediatr.* **117**:85–89.
99. Rotbart, H. A., J. P. Kinsella, and R. L. Wasserman. 1990. Persistent enterovirus infection in culture-negative meningoencephalitis: Demonstration by enzymatic RNA amplification. *J. Infect. Dis.* **161**:787–791.
100. Sabin, A. B. 1991. Perspectives on rapid elimination and ultimate global eradication of paralytic poliomyelitis caused by polioviruses. *Eur. J. Epidemiol.* **7**:95–120.
101. Spigland, I., J. P. Fox, L. R. Elveback, et al. 1966. The Virus Watch program: a continuing surveillance of virus infections in metropolitan New York families. II. Laboratory methods and preliminary report on infections revealed by virus isolation. *Am. J. Epidemiol.* **83**:413–435.
102. Sutter, R. W., P. A. Patriarca, S. Brogan, et al. 1991. Outbreak of paralytic poliomyelitis in Oman: evidence for widespread transmission among fully vaccinated children. *Lancet* **338**:715–720.
103. Takeda, N., K. Miyamura, T. Ogino, et al. 1984. Evolution of enterovirus type 70: oligonucleotide mapping analysis of RNA genome. *Virology* **134**:375–388.
104. Takeda, N., M. Tanimura, and K. Miyamura. 1994. Molecular evolution of the major capsid protein VP1 of enterovirus 70. *J. Virol.* **68**:854–862.
105. Thoren, A., A. J. Robinson, T. Maguire, and R. Jenkins. 1992. Two-step PCR in the retrospective diagnosis of enteroviral viraemia. *Scand. J. Infect. Dis.* **24**:137–141.
106. Tsilimigras, C. W. A., E. Rossouw, and B. D. Schoub. 1989. Outbreak of poliomyelitis in South Africa investigated by oligonucleotide mapping. *J. Med. Virol.* **28**:52–56.
107. Tsilimigras, C. W. A., E. Rossouw, and B. D. Schoub. 1991. Molecular epidemiology of an outbreak of poliomyelitis in South Africa in 1987/1988. *J. Med. Virol.* **35**:121–127.
108. van Niekerk, A. B. W., B. D. Schoub, C. Chezzi, et al. 1994. Outbreak of poliomyelitis in Namibia. *Lancet* **343**:51.
109. Vonsover, A., R. Handsher, M. Neuman, et al. 1993. Molecular epidemiology of type 1 polioviruses isolated in Israel and defined by restriction fragment length polymorphism assay. *J. Infect. Dis.* **167**:199–203.
110. Ward, N., J. Milstien, H. Hull, and B. Hull. 1993. A global overview and hope for the eradication of poliomyelitis by the year 2000. *Trop. Geogr. Med.* **45**:198–202.
111. Wong, C. Y., J. J. Woodruff, and J. F. Woodruff. 1977. Generation of cytotoxic lymphocytes during coxsackievirus B-3 infection. III. Role of sex. *J. Immunol.* **119**:591–597.
112. Wright, P. F., R. J. Kim-Farley, C. A. de Quadros, S. E. Robertson, R. M. Scott, N. A. Ward, and R. H. Henderson. 1991. Strategies for the global eradication of poliomyelitis by the year 2000. *N. Engl. J. Med.* **325**:1774–1779.
113. Zheng, D. P., L. B. Zhang, Z. Y. Fang, et al. 1993. Distribution of wild type 1 poliovirus genotypes in China. *J. Infect. Dis.* **168**:1361–1367.

ENTEROVIRUS GENETICS

Christopher U. T. Hellen and Eckard Wimmer

2

The genus *Enterovirus* of the family *Picornaviridae* consists of over 100 mammalian and insect viruses (262, 288). The prototype enterovirus is poliovirus, the causative agent of poliomyelitis (223, 318), and the genus includes many important human and animal pathogens (28, 123, 262). The viral etiology of poliomyelitis was discovered in 1909 (223), but genetic studies did not begin to contribute to an understanding of the biology of enteroviruses for another half century (76). This state of affairs changed radically following the development of techniques for the growth of poliovirus in cultured mammalian cells (108), for its purification (375, 376), and for the isolation and characterization of clonal strains by plaque assay (98, 99). These technical advances were rapidly applied to studies of other enteroviruses (150, 151, 383) and yielded a number of fundamental insights.

Enterovirus genomes are composed of RNA (375) and are infectious (10, 65, 254, 390). Phenotypic variants can be readily selected from clonal enteroviral populations, and, significantly, mutation of a single nucleotide within the genome is sufficient to cause a phenotypic change (39). Early attempts at genetic analysis of enteroviruses were complicated by difficulties in identifying mutants that bore single defined genetic lesions and by the instability of the mutants (i.e., high reversion rates). Nevertheless, isolation of a number of temperature-sensitive (*ts*) poliovirus mutants led to the discovery that the genomes of these viruses can undergo genetic recombination, and this phenomenon was in turn used to separate and map poliovirus genetic functions (69, 140, 229).

The genetic analysis of enteroviruses was revolutionized by the advent of genetic engineering techniques and more specifically by two discoveries. First, the genetic map of the poliovirus genome was determined through sequence analysis of viral RNA and virus-encoded proteins (202, 342). The complete nucleotide sequences of over 25 enterovirus genomes and partial nucleotide sequences of many more are now known (Table 1). Second, cDNA copies of picornavirus genomes were found to yield infectious virus when they were introduced into mammalian cells either as DNA or, more efficiently, as RNA transcripts (341, 426). This development has permitted facile generation and analysis of

---

Christopher U. T. Hellen, Department of Microbiology and Immunology, State University of New York Health Sciences Center at Brooklyn, 450 Clarkson Avenue, Box 44, Brooklyn, New York 11203-2098. *Eckard Wimmer*, Department of Microbiology, State University of New York at Stony Brook, Stony Brook, New York 11794-8621.

TABLE 1 Nucleotide sequences and organization of enterovirus genomes

Virus	Serotype or strain	No. of nt 5' NTR	No. of nt 3' NTR	Total	Reference
Poliovirus	1 Mahoney	742	72	7,433	202
					342
	1 LS-a	742	72	7,433	241
	1 Sabin	742	72	7,441	305
					417
	2 Lansing	744	72	7,437	222
	2 Sabin				417
					334
	2-117	747	71	7,439	334
	2-712	747	71	7,439	289
	2W-2	747	72	7,434	325
	3 Leon/37	742	71	7,431	393
	3 Sabin	742	72	7,432	392
					417
					409
	3 Saukett				157
	3 119	742	72	7,432	47
	3 Finland	746	71	7,435	154
Coxsackievirus	A2				335
	A9	743	106	7,452	49
	A16	750	81	7,413	335
	A21	711	72	7,401	155
	A24	750	69	7,461	398
	B1	742	102	7,389	161
	B3	740	98	7,396	239
					52
					421
	B4	742	100	7,395	178
					344
					153
					414
	B5	743	101	7,402	444
Swine vesicular disease virus	H/3'76	742	102	7,400	164
	J1'73	743	102	7,400	165
	UKG/27/72	742	103	7,400	377
Echovirus	6		102		22, 122
	9				434
	11		101		21
	12	740	97	7,421	212
Enterovirus	70	727	82	7,391	403, 366
	71				335, 445
Bovine enterovirus	Vg/5/27	818	71	7,414	102
	RM-2	822			257
	PS-87	822			257
Cricket paralysis virus			242		195, 196

mutant viruses at the molecular level. Full-length infectious cDNA clones of several other enteroviruses, including bovine enterovirus (BEV) (102); echovirus 6 (36, 122); and coxsackieviruses B1 (162), B3 (52, 184, 204, 420), and B4 (345), have since been constructed. Genetic studies based on these two developments have contributed substantially to our understanding of the biology and pathogenic properties of enteroviruses.

CLASSIFICATION

The genus *Enterovirus* is defined on the basis of genetic and physicochemical properties such as density (1.32–1.35 g/cm3 in CsCl), sedimentation coefficient (150S to 165S), weight of virions (8×10^6 to 9×10^6 D), absence of a lipid envelope, ether resistance, and stability over a pH range of 3 to 10 (263, 265, 266). More recently, it has become clear that all enteroviruses have the same genetic organization (Fig. 1). Therefore, genetic criteria are also used now to classify these viruses (314) and have led to reclassification of some picornaviruses, such as hepatitis A virus and (probably) echoviruses 22 and 23, that had previously been assigned to the genus *Enterovirus* (158, 413). Rhinoviruses are not acid stable, but they share many biophysical properties with enteroviruses and are genetically so closely related to them that there are grounds for suggesting that these two genera could reasonably be combined (314).

Identification of enterovirus isolates depends on neutralization of cytopathic effects by specific antisera (183, 205, 267, 433), but different isolates of the same virus type can exhibit tremendous diversity in neutralization epitopes, host range, tissue tropism, and virulence. The majority of human enteroviruses have been allocated to either the poliovirus group (3 serotypes), the enteric cytopathogenic human orphan virus group (32 serotypes), or the coxsackie A virus and coxsackie B virus subgroups (6 and 23 serotypes, respectively). These divisions are somewhat arbitrary, and more recently discovered human enteroviruses are simply numbered (266).

POLIOVIRUS GENOME STRUCTURE, ORGANIZATION, AND FUNCTIONS

Poliovirus has a single-stranded 7,441-nucleotide (nt) RNA genome that is 3' polyadenylated and covalently linked to a virus-encoded oligopeptide (VPg) at its 5' terminus (113, 138, 231). These and all other properties of the poliovirus genome described in this section are representative of all enteroviruses. Poliovirus genomic RNA and mRNA are identical molecules except that VPg is absent from the 5' end of mRNA (the 5' end of mRNA is pUUAAA......[301]). Lytic RNA viruses whose genomes and mRNAs are of the same polarity are classified as plus-strand RNA viruses; their genomes function as mRNA on entry into the cytoplasm and are translated to yield all viral polypeptides necessary for replication (25). The enteroviral genome is monocistronic and has a long 5' nontranslated region (NTR) of 711 to 822 nt; the single large open reading frame (ORF) encodes a polyprotein of about 250 kDa that is proteolytically processed by virus-encoded proteinases to yield structural and nonstructural

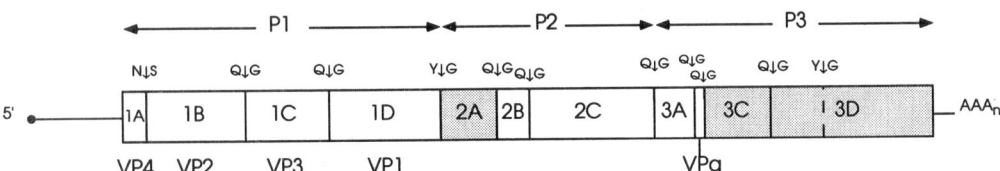

FIGURE 1 Genetic organization of poliovirus type 1 (Mahoney), the type member of genus *Enterovirus* of *Picornaviridae*. The polyprotein encoded by the single ORF is shown as an elongated rectangle, the 5' and 3' noncoding regions are shown as lines, and the genome-linked protein (VPg) is indicated by a black circle. Cleavage sites between individual viral proteins are shown above the genome at appropriate locations; these proteins are described within the rectangle according to the L434 nomenclature (365); the capsid proteins 1AB, 1A, 1B, 1C, and 1D are commonly referred to as VP0, VP4, VP2, VP3, and VP1, respectively. The proteinases 2A^{pro}, 3C^{pro}, and 3CD^{pro} are represented by shaded boxes. The structural protein precursor P1 and the nonstructural protein precursors P2 and P3 are indicated above the polyprotein.

proteins (Fig. 1) (see chapter 5). Subgenomic mRNAs are not synthesized during infection.

RNA viruses cannot use cellular proofreading or editing functions to eliminate errors that occur during genome replication, and they therefore have high mutation rates (147). This has the consequence that a "clonal" preparation of an RNA virus is not homogeneous but instead consists of a collection of genomes with slightly divergent nucleotide sequences and is therefore referred to as a "quasispecies" (90, 105). Although a high mutation rate allows for rapid genetic adaptation to environmental changes, it also strongly favors minimization of genome size, so that picornaviruses exist under conditions of genetic austerity (348). The monocistronic nature of the enteroviral genome limits the number of regulatory sequence elements that the genome contains, and its relatively small size limits the number of proteins that can be encoded. The bifunctional nature of several nonstructural enteroviral proteins and some aspects of the expression mechanism (such as the regulated proteolytic processing of the capsid protein precursor during morphogenesis) may be evolutionary responses to these limitations.

Cloverleaf

The 5' end of the poliovirus genome (nt 1 to 88) forms a characteristic cloverleaf or tRNA-like structure (Fig. 2) (15, 225, 228, 356). Most mutations in this structure confer defects in RNA synthesis on poliovirus (15, 16, 343), although there is one report of a resulting defect in protein synthesis (384). A second-site suppressor of a linker insertion mutation at nt 70 in the cloverleaf mapped downstream to 3C^{pro}, the viral proteinase (16). A ribonucleoprotein complex consisting of the 3CD^{pro} proprecursor of this proteinase and either a host factor or the viral polypeptide 3AB can form around the cloverleaf and may play a role in initiation of plus-strand RNA synthesis (14, 15, 132). tRNA-like structures play key roles in a variety of replicative processes involving RNA molecules, and it has been suggested

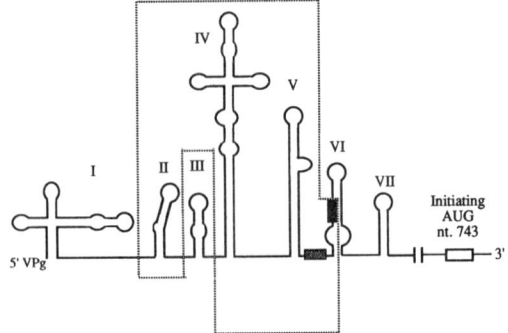

FIGURE 2 Schematic depiction of the secondary structure of the 5' nontranslated region of poliovirus based on previous models (15, 135, 327, 385). The nomenclature of structural elements is described elsewhere (135, 436a). Boundaries of IRES are indicated by a dotted line; the Y_n and AUG elements of the Y_n-X_m-AUG motif are represented by shaded and black rectangles, respectively; and the initiating codon of the viral polyprotein is represented by an open rectangle.

that they are "molecular fossils," that is, structural motifs that played an essential role in the earliest self-replicating systems and have been retained throughout subsequent evolution (251).

IRES

Translation of synthetic bicistronic mRNAs has revealed that a function of the enterovirus 5' NTR downstream of the cloverleaf is to promote initiation of translation by internal ribosomal entry (54, 320). This segment of the 5' NTR is separated from the cloverleaf by an unstructured pyrimidine-rich tract and is termed the internal ribosomal entry site (IRES) (174). All picornaviruses contain functionally related IRES elements, but there is surprisingly little sequence or structural similarity between the (type 1) IRES elements of entero- and rhinoviruses on the one hand and the (type 2) IRES elements of cardio- and aphthoviruses on the other. Roles for sequences within the poliovirus IRES in viral RNA synthesis and for sequences within the cloverleaf in IRES-dependent translation have been suggested (41, 384), although other experimental observations indicate that the 5' NTR has a modular organization in which the cloverleaf is involved exclusively in RNA synthesis and the IRES is involved exclusively in translation (11, 358).

The primary structure of the 5' NTR is strongly conserved between different enteroviruses, particularly within the first 650 nt (see below). The length of the spacer downstream of these residues is also conserved in polioviruses, but its sequence is the most variable region within the enteroviral genome (417). The boundaries of the poliovirus IRES have been defined by deletion analysis; the 5' and 3' borders are at about nt 134 and 556, respectively (Fig. 2; 160, 215, 298). Analysis of a pseudorevertant virus and subsequent deletion analysis showed that domain III is not required for IRES function (88, 298, 322). Mutant viruses lacking nucleotides downstream of the 3' border of the IRES are viable but have slightly impaired growth properties and significantly reduced virulence (119, 125, 126, 160, 162, 324, 328). These and other observations suggest that the spacer contains cis-acting elements that may influence the efficiency of initiation (136, 324).

The influence of single substitutions and small insertions or deletions within the IRES on the attenuation phenotype and on IRES-dependent translation suggested that the structure of the 5' NTR might be important for its function (111, 423, 436a). Various models for the secondary structure of the poliovirus 5' NTR have been derived by biochemical and computational analysis (135, 228, 327, 356, 385); the structure shown in Fig. 2 is a consensus model. Most sequence variation in the IRES takes the form of compensatory mutations that serve to maintain its secondary structure. Some pseudorevertant viruses contain compensating mutations that restore base pairing within domain V, providing genetic support for the proposed secondary structure of this domain (246, 276, 385). Some preliminary attempts to elucidate tertiary interactions within the 5' NTR have also been made (227, 296); the identification of second-site mutations in domain V that suppressed the effects of a 4-nt insertion in domain III suggests that there are long-range interactions between these two loci (215).

The structural conservation of type 1 IRES elements and the sensitivity of IRES function to subtle mutations suggest that much of the IRES is required either for direct interaction with trans-acting factors or for maintaining the conformation of the cis-acting elements necessary for such interactions. Binding sites for four cytoplasmic proteins that associate with the poliovirus IRES have been identified. The α subunit of eIF-2 has been detected in protein complexes associated with nt 97 to 182 and 510 to 629 of the 5' NTR (78), p50 binds to domain III (297), p52 binds to domain VI (259), and p57 binds to three noncontiguous sites at the 5' border of the IRES within domain V and downstream of the IRES (135, 137, 323). p52 and p57 have been identified as the La autoantigen and the pyrimidine tract-binding protein, respectively (40, 137, 260), but the molecular basis for their involvement in picornavirus translation has not yet been established. Fractionation of murine ribosomal salt wash fractions yielded a protein complex (initiation correction factor) of about 450 kDa that promoted accurate and efficient translation of poliovirus RNA in rabbit reticulocyte lysate (401), in which poliovirus mRNA is otherwise translated inefficiently and aberrantly (92). This complex may contain eIF2/2B and p57. A correlation between reduced translation efficiency and reduced binding of p52 as a result of nucleotide substitutions within domain VI has been established (259). Similarly, attenuating mutations within domain V that impair translation are associated with a reduced response to initiation correction factor activity (399, 401). Mutations in 2A^{pro} suppress ts phenotypes caused by destabilizing mutations in domain V, which suggests that 2A^{pro} may interact with this domain directly or indirectly (247). The precise role of these various viral and cellular trans-acting factors in IRES-dependent translation has not yet been elucidated.

Conservation of specific sequence motifs in type 1 IRES elements suggests that they contain several *cis*-acting RNA elements, but only one has been characterized in detail. The 3' border of type 1 IRES elements is about 160 nt upstream of the initiation codon, whereas the 3' border of type 2 IRES elements is at or close to the initiation codon. However, a strikingly conserved motif is present at the 3' border of all picornavirus IRES elements (175): a pyrimidine-rich (Y_n) tract ($n = 6$ to 9 nt) close to the IRES 3' boundary is separated by a nonconserved sequence (X_m, where $m = 15$ to 20 nt) from an AUG triplet. This AUG triplet is the initiation codon in type 2 IRES elements but is cryptic in type 1 IRES elements. The importance of the Y_n-X_m-AUG motif was first suggested by deletion analysis, and the importance of individual elements within it has subsequently been demonstrated by mutational analysis (162, 258, 298, 319, 323, 324, 328). Further evidence for the importance of this motif was obtained by analysis of phenotypic revertants of mutants containing lesions in this region of the 5' NTR: all were found to have regenerated correctly spaced Y_n and AUG elements by substitution, deletion, or insertion (119, 328).

Polyprotein

Analysis of poliovirus translation revealed a fundamental property of almost all eukaryotic mRNAs: initiation of translation is limited to a single 5'-proximal site, indicating that its genome is functionally monocistronic (172). Sequence analysis of poliovirus RNA confirmed this conclusion: the genome contains a single large ORF and up to 15 AUG triplets upstream of the initiation codon (202, 336, 342, 417). The large poliovirus ORF encodes a 250-kDa polyprotein that is proteolytically processed by virus-encoded proteinases, yielding proteins with diverse functions (131, 134) (see chapter 5).

The genetic map of poliovirus was established by mapping amino- and carboxy-terminal residues of virus-encoded proteins onto the sequence of the viral genome (2, 106, 201, 224, 378, 380). All entero- and rhinoviruses encode the same complement of polypeptides, which are described according to a systematic nomenclature (Fig. 1) (365). The genetic units 5'-virion proteins-RNA synthesis II-RNA synthesis I-3' described by Cooper (68, 69) correspond to the P1 (1ABCD), P2 (2ABC), and P3 (3ABCD) regions of the genome, which are processed to yield four (1A through 1D), three (2A through 2C), or four (3A through 3D) cleavage products. The terms VP0, VP4, VP2, VP3, and VP1 are still widely used to describe the capsid proteins 1AB, 1A, 1B, 1C, and 1D, respectively; the term VPg is used to describe the genome-linked protein 3B.

3' NTR

The 3' NTRs of enteroviruses are about 70 to 100 nt long (Table 1) (22) and are thought to form a pseudoknot or tRNA-like structure (161, 173, 329). The apparent deletion of about 30 nt in poliovirus and related enteroviruses corresponds to the loss of a complete hairpin present in the 3' NTRs of coxsackie B viruses (22). Insertion of 8 nt at nt 7387 yielded a virus with a *ts* phenotype that was defective in minus-strand RNA synthesis at the restrictive temperature; sequence alterations in the vicinity of nt 7387 could restore base pairing in the pseudoknot in pseudorevertants that synthesize RNA normally at the restrictive temperature (173, 372). These observations are consistent with the hypothesis that tRNA-like structures act as recognition signals in RNA replication.

3' Terminal Polyadenylic Acid

Most mammalian mRNAs have 3'-terminal poly(A) tails whose function may be to stabilize mRNAs or that could be involved in the regulation of translation (171). Poliovirus is also adenylated (20, 439); the mean length of the poly(A) tail is 60 nt (9), and it appears to be required for infectivity (371, 387). The observation that binding of 3D of human rhinovirus type 14 to the 3' end of its genome requires the 3' poly(A) sequence may indicate that the poly(A) tail plays a role in the formation of a replication complex at the 3' end of the template strand (74). The poly(A) tail is genetically encoded, i.e., it is transcribed from poly(U) in minus strands (93, 438a, 440). Progeny viruses with homopolymeric tails of normal length were recovered after transfection of poliovirus RNA transcripts containing short (12-nt) poly(A) tails into cells (309). This change could be due to incorporation of nontemplated residues during replication, which has been described following analysis of progeny derived from transcripts of other enteroviruses (130, 204).

Biological Functions of Viral Proteins
The P1 region of the enteroviral genome encodes the P1 precursor of the structural proteins VP4, VP2, VP3, and VP1. This precursor is cotranslationally myristoylated at its amino terminus (57) and is then processed by a regulated series of proteolytic cleavage reactions to yield the individual capsid proteins in a manner that is intimately connected to their assembly into virions (see chapter 7). The poliovirus capsid is an icosahedron assembled from 60 copies of the four capsid proteins (141). VP1, VP2, and VP3 are the main structural components of the virion, whereas VP4 is relatively unstructured and wholly internal. VP1, VP2, and VP3 each adopt an eight-stranded antiparallel β-barrel fold, and the disposition of these domains is responsible for the surface topography of the virus. A canyon 24 Å (2.4 nm) deep and 12 to 30 Å (1.2 to 3.0 nm) wide separates a peak formed by VP1 molecules at the fivefold axis of symmetry from a broad plateau formed by alternating VP2 and VP3 molecules at the pseudo sixfold axis of symmetry. In an immune response to an infection, antibodies capable of neutralizing viral infectivity are usually elicited against the exposed loops that connect the β strands within these barrels and that are therefore major components of the neutralizing antigenic sites (N-Ags). Poliovirus escape mutants resistant to neutralizing monoclonal antibodies can readily be selected (37, 86, 107, 279), and most have been found to map to these loops (312). Antigenic variants of other enteroviruses have been identified (56, 100, 205, 337, 338, 430), but the antigenic structures of these viruses and the locations and identities of variable residues have not yet been characterized in detail. However, the antigenic structure of human rhinovirus type 14 is nearly identical to that of poliovirus (362), and it is therefore reasonable to assume that other enteroviruses will also be similar. Poliovirus has four major N-Ags (142, 273) and only three unique sets of these sites, so there are only three poliovirus serotypes. Natural isolates in which the type-specific N-Ags are mixed have not been isolated, and a "tritypic" poliovirus constructed by using recombinant DNA techniques grew poorly (294).

The importance of myristoylation and proteolytic processing to virus assembly has been confirmed by analysis of mutants in which these processes have been impaired (e.g., see references 18, 66, and 252). A mutation in VP3 of poliovirus type 3 (Sabin) [PV3(S)] is responsible for its *ts* phenotype, and analysis of suppressor mutations elsewhere in the P1 region has identified residues that are probably involved in conformational transitions during assembly (112, 245, 277). Analysis of poliovirus mutants has also resulted in the identification of residues involved in encapsidation of RNA (17), interaction with the poliovirus receptor (PVR) (see chapter 3), uptake and disassembly of virions (185, 197), host range (72, 253, 290, 295), and the attenuation phenotype (249, 351, 409, 435). The capsid proteins of other enteroviruses are likely to contribute to an equally diverse number of biological properties: VP1 of CB4 contains a determinant of virulence (44), and VP1 of CB3 is altered in an isolate with an altered host range (347).

The P2 region of the genome encodes polypeptides 2A, 2B, and 2C; the processing intermediate 2BC is stable and may have functions that are distinct from those of its cleavage products. 2A is a small trypsinlike proteinase that catalyzes cleavage at its own amino terminus, releasing the P1 capsid protein precursor (418). Genetic analysis has implicated 2A^{pro} in the shutoff of host cell protein synthesis that occurs some hours after enteroviral infection (33, 310); this is the result of proteolytic cleavage of the translation initiation factor eIF-4γ (386). A direct role for 2A^{pro} in initiation of IRES-dependent translation is suggested by the observation that mutations in 2A^{pro} can suppress the inhibitory effects of substitutions in domain V of the poliovirus 5' NTR (247). Deletion analysis of subgenomic RNA genomes and analysis of dicistronic and other mutant polioviruses have also implicated 2A^{pro} in viral RNA synthesis (64, 285, 443). 2B mutants exhibit noncomplementable defects in RNA synthesis, and some exhibit partial *trans* dominance over wild-type (*wt*) poliovirus (32, 179, 235), but nothing else is known about the role of this polypeptide in enterovirus replication. 2C is the most strongly conserved of all enterovirus proteins (19), and it contains three well-characterized sequence motifs: an amino-terminal amphipathic helix (317), a nucleoside triphosphate (NTP)-binding site (83), and a putative zinc finger in the carboxy-terminal third of the polypeptide (285a). The zinc finger motif is also present in rhinovirus 2C polypeptides but is absent from 2C encoded by cardio- and aphthoviruses. 2C has nucleoside triphosphatase activity (281, 357), and mutations in a conserved sequence motif associated with this activity confirm its importance for virus viability (280, 411). Guanidine hydrochloride can completely inhibit enterovirus replication at millimolar concentrations (73, 264, 355). The major effect of guanidine appears to be blockage of single-stranded RNA synthesis with a concomitant accumulation of double-stranded RNA, although the molecular basis for this effect remains obscure (45). Drug-resistant (g^r) and drug-dependent (g^d) mutants are readily selected and have been found to map to 2C (13, 23, 330–332, 416). A conditional lethal mutation in 2C is severely temperature sensitive in RNA synthesis (235) and, in contrast to the g^s phenotype is readily complemented.

This observation suggests that 2C may perform separate functions in RNA replication. A third function for 2C, RNA encapsidation, has been suggested (236).

The P3 region of the enterovirus genome consists of the polypeptides 3A, 3B, 3C, and 3D; 3AB and 3CD are stable processing intermediates, and the latter is known to have functions distinct from its cleavage products 3C and 3D. 3A is tightly associated with membrane-associated replication complexes in infected cells (407), and genetic evidence suggests that 3A or 3A-containing polypeptides may be involved in the assembly of functional initiation complexes (31, 117, 118). 3A is part of the stable precursor 3AB, which also contains the sequence of VPg, the 22-amino-acid oligopeptide that is linked to the 5' ends of positive- and negative-stranded viral RNAs. 3AB is therefore a candidate donor of uridylylated VPg to the replication complex (404). Extensive mutagenesis of poliovirus 3B (VPg) has revealed that residues Y4 (which is normally the site of covalent attachment to RNA) and R17 are essential for viability but that many other substitutions are tolerated (217, 218, 352). Uridylylation of VPg is temperature sensitive in enterovirus 70 (EV70) and PV3(S) and is associated with impaired RNA replication at the restrictive temperature (405, 419). The *ts* defect in uridylylation of poliovirus VPg is associated with a point mutation in the 3D coding sequence; the location of the lesion responsible for the *ts* defect in EV70 RNA replication is not known.

The polypeptide 3CD is proteolytically cleaved between either Glu-Gly (Q-G) or Tyr-Gly (Y-G) dipeptides, yielding the cleavage products 3C and 3D or 3C' and 3D', respectively. The polypeptides 3C' and 3D' are not necessary for virus viability, and their functions are not known (230). 3CD is the proteinase that cleaves the P1 precursor between Q-G dipeptides to release the capsid proteins VP0, VP3, and VP1 (181, 442); 3C is the catalytic core of this proteinase (129), and 3D is the viral RNA-dependent RNA polymerase (427). 3C^{pro} can cleave peptide substrates that correspond to some cleavage sites within the polyprotein (299, 313), but it is likely that cleavage in vivo is catalyzed by larger 3C-containing precursors (218). Additional interactions between such precursors and structural domains of polyprotein substrates are thus likely to be determinants of cleavage (e.g., see reference 442a). Genetic and biochemical evidence supports predictions (27, 121) that 3C proteinases contain a cysteine nucleophile but that the active-site geometry otherwise resembles that of trypsinlike serine proteinases (127, 188, 226). These observations are consistent with structural analyses of hepatitis A virus and human rhinovirus type 14 3C proteinases (11a, 255). A number of amino acid residues that alter cleavage of 3CD have been identified (14, 84, 85, 128, 187a); many of the residues in $3C^{pro}$, such as H31, V54, K60, I74, D85, and R87, map outside the enzyme active site. The crystallographic model of human rhinovirus type 14 $3C^{pro}$ suggests that these residues form part of an intermolecular interface between two adjacent proteinase molecules and that this interaction promotes cleavage of the 3CD bond in trans (255).

Analysis of a pseudorevertant poliovirus indicates that mutations in $3C^{pro}$ suppressed a defect in RNA replication caused by an insertion into the 5' terminal cloverleaf (16), and detailed mutational analysis identified residues in $3C^{pro}$ that are involved in its ability to bind RNA (14, 233). Interestingly, these amino acid residues are located near the putative $3C^{pro}$ dimer interface, an observation that suggests that the interaction between 3CD and the cloverleaf may promote formation of the complex that cleaves 3D from 3CD. 3D is a template-dependent RNA polymerase, whereas 3CD has no such activity, so cleavage of 3CD results in activation of the polymerase (427). Purified $3D^{pol}$ is capable of RNA chain elongation but is unable to initiate RNA synthesis and does not provide the specificity for RNA synthesis in vitro that is observed in infected cells (77, 425). It is therefore likely that $3D^{pol}$ associates with viral (and possibly cellular) factors to form a replication complex. Mutations within the poliovirus coding region 2A, 2B, 2C, 3A, 3B, 3C, and 3D all cause primary defects in RNA replication, and they are therefore all potentially components of such a complex. Interactions between some of these proteins are suggested by the results of genetic analysis (419), functional assays (132, 219, 283), biochemical fractionation (407), and subcellular localization (34).

Some progress has been made in relating the structure of $3D^{pol}$ to its functions. Enteroviral 3D polymerases share four highly conserved regions of sequence similarity (termed motifs A, B, C, and D) with viral RNA polymerases, reverse transcriptases, and DNA polymerases (79, 333). Some residues within these conserved regions are essential for polymerase activity and/or virus viability; thus, a Y326M substitution within motif C impaired virus replication but did not affect polymerase elongation capacity. The replication defect was suppressed by an additional E108D substitution (169, 170). These two residues, and possibly Y-424 (8, 43), may be involved in the initiation of RNA synthesis; insertion of a Leu residue after D-257 yielded a polymerase that was defective in RNA chain elongation (53). Several other conditional poliovirus mutants bearing mutations in the $3D^{pol}$ coding region have been identified (33, 87), and further analysis may identify specific residues in 3D that are involved in its various functions and may help reveal specific interactions between 3D and other viral and cellular proteins.

GENETIC CONSERVATION AND DIVERSITY IN ENTEROVIRAL GENOMES

Complete or partial nucleotide sequences of many enteroviruses have been determined (Table 1), and it has become apparent that these sequences can be described in terms of a common organizational pattern despite considerable sequence variation between virus types and strains (Fig. 1). The number of nucleotide differences between sequences reflects the genetic distance between genomes with a common origin, and this information can be used to construct an approximate phylogeny: cardio-, aphtho-, and hepatoviruses form distinct groups, whereas rhino- and enteroviruses overlap considerably (314, 391). There is a considerable degree of nucleotide identity (<50%) between viruses within each of these genera. The conventional subdivision of enteroviruses into various groups has been described above, and this classification holds well at the molecular level for the poliovirus group and the coxsackie B virus subgroup (which includes swine vesicular disease virus (SVDV)) (Fig. 3) (164, 165, 377). However, the molecular relationships between other members of the enterovirus genus are more complex. Some echoviruses and coxsackie A viruses (e.g., CAV-9, -10, and -12 as well as most echoviruses [21, 22, 49, 391, 434]) can be considered candidate members of the coxsackie B virus subgroup, and others (e.g., CAV-11, -18, -21, and -24 [22, 155, 156, 166, 391, 398]) are clearly related to the poliovirus group. Some enteroviruses, such as CAV-2, CAV-16, BEV, EV70, and EV71, do not clearly fall into any previously recognized nucleotide identity group (102, 159, 257, 335, 403). Extensive regions of sequence homology with poliovirus have been identified within the genomes of CAV-21 and EV70, and these and other enteroviruses (such as EV22) may have recombinant genomes (155, 156, 158, 366). The evolutionary role of recombination in the generation of enterovirus genomes is discussed in greater detail below.

Enteroviral genomes are more strongly conserved in the P2 and P3 regions (which encode nonstructural proteins) than in the P1 region (which encodes structural proteins). Similar differences in the rates of accepted point mutations are apparent in the genomes of all RNA viruses. The rate of mutation is constant throughout the genome, and this phenomenon must therefore reflect differing effects of selection on different genes. Sequence variation between different isolates or strains of the same virus type is usually small, but comparison of their nucleotide sequences can provide useful information concerning the genetic basis of phenotypic properties and the phylogenetic relationship between virus isolates. Extensive microheterogeneity has been identified in regions of the poliovirus genome corresponding to the neutralizing antigenic sites (37, 86, 107, 279) and to the sequence between domain VI of the 5' NTR and the initiation codon of the polyprotein (417). The length of this spacer varies from about 75 to 115 nt in different enteroviruses (Table 1). A number of other probable deletions and insertions in enterovirus genomes, including duplication of the 5'-terminal cloverleaf in BEV;

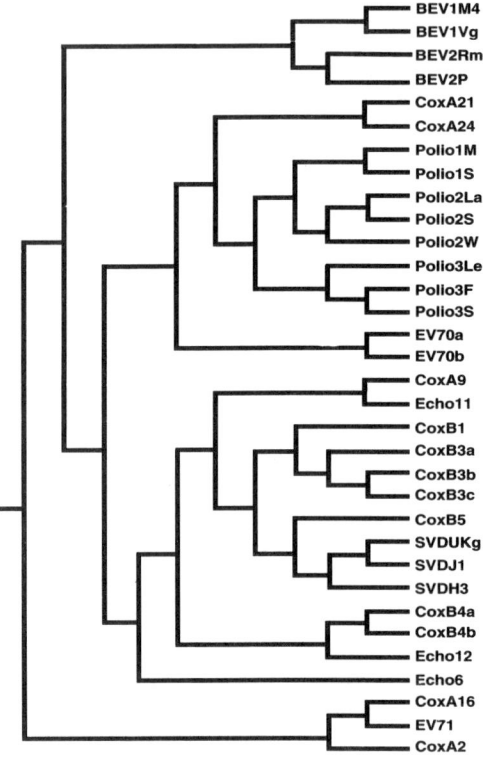

FIGURE 3 Relationship among members of the *Enterovirus* genus, according to aligned sequences of their genomic RNAs. Relationships are presented graphically as a minimum length, binary parsimonious rooted cladogram, calculated by using heuristic methods. Abbreviations: BEV, bovine enterovirus; CoxA, coxsackie A virus; CoxB, coxsackie B virus; Echo, echovirus; EV, enterovirus; Polio, poliovirus; SVD, swine vesicular disease virus.

deletion of domain III of the IRES in CAV-9, CB1, CB2, CB4, CB5, SVDV, and BEV; possible transduction of cellular sequences into the C terminus of VP1 in CAV-9; and deletion of 3' noncoding sequences in all polioviruslike enteroviruses (see Table 1 for references), have been noted. Sufficient data to evaluate molecular relationships can be derived from relatively short sequences, and this approach has therefore been used extensively in epidemiologic studies to document the origin and transmission of enteroviruses (156a, 166, 167, 237, 238, 282, 354, 406, 437, 447). The sequence similarity between different enteroviruses is greater, but analysis of invariant residues has resulted in the identification of specific sequence motifs in noncoding and coding regions of the genome. The former include elements involved in RNA replication and translation (228, 327, 328, 356), and the latter are characteristic of specific functional domains such as NTP-binding sites and the active sites of proteinases and polymerases (19, 27, 83, 114, 120, 121, 333, 446).

The arrangement of these and other domains is identical within all enteroviral genomes (Fig. 1) and is only slightly modified in other picornaviruses (364, 391). Sequence homologies between these and functionally equivalent polypeptides were first identified in three groups of plant RNA viruses that on first inspection appeared to be unrelated to picornaviruses, because two groups (comoviruses and nepoviruses) have bipartite genomes, and one group (potyvirus) forms long flexuous particles (19, 89, 114). Related protein sequences have subsequently been identified in a much broader range of RNA viruses, although they often occur in a different order or on separate genomic segments (27, 120, 121, 333, 396). Picornaviruses and members of the three plant virus groups contain the same module of related genes (nucleoside triphosphatase, VPg, trypsinlike protease, and polymerase, which correspond to the picornavirus 2C, 3B, 3C, and 3D polypeptides, respectively) and a varying complement of ancillary genes. These observations suggest that the genomes of RNA viruses have a modular construction and that they arise by shuffling of functional units. Reassortment of viral genes almost certainly occurs by a process of recombination, which has been well documented in picornaviruses and is the likely mechanism by which the 5'-terminal cloverleaf was duplicated in BEV (102, 257) and by which the "hybrid" genomes of CAV-21 and EV70 arose (155, 366, 403). The origin of the functional modules found in RNA virus genomes is not known, but they may be evolutionary descendants of captured cellular genes. There is evidence for the transduction of cellular sequences into the genomes of RNA viruses (192, 271, 286, 293), possibly including enteroviruses (49, 50, 53a). Several of the sequence motifs that occur in enteroviral genomes (such as the NTP-binding site in 2C and the proteinase active sites of 2A and 3C) closely resemble motifs found in functionally related cellular polypeptides, and recent structural studies of two picornavirus 3C moieties have confirmed predictions that they have a trypsinlike fold (11a, 255).

GENETIC DISSECTION OF THE GENOME

Infectious cDNA Clones and Transcription of Infectious Viral RNA

Genetic studies of enteroviruses were revolutionized by the finding that full-length cDNA clones of poliovirus produced progeny virus after transfection into HeLa cells (341). This approach permitted genetic manipulation of the poliovirus genome, but the utility of the method was limited by the low specific infectivity of these cDNA clones, particularly if poliovirus derivatives had impaired growth properties (207, 379). However, the use of T7 polymerase to transcribe full-length cDNA clones yielded poliovirus RNAs whose specific infectivity is similar to that of virion RNA (371, 426). Enteroviral RNAs remain infectious after various modifications at their 5' termini, but the proper 5' terminus is always restored in viral RNA recovered from progeny virions (130, 184, 304, 426). Transcription vectors containing full-length cDNA clones of numerous enteroviral genomes controlled by the bacteriophage T7 promoter have successfully been constructed (36, 52, 102, 122, 162, 204, 345, 420).

Selection and Generation of Mutants
Generation of enterovirus mutants is the first critical step in their genetic analysis. The first mutant viruses were selected from virus stocks with or without prior chemical mutagenesis of the inoculant (39, 140, 229), but further genetic analysis was frequently complicated by difficulties in ensuring the complete removal of mutants with multiple lesions. Mutants with single defined genetic alterations are preferred starting materials for genetic experiments, and they can now be generated readily by manipulation of infectious cDNA clones, and genotypes can be confirmed by recloning and sequencing. Enteroviral mutants have been generated by a variety of strategies, as described below.

Mutant viruses can easily be selected from a quasispecies population when host cells are infected with a low multiplicity under conditions restricting *wt* virus proliferation. Early genetic studies used poliovirus mutants with markers (such as *ho* and *bo*) that represent sensitivity to constituents of growth media (68, 69, 206). The genetic lesions responsible for these phenotypes have not been characterized; subsequent genetic studies have used mutants isolated on the basis of resistance to inhibition by 2 mM guanidine (g^r, which maps to 2C [107a, 330]), to neutralizing monoclonal antibodies (which led to the identification of the poliovirus N-Ags [37, 86, 107, 279]), and to other clearly defined and characterized criteria. A number of *ts* poliovirus mutants have been generated by chemical mutagenesis and were used to establish a recombination map and to assign gene function despite the difficulties (i.e., the high reversion rate) of selecting and maintaining mutants that contain single defined lesions (68, 69). Precise changes can now be introduced into enteroviral genomes by using PCR and oligonucleotide-mediated techniques for site-directed mutagenesis. These powerful methods have been used to investigate the roles of *cis*-acting elements within noncoding regions of the genome, cleavage sites within the polyprotein, and specific sequence motifs within nonstructural proteins (summarized in reference 436a). Substitutions have been introduced into the 5' NTR (248) and the coding sequence of the viral polymerase 3D (87) with the intention of generating mutants with *ts* phenotypes; isolation of revertants and characterization of altered coding and noncoding sequences containing suppressor mutations are likely to yield insights into the functions and interactions of the mutated targets (e.g., see references 16, 170, and 247).

A quasispecies population contains a large spectrum of genotypes, most of which differ from one another by a small number of substitutions, so that methods that make possible the construction of mutants containing random or semirandom insertions and deletions (which are much less common) are of special interest (31, 85, 200). Numerous mutants have been derived in this way, and they have provided insights into various aspects of enterovirus replication (summarized in reference 436a). Some of these methods have utilized restriction enzyme sites within infectious cDNA clones that have been filled in or chewed back. A related mutagenesis method involves the insertion of selected or randomized DNA cartridges between restriction sites (217, 253, 295). Large genomic segments can be exchanged between enteroviruses by recombination in vivo, and this phenomenon can be mimicked in vitro by using existing or engineered restriction sites to exchange cDNA segments of any size between genomes. This approach has been instrumental in mapping determinants of the attenuation phenotype of Sabin vaccine strains of poliovirus (see below) and has also provided insight into the compatibility of picornavirus genetic elements (11, 180, 358, 381).

Dicistronic Viruses

The enteroviral genome is monocistronic and encodes a single polyprotein that is proteolytically processed to release various structural and nonstructural polypeptides. These properties have consequences that may complicate genetic analysis, because a point mutation within a coding region may have multiple effects on phenotype. For example, a substitution could (i) alter the primary structure of a polypeptide and also affect a function dependent on RNA structure, (ii) affect the (potentially distinct) functions of the polypeptide in which it occurs and those of its precursors, and (iii) affect the global folding and consequently the proteolytic processing of the polyprotein. Genetic dissection of the enteroviral 5' NTR and polyprotein has been facilitated by the recent development of a strategy that involves insertion of an IRES element into the enteroviral genome (284). The encephalomyocarditis virus (EMCV) IRES has been used in all constructs to date, because its low sequence similarity to enteroviral IRES elements reduces the possibility of recombination. An insertion of this type generates a dicistronic genome that should be a viable entity, provided the insertion does not disrupt the coding sequence of an essential gene product and does not interfere with proteolytic processing of the polyprotein. Three insertion sites that meet these criteria have been identified and have yielded viable dicistronic polioviruses (Fig. 4). The scissile bond between the P1 (capsid protein) and P2-P3 (nonstructural protein) regions was chosen as the first insertion site for the EMCV IRES because this bond is cleaved cotranslationally, and the P1 partial polyprotein is subsequently cleaved in *trans*. The resulting virus, W1-P1/E/P2,3-1, was genetically stable, but its replication was impaired; partial deletion of the EMCV IRES abolished viral replication (284). A similar dicistronic virus was subsequently reported elsewhere (41). Insertion of the EMCV IRES between 2A^{pro} and 2B yielded a viable virus, W1-P1, 2A/E/2BC, P3-1, with impaired replication characteristics, indicating that 2A^{pro} can function in *trans* in all events subsequent to its separation from P1 (284). Dicistronic genomes lacking 2A^{pro} failed to replicate, as did genomes in which 2A^{pro} had been modified by partial deletion or active-site substitution, suggesting a role for this polypeptide in genome replication (see above). Insertion of the EMCV IRES into all other cleavage sites of the polyprotein abolished viral replication, possibly because of aberrant proteolytic processing of the P2-P3 region and/or disruption of an active precursor (e.g., 2BC, 3AB, or 3CD [436a]). However, insertion of the EMCV IRES at nt 630 in the poliovirus 5' NTR produced the viable, genetically stable virus W1-PNENPO, which has two different IRES elements arranged in tandem (Fig. 4); replacement of the poliovirus IRES with the EMCV IRES yielded the virus W1-P108ENPO, in which translation is dependent solely on the heterologous EMCV IRES (11). The dicistronic poliovirus genome pDICAT (Fig. 4) stably expressed the chloramphenicol acetyltransferase coding sequence in vivo (11), confirming the utility of such viruses as expression vectors. Other coding sequences could be substituted for this reporter gene: expression of a duplicated enterovirus gene could be used to complement genetic defects in mutant enteroviral genomes (436a).

Characterization of Revertants

Isolation and characterization of revertant viruses from cells infected with mutant viral genomes can contribute substantially toward elucidation of the molecular basis of mutant phenotypes. Several kinds of revertant have been identified. First, reversion to the *wt* sequence indicates that the substituted nucleotide or amino acid residue is crucial for the *wt* phenotype. For example, the mutation CAA→AAA (Lys-135-Gln) within the NTP-binding site of 2C always reverted to the *wt* sequence by an infrequent transversion mutation, AAA→CAA (280); reversion of this type within the 5' NTR may indicate the importance of specific sequence or structural elements. Second, some positions within a

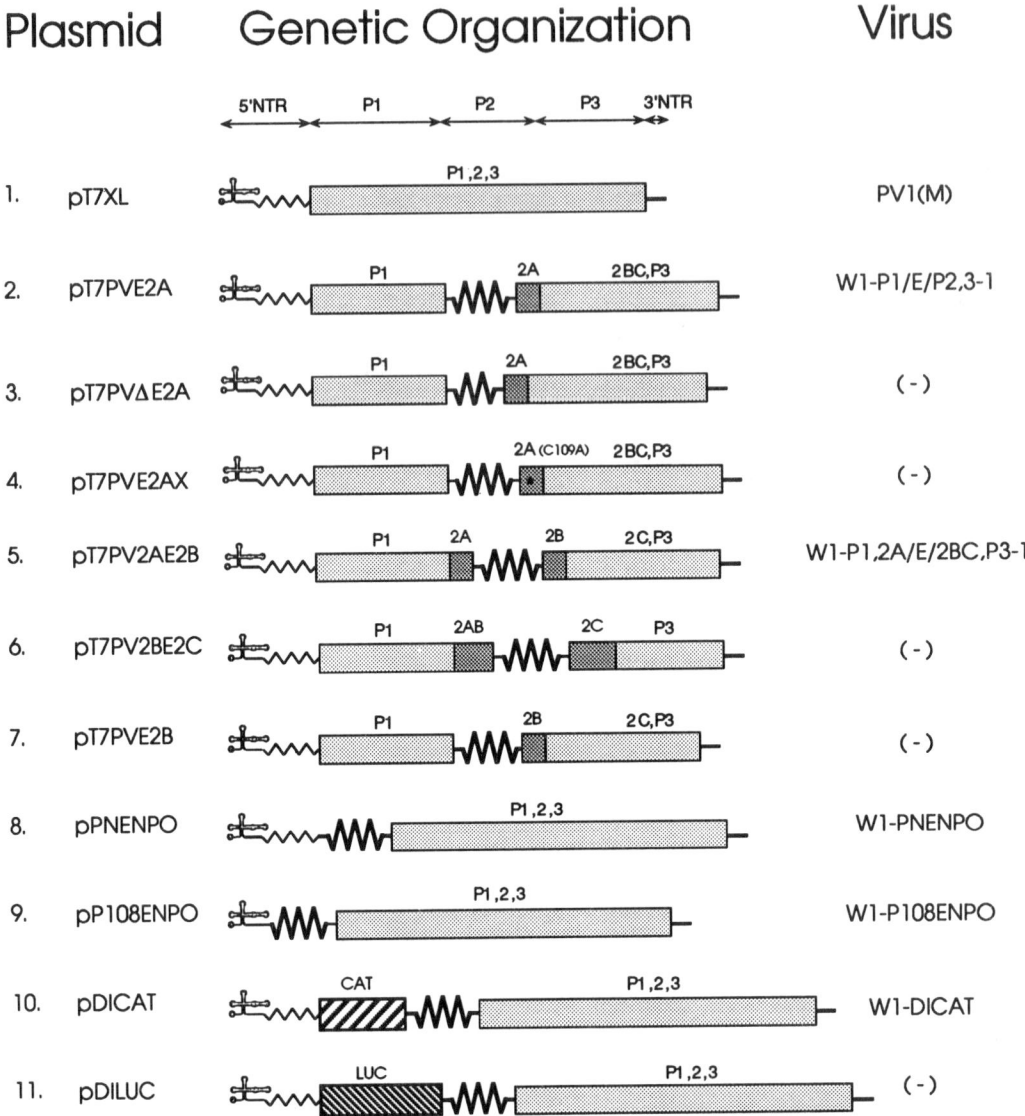

FIGURE 4 Genetic organization of dicistronic poliovirus mRNA genomes. The 5'-terminal 108-nt fragment of the PV1(M) 5' NTR is shown as a cloverleaf, the downstream segments of the 5' NTR (including the IRES) are shown as thin zigzag lines, and the segments of the EMCV 5' NTR inserted into the poliovirus genome are shown as thick zigzag lines. EMCV segments correspond to nt 260 to 848 (in plasmids 1 and 4), 260 to 833 (in plasmids 5 to 11), and 435 to 833 (in plasmid 3). Stippled rectangles represent poliovirus coding regions, and the cross-hatched rectangles represent the chloramphenicol acetyltransferase (CAT) and luciferase (LUC) coding regions. Viruses recovered after transfection of mRNA transcripts into HeLa cells are described with standard nomenclature; (−) indicates that a viable virus was not recovered.

polypeptide may tolerate the presence of several non-*wt* amino acid residues; thus, the substitution Lys-82-Gln within 3C^{pro} reverted by replacement of the Gln residue with an Arg residue (128). Third, reversion may occur by deletion of the mutation and of flanking residues. This phenomenon has been observed in studies of the poliovirus 5'NTR (88, 119, 126,

329). Fourth, mutation at a second site (which may be thousands of nucleotides distant from the original substitution) may result in reversion to a *wt* phenotype. Such second-site reversions can reveal interacting residues in the three-dimensional arrangement of a polypeptide or nucleotide sequence or in larger complexes. This is the rationale behind the development of site-directed mutational methods for the generation of enteroviruses with *ts* phenotypes (87). Numerous second-site revertants have been identified in the poliovirus 5' NTR, particularly in domain V of the IRES (436a); other suppressor mutations indicate longer-range interactions within the 5' NTR (215). Intra-allelic suppressor mutations have been identified within $3D^{pol}$ (170); interallelic suppression of mutations within the cloverleaf and IRES elements of the 5' NTR by substitutions within $3C^{pro}$ and $2A^{pro}$ indicate a role for these polypeptides in RNA replication and IRES-dependent translation, respectively (16, 247).

GENETIC COMPLEMENTATION

Genetic Complementation in Poliovirus Replication

Genetic complementation is the compensatory actions of the gene products of two homologous genetic systems in cells with mixed infections that alleviate defects in mutant genes without causing genotypic change. For example, two polioviruses may grow to *wt* levels in mixed infections if the product of the normal gene of one virus can compensate for the defective product of the mutant virus. Mutations that fail to complement a specific defect have been defined as affecting the same unit of function and can be combined into a complementation group (see, e.g., reference 424). The monocistronic enteroviral genome encodes a single polyprotein, so complementation groups may not necessarily indicate separate coding sequences but could represent different functions of a polypeptide precursor and its cleavage products or distinct functions of the same protein. Moreover, a recent report concerning complementation of mutants in the poliovirus IRES suggests that a complementation group may even map to a noncoding region of the genome if it has a function that can act in *trans* (395).

The most typical form of complementation is nonallelic (intergenic) complementation, in which mutants defective in different functions assist each other's growth by supplying the function that is defective in the other virus. Allelic (intragenic) complementation is less frequent; it normally occurs when the two parental viruses have defects in different domains of the same protein. Symmetric complementation occurs when the yield of both mutants defective in different functions is enhanced during a mixed infection; it was first conclusively demonstrated by using linker-insertion mutants that contained lesions in polypeptides 2A and 3A (32). Complementation can also be asymmetric; this occurs when only one of the polioviruses grows to increased titers. Such unidirectional complementation is referred to as "rescue" and can occur during a mixed infection with two mutant viruses (32, 67) or when a *wt* virus supplies a gene product needed by the mutant (e.g., the rescue of defective interfering [DI] particles, which lack part of the P1 capsid protein coding sequence) (63, 302). Complementation tests involve determination of the virus yield by plaque assay of mutants produced during a single cycle of cells infected either singly or multiply under nonpermissive conditions. A complementation index for a mutant is calculated as the yield of the mutant in a mixed infection divided by the yield of the mutant in a single infection; this value must be corrected for reversion, which may contribute substantially to the apparent yield of a mutant. However, an apparent decrease in the yield of some revertants (compared to that which occurs during a single infection) has been noted when virus stocks were grown under conditions of complementation, presumably because of decreased selection for revertants (32). Analysis of this type indicates that the efficiency of complementation within the same genome and even within the same coding sequence can be very variable.

The first enteroviral mutants to be used for studies of genetic complementation were polioviruses whose replication was sensitive to (the *wt* phenotype), resistant to, or dependent on the presence of guanidine (g^s, g^r, and g^d, respectively) (6, 70, 71, 163, 431). In these experiments, complementation was asymmetrical (e.g., g^s mutants were rescued by g^r or g^d mutants in the presence of the drug), but symmetrical intra-allelic complementation between g^s and g^d mutants under conditions restrictive for growth of both mutants has also been reported (416). However, the complementation index score was always low (i.e., complementation was inefficient), which has permitted the widespread use of *g* mutants in experiments involving selection for recombinants (199, 415). The observation that a linker insertion mutation in 2C with a *ts* phenotype is complemented very efficiently (235) suggests that 2C has more than one function in viral replication.

Coinfection of cells with poliovirus *g* mutants of different serotypes led to the discovery of a phenomenon variously referred to as genomic masking or phenotypic mixing, in which the genome of the rescued virus is enclosed within capsid proteins that were encoded by the helper virus. Such pseudotypic enteroviruses have been detected after coinfection of cells with either echovirus type 7 and CA-9 (168) or poliovirus types 1 and 2, CB1, CB5, or echovirus type 1 (29, 70, 71, 149, 163, 261, 388, 389, 431). One report even indicates that the genome of the aphthovirus foot-and-mouth disease virus can be encapsidated by BEV coat proteins (422). It is not yet apparent whether the formation of such a variety of pseudotypes indicates that picornaviruses contain conserved determinants of encapsidation (see chapter 7).

A number of mutants that could not be complemented, including four with lesions in 2B, one with a lesion in 3A, one with a lesion in 3D, and one with a lesion in the 3' NTR, have been identified (32, 179, 235). Some of the mutations in these and other nonstructural proteins (3A and 3C) are *cis* dominant (Fig. 5 [16, 117]). The lesion mapping to a structural element in the 3' NTR can probably not be complemented, because it has a *cis*-acting function in RNA synthesis (173). Lack of complementation of 2B, 3A, and 3D mutants is more difficult to explain, particularly since other mutants in 3D are complementable (8, 53, 307), because some mutants in 2B are *trans* dominant (i.e., capable of acting in *trans* to inhibit replication of *wt* virus [179]), and because a lethal mutation in VPg could be complemented intragenomically by *wt* 3AB in a dicistronic virus (see below). However, the lack of complementation of these mutants may be related to observations that a large segment of the P2-P3 region of the poliovirus genome must be translatable in replication-competent genomes. Deletions within natural DI particles occur exclusively within the 5' NTR and P1 regions of the genome and always maintain the reading frame of the largest potential ORF (see below). Moreover, DI replicons that contained deletions within the P2 and P3 regions or in which these regions had been placed out of frame with respect to the initiation codon of the viral polyprotein were not actively replicated (64, 124). Several mechanisms could account for the dependence of poliovirus replication on translation in *cis*. For example, these nonstructural proteins could have activities that function exclusively in *cis* on the genomes from which they were translated either because of direct binding to the RNA or because of rapid inactivation or other limits on their free diffusion in active form. Alternatively, replication could be coupled directly to the process of translation, either because ribosomal transit causes structural alterations in the conformation of RNA structures downstream of the P1 coding sequence that are required for replication or because a ribosome-associated protein required for replication becomes associated with the genome only after ribosomal passage through the critical segment of the P2-P3 region. Other mechanisms are clearly possible, but all would have the effect of limiting the spread of "selfish" mutants that contain

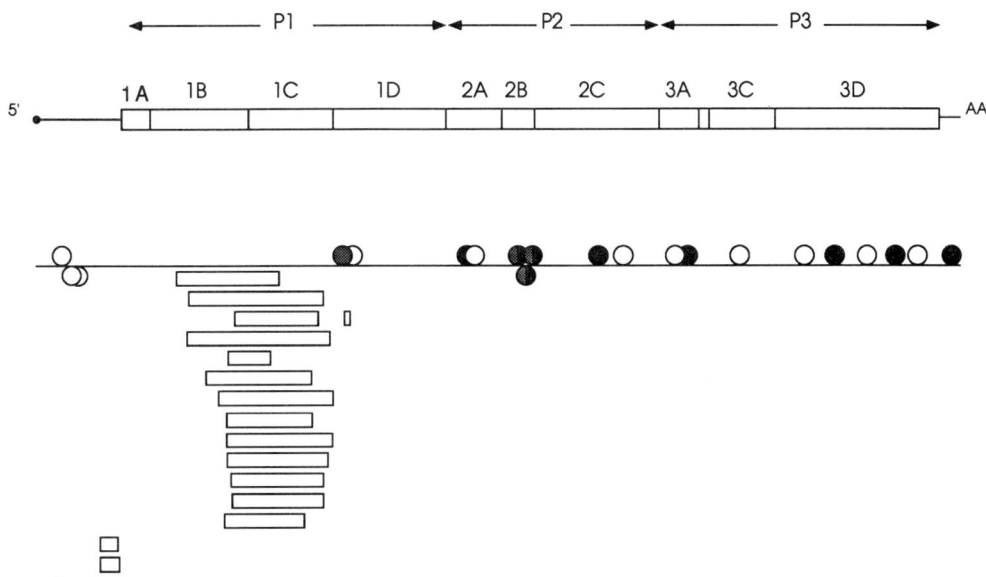

FIGURE 5 Complementation map of poliovirus. Deletions identified in DI particles (88, 119, 126, 182, 216, 328) are shown as rectangles; other mutations are shown as circles. Open circles represent recessive mutations that can be complemented by *wt* or other mutant viruses (8, 33, 53, 235, 307, 373, 416), black circles represent *cis*-dominant mutations that cannot be complemented or rescued (16, 33, 117, 179, 235, 307, 373, 423), and gray circles represent *trans*-dominant mutations that can inhibit the growth of coinfecting virus (33, 179, 373). Adapted from a figure by Kirkegaard (198).

frameshift, deletion, or nonsense mutations in the P2-P3 region and that might otherwise enjoy a replicative advantage over *wt* viruses and interfere with their growth (63, 307).

Intragenomic Complementation

A novel strategy of complementation has been developed by using dicistronic viruses that have the genetic structure poliovirus 5' NTR - X - EMCV IRES - poliovirus P1,P2,P3' - poliovirus 3' NTR (436a). They resemble the dicistronic viruses described above except that the reporter gene has been replaced by genetic unit X, which encodes a viral polypeptide (Fig. 4). The presence of a duplicated coding segment of the poliovirus genome may complement lethal mutations mapping to different genetic units of the polyprotein. This strategy has so far resulted in complementation in one instance: genomic RNAs with a lethal double substitution in VPg (Y3F-T4A) could be complemented to yield viable virus if the PVG unit was *wt* 3AB (48a).

REVERSION

A high rate of misincorporation of bases and thus of genotypic change (i.e., mutation) is intrinsic to the replication of RNA viruses (94, 143, 147). Analysis of revertant poliovirus genomes derived from a viable insertion mutant indicated that the poliovirus replicase has a strong inclination toward transition (i.e., purine to purine or pyrimidine to pyrimidine) over transversion (purine to pyrimidine or vice versa) mutation in nucleotide substitutions (213). Various experimental approaches have been taken to determine the mutation rates of enteroviruses: estimates for poliovirus have ranged from 3×10^{-3} (429) to 2×10^{-6} (316). Determination of mutation rates is complicated by the possibility of additional experimental artifacts, which may partly explain the large differences between estimates of mutation rates. Moreover, it is not always apparent whether an experiment was designed to measure rates or frequencies of mutation (436a). The mutation rate is defined as the average number of mutations per replication, and the mutation frequency is the fraction at which a specific base change is found in the population of product RNAs. Using published data, Drake (94) calculated the values of u_b (the average rate of mutation per base pair per replication) and u_g (the genomic mutation rate [$u_g = Gu_b$ for a genome of G bases]) for several RNA viruses, including poliovirus, for which the mean values are $u_b = 6 \times 10^{-6}$ and $u_g = 5$. An optimal experiment for determining the frequency of mutation used poliovirus mutants with a guanidine phenotype mapping to 2C and measured the frequency of mutants that changed from g^d to g^r in the absence of the drug (82). The target size for mutational events (the codon for amino acid 227 of 2C) in this experiment was known precisely, the sensitivity for identification of mutants is high, and mutants were isolated without selection (since g^d and g^r mutants replicate equally well and do not interfere with one another). The minimal corrected base substitution frequency per single nucleotide position in codon 227 of 2C was $(2.1 \pm 1.9) \times 10^{-4}$; $u_b = 1.6 \times 10^{-4}$, and $u_g = 1.21$ (82, 94). Mutation frequencies for poliovirus in the range of 10^{-5} to 10^{-4} have generally been obtained when viable progeny were scored. These studies include the detection of (i) neutralization escape mutants resistant to neutralizing monoclonal antibodies (37, 86, 106a, 107, 273), (ii) resistance to 0.5 mM guanidine (330), and (iii) guanidine dependence (199, 331). Similar results have been obtained for CAV-9 by screening revertants from dependence on (2-(alpha-hydroxybenzyl)-benzimidazole) to independence (104) and for echovirus 11 by screening for nonhemagglutinating mutants derived from hemagglutinating clones (382).

Enteroviruses thus exhibit high mutation frequencies that generate genetically heterogeneous populations known as quasispecies (105). The genetic diversity present in a large quasispecies population provides enteroviruses with great adaptability, because the population consists of entities with a range of phenotypes that is continuously being tested under varying environmental conditions. The genetic plasticity of enteroviral genomes explains the ease with which mutants with altered biological properties can be selected. However, high mutation frequencies also generate a large number of lethal or deleterious mutations, so enteroviruses replicate near the threshold of error catastrophe: an increase in error frequency (for example, by chemical mutagenesis) would lead to a loss of information and a decline in viability (144). A high mutation rate can be detrimental to the fitness of RNA viruses if selection does not occur (for example, during a genetic bottleneck, which can occur when only a few viruses are transferred from one host to another) because of the accumulation of deleterious mutations (51, 97, 292).

The genetic plasticity of enteroviral genomes appears to preclude the conservation of distinct viral genotypes, but analysis of the genomic RNAs of various laboratory stocks of poliovirus type 1 (Mahoney) has revealed that the genotype of this virus has been strongly conserved after repeated passage (95, 202, 342); such conservation is particularly striking when it occurs in highly degenerate codons, because such substitutions would be silent at the coding level (436a). Genotype conservation may reflect the influence of selective forces, the most obvious of which is maintenance of protein structure and function but which may also include maintenance of higher-order RNA structures and accommodation of tissue- and species-specific biases in codon utilization (133). Precise genotypic changes have been documented following growth of poliovirus in cell culture. First, four silent base reversions to the *wt* sequence near the *ts* locus always accompanied reversion of a fifth base that determined the *ts* phenotype of the mutant (80); second, passage of PV3(S) in Vero cells resulted in the selection of two silent mutations at nt 1127 and 1141 in the VP2 coding sequence (352a); and third, two different isolates of PV1(S) strains that had stably acquired the ability to establish persistent infections in cells of neural and nonneural origin gained the same 31 point mutations during cultivation, and of these, 16 were silent mutations within the polyprotein ORF (42). The maintenance of a specific genotype is also likely to be influenced by the mode of transmission: as discussed above, repeated passage of an RNA virus through a genetic bottleneck results in a decline in fitness, as predicted by Müller's ratchet hypothesis (292). Repeated passage of a large spectrum of a quasispecies allows the operation of natural selection, so that noncompetitive (inferior) genotypes are eliminated, but under these conditions, high-relative-fitness variants may also be suppressed within populations of lower mean fitness (81, 96, 97). These observations may help explain the apparently paradoxical maintenance of *wt* enteroviral genomes.

RECOMBINATION

Homologous Recombination

Picornavirus recombination involves the exchange of genetic elements between two genomes during their replication in the same cell. Poliovirus recombinants were initially detected because they acquired genetic traits from their parental strains and were thus able to proliferate under conditions that restricted the growth of both parents (140, 229). An elegant method of studying recombination without the necessity for selection based on direct and quantitative detection of recombinant RNA molecules by reverse transcription and PCR has recently been developed (177). The frequency of recombination is proportional to the distance between genetic loci and can therefore be used to construct a genetic map. *ts* and g^r mutants were used to establish that the order of genetic units in the poliovirus genome is RNA synthesis I–RNA synthesis II–virion proteins (68, 69). The orientation of the map (5' → 3') was established independently by protein labeling studies in the presence of the inhibitor pactamycin (349, 397a, 402), and it is now apparent that these three genetic units correspond to the P3, P2, and P1 regions of the genome. Biochemical evidence for recombination between picornavirus genomes was derived first by analyses of poliovirus proteins (361, 415) and subsequently by fingerprinting of genomic RNAs of parental and recombinant strains of aphthovirus strains (194).

Strand switching during picornavirus RNA recombination is precise (so that nucleotides are neither inserted nor deleted at the crossover site) (177, 199, 360, 415) and homologous (the sequences of crossover sites or regions of strand switching in parental genomes are highly homologous) (199). The precision of strand switching has been confirmed by analysis of recombination in noncoding regions of the genome, eliminating the possibility that selection (e.g., for maintenance of the correct reading frame) masked some sloppy crossover events (177). The observation that recombination frequencies are lower between different serotypes of poliovirus (whose nucleotide sequences can vary by 15%) than between isogenic parents is consistent with a requirement that regions of strand switching be homologous (199, 415). Homologous recombination can occur throughout the genome, but it is likely that some recombinants have reduced fitness: indeed, naturally existing mixed poliovirus serotypes are not known. Recombination is very efficient, to the extent that 10 to 20% of viral RNA molecules undergo recombination during a single infectious cycle (199). Analysis of reciprocal recombination frequencies in the absence of selection by quantitative PCR indicated that they depend on the input ratio of parental virus strains (177). This result suggests that the frequency of recombination depends on the acceptor template concentration.

Mechanistically, picornavirus RNA recombination differs from the strand scission and religation pathway that is characteristic of

DNA recombination. The use of defined conditional mutants to selectively inhibit replication of one parent in a recombinant cross showed that poliovirus recombination occurs instead by a copy choice mechanism in which the viral polymerase and associated nascent strand switch templates during RNA synthesis (199). Inspection of crossover sites has not revealed a consensus sequence motif(s) for recombination (177, 193, 199, 415), but strand switching would probably be promoted by sequences or structures that promote transcriptional pausing, such as intrastrand secondary structure (272) or intermolecular duplexes (360). Some propensity for recombination to occur in regions of the genome with a potential to form secondary structure has been noted (193, 360, 415, 436), although other reports indicate that template switching occurs at random locations throughout the genome (177). Recombination does not result in deletion of nucleotides, so a nonprocessive mechanism for recombination (in which the nascent and/or template strands dissociate from the replication complex) is unlikely.

Template switching occurs during minus-strand synthesis (199), so a central issue in elucidating the mechanism of recombination concerns the structure of the RNA intermediate in negative-strand synthesis. Minus-strand intermediates with several nascent minus strands (Fig. 6A) have not been detected and may not exist (35). The asymmetry of plus- to minus-strand synthesis (50:1) (139, 306a) is likely to result from initiation of minus-strand synthesis at a relatively lower rate than initiation of plus-strand synthesis, with the consequence that intermediates in minus-strand synthesis may have only a single nascent strand and contain a transcribed region that is either mainly single stranded (Fig. 6B) or double stranded (Fig. 6C). One of these two structures is likely to be involved in homologous recombination. Structure 6C may be more likely if poliovirus double-stranded RNA (replicative form [RF]; Fig. 6D) is a true replication intermediate and not simply an artifact of isolation. However, the role (if any) of RF RNA in RNA replication is uncertain. Recent evidence that binding of $3CD^{pro}$ to the 5' end of virion RNA is important for positive-strand RNA synthesis (14, 15) indicates that this complex must be close to the 3' end of a minus strand, which is clearly so in RF molecules. Multiple initiation prior to completion of one plus strand would then result in a positive-strand replication intermediate molecule being mainly double stranded (Fig. 6F). Experimental evidence supporting both the closed structure (6F [24, 26, 270, 300, 440]) and the open structure (6G [353]) has been presented elsewhere. A model involving replication via the closed structure (6F) would explain why strand switching occurs during minus-strand synthesis (436a).

Two models for poliovirus recombination that involve a processive replication mechanism in which the replication complex remains associated with the RNA have been proposed (Fig. 7): (i) the polymerase-template complex comes to a transcriptional pause, slides backwards, and thus unpairs a few bases of the nascent strand, which then hybridize with an invading acceptor RNA strand (177); or (ii) homologous regions of two plus-strand RNA molecules form intermolecular duplexes that may either be dissociated by the advancing replication complex or cause it to pause, leading to the possibility of strand switching (360).

Recombination of poliovirus occurs in human vaccine recipients and can lead to the evolution of highly virulent strains (46, 115, 189, 190, 240, 244, 278, 410); recombination has also been detected in *wt* poliovirus populations (191). All recombinants had genetic exchanges in or downstream of 2C that may be due to selection of recombinants at the level of RNA replication (274).

A high rate of recombination may confer a variety of advantages on enterovirus genomes (176, 193), such as (i) providing a homeostatic mechanism for eliminating errors accumulated during RNA synthesis, thereby conserving the *wt* genotype; and (ii) enabling virus variants that are better suited for survival to appear by exchanging entire genetic units between strains

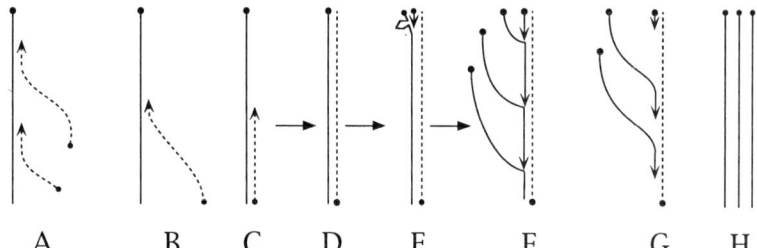

FIGURE 6 Steps in the replication of poliovirus RNA. Parental positive-sense virion RNA is transcribed in a primer-dependent manner. A replicative intermediate (RI) form (A) consisting of a single positive-sense template (solid line) and multiple nascent negative-strands (dashed lines) has not been detected, so that more probable intermediates in negative-strand synthesis could be mainly single stranded (B) or double stranded (C). Elongation of nascent negative-sense strand (C) yields RF double-stranded RNA (D). This product of replication may be an intermediate in the synthesis of positive-sense replicative intermediate structure F or G. The first step in this process may be the partial melting of RF RNA, leading to the formation of terminal cloverleaf structures; the cloverleaf formed on the positive-sense strand may be stabilized by a complex consisting of 3CD^{pro} and host factors or other viral polypeptides (E). The final product is single-stranded positive-sense genomic virion RNA (H). The generation of free negative-sense strands is unlikely. The 5'-terminal VPg moieties are represented by solid circles.

of the same genus or even between strains of different genera. The viability of some chimeric enteroviruses constructed in vitro indicates that genetic elements within different enteroviruses are compatible and can be exchanged (180, 381). The 3' part of the coxsackievirus A21 genome is remarkably homologous (>90% at the amino acid level) to that of poliovirus (155), whereas the genome of echovirus 22 appears to be a mixture of genetic units of entero- and cardioviruses (158).

Nonhomologous Recombination

The most commonly observed occurrence of nonhomologous recombination is the production of DI particles during high-multiplicity passages. DI particles are subgenomic deletion mutants derived from infectious virus genomes that require a homologous parental virus for replication (152, 363). They replicate preferentially at the expense of the helper virus by competing for helper virus-encoded replication and structural proteins and can facilitate the establishment and maintenance of persistent infections of cells. Deletions are located in the region of the genome that encodes the capsid proteins (63, 182, 216, 302) and constitute up to 20% of the genome (Fig. 5). Subgenomic replicons containing larger deletions that can replicate in vivo have been constructed, but some of them are not encapsidated, and a 20% reduction in genome size may therefore represent the largest deletion compatible with virion stability (64, 124, 186). DI genomes are probably generated by a template-switching mechanism during replication (i.e., by nonhomologous recombination). Sequence analysis rules out a simple model in which deletions arise by synthesis of RNA across the base of hairpin structures, but more complicated recombinational intermediates cannot be ruled out (216). DI genomes are not static and can undergo additional changes in structure during further rounds of replication; mosaic genomes resulting from multiple deletion events have been characterized (7, 216, 242). The structures of viable DI genomes reflect selective pressures encountered during different stages of the replication cycle, one of which may be a minimum size compatible with virion stability. Genomic deletions

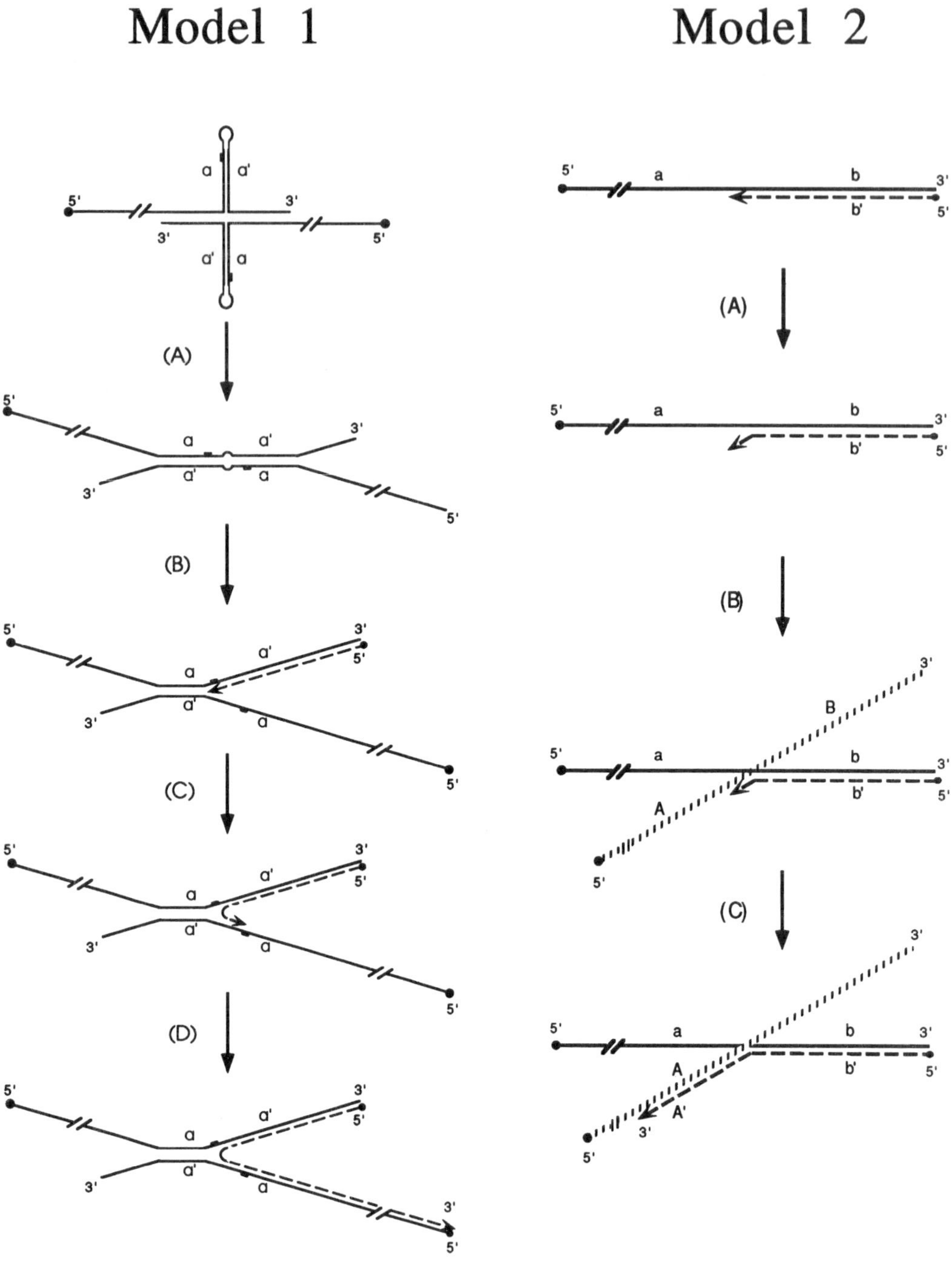

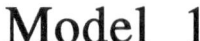

FIGURE 7 Two models for recombination between poliovirus genomes based on proposals by Romanova et al. (360) and (model 1) Jarvis and Kirkegaard (176, 177) (model 2). In model 1, self-complementary regions are denoted as a and a'. Solid lines correspond to genomic template RNA molecules, and dashed lines correspond to the complementary RNA strand. Homologous recombination sites are represented by black rectangles. Heteroduplex formation results in base pairing of two genome molecules that are brought close together (step

are restricted to the P1 region and parts of the 5' NTR; they all maintain the ORF of the P2 and P3 regions of the polyprotein (216), and DI genomes in which the P2-P3 region is engineered to be out of frame with respect to the initiation codon are not viable (64, 124). These observations suggest that translation may be *cis* dominant with respect to genome replication either because at least one nonstructural protein is *cis* acting and cannot be supplied by the helper virus or because initiation of RNA replication requires concurrent translation of the RNA. DI particles contain all the information required for replication, and they are therefore potentially useful tools for investigating different aspects of this process (such as translation, RNA replication, and encapsidation) and for expressing foreign genes in place of capsid proteins (55, 64, 124, 186, 321).

Spontaneous insertions and deletions have also been identified at two locations in rapidly replicating genomes selected after replication of mutated RNAs in cells. Deletion of four nucleotides at nt 220 in the 5' NTR yielded a virus with a *ts* phenotype, but analysis of a pseudorevertant virus that grew well at 37°C revealed deletion of about 40 additional nucleotides, eliminating almost all of domain III of the IRES (88). Mutations in the IRES within domain VI and the upstream pyrimidine-rich tract (i.e., the Y_n-X_m-AUG motif) severely impaired virus growth, but a number of pseudorevertant viruses in which the Y_n-X_m-AUG motif was restored as a result of point mutations and, on occasion, of either deletion or insertion were recovered (119, 126, 328). A mutant poliovirus genome in which the VPg genetic unit was duplicated (....3A-$3B_1$-$3B_2$-$3C^{pro}$.....) rapidly lost the 3C-proximal VPg on replication in HeLa cells (48). The mechanism by which this precise deletion event occurred is not known.

Nonhomologous recombination is less frequent than homologous recombination, but both may occur by the same general mechanism such that intratypic, intertypic, and nonhomologous recombinations occur with decreasing frequency because of the decreasing probability of base pairing between donor and acceptor strands (176). Nonhomologous recombination can even result in the transduction of cellular sequences (192, 271, 286, 293) and may contribute to the genetic repertoire of viral RNA genomes.

GENETICS OF PATHOGENESIS

Enteroviruses multiply throughout the alimentary tract, and most enteric infections in human and animal populations are characterized by subclinical manifestations. Viremia may occur after continuing replication in the gut, leading to the infection of specific target organs, which vary according to the identity of the infecting enterovirus. Infection by different enterovirus strains and isolates can therefore cause any of a wide spectrum of clinical diseases, including aseptic meningitis, common cold, conjunctivitis, encephalitis, exanthema, flaccid paralysis, herpangina, myocarditis, and pleurodynia (123, 262, 287). Some enteroviruses [e.g., CB3, echovirus 6, and PV1(S)] can also cause persistent infections in cell culture and in vivo and may have clinical manifestations such as chronic myocarditis (42, 62, 72a, 122, 203) (see chapter 14).

The genetic heterogeneity of enteroviral quasispecies populations enables new variants to be tested after each round of replication, and selective pressure can lead to the evolu-

---

A). The viral RNA polymerase copies one RNA molecule from the 3' end and may pause within the region of intermolecular base pairing (step B), dissociate, and reassociate with a homologous site in the second RNA molecule (step C). Synthesis of a recombinant minus-strand molecule then continues (step D). In model 2, solid lines represent genomic template RNA molecules, broken lines correspond to nascent minus strands, and dashed lines correspond to invading positive-sense template RNA molecule. The viral RNA polymerase copies one RNA molecule from the 3' end and may pause, slide backward, and unpair a few bases of the nascent strand (step A), which then associates with an invading acceptor RNA strand (step B). Synthesis of a recombinant minus-strand molecule then continues (step C).

tion of variants with altered pathogenic properties such as virulence, tissue specificity, and host range. Variants of many different enteroviruses have been obtained after serial passage of *wt* isolates that exhibited altered patterns of virulence in different animal hosts and tissues, and analysis of such variants has yielded many valuable insights into the genetics of pathogenesis.

Host Range and Tissue Tropism

The host ranges of enteroviruses differ from one virus type to another (75, 261, 265, 374), and this characteristic property of host range has been used in their classification. However, many enteroviral variants with host range alterations have been described. For example, polioviruses have a very restricted (primate) host range, but variants that grow well in mice have been identified, and others have been adapted to grow in chick embryos and suckling hamsters (reviewed in reference 340). Similarly, infection of domestic animals with human coxsackie A and B viruses has been documented (reviewed in reference 250), and experimental selection of host range variants of echovirus 9 and coxsackievirus types B1 through B6 has been reported (103, 116, 347).

Enterovirus replication in the intestinal mucosa is followed by a primary viremia during which the virus circulates in the bloodstream, but although the virus has access to a broad range of tissues in the body, only a very restricted number of cell types are infected (368). However, a wide range of normally nonsusceptible cultured cells and living animals can support a single round of replication initiated by viral RNA, for example from PV1(M), CAV-9, CB1, and echovirus 8, but these cells are not infected by the resulting infectious virus (145, 146). The major determinant of the cell tropism of enteroviruses is the presence of an appropriate cellular receptor (148, 256) (see chapter 3). Cellular receptors for poliovirus (PVR), echovirus 1 (integrin VLA-2), and possibly CAV-9 ($\alpha_v\beta_3$ integrin) have been identified (30, 269, 359), and some enteroviruses (CAV-3, -18, and -21) are known to attach to intercellular adhesion molecule 1, which is the major rhinovirus receptor (1). Transformation of murine cells with the PVR gene and introduction of this gene into the germ lines of mice is sufficient to overcome the host range restriction of poliovirus type 1 (Mahoney) [PV1(M)] for murine cells (208, 268, 269, 350) (see chapter 3).

The host range restriction of an enterovirus can be overcome by the acquisition of a second receptor binding site on virions. For example, adaptation of CB3 to growth on rhabdomyosarcoma cells is the result of selection for a virus variant that had gained the ability to attach to a virus receptor on these cells (possibly due to mutations in VP1) without losing the ability to bind to and infect HeLa cells (347). A large number of poliovirus host range variants have been identified, and a few, including mouse neurovirulent type 1 LS-a, type 2 Lansing, and type 2 W-2, have been characterized at the molecular level (222, 241, 325). Initial experiments showed that the capsid coding region of poliovirus type 2 (Lansing) [PV2(L)] was sufficient to confer the mouse neurovirulence phenotype on PV1(M) and that escape mutants of PV2(L) (selected by resistance to neutralizing monoclonal antibodies) that contain substitutions in N-Ag1 have reduced mouse neurovirulence (220–222). Replacement of amino acid residues from the exposed loop between the B and C β-strands of VP1 in PV1(M) (i.e., N-Ag1) with those of PV2(L) is sufficient to confer mouse neurovirulence on the recombinant virus (253, 295). The reciprocal recombinant was attenuated in normal mice and virulent in PVR transgenic mice (290). The BC loop is therefore the primary determinant of the mouse virulence of PV2(L) and, conversely, of the host restriction of PV1(M). The reciprocal recombinant variants are able to replicate in human cells and in PVR transgenic mice, so this determinant must differ from the site used by the virus to recognize the human PVR.

Restriction of enterovirus replication is not solely due to the lack of appropriate receptors.

Studies of poliovirus variants suggest that cellular factors involved in other stages of replication (entry into cells, uncoating, translation, and RNA synthesis) may influence cell susceptibility (see below). Two mutations located in the N terminus of VP1 each suppress the requirement for the PV2(L)-specific BC loop for infection of mice (290). These residues are located on the interior surface of the virus, and structural analysis suggested that these residues and the BC loop in VP1 may regulate mouse neurovirulence by mediating the ability of the murine receptor to induce conformational changes required for entry and uncoating (438). Characterization of virulent PV1(M) isolates that had been adapted to growth in the mouse central nervous system resulted in the identification of additional residues (in VP1 and VP2) located on the inner surface of the virion that overcome the host restriction of PV1(M) (72).

Enteroviral Variants with Altered Pathogenic Properties

Adaptation of a virus subpopulation to efficient growth in a new type of cell is usually the result of numerous mutations in the viral genome, and alterations in host range and tissue specificity may increase virulence and cause disease syndromes not ordinarily associated with the prototype virus (315, 346, 441). Alternatively, an attenuated virus variant that still grows well in the original host but is less virulent can occasionally emerge from the adapted subpopulation. Attenuated variants of several enteroviruses, including echoviruses 2 and 12 (428); coxsackie A virus, types A7, A14, A16, and A21 (210, 211, 232, 291); coxsackieviruses B3 and B4 (116, 232, 339); and poliovirus types 1, 2, and 3 (109, 209, 234, 370, 412), have been isolated. Expression of the virulence phenotype varies widely between virus isolates and also depends on both the host and the route of inoculation (367, 368), so virulence cannot be regarded as a single biological property. Taking poliovirus as an example, the virus titer required to establish an enteric infection may vary many thousandfold between strains, and there may also be differences in the abilities of the strains to invade the central nervous system and to infect different neural tissue (e.g., anterior horn cells, meninges, cranial nerve nuclei, etc.) and in the degree of neuronal damage that they cause (38). These observations suggest that virulence has multiple genetic determinants and that attenuation is therefore likely to involve multiple genetic changes. Many of the variants described above have probably been lost, but genetic differences between some virulent and avirulent poliovirus and coxsackie B virus (CB3, CB4, and SVDV) isolates have been identified by sequence analysis (Table 1). Analysis of chimeric recombinant CB3 and CB4 viruses indicates that determinants of virulence may occur in coding and noncoding regions in the 5' half of the genome (44). Genetic analysis of attenuated poliovirus strains and assorted neurovirulent revertants has been more extensive and has yielded detailed insights into the genetic basis of attenuation.

The Molecular Basis of Poliovirus Attenuation

The attenuated poliovirus vaccine strains of types 1 and 3 were derived from the virulent type 1 (Mahoney) and type 3 (Leon) strains by multiple passage in simian extraneural cells, whereas the parent of the type 2 vaccine strain already had low intraspinal monkey neurovirulence (369). The type 1 PV1(M) and type 2 (P712) progenitor isolates were obtained from the feces of healthy children, whereas the type 3 progenitor was isolated from the central nervous system of a patient with fatal poliomyelitis. Studies to identify properties that correlated with reduced neurovirulence indicated that attenuated poliovirus strains had a *ts* phenotype (243). Other in vitro tests to differentiate neurovirulent from attenuated strains have not been useful in elucidating the molecular mechanism of expression of the attenuation (*att*) phenotype.

Genetic differences between attenuated polioviruses and their neurovirulent parents were first detected by RNA fingerprinting

(303). Comparison of the complete genomic sequences of the type 1 and type 3 Sabin strains and of a neurovirulent type 3 revertant from a vaccine recipient (47, 305, 393, 417, 432) with those of the neurovirulent progenitor strains PV1(M) and PV3 (Leon) (202, 341, 393) allowed the mutations that had accumulated during attenuation to be identified (Fig. 8). The relationship between these mutations and the *att* phenotype was subsequently determined by genetic analyses (reviewed in references 12, 274, 306, and 340).

The first experiments to elucidate this relationship used intertypic recombinants between *wt* and *att* strains and led to the conclusion that the 5' half of the genome contains a major determinant of attenuation in PV3(S) and that the 3' half of the genome also contains attenuating mutations in PV1(S) (3–5). Construction of defined chimeric recombinant genomes facilitated more detailed analysis of the *att* phenotype. The genomes of the type 3 Sabin vaccine strain and its neurovirulent precursor poliovirus type 3 (Leon) differ by 11

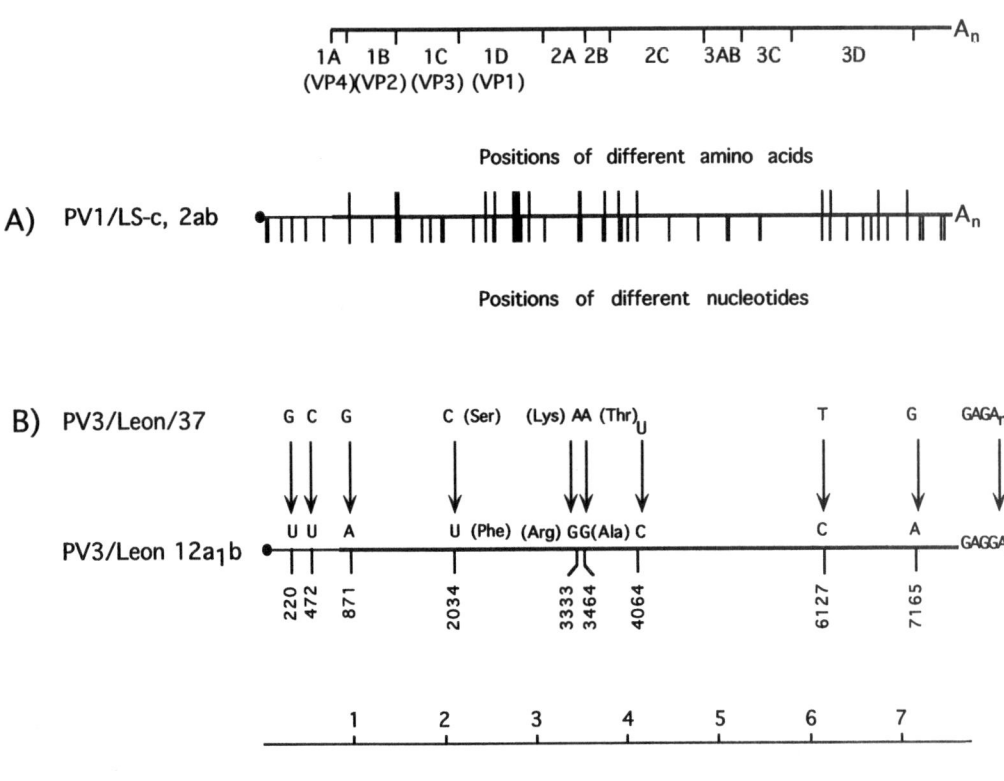

FIGURE 8 Locations of attenuating mutations in poliovirus types 1 and 3 (Sabin) strains. (A) Locations of nucleotide and amino acid differences between the P1/Mahoney/41 (parent) and P1/LS-c, 2ab (vaccine) strains are indicated by lines above and below the genomic RNA, respectively. There are 55 nucleotide differences between the genomes of these two PV type 1 strains (305). (B) Nucleotide and predicted amino acid sequence differences between P3/Leon/37 (parent) and P3/Leon 12a$_1$b (Sabin vaccine) poliovirus type 3 strains (47, 394). Genomic RNA and its genetic organization are shown at the top, and the length of the poliovirus genome from the 5' terminus is indicated at the bottom. An additional recently reported difference between these two strains (409, 432) at nt 2493, producing an amino acid change at residue 6 of the capsid protein VP1, is not shown.

nt (Fig. 8), and the genome of a virulent revertant differs from its precursor [i.e., PV3(S)] at only six nucleotide positions. The base at nt 472 was the only simple backmutation in the revertant, and it is the major determinant of virulence; a *ts* mutation mapping to VP3 and a mutation in VP1 also contribute to the *att* phenotype (111, 394, 409, 435). The progenitor of the type 2 Sabin vaccine strain is not generally available, so direct comparison of its genome with that of PV2(S) is not possible. However, the sequence of a neurovirulent revertant isolated from a patient with vaccine-associated poliomyelitis differed from that of its parent at 23 nucleotide positions (334). Reversion may be due to as few as three mutations, including one in the 5' NTR at nt 481 and a second in VP1 (248, 249, 351). Attenuation of poliovirus type 1 appears to be more complex than that of the other two vaccine strains. A major determinant of the *att* phenotype is nt 480 within the 5' NTR, but many other attenuating mutations occurred throughout the genome (308). PV1(S) passaged at supraoptimal temperatures became increasingly neurovirulent, and almost total reversion to neurovirulence appeared to be caused by only two or three mutations, including one at nt 525 and another at nt 6203 within the $3D^{pol}$ coding sequence. Reversion at nt 480 (G480A) and nt 6203 (C6203U) has been detected in naturally occurring neurovirulent revertants of PV1(S) isolated from patients with vaccine-associated paralytic poliomyelitis (115, 311).

The three Sabin vaccine strains were isolated by different routes, but all have attenuating mutations within the same short sequence in the 5' NTR. Notably, other attenuated poliovirus strains that were considered as candidate live vaccines are genetically less stable than the Sabin strains and lack base changes in this region (276). Analysis of poliovirus type 3 isolates from patients with vaccine-associated cases of poliomyelitis revealed that nt 472 had consistently reverted, which suggested that this residue likely plays an important role in attenuation (111). This hypothesis was supported by analysis of recombinant viruses containing single substitutions of this residue in the genetic background of the *wt* type 3 5' NTR (220, 435). Similar experiments with type 1 and type 2 polioviruses revealed corresponding *att* mutations (187, 246, 351). The attenuating mutations in the 5' NTRs, of the vaccine strains of three poliovirus serotypes map to domain V of the IRES, albeit to different bases, and are likely to destabilize the structure of this element. Some neurovirulent revertants of PV3(S) had acquired a U525C substitution that would stabilize the base pair nt 480 to 525 (Fig. 9) (58, 352a); moreover, mutational analysis of domain V showed a correlation between its secondary structure and the attenuation of mutant viruses in tissue culture cells (246, 385). Expression of the attenuating mutations may reside in the translational efficiency of the viral RNAs (399–401). The restricted growth of attenuated strains in neural tissue may result from impairment of IRES function; the mechanism of restriction is not understood, but it may involve the interaction of *trans*-acting factors with this domain.

Almost 160 nt have been deleted from the 3' end of the 5' NTRs of poliovirus and coxsackie virus B1 without loss of viability (160, 162, 215, 324), but viruses containing such mutations are less virulent than *wt* viruses. These *att* mutations are likely to be more stable genetically than the attenuating substitutions within domain V of the IRES, and their incorporation into enteroviral vaccines would therefore be beneficial.

In contrast to mutations in the 5' NTR, attenuating mutations in the ORF show no common pattern. Genetic analyses identified an S3091F substitution within VP3 caused by a missense mutation at nt 2034 as a major *att* mutation (435). This mutation confers a *ts* phenotype on PV3(S), possibly by destabilizing protomer interactions and affecting viral assembly (112, 245, 248, 277). The effects of the mutations in VP1 (at nt 2692) in PV3(S) and in VP1 (at nt 2908) in PV2(S) on virus stability and replication have not yet been

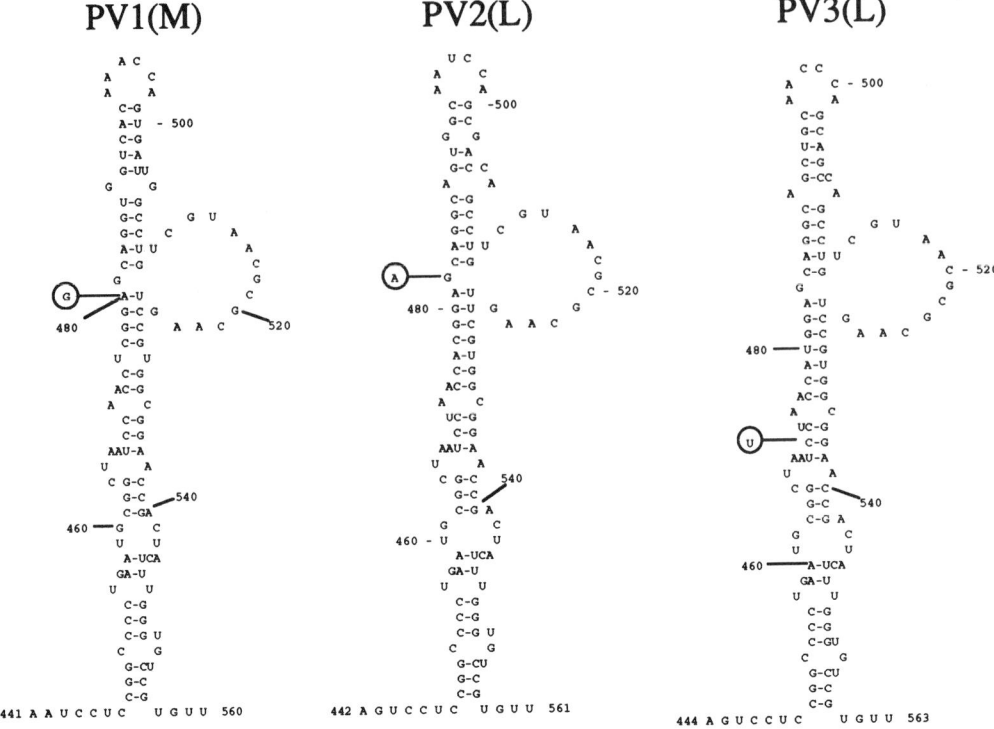

FIGURE 9 Domain V of the 5' noncoding regions of poliovirus types 1 (Mahoney), 2 (Lansing), and 3 (Leon), based on the structure proposed by Pilipenko et al. (327). The nucleotide substitutions that attenuate the Sabin vaccine strains of these three serotypes are circled, and their locations are indicated.

analyzed in detail. Studies with PV1(S) are more complicated, because multiple determinants mapping to the ORF contribute to its *att* phenotype. A missense mutation at nt 6203 that results in an H70F substitution in 3D^{pol} has been implicated in the *att* phenotype (58, 115, 408) and is responsible for a *ts* phenotype in studies of initiation of plus-strand RNA synthesis in vitro (419).

In Vivo Variation of *att* Mutations

The live Sabin strains of poliovirus have been safe and effective vaccines and have contributed considerably to the eradication of poliomyelitis in many regions of the world (see chapter 9). However, vaccine-associated cases of poliomyelitis do occur, albeit very rarely (ca. 1 case per 2.5 million doses of oral poliovirus vaccine [397]). The incidence of vaccine-associated poliomyelitis is in fact surprisingly low given the high propensity of vaccine strains of poliovirus to revert to neurovirulence (see below); this observation suggests that animal models for poliovirus neurovirulence may overestimate its virulence in humans. Most vaccine-associated cases are attributable to types 2 and 3, and PV1(S) accounts for only 10% of all cases, even though the PV1(M) progenitor is the most neurovirulent strain.

Reversion of poliovaccines to neurovirulence is almost invariably the result of reversion to the *wt* sequence by point mutation. The most consistent point mutation is reversion of nt 472 in PV3(S) (47, 111, 244, 410), which has been observed upon passaging of virus in cell culture (60, 61) and can be complete in a vaccine recipient in as few as 2 days (278). Corresponding reversion of nt 481 in type 2 and of nt 480 in type 1 has also been detected in cell culture (59, 352a) and in vaccinees (101, 110, 249, 276, 311, 334). The mechanism for selection against U-472 of PV3(S) in the gut is obscure; it operates much less strongly against corresponding *att* mutations in PV1(S) and PV2(S) (101) and may involve interaction with cell type-specific factors (59, 352a). A *ts* phenotype is associated with the corresponding *att* mutation in PV2(S) and has a cell type-specific pattern of expression (275). The *att* mutation of VP1 in PV3(S) at nt 2493 can also revert rapidly (2 to 4 days) in vaccinees, whereas the *ts* phenotype of PV3(S) due to the *att* mutation at nt 2034 in VP3 is lost after 11 or 12 days (101, 244, 274). Interestingly, the *att* phenotype associated with the VP3 capsid protein can be suppressed by second-site mutations (277), whereas reversion of the *att* phenotype associated with Ile-143 in VP1 of PV2(S) occurs exclusively by substitution (110, 249).

Recombination is a frequent phenomenon in the evolution of poliovirus vaccine strains (46, 101, 110, 115, 189, 191, 240, 278, 354, 410), and whereas intertypic recombinants generated in tissue culture can be detected only under conditions of stringent selection, intertypic recombinants generated in vaccinees appear to readily outcompete the parental strain in the human gut. The nature of the competitive advantage of intertypic recombinants is unknown.

ACKNOWLEDGMENT

We thank Ann Palmenberg for generously providing Fig. 3.

REFERENCES

1. **Abraham, G., and R. J. Colonno.** 1984. Many rhinovirus serotypes share the same cellular receptor. *J. Virol.* **51:**340–345.
2. **Adler, C. J., M. Elzinga, and E. Wimmer.** 1983. The genome-linked protein of picornavirus. VIII. Complete amino acid sequence of poliovirus VPg and carboxy-terminal analysis of its precursor, P3-9. *J. Gen. Virol.* **64:**349–355.
3. **Agol, V. I., S. G. Drozdov, M. P. Frolova, V. P. Grachev, M. S. Kolesnikova, V. G. Kozlov, N. M. Ralph, L. I. Romanova, E. A. Tolskaya, and E. G. Viktorova.** 1985. Neurovirulence of the intertypic poliovirus recombinant $v^3/a1$-25: characterization of strains isolated from the spinal cord of diseased monkeys and evaluation of the contribution of the 3' half of the genome. *J. Gen. Virol.* **66:**309–316.
4. **Agol, V. I., S. G. Drozdov, V. P. Grachev, M. S. Kolesnikova, V. G. Kozlov, N. M. Ralph, L. I. Romanova, E. A. Tolskaya, A. V. Tyufanov, and E. G. Viktorova.** 1985. Recombination between attenuated and virulent strains of poliovirus type 1: derivation and characterization of recombinants with centrally located crossover points. *Virology* **143:**467–477.
5. **Agol, V. I., V. P. Grachev, S. G. Drozdov, M. S. Kolesnikova, V. G. Kozlov, N. M. Ralph, L. I. Romanova, E. A. Tolskaya, A. V. Tyufanov, and E. G. Viktorova.** 1984. Construction and properties of intertypic poliovirus recombinants: first approximate mapping of the major determinants of neurovirulence. *Virology* **136:**41–55.
6. **Agol, V. I., and G. Shirman.** 1964. Interaction of guanidine-sensitive and guanidine-dependent variants of poliovirus in mixedly infected cells. *Biochem. Biophys. Res. Commun.* **17:**28.
7. **Agut, H., K. M. Kean, C. Bellocq, O. Fichot, and M. Girard.** 1987. Intratypic recombination of polioviruses: evidence for multiple crossing-over sites on the viral genome. *J. Virol.* **61:**1722–1725.
8. **Agut, H., K. M. Kean, O. Fichot, J. Morasco, J. B. Flanegan, and M. Girard.** 1989. A point mutation in the poliovirus polymerase gene determines a complementable temperature-sensitive defect of RNA replication. *Virology* **168:**302–311.
9. **Ahlquist, P., and P. Kaesberg.** 1979. Determination of the length distribution of poly(A) at the 3' terminus of the virion RNAs of EMC virus, poliovirus, rhinovirus, RAV-61 and CPMV and of mouse globin mRNA. *Nucleic Acids Res.* **7:**1195–1204.
10. **Alexander, H., G. Koch, I. Mountain, K. Sprunt, and O. van Damme.** 1958. Infectivity of ribonucleic acid of poliovirus on HeLa cell monolayers. *Virology* **5:**172.
11. **Alexander, L., H. H. Lu, and E. Wimmer.** 1994. Polioviruses containing picornavirus type 1 and/or type 2 internal ribosomal entry site elements: genetic hybrids and the expression of a foreign gene. *Proc. Natl. Acad. Sci. USA* **91:**1406–1410.
11a. **Allaire, M., M. M. Chernaia, B. A. Malcolm, and M. N. G. James.** 1994. Picornaviral 3C proteinases have a fold similar to the chymotrypsin-like serine proteinases.

Nature (London) **369**:72–76.
12. **Almond, J. W.** 1987. The attenuation of poliovirus neurovirulence. *Annu. Rev. Microbiol.* **41**:153–180.
13. **Anderson-Sillman, K., S. Bartal, and D. R. Tershak.** 1984. Guanidine-resistant poliovirus mutants produce modified 37-kilodalton proteins. *J. Virol.* **50**:922–928.
14. **Andino, R., G. E. Rieckhof, P. L. Achahoso, and D. Baltimore.** 1993. Poliovirus RNA synthesis utilizes an RNP complex formed around the 5'-end of viral RNA. *EMBO J.* **12**:3587–3598.
15. **Andino, R., G. E. Rieckhof, and D. Baltimore.** 1990. A functional ribonucleoprotein complex forms around the 5' end of poliovirus RNA. *Cell* **63**:369–380.
16. **Andino, R., G. E. Rieckhof, D. Trono, and D. Baltimore.** 1990. Substitutions in the protease (3C^{pro}) gene of poliovirus can suppress a mutation in the 5' noncoding region. *J. Virol.* **64**:607–612.
17. **Ansardi, D. C., M. Luo, and C. D. Morrow.** 1994. Mutations in the poliovirus P1 capsid precursor at arginine residues VP4-ARG34, VP3-ARG223, and VP1-ARG129 affect virus assembly and encapsidation of genomic RNA. *Virology* **199**:20–34.
18. **Ansardi, D. C., and C. D. Morrow.** 1993. Poliovirus capsid proteins derived from P1 precursors with glutamine-valine cleavage sites have defects in assembly and RNA encapsidation. *J. Virol.* **67**:7284–7297.
19. **Argos, P., G. Kamer, M. J. H. Nicklin, and E. Wimmer.** 1984. Similarity in gene organization and homology between proteins of animal picornaviruses and plant comovirus suggest common ancestry of these virus families. *Nucleic Acids Res.* **12**:7251–7267.
20. **Armstrong, J. A., M. Edmonds, H. Nakazato, B. A. Philips, and M. H. Vaughan.** 1972. Polyadenylic acid sequences in the virion RNA of poliovirus and eastern equine encephalitis virus. *Science* **176**:526–528.
21. **Auvinnen, P., and T. Hyppia.** 1990. Echoviruses include genetically distinct serotypes. *J. Gen. Virol.* **71**:2133–2139.
22. **Auvinnen, P., G. Stanway, and T. Hyppia.** 1989. Genetic diversity of enterovirus subgroups. *Arch. Virol.* **104**:175–186.
23. **Baltera, R. F., and D. R. Tershak.** 1989. Guanidine-resistant mutants of poliovirus have distinct mutations in peptide 2C. *J. Virol.* **63**:4441–4444.
24. **Baltimore, D.** 1968. Structure of the poliovirus replicative intermediate RNA. *J. Mol. Biol.* **32**:359–368.
25. **Baltimore, D.** 1971. Expression of animal viral genomes. *Bacteriol. Rev.* **35**:235–241.
26. **Baltimore, D., and M. Girard.** 1966. An intermediate in the synthesis of poliovirus RNA. *Proc. Natl. Acad. Sci. USA* **56**:741–746.
27. **Bazan, J. F., and R. F. Fletterick.** 1988. Viral cysteine proteinases are homologous to the trypsin-like family of serine proteases: structural and functional implications. *Proc. Natl. Acad. Sci. USA* **85**:7872–7876.
28. **Bendinelli, M., and H. Friedman.** 1988. *Coxsackieviruses: a General Update*. Plenum Press, New York.
29. **Benyesh, M., H. Itoh, G. D. Hsiung, and J. L. Melnick.** 1957. Mixed infections between ECHO and polioviruses. *Fed. Proc.* **16**:365.
30. **Bergelson, J. M., M. P. Shepley, B. M. C. Chan, M. E. Hemler, and R. W. Finberg.** 1992. The integrin VL-2: an echovirus receptor. *Science* **255**:1718–1720.
31. **Bernstein, H. D., and D. Baltimore.** 1988. Poliovirus mutant that contains a cold-sensitive defect in viral RNA synthesis. *J. Virol.* **62**:2922–2928.
32. **Bernstein, H. D., P. Sarnow, and D. Baltimore.** 1986. Genetic complementation among poliovirus mutants derived from an infectious cDNA clone. *J. Virol.* **60**:1040–1049.
33. **Bernstein, H. D., N. Sonenberg, and D. Baltimore.** 1986. Poliovirus mutant that does not selectively inhibit host cell protein synthesis. *Mol. Cell. Biol.* **5**:2913–2923.
34. **Bienz, K., D. Egger, T. Pfister, and M. Troxler.** 1992. Structural and functional characterization of the poliovirus replication complex. *J. Virol.* **66**:2740–2747.
35. **Bishop, J. M., and G. Koch.** 1969. Infectious replicative intermediate of poliovirus: purification and characterization. *Virology* **37**:521–534.
36. **Blackburn, R. V., V. R. Racaniello, and V. F. Righthand.** 1991. Construction of an infectious cDNA clone of echovirus 6. *Virus Res.* **22**:71–78.
37. **Blondel, B., R. Crainic, O. Fichot, G. Dufraisse, A. Candrea, D. Diamond, M. Girard, and F. Horaud.** 1986. Mutations conferring resistance to neutralization with monoclonal antibodies in type 1 poliovirus can be located outside or inside the antibody-binding site. *J. Virol.* **57**:81–90.
38. **Bodian, D., and D. M. Horstmann.** 1965. Polioviruses, p. 430–473. *In* F. Horsfall and I. Tamm (ed.), *Viral and Rickettsial Diseases of Man*, 4th ed. J. B. Lippincott, Philadelphia.
39. **Boeye, A.** 1959. Induction of mutation in poliovirus by nitrous acid. *Virology* **9**:691–700.

40. **Borman, A., M. T. Howell, J. G. Patton, and R. J. Jackson.** 1993. The involvement of a spliceosome component in internal initiation of human rhinovirus RNA translation. *J. Gen. Virol.* **74:**1775–1788.
41. **Borman, A. M., F. G. Deliat, and K. M. Kean.** 1994. Sequences within the poliovirus internal ribosome entry segment control viral RNA synthesis. *EMBO J.* **13:**3149–3157.
42. **Bozarkian, S., I. Pelletier, V. Calvez, and F. Colbere-Garapin.** 1993. Precise missense and silent mutations are fixed in the genomes of poliovirus mutants from persistently infected cells. *J. Virol.* **67:**2914–2917.
43. **Burns, C. C., O. C. Richards, and E. Ehrenfeld.** 1992. Temperature-sensitive polioviruses containing mutations in RNA polymerase. *Virology* **189:**568–582.
44. **Caggana, M., P. Chan, and A. Ramsingh.** 1993. Identification of a single amino acid residue in the capsid protein VP1 of coxsackievirus B4 that determines the virulent phenotype. *J. Virol.* **67:**4797–4803.
45. **Caliguiri, L. A., and I. Tamm.** 1973. Guanidine and 2-(α-hydroxybenzyl)-benzimidazole (HBB): selective inhibitors of picornavirus multiplication, p. 257–294. *In* W. Carter (ed.), *Selective Inhibitors of Viral Function.* CRC Press, Cleveland.
46. **Cammack, N., A. Phillips, G. Dunn, V. Patel, and P. D. Minor.** 1988. Intertypic genomic rearrangements of poliovirus vaccine strains in vaccinees. *Virology* **167:**507–514.
47. **Cann, A. J., G. Stanway, P. J. Hughes, P. D. Minor, D. M. A. Evans, G. C. Schild, and J. W. Almond.** 1984. Reversion to neurovirulence of the live attenuated Sabin type 3 oral poliovirus vaccine. *Nucleic Acids Res.* **12:**7787–7792.
48. **Cao, X.-M., R. J. Kuhn, and E. Wimmer.** 1993. Replication of poliovirus RNA containing two VPg coding sequences leads to a specific deletion event. *J. Virol.* **67:**5572–5578.
48a. **Cao, X.-M., and E. Wimmer.** Unpublished results.
49. **Chang, K. H., P. Auvinen, T. Hyppiä, and G. Stanway.** 1989. The nucleotide sequence of coxsackievirus A9: implications for receptor binding and enterovirus classification. *J. Gen. Virol.* **70:**3269–3280.
50. **Chang, K. H., C. Day, J. Walker, T. Hyppiä, and G. Stanway.** 1992. The nucleotide sequences of wild-type coxsackievirus A9 strains imply that an RGD motif in VP1 is functionally significant. *J. Gen. Virol.* **73:**621–626.
51. **Chao, L.** 1990. Fitness of RNA virus decreased by Müller's ratchet. *Nature* (London) **348:**454–455.
52. **Chapman, N. M., Z. Tu, S. Tracy, and C. J. Gauntt.** 1994. An infectious cDNA copy of the genome of a non-cardiovirulent coxsackievirus B3 strain: its complete sequence analysis and comparison to the genomes of other cardiovirulent coxsackieviruses. *Arch. Virol.* **135:**115–130.
53. **Charini, W. A., C. C. Burns, E. Ehrenfeld, and B. L. Semler.** 1991. *trans* rescue of a mutant poliovirus RNA polymerase function. *J. Virol.* **65:**2655–2665.
53a. **Charini, W. A., S. Todd, G. A. Gutman, and B. L. Semler.** 1994. Transduction of a human RNA sequence by poliovirus. *J. Virol.* **68:**6547–6552.
54. **Chen, B.-F., L.-H. Hwang, and D. S. Chen.** 1993. Characterization of a bicistronic retroviral vector composed of the swine vesicular disease virus internal ribosome entry site. *J. Virol.* **67:**2142–2148.
55. **Choi, W. S., R. Pal-Ghosh, and C. D. Morrow.** 1991. Expression of human immunodeficiency virus type 1 (HIV-1) *gag*, *pol* and *env* proteins from chimeric HIV-1-poliovirus minireplicons. *J. Virol.* **65:**2875–2883.
56. **Choppin, P. W., and H. J. Eggers.** 1962. Heterogeneity of coxsackievirus B4 virus: two kinds of particles which differ in antibody sensitivity, growth rate, and plaque size. *Virology* **18:**470–476.
57. **Chow, M., J. F. E. Newman, D. Filman, J. M. Hogle, D. J. Rowlands, and F. Brown.** 1987. Myristylation of picornavirus capsid protein VP4 and its structural significance. *Nature* (London) **327:**482–486.
58. **Christodoulou, C., F. Colbere-Garapin, A. Macadam, L. F. Taffs, S. Marsden, P. D. Minor, and F. Horaud.** 1990. Mapping of mutations associated with monkey neurovirulence of Sabin 1 poliovirus revertants selected at high temperature. *J. Virol.* **64:**4922–4929.
59. **Chumakov, K. M., E. M. Dragunsky, L. P. Norwood, M. P. Douthitt, Y. Ran, R. E. Taffs, J. Ridge, and I. S. Levenbrook.** 1994. Consistent selection of mutations in the 5'-untranslated region of oral poliovirus vaccine upon passaging in vitro. *J. Med. Virol.* **42:**79–85.
60. **Chumakov, K. M., L. P. Norwood, M. Parker, E. Dragunsky, R. Taffs, Y. Ran, J. Ridge, and I. Levenbrook.** 1992. RNA sequence variants in live poliovaccine and their relation to neurovirulence. *J. Virol.* **66:**966–970.
61. **Chumakov, K. M., L. B. Powers, K. E. Noonan, I. B. Roninson, and I. S. Levenbrook.** 1991. Correlation between amount of

virus with altered nucleotide sequence and the monkey test for acceptance of oral poliovaccine. *Proc. Natl. Acad. Sci. USA* **88**:199–203.

62. **Colbere-Garapin, F., C. Christodolou, R. Crainic, and I. Pelletier.** 1989. Persistent poliovirus infection of human neuroblastoma cells. *Proc. Natl. Acad. Sci. USA* **86**:7590–7594.

63. **Cole, C. N., and D. Baltimore.** 1973. Defective interfering particles of poliovirus. II. Nature of the defect. *J. Mol. Biol.* **76**:325–343.

64. **Collis, P. S., B. J. O'Donnell, D. J. Barton, J. A. Rogers, and J. B. Flanegan.** 1992. Replication of poliovirus RNA and subgenomic RNA transcripts in transfected cells. *J. Virol.* **66**:6480–6488.

65. **Colter, J. S., H. H. Bird, A. W. Moyer, and R. A. Brown.** 1957. Infectivity of ribonucleic acid from virus infected tissues *Virology* **4**:522.

66. **Compton, S. R., B Nelsen, and K. Kirkegaard.** 1990. Temperature-sensitive poliovirus mutant fails to cleave VP0 and accumulates provirions. *J. Virol.* **64**:4067–4075.

67. **Cooper, P. D.** 1965. Rescue of one phenotype in mixed infections with heat-defective mutants of poliovirus type 1. *Virology* **25**:431–438.

68. **Cooper, P. D.** 1968. A genetic map of poliovirus temperature-sensitive mutants. *Virology* **35**:584–596.

69. **Cooper, P. D.** 1977. Genetics of picornaviruses. *Comp. Virol.* **9**:133–207.

70. **Cords, C. E., and J. J. Holland.** 1964. Replication of poliovirus RNA induced by a heterologous virus. *Proc. Natl. Acad. Sci. USA* **51**:1080–1082.

71. **Cords, C. E., and J. J. Holland.** 1964. Alteration of the species and tissue specificity of poliovirus by enclosure of its RNA within the protein capsid of coxsackie B1 virus. *Virology* **24**:492–495.

72. **Couderc, T., J. Hogle, H. Le Blay, F. Horaud, and B. Blondel.** 1993. Molecular characterization of mouse-virulent poliovirus type 1 Mahoney mutants: involvement of residues of polypeptides VP1 and VP2 located on the inner surface of the capsid protein shell. *J. Virol.* **67**:3808–3817.

72a. **Crowell, R. L., and J. T. Syverton.** 1961. The mammalian cell-virus relationship. VI. Sustained infection of HeLa cells by coxsackievirus B3 virus and effect on superinfection. *J. Exp. Med.* **113**:419–435.

73. **Crowther, D., and J. L. Melnick.** 1961. Studies on the inhibitory action of guanidine on poliovirus multiplication in cell cultures. *Virology* **15**:65–74.

74. **Cui, T., S. Sankar, and A. G. Porter.** 1994. Binding of EMC virus RNA polymerase to the 3'-noncoding region of the viral RNA is specific and requires the 3'-poly(A) tail. *J. Biol. Chem.* **268**:26093–26098.

75. **Dalldorf, G.** 1950. The Coxsackie viruses. *Bull. N.Y. Acad. Med.* **26**:329–335.

76. **Darnell, J. E., and H. Eagle.** 1960. The biosynthesis of poliovirus in cell cultures. *Adv. Virus Res.* **6**:1–26.

77. **Dasgupta, A., M. H. Baron, and D. Baltimore.** 1979. Poliovirus replicase: a soluble enzyme able to initiate copying of poliovirus RNA. *Proc. Natl. Acad. Sci. USA* **76**:2679–2683.

78. **Del Angel, R. M., A. G. Papavassiliou, C. Fernandez-Thomas, S. J. Silverstein, and V. R. Racaniello.** 1989. Cell proteins bind to multiple sites within the 5' untranslated region of poliovirus RNA. *Proc. Natl. Acad. Sci. USA* **86**:8299–8303.

79. **Delarue, M., O. Poch, N. Tordo, D. Moras, and P. Argos.** 1990. An attempt to unify the structure of polymerases. *Protein Eng.* **3**:461–467.

80. **de la Torre, J. C., C. Giachetti, B. L. Semler, and J. J. Holland.** 1992. High frequency of single-base transitions and extreme frequency of precise multiple-base reversion mutations in poliovirus. *Proc. Natl. Acad. Sci. USA* **89**:2351–2355.

81. **de la Torre, J. C., and J. J. Holland.** 1990. RNA virus quasispecies populations can suppress vastly superior mutant progeny. *J. Virol.* **64**:6278–6281.

82. **de la Torre, J. C., E. Wimmer, and J. J. Holland.** 1990. Very high frequency of reversion to guanidine resistance in clonal pools of guanidine-dependent type 1 poliovirus. *J. Virol.* **64**:664–671.

83. **Dever, T. E., M. J. Glynias, and W. C. Merrick.** 1987. GTP-binding domain: three consensus sequence elements with distinct spacing. *Proc. Natl. Acad. Sci. USA* **84**:1814–1818.

84. **Dewalt, P. G., W. S. Blair, and B. L. Semler.** 1989. A genetic locus in mutant poliovirus genomes involved in over-production of RNA polymerase and 3C proteinase. *Virology* **174**:504–514.

85. **Dewalt, P. G., and B. L. Semler.** 1987. Site-directed mutagenesis of proteinase 3C results in a poliovirus deficient in synthesis of viral RNA polymerase. *J. Virol.* **61**:2162–2170.

86. **Diamond, D., B. A. Jameson, J. Bonin, M. Kohara, S. Abe, H. Itoh, T. Komatsu, M. Arita, S. Kuge, A. Nomoto, A. D. M. E. Osterhaus, R. Crainic, and E. Wimmer.** 1985. Antigenic variation and resistance to neu-

tralization of poliovirus type 1. *Science* **229**:1090–1093.
87. Diamond, S. E., and K. Kirkegaard. 1994. Clustered charged-to-alanine mutagenesis of poliovirus RNA-dependent RNA polymerase yields multiple temperature-sensitive mutants defective in RNA synthesis. *J. Virol.* **68**:863–876.
88. Dildine, S., and B. L. Semler. 1989. The deletion of 41 proximal nucleotides reverts a poliovirus mutant containing a temperature-sensitive lesion in the 5' noncoding region of genomic RNA. *J. Virol.* **63**:847–862.
89. Domier, L. L., J. G. Shaw, and R. E. Rhoads. 1987. Potyviral proteins share amino acid sequence homology with picorna-, como-, and caulimoviral proteins. *Virology* **158**:20–27.
90. Domingo, E., E. Martinez-Salas, F. Sobrino, J. C. de la Torre, A. Portela, J. Ortin, C. Lopez-Galindez, P. Peres-Brena, N. Villanueva, R. Najera, S. VandePol, D. Steinhauer, N. DePolo, and J. J. Holland. 1985. The quasispecies (extremely heterogenous) nature of viral RNA genome populations: biological relevance—a review. *Gene* **40**:1–8.
91. Dorner, A. J., L. F. Dorner, G. R. Larsen, E. Wimmer, and C. W. Anderson. 1982. Identification of the initiation site of poliovirus polyprotein synthesis. *J. Virol.* **42**:1017–1028.
92. Dorner, A. J., B. L. Semler, R. J. Jackson, R. Hanecak, E. Duprey, and E. Wimmer. 1984. In vitro translation of poliovirus RNA: utilization of internal initiation sites in reticulocyte lysate. *J. Virol.* **50**:507–514.
93. Dorsch-Haesler, K., Y. Yogo, and E. Wimmer. 1975. Replication of picornaviruses. I. Evidence from in vitro RNA synthesis that poly(A) of the poliovirus genome is genetically coded. *J. Virol.* **16**:1512–1517.
94. Drake, J. W. 1993. Rates of spontaneous mutation among RNA viruses. *Proc. Natl. Acad. Sci. USA* **90**:4171–4175.
95. Dreano, M. C., C. Bellocq, O. Fichot, S. van der Werf, and M. Girard. 1985. Genetic variations in the Mahoney strain of poliovirus type 1. *Ann. Inst. Pasteur/Virol.* **136**:102–114.
96. Duarte, E. A., D. K. Clarke, A. Moya, S. F. Elena, E. Domingo, and J. J. Holland. 1993. Many-trillionfold amplifications of single RNA virus particles fail to overcome the Müller's ratchet effect. *J. Virol.* **67**:3620–3623.
97. Duarte, E. A., I. S. Novella, S. Ledesma, D. K. Clarke, A. Moya, S. F. Elena, E. Domingo, and J. J. Holland. 1994. Subclonal components of consensus fitness in an RNA virus clone. *J. Virol.* **68**:4295–4301.
98. Dulbecco, R. 1952. Production of plaques in monolayer tissue cultures by single particles of an animal virus. *Proc. Natl. Acad. Sci. USA* **38**:747–752.
99. Dulbecco, R., and M. Vogt. 1954. Plaque formation and isolation of pure lines with poliomyelitis viruses. *J. Exp. Med.* **99**:167–182.
100. Duncan, I. R. B. 1968. A comparative study of 63 strains of ECHO virus type 30. *Arch. Ges. Virusforsch.* **25**:93–104.
101. Dunn, G., N. T. Begg, N. Cammack, and P. D. Minor. 1990. Virus excretion and mutation by infants following primary vaccination with live oral poliovaccine from two sources. *J. Med. Virol.* **32**:92–95.
102. Earle, J. A. P., R. A. Skuce, C. S. Fleming, E. M. Hoey, and S. J. Martin. 1988. The complete nucleotide sequence of a bovine enterovirus. *J. Gen. Virol.* **69**:253–263.
103. Eggers, H. J., and A. B. Sabin. 1959. Factors determining pathogenicity of variants of ECHO 9 virus for newborn mice. *J. Exp. Med.* **110**:951–967.
104. Eggers, H. J., and I. Tamm. 1962. On the mechanism of selective inhibition of enterovirus multiplication by 2-(a-hydroxybenzyl)-benzimidazole. *Virology* **18**:426–438.
105. Eigen, M., and C. K. Biebricher. 1988. Sequence space and quasispecies distribution, p. 211–245. In E. Domingo, J. J. Holland, and P. Ahlquist (ed.), *RNA Genetics*, vol. 3. CRC Press, Boca Raton.
106. Emini, E., M. Elzinga, and E. Wimmer. 1982. Carboxy-terminal analysis of poliovirus proteins: termination of poliovirus RNA translation and location of unique poliovirus polyprotein cleavage sites. *J. Virol.* **42**:194–199.
106a. Emini, E. A., B. A. Jameson, A. J. Lewis, G. R. Larsen, and E. Wimmer. 1982. Poliovirus neutralization epitopes: analysis and localization with neutralizing monoclonal antibodies. *J. Virol.* **43**:997–1005.
107. Emini, E., S. Y. Kao, A. J. Lewis, R. Crainic, and E. Wimmer. 1983. Functional basis of poliovirus neutralization determined with monospecific neutralizing antibodies. *J. Virol.* **46**:466–474.
107a. Emini, E. A., J. Leibowitz, D. C. Diamond, J. Bonin, and E. Wimmer. 1984. Recombinants of Mahoney and Sabin strain poliovirus type 1: analysis of in vitro phenotypic markers and evidence that resistance to guanidine maps in the nonstructural proteins. *Virology* **137**:74–85.
108. Enders, J. F., T. H. Weller, and F. C. Robbins. 1949. Cultivation of the Lansing

strain of poliomyelitis virus in cultures of various human embryonic tissues. *Science* **109:**85–87.
109. **Enders, J. F., T. H. Weller, and F. C. Robbins.** 1952. Alteration in pathogenicity of Brunhilde strain of poliomyelitis virus following cultivation in human tissues. *Fed. Proc.* **11:**467.
110. **Equestre, M., D. Genovese, F. Valiere, L. Fiore, R. Santoro, and R. Perez-Bercoff.** 1991. Identification of a consistent pattern of mutations in neurovirulent variants derived from the Sabin vaccine strain of poliovirus type 2. *J. Virol.* **65:**2707–2710.
111. **Evans, D. M., G. Dunn, P. D. Minor, G. C. Schild, A. J. Cann, G. Stanway, J. W. Almond, K. Currey, and J. V. Maizel.** 1985. Increased neurovirulence associated with a single nucleotide change in a noncoding region of the Sabin type 3 poliovaccine genome. *Nature* (London) **314:**548–550.
112. **Filman, D. J., R. Syed, M. Chow, A. J. Macadam, P. D. Minor, and J. M. Hogle.** 1989. Structural factors that control conformational transitions and serotype specificity in type 3 poliovirus. *EMBO J.* **8:**1567–1579.
113. **Flanegan, J. B., R. F. Pettersson, V. Ambros, M. J. Hewlett, and D. Baltimore.** 1977. Covalent linkage of a protein to a defined nucleotide sequence at the 5'-terminus of virion and replicative intermediate RNAs of poliovirus. *Proc. Natl. Acad. Sci. USA* **74:**961–965.
114. **Franssen, H., J. Leunissen, R. Goldbach, G. P. Lomonossoff, and D. Zimmern.** 1984. Homologous sequences in non-structural proteins from cowpea mosaic virus and picornaviruses. *EMBO J.* **3:**855–861.
115. **Furione, M., S. Guillot, D. Otelea, J. Balanant, A. Candrea, and R. Crainic.** 1993. Polioviruses with natural recombinant genomes isolated from vaccine-associated paralytic poliomyelitis. *Virology* **196:**199–208.
116. **Gauntt, C. J., M. D. Trousdale, D. R. L. LaBadie, R. E. Paque, and T. Nealon.** 1979. Properties of coxsackievirus B3 variants which are amyocarditic or myocarditic for mice. *J. Med. Virol.* **3:**207–220.
117. **Giachetti, C., S. S. Hwang, and B. L. Semler.** 1992. cis-Acting lesions targeted to the hydrophobic domain of a poliovirus membrane protein involved in RNA replication. *J. Virol.* **66:**6045–6057.
118. **Giachetti, C., and B. L. Semler.** 1991. Role of a viral membrane polypeptide in strand-specific initiation of poliovirus RNA synthesis. *J. Virol.* **65:**2647–2654.
119. **Gmyl, A. P., E. V. Pilipenko, S. V. Maslova, G. A. Belov, and V. I. Agol.** 1993. Functional and genetic plasticities of the poliovirus genome: quasi-infectious RNAs modified in the 5'-untranslated region yield a variety of pseudorevertants. *J. Virol.* **67:**6309–6316.
120. **Gorbalenya, A. E., V. M. Blinov, and E. Koonin.** 1985. Prediction of nucleotide-binding properties of virus-specific proteins from their primary structure. *Mol. Genet.* **11:**30–36.
121. **Gorbalenya, A. E., A. P. Donchenko, V. M. Blinov, and E. Koonin.** 1989. Cysteine proteases of positive strand RNA viruses and chymotrypsin-like serine proteases. A distinct protein superfamily with a distinct protein fold. *FEBS Lett.* **243:**103–114.
122. **Gratsch, T. E., and V. F. Righthand.** 1994. Construction of a recombinant cDNA of echovirus 6 that established a persistent in vitro infection. *Virology* **201:**341–348.
123. **Grist, N. R., E. J. Bell, and F. Assad.** 1978. Enteroviruses in human disease. *Prog. Med. Virol.* **24:**114–157.
124. **Hagino-Yamagishi, K., and A. Nomoto.** 1989. In vitro construction of poliovirus defective interfering particles. *J. Virol.* **63:**5386–5392.
125. **Haller, A. A., J. H. C. Nguyen, and B. L. Semler.** 1994. Minimum internal ribosome entry site required for poliovirus infectivity. *J. Virol.* **67:**7461–7471.
126. **Haller, A. A., and B. L. Semler.** 1992. Linker scanning mutagenesis of the internal ribosome entry site of poliovirus RNA. *J. Virol.* **66:**5075–5086.
127. **Hämmerle, T., C. U. T. Hellen, and E. Wimmer.** 1991. Site-directed mutagenesis of the catalytic triad of poliovirus 3C proteinase. *J. Biol. Chem.* **266:**5412–5416.
128. **Hämmerle, T., A. Molla, and E. Wimmer.** 1992. Mutational analysis of the proposed FG loop of poliovirus proteinase 3C identifies amino acids that are necessary for 3CD cleavage and might be determinants of a function distinct from proteolytic activity. *J. Virol.* **66:**6028–6034.
129. **Hanecak, R., B. L. Semler, C. W. Anderson, and E. Wimmer.** 1982. Proteolytic processing of poliovirus polypeptides: antibodies to polypeptide P3-7c inhibit cleavage at glutamine-glycine pairs. *Proc. Natl. Acad. Sci. USA* **79:**3973–3977.
130. **Harmon, S. A., O. C. Richards, D. F. Summers, and E. Ehrenfeld.** 1991. The 5'-terminal nucleotides of hepatitis A virus RNA, but not poliovirus RNA, are required for infectivity. *J. Virol.* **65:**2757–2760.
131. **Harris, K. S., C. U. T. Hellen, and E.**

Wimmer. 1990. Proteolytic processing in the replication of picornaviruses. *Semin. Virol.* **1**:323–333.
132. Harris, K. S., W. Xiang, L. Alexander, W. C. Lane, A. V. Paul, and E. Wimmer. 1994. Interaction of the polioviral polypeptide 3CD^{pro} with the 5' and 3' termini of the poliovirus genome: identification of viral and cellular cofactors needed for efficient binding. *J. Biol. Chem.* **269**:27004–27014.
133. Hatfield, G. W., and G. A. Gutman. 1993. Codon pair utilization bias in bacteria, yeast, and mammals, p. 157–189. *In* D. L. Hatfield, B. J. Lee, and R. M. Pirtle (ed.), *Transfer RNA in Protein Synthesis.* CRC Press, Inc., Boca Raton, Fla.
134. Hellen, C. U. T., H.-G. Kräusslich, and E. Wimmer. 1989. Proteolytic processing of polyprotein in the replication of RNA viruses. *Biochemistry* **28**:9881–9890.
135. Hellen, C. U. T., T. V. Pestova, M. Litterst, and E. Wimmer. 1994. The cellular polypeptide p57 (pyrimidine-tract binding protein) binds to multiple sites in the poliovirus 5' nontranslated region. *J. Virol.* **68**:941–950.
136. Hellen, C. U. T., T. V. Pestova, and E. Wimmer. 1994. Effect of mutations downstream of the internal ribosome entry site on initiation of poliovirus protein synthesis. *J. Virol.* **68**:6312–6322.
137. Hellen, C. U. T., G. W. Witherell, M. Schmidt, S. H. Shin, T. V. Pestova, A. Gil, and E. Wimmer. 1993. A cytoplasmic 57kDa protein (p57) that is required for translation of picornavirus RNA by internal ribosomal entry is identical to the nuclear pyrimidine-tract binding protein. *Proc. Natl. Acad. Sci. USA* **90**:7642–7646.
138. Hewlett, M. J., and R. Z. Florkiewicz. 1980. Sequence of picornavirus RNAs containing a radioiodinated 5'-linked peptide reveals a conserved 5' sequence. *Proc. Natl. Acad. Sci. USA* **77**:303–307.
139. Hewlett, S., S. Rosenblatt, V. Ambros, and D. Baltimore. 1977. Separation and quantitation of intracellular forms of poliovirus RAN by agarose gel electrophoresis. *Biochemistry* **16**:2763–2767.
140. Hirst, G. 1962. Genetic recombination with Newcastle disease virus, polioviruses and influenza. *Cold Spring Harbor Symp. Quant. Biol.* **27**:303–308.
141. Hogle, J. M., M. Chow, and D. J. Filman. 1985. The three-dimensional structure of poliovirus at 2.9Å resolution. *Science* **229**:1358–1365.
142. Hogle, J. M., and D. J. Filman. 1989. The antigenic structure of poliovirus. *Phil. Trans. R. Soc. Lond. Ser. B* **323**:467–478.
143. Holland, J., J. C. de la Torre, and D. A. Steinhauer. 1990. RNA virus populations as quasispecies. *Curr. Top. Microbiol. Immunol.* **176**:1–20.
144. Holland, J., E. Domingo, J. C. de la Torre, and D. A. Steinhauer. 1990. Mutation frequencies at defined single codon sites in vesicular stomatitis virus can be increased only slightly by chemical mutagenesis. *J. Virol.* **64**:3960–3962.
145. Holland, J., L. C. McLaren, and J. T. Syverton. 1959. The mammalian cell-virus relationship. IV. Infection of naturally insusceptible cells with enterovirus ribonucleic acid. *J. Exp. Med.* **110**:65–80.
146. Holland, J., L. C. McLaren, and J. T. Syverton. 1959. The mammalian cell-virus relationship. III. Non-primate cells exposed to poliovirus ribonucleic acid. *Proc. Soc. Exp. Biol. Med.* **100**:843–845.
147. Holland, J., K. Spindler, F. Horodyski, B. Garabau, S. Nichol, and S. Vandenpol. 1982. Rapid evolution of RNA genomes. *Science* **215**:1577–1585.
148. Holland, J. J. 1961. Receptor affinities as major determinants of enterovirus tissue tropism in humans. *Virology* **15**:312–326.
149. Holland, J. J., and C. E. Cords. 1964. Maturation of poliovirus RNA with capsid protein coded by heterologous enteroviruses. *Proc. Natl. Acad. Sci. USA* **51**:1082–1085.
150. Hsiung, G. D., and J. L. Melnick. 1957. Morphologic characteristics of plaques produced on monkey kidney monolayer cultures by enteric viruses (poliomyelitis, Coxsackie, and ECHO groups). *J. Immunol.* **78**:128–136.
151. Hsiung, G. D., and J. L. Melnick. 1957. Comparative susceptibility of kidney cells from different monkey species to enteric viruses (poliomyelitis, Coxsackie, and ECHO groups). *J. Immunol.* **78**:137–146.
152. Huang, A. S. 1973. Defective interfering viruses. *Annu. Rev. Microbiol.* **27**:101–117.
153. Hughes, M. S., E. M. Hoey, and P. V. Coyle. 1993. A nucleotide sequence comparison of coxsackievirus B4 isolates from aquatic samples and clinical specimens. *Epidemiol. Infect.* **110**:389–398.
154. Hughes, P. J., D. M. A. Evans, P. D. Minor, G. C. Schild, J. W. Almond, and G. Stanway. 1986. The nucleotide sequence of a type 3 poliovirus isolated during a recent outbreak of poliomyelitis in Finland. *J. Gen. Virol.* **67**:2093–2102.
155. Hughes, P. J., C. North, P. D. Minor, and

G. Stanway. 1989. The complete nucleotide sequence of coxsackievirus A21. *J. Gen. Virol.* **70:**2943–2952.
156. Hughes, P. J., A. Phillips, P. D. Minor, and G. Stanway. 1987. The sequence of the coxsackievirus A21 polymerase gene indicates a remarkably close relationship to the poliovirus. *Arch. Virol.* **94:**141–147.
156a. Huovilainen, A., T. Hovi, L. Kinnunen, K. Takkinen, M. Ferguson, and P. Minor. 1987. Evolution of poliovirus during an outbreak: sequential type 3 poliovirus isolates from several persons show shifts of neutralization determinants. *J. Gen. Virol.* **68:**1373–1378.
157. Huovilainen, A., L. Kinnunen, T. Pöyry, L. Laaksonen, M. Roivainen, and T. Hovi. 1994. Poliovirus type 3/Saukett: antigenic and structural correlates of sequence variation in the capsid proteins. *Virology* **199:**228–232.
158. Hyppia, T., C. Horsnell, M. Maaronen, M. Khan, N. Kalkkinen, T. Auvinen, L. Kinnunen, and G. Stanway. 1992. A distinct picornavirus group identified by sequence analysis. *Proc. Natl. Acad. Sci. USA* **89:**8847–8851.
159. Hyppia, T., and G. Stanway. 1992. Biology of coxsackie A viruses. *Adv. Virus. Res.* **42:**343–373.
160. Iizuka, N., M. Kohara, M., K. Hagino-Yamagishi, S. Abe, T. Komatsu, K. Tago, M. Arita, and A. Nomoto. 1989. Construction of less neurovirulent polioviruses by introducing deletions into the 5' noncoding sequence of the genome. *J. Virol.* **63:**5354–5363.
161. Iizuka, N., S. Kuge, and A. Nomoto. 1987. Complete nucleotide sequence of the genome of coxsackievirus B1. *Virology* **156:**64–73.
162. Iizuka, N., H. Yonekawa, and A. Nomoto. 1991. Nucleotide sequences important for translation initiation of enterovirus RNA. *J. Virol.* **65:**4867–4873.
163. Ikegami, N., H. J. Eggers, and I. Tamm. 1964. Rescue of drug-requiring and drug-inhibited enteroviruses. *Proc. Natl. Acad. Sci. USA* **52:**1419–1426.
164. Inoue, T., T. Suzuki, and K. Sekiguchi. 1989. The complete nucleotide sequence of swine vesicular disease virus. *J. Gen. Virol.* **70:**919–934.
165. Inoue, T., S. Yamaguchi, T. Kanno, S. Sugita, and T. Saeki. 1993. The complete nucleotide sequence of a pathogenic swine vesicular disease virus isolated in Japan (J1'73) and phylogenetic analysis. *Nucleic Acids Res.* **21:**3896.
166. Ishiko, H., N. Takeda, K. Miyamura, N. Kato, M. Tanimura, K. H. Lin, M. Yin-Murphy, J. S. Tam, G. F. Mu, and S. Yamazaki. 1992. Phylogenetic analysis of a coxsackievirus A24 variant: the most recent worldwide pandemic was caused by progenies of a common virus prevalent around 1981. *Virology* **187:**748–759.
167. Ishiko, H., N. Takeda, K. Miyamura, M. Tanimura, T. Yamanaka, K. Kasuga, K. Oda, K. Imai, Y. Yamamoto, Y. Mochida, K. Uchida, H. Nakagawa, and S. Yamazaki. 1992. Phylogenetically different strains of a variant of coxsackievirus A24 were repeatedly introduced but discontinuously circulating in Japan. *Arch. Virol.* **126:**179–193.
168. Itoh, H., and J. D. Melnick. 1959. Double infections of single cells with ECHO 7 and coxsackie A9 viruses. *J. Exp. Med.* **109:**393–406.
169. Jablonski, S. A., M. Luo, and C. D. Morrow. 1991. Enzymatic activity of poliovirus RNA polymerase mutants with single amino acid changes in the conserved YGDD amino acid motif. *J. Virol.* **65:**4565–4572.
170. Jablonski, S. A., and C. D. Morrow. 1993. Enzymatic activity of poliovirus RNA polymerases with mutations at the tyrosine residue of the conserved YGDD motif: isolation and characterization of polioviruses containing RNA polymerases with FGDD and MGDD sequences. *J. Virol.* **67:**373–381.
171. Jackson, R. J., and N. Standart. 1990. Do the poly(A) tail and 3' untranslated region control mRNA translation? *Cell* **62:**15–24.
172. Jacobson, M. F., and D. Baltimore. 1968. Polypeptide cleavages in the formation of poliovirus proteins. *Proc. Natl. Acad. Sci. USA* **61:**77–84.
173. Jacobson, S. J., D. A. M. Konings, and P. Sarnow. 1993. Biochemical and genetic evidence for a pseudoknot structure at the 3' terminus of the poliovirus RNA genome and its role in viral RNA amplification. *J. Virol.* **67:**2961–2971.
174. Jang, S. K., H.-G. Kräusslich, M. J. H. Nicklin, G. M. Duke, A. C. Palmenberg, and E. Wimmer. 1988. A segment of the 5' nontranslated region of encephalomyocarditis virus RNA directs internal entry of ribosomes during in vitro translation. *J. Virol.* **62:**2636–2643.
175. Jang, S. K., T. V. Pestova, C. U. T. Hellen, G. W. Witherell, and E. Wimmer. 1990. Cap-independent translation of picornavirus RNAs: structure and function of the internal ribosomal entry site. *Enzyme* **44:**292–309.
176. Jarvis, T. C., and K. Kirkegaard. 1991. The

polymerase in its labyrinth. *Trends Genet.* **7**:186–191.
177. Jarvis, T. C., and K. Kirkegaard. 1992. Poliovirus RNA recombination: mechanistic studies in the absence of selection. *EMBO J.* **11**:3135–3145.
178. Jenkins, O., J. D. Booth, P. D. Minor, and J. W. Almond. 1987. The complete nucleotide sequence of coxsackievirus B4 and its comparison to other members of the Picornaviridae. *J. Gen. Virol.* **68**:1835–1848.
179. Johnson, K. L., and P. Sarnow. 1991. Three poliovirus 2B mutants exhibit noncomplementable defects in viral RNA amplification and display dosage-dependent dominance over wild-type poliovirus. *J. Virol.* **65**:4341–4349.
180. Johnson, V. H., and B. L. Semler. 1988. Defined recombinants of poliovirus and coxsackievirus: sequence-specific deletions and functional substitutions in the 5'-noncoding regions of viral RNAs. *Virology* **162**:47–57.
181. Jore, J., B. de Geus, R. J. Jackson, P. H. Pouwels, and B. E. Enger-Valk. 1988. Poliovirus protein 3CD is the active protease for processing of the precursor protein P1 in vitro. *J. Gen. Virol.* **69**:1627–1636.
182. Kajigaya, S., H. Arakawa, S. Kuge, T. Koi, N. Imura, and A. Nomoto. 1985. Isolation and characterization of defective-interfering particles of poliovirus Sabin 1 strain. *Virology* **142**:307–316.
183. Kamitsuka, P. S., T. Y. Lon, A. Fabiyi, and H. A. Wenner. 1965. Preparation and standardization of coxsackievirus reference antisera. I. For twenty-four group A viruses. *Am. J. Epidemiol.* **81**:283–305.
184. Kandolf, R., and P. H. Hofschneider. 1985. Molecular cloning of the genome of cardiotropic coxsackie B3 virus: full-length reverse-transcribed recombinant cDNA generates infectious virus in mammalian cells. *Proc. Natl. Acad. Sci. USA* **82**:4818–4822.
185. Kaplan, G., D. Peters, and V. R. Racaniello. 1990. Poliovirus mutants resistant to neutralization with soluble cell receptors. *Science* **250**:1596–1599.
186. Kaplan, G., and V. R. Racaniello. 1988. Construction and characterization of poliovirus subgenomic replicons. *J. Virol.* **62**:1687–1696.
187. Kawamura, N., M. Kohara, S. Abe, T. Komatsu, K. Tago, M. Arita, and A. Nomoto. 1989. Determinants in the 5' noncoding region of poliovirus Sabin 1 RNA that influence the attenuation phenotype. *J. Virol.* **63**:1302–1309.
187a. Kean, K. M., H. Agut, O. Fichot, E. Wimmer, and M. Girard. 1988. A poliovirus mutant defective for self-cleavage at the COH-terminus of the 3C protease exhibits secondary processing defects. *Virology* **163**:330–340.
188. Kean, K. M., N. L. Teterina, D. Marc, and M. Girard. 1991. Analysis of the putative active site residues of the poliovirus 3C proteinase. *Virology* **181**:330–340.
189. Kew, O. M., and B. K. Nottay. 1984. Evolution of the oral polio vaccine in humans occurs by both mutation and intramolecular recombination, p. 357–362. *In* R. A. Lerner, R. M. Chanock, and F. Brown (ed.), *Vaccines '86*. Cold Spring Harbor Laboratory Press, Plainview, N.Y.
190. Kew, O. M., B. K. Nottay, M. H. Hatch, J. H. Nakano, and J. F. Obijeski. 1981. Multiple genetic changes can occur in oral polio vaccines upon replication in humans. *J. Gen. Virol.* **56**:337–347.
191. Kew, O. M., M. Pallansch, B. K. Nottay, R. Rico-Hesse, L. De, and D. L. Yang. 1990. Genotypic relationships among wild polioviruses from different regions of the world, p. 357–365. *In* M. A. Brinton and F. X. Heinz (ed.), *New Aspects of Positive-Strand Viruses*. American Society for Microbiology, Washington, D.C.
192. Khatchikian, D., M. Orlich, and R. Rott. 1989. Increased viral pathogenicity after insertion of a 28S ribosomal RNA sequence into the haemagglutinin gene of an influenza virus. *Nature* (London) **340**:156–157.
193. King, A. M. Q. 1988. Preferred sites of recombination in poliovirus RNA: an analysis of 40 intertypic cross-over sequences. *Nucleic Acids Res.* **16**:11705–11723.
194. King, A. M. Q., D. McCahon, W. R. Slade, and J. W. I. Newman. 1982. Recombination in RNA. *Cell* **29**:921–928.
195. King, L. A. 1986. Molecular biology of insect picornaviruses. Ph.D. thesis. University of Oxford, Oxford, United Kingdom.
196. King, L. A., J. S. K. Pullin, G. Stanway, J. W. Almond, and N. F. Moore. 1987. Cloning of the genome of cricket paralysis virus: sequence of the 3' end. *Virus Res.* **6**:331–344.
197. Kirkegaard, K. 1990. Mutations in VP1 of poliovirus specifically affect both encapsidation and release of viral RNA. *J. Virol.* **64**:195–206.
198. Kirkegaard, K. 1992. Genetic analysis of picornaviruses. *Curr. Top. Genet. Dev.* **2**:64–70.
199. Kirkegaard, K., and D. Baltimore. 1986. The mechanism of RNA recombination in poliovirus. *Cell* **47**:433–443.

200. **Kirkegaard, K., and B. Nelsen.** 1990. Conditional poliovirus mutants made by random deletion mutagenesis of infectious cDNA. *J. Virol.* **64**:185–194.
201. **Kitamura, N., C. Adler, J. Martinko, S. Nathenson, and E. Wimmer.** 1980. The genome-linked protein of picornaviruses. VII. Genetic mapping of poliovirus VPg by protein and RNA sequence studies. *Cell* **21**:295–302.
202. **Kitamura, N., B. L. Semler, P. G. Rothberg, G. R. Larsen, C. J. Adler, A. J. Dorner, E. A. Emini, R. Hanecak, J. Lee, S. van der Werf, C. W. Anderson, and E. Wimmer.** 1981. Primary structure, gene organization and polypeptide expression of poliovirus RNA. *Nature* (London) **291**:547–553.
203. **Klingel, K., C. Hohenadl, A. Canu, M. Albrecht, M. Seemann, G. Mall, and R. Kandolf.** 1992. Ongoing enterovirus-induced myocarditis is associated with persistent heart muscle infection: quantitative analysis of virus replication, tissue damage, and inflammation. *Proc. Natl. Acad. Sci. USA* **89**:314–318.
204. **Klump, W. M., I. Bergmann, B. C. Müller, D. Ameis, and R. Kandolf.** 1990. Complete nucleotide sequence of infectious coxsackievirus B3 cDNA: two initial 5' uridine residues are regained during plus-strand RNA synthesis. *J. Virol.* **64**:1573–1583.
205. **Knowles, N. J., and I. T. R. Barnett.** 1985. A serological classification of bovine enteroviruses. *Arch. Virol.* **83**:141–155.
206. **Koch, F., and G. Koch.** 1985. *The Molecular Biology of Poliovirus.* Springer Verlag, Vienna.
207. **Kohara, M., S. Abe, S. Kuge, B. L. Semler, T. Komatsu, M. Arita, H. Itoh, and A. Nomoto.** 1986. An infectious cDNA clone of the poliovirus Sabin strain could be used as a stable repository and inoculum for the oral polio live vaccine. *Virology* **151**:21–30.
208. **Koike, S., C. Taya, T. Kurata, S. Abe, I. Ise, H. Yonekawa, and A. Nomoto.** 1991. Transgenic mice susceptible to poliovirus. *Proc. Natl. Acad. Sci. USA* **88**:951–955.
209. **Koprowski, H., G. A. Jervis, and T. W. Norton.** 1952. Immune responses in human volunteers upon oral administration of a rodent-adapted strain of poliomyelitis virus. *Am. J. Hyg.* **55**:108–126.
210. **Koroleva, G. A., and M. P. Frolova.** 1964. Investigations on coxsackievirus A7, A14 and A16 viruses in tissue culture and in animals. *Acta Virol.* **8**:532–540.
211. **Koroleva, G. A., M. P. Frolova, M. K. Voroshilova, and I. A. Robinzon.** 1967. Changes in neurovirulence of coxsackieviruses A7, A14 and A16 dependent on passaging in cell cultures and animals. *Acta Virol.* **11**:78–88.
212. **Kraus, W., and B. E. Nelsen-Salz.** 1994. Echovirus type 12, prototype Travis wild type genome. GenBank accession number X79047.
213. **Kuge, S., N. Kawamura, and A. Nomoto.** 1989. Strong inclination toward transition mutation in nucleotide substitutions by poliovirus replicase. *J. Mol. Biol.* **207**:175–182.
214. **Kuge, S., N. Kawamura, and A. Nomoto.** 1989. Genetic variation occurring in the genome of an in vitro insertion mutant of poliovirus type 1. *J. Virol.* **63**:1069–1075.
215. **Kuge, S., and A. Nomoto.** 1987. Construction of viable deletion and insertion mutants of the Sabin strain type 1 poliovirus: function of the 5' noncoding sequence in viral replication. *J. Virol.* **61**:1478–1487.
216. **Kuge, S., L. Saito, and A. Nomoto.** 1986. Primary structure of poliovirus defective interfering particle genomes and possible generation mechanism of the particles. *J. Mol. Biol.* **192**:473–487.
217. **Kuhn, R. J., H. Tada, M.-F. Ypma-Wong, J. J. Dunn, B. L. Semler, and E. Wimmer.** 1988. Construction of a "mutagenesis cartridge" for poliovirus genome-linked protein: isolation and characterization of viable and nonviable mutants. *Proc. Natl. Acad. Sci. USA* **85**:519–523.
218. **Kuhn, R. J., H. Tada, M.-F. Ypma-Wong, B. L. Semler, and E. Wimmer.** 1988. Mutational analysis of the genome-linked protein VPg of poliovirus. *J. Virol.* **62**:4207–4215.
219. **Lama, J., A. V. Paul, K. S. Harris, and E. Wimmer.** 1994. Properties of purified recombinant poliovirus protein 3AB as substrate for viral proteinases and as co-factor for RNA polymerase 3D^{pol}. *J. Biol. Chem.* **269**:66–70.
220. **La Monica, N., J. W. Almond, and V. R. Racaniello.** 1987. A mouse model for poliovirus neurovirulence identifies mutations that attenuate the virus for humans. *J. Virol.* **61**:2917–2920.
221. **La Monica, N., N. Kupsky, and V. R. Racaniello.** 1987. Reduced mouse neuorvirulence of poliovirus type 2 Lansing antigenic variants selected with monoclonal antibodies. *Virology* **161**:429–437.
222. **La Monica, N., C. Meriam, and V. R. Racaniello.** 1986. Mapping of sequences required for mouse neurovirulence of poliovirus type 2 Lansing. *J. Virol.* **57**:515–525.
223. **Landsteiner, K., and E. Popper.** 1909. Übertragung der Poliomyelitis acuta auf Affen. *Z. Immunitätsforsch. Orig.* **2**:377–390.
224. **Larsen, G., C. W. Anderson, A. Dorner, B. L. Semler, and E. Wimmer.** 1982.

Cleavage sites within the poliovirus capsid protein precursors. *J. Virol.* **41**:340–344.
225. **Larsen, G. R., B. L. Semler, and E. Wimmer.** 1981. Stable hairpin structure within the 5' terminal 85 nucleotides of poliovirus RNA. *J. Virol.* **37**:328–335.
226. **Lawson, M. A., and B. L. Semler.** 1991. Poliovirus thiol proteinase 3C can utilize a serine nucleophile within the putative catalytic triad. *Proc. Natl. Acad. Sci. USA* **88**:9919–9923.
227. **Le, S.-Y., J. H. Chen, N. Sonenberg, and J. V. Maizel.** 1992. Conserved tertiary structure elements in the 5' untranslated region of human enteroviruses and rhinoviruses. *Virology* **191**:858–866.
228. **Le, S.-Y., and M. Zuker.** 1990. Common structures of the 5'-noncoding RNA in enteroviruses and rhinoviruses. *J. Mol. Biol.* **216**:729–741.
229. **Ledinko, N.** 1963. Genetic recombination with poliovirus type 1. Studies of crosses between a normal horse serum-resistant mutant and several guanidine-resistant mutants of the same strain. *Virology* **20**:107–119.
230. **Lee, C.-K., and E. Wimmer.** 1988. Proteolytic processing of poliovirus polyprotein: elimination of 2A^{pro}-mediated, alternative cleavage of polypeptide 3CD by in vitro mutagenesis. *Virology* **166**:405–414.
231. **Lee, Y. F., A. Nomoto, B. M. Detjen, and E. Wimmer.** 1977. The genome-linked protein of picornaviruses. I. A protein covalently linked to poliovirus genome RNA. *Proc. Natl. Acad. Sci. USA* **74**:59–63.
232. **Lehmann-Grube, F., and J. T. Syverton.** 1961. Pathogenicity for suckling mice of coxsackie viruses adapted to human amnion cells. *J. Exp. Med.* **113**:811–829.
233. **Leong, L. E.-C., P. A. Walker, and A. G. Porter.** 1993. Human rhinovirus-14 protease 3C (3C^{pro}) binds specifically to the 5'-noncoding region of the viral RNA. *J. Biol. Chem.* **268**:25735–25739.
234. **Li, C. P., and W. G. Jahnes.** 1956. Studies on variation in virulence of poliomyelitis virus. I. The loss and gain of virulence of the mouse-adapted type III virus. *Virology* **2**:828–835.
235. **Li, J.-P., and D. Baltimore.** 1988. Isolation of poliovirus 2C mutants defective in viral RNA synthesis. *J. Virol.* **62**:4016–4021.
236. **Li, J.-P., and D. Baltimore.** 1990. An intragenic revertant of a poliovirus 2C mutant has an uncoating defect. *J. Virol.* **64**:1102–1107.
237. **Lin, K. H., N. Takeda, K. Miyamura, S. Yamakazi, and W. C. Chen.** 1991. The nucleotide sequence of 3C proteinase region of coxsackievirus A24 variant: comparison of the isolates in Taiwan in 1985–1988. *Virus Genes* **5**:121–131.
238. **Lin, K. H., H.-L. Wang, M.-M. Sheu, W.-L. Huang, C. W. Chen, C.-S. Yang, N. Takeda, N. Kato, K. Miyamura, and S. Yamakazi.** 1993. Molecular epidemiology of a variant of coxsackievirus A24 in Taiwan: two epidemics caused by phylogenetically distinct viruses from 1985 to 1989. *J. Clin. Microbiol.* **31**:1160–1166.
239. **Lindberg, A. M., P. O. K. Ståhlhandske, and U. Petterson.** 1987. Genome of coxsackievirus B3. *Virology* **156**:50–63.
240. **Lipskaya, G. Y., A. R. Muzychenko, O. K. Kutitova, S. V. Maslova, M. Equestre, S. G. Drozdov, R. Perez-Bercoff, and V. I. Agol.** 1991. Frequent recombination of intertypic poliovirus recombinants with serotype 2 specificity from vaccine-associated polio cases. *J. Med. Virol.* **35**:290–296.
241. **Lu, H.-H., C.-F. Yang, A. D. Murdin, M. H. Klein, J. J. Harber, O. M. Kew, and E. Wimmer.** 1994. Mouse neurovirulence determinants of poliovirus type 1 strain LS-a map to the coding regions of capsid protein VP1 and proteinase 2A^{pro}. *J. Virol.* **68**:7507–7515.
242. **Lundquist, R., M. Sullivan, and J. V. Maizel.** 1979. Characterization of a new isolate of poliovirus defective interfering particles. *Cell* **18**:759–769.
243. **Lwoff, A., and M. Lwoff.** 1958. Inhibition du development du virus poliomyelitique a 39°C et le probleme de role de l'hypothermie dans l'evolution des infections virales. *C.R. Acad. Sci.* (Paris) **246**:190–192.
244. **Macadam, A. J., C. Arnold, J. Howlett, A. John., S. Marsden, F. Taffs, P. Reeve, N. Hamada, K. Wareham, J. Almond, N. Cammack, and P. D. Minor.** 1989. Reversion of the attenuated and temperature-sensitive phenotypes of the Sabin type strain of poliovirus in vaccinees. *Virology* **174**:408–414.
245. **Macadam, A. J., G. Ferguson, C. Arnold, and P. D. Minor.** 1991. An assembly defect as a result of an attenuating mutation in the capsid proteins of the poliovirus type 3 vaccine strain. *J. Virol.* **65**:5225–5231.
246. **Macadam, A. J., G. Ferguson, J. Burlison, D. Stone, R. Skuce, J. W. Almond, and P. D. Minor.** 1992. Correlation of RNA secondary structure and attenuation of Sabin vaccine strains of poliovirus in tissue culture. *Virology* **189**:415–422.
247. **Macadam, A. J., G. Ferguson, T. Fleming, D. M. Stone, J. W. Almond, and P. D. Minor.** 1994. Role for poliovirus protease 2A

in cap independent translation. *EMBO J.* **13:**924–927.
248. **Macadam, A. J., S. R. Pollard, G. Ferguson, G. Dunn, R. Skuce, J. W. Almond, and P. D. Minor.** 1991. The 5' noncoding region of the type 2 poliovirus vaccine strain contains determinants of attenuation and temperature sensitivity. *Virology* **181:**451–458.
249. **Macadam, A. J., S. R. Pollard, G. Ferguson, R. Skuce, D. Wood, J. W. Almond, and P. D. Minor.** 1993. Genetic basis of attenuation of Sabin type 2 vaccine strain of poliovirus in primates. *Virology* **192:**18–26.
250. **Mahy, B. W. J.** 1988. Classification and general properties, p. 1–18. *In* M. Bendinelli and H. Friedman (ed.), *Coxsackieviruses: a General Update.* Plenum Press, New York.
251. **Maizels, N., and A. M. Weiner.** 1993. The genomic tag hypothesis: modern viruses as molecular fossils of ancient strategies for genomic replication, p. 577–602. *In* R. F. Gesteland and J. F. Atkins (ed.), *The RNA World.* Cold Spring Harbor Laboratory Press, Plainview, N.Y.
252. **Marc, D., G. Masson, M. Girard, and S. van der Werf.** 1990. Lack of myristoylation of poliovirus capsid polypeptide VP0 prevents the formation of virions or results in the assembly of noninfectious virus particles. *J. Virol.* **64:**4099–4107.
253. **Martin, A., C. Wychowski, T. Couderc, R. Crainic, J. Hogle, and M. Girard.** 1988. Engineering a poliovirus type 2 antigenic site on a type 1 capsid results in a chimaeric virus which is neurovirulent for mice. *EMBO J.* **7:**2839–2847.
254. **Mattern, C. F. T.** 1962. Some physical and chemical properties of coxsackieviruses A9 and A10. *Virology* **17:**520–532.
255. **Matthews, D. A., W. S. Smith, R. A. Ferre, B. Condon, G. Budahazi, W. Sisson, J. E. Villafranca, C. A. Janson, H. E. McElroy, C. L. Gribskov, and S. Worland.** 1994. Structure of human rhinovirus 3C protease reveals a trypsin-like polypeptide fold, RNA-binding site, and means for cleaving precursor polyprotein. *Cell* **77:**761–771.
256. **McLaren, L. C., J. J. Holland, and J. T. Syverton.** 1959. The mammalian cell-virus relationship. I. Attachment of poliovirus to cultivated cells of primate and non-primate origin. *J. Exp. Med.* **109:**475–485.
257. **McNally, R. M., J. A. P. Earle, M. McIlhatton, E. M. Hoey, and S. J. Martin.** 1994. Nucleotide sequence of the 5' noncoding and capsid coding regions of two bovine enterovirus strains. GenBank accession number X79368.
258. **Meerovitch, K., R. Nicholson, and N. Sonenberg.** 1991. In vitro mutational analysis of *cis*-acting RNA translational elements within the poliovirus type 2 5' untranslated region. *J. Virol.* **65:**5895–5901.
259. **Meerovitch, K., J. Pelletier, and N. Sonenberg.** 1989. A cellular protein that binds to the 5'-noncoding region of poliovirus RNA: implications for internal translation initiation. *Genes Dev.* **3:**1026–1034.
260. **Meerovitch, K., Y. V. Svitkin, H. S. Lee, F. Lejbkowicz, D. J. Kenan, E. K. L. Chan, V. I. Agol, J. D. Keene, and N. Sonenberg.** 1993. La autoantigen enhances and corrects aberrant translation of poliovirus RNA in reticulocyte lysate. *J. Virol.* **67:**3798–3807.
261. **Melnick, J. L.** 1957. ECHO viruses. *Spec. Publ. N.Y. Acad. Sci.* **5:**365.
262. **Melnick, J. L.** 1990. Enteroviruses: poliovirus, coxsackievirus, echoviruses and newer enteroviruses, p. 549–606. *In* B. N. Fields, D. M. Knipe, R. M. Chanock, M. S. Hirsch, J. L. Melnick, T. P. Monath, and B. Roizman (ed.), *Virology,* 2nd ed. Raven Press, New York.
263. **Melnick, J. L., V. I. Agol, H. L. Bachrach, F. Brown, P. D. Cooper, W. Fiers, S. Gard, J. H. S. Gear, Y. Ghendon, L. Kasza, M. LaPlaca, B. Mandel, S. McGregor, S. B. Mohanty, G. Plummer, R. R. Rueckert, F. L. Schaeffer, I. Tagaya, D. A. J. Tyrell, M. Voroshilova, and H. A. Wenner.** 1974. Picornaviridae. *Intervirology* **4:**303–316.
264. **Melnick, J. L., D. Crowther, and J. Barrera-Oro.** 1961. Rapid development of drug-resistant mutants of poliovirus. *Science* **134:**557.
265. **Melnick, J. L., G. Dalldorf, J. F. Enders, H. M. Gelfand, W. M. Hammon, R. J. Huebner, L. Rosen, A. B. Sabin, J. T. Syverton, and H. A. Wenner.** 1957. The enteroviruses. *Am. J. Public Health* **47:**1556–1566.
266. **Melnick, J. L., G. Dalldorf, J. F. Enders, H. M. Gelfand, W. M. Hammon, R. J. Huebner, L. Rosen, A. B. Sabin, J. T. Syverton, and H. A. Wenner.** 1962. Classification of enteroviruses. *Virology* **16:**501–504.
267. **Melnick, J. L., V. Rennick, B. Hampil, N. J. Schmidt, and H. H. Ho.** 1973. Lyophilised combination pools of enterovirus equine sera: preparation and test procedures for the identification of field strains of 42 enteroviruses. *Bull. W.H.O.* **48:**263–268.
268. **Mendelsohn, C. L., B. Johnson, K. A.**

Lionetti, P. Nobis, E. Wimmer, and V. R. Racaniello. 1986. Transformation of a human poliovirus receptor gene into mouse cells. *Proc. Natl. Acad. Sci. USA* **83**:7845–7849.
269. Mendelsohn, C. L., E. Wimmer, and V. R. Racaniello. 1989. Cellular receptor for poliovirus: molecular cloning, nucleotide sequence, and expression of a new member of immunoglobulin superfamily. *Cell* **56**:855–865.
270. Meyer, J., R. E. Lundquist, and J. V. Maizel. 1978. Structural studies of the RNA component of the poliovirus replication complex. *Virology* **85**:445–455.
271. Meyers, G., T. Rümenapf, and H.-J. Thiel. 1989. Ubiquitin in a togavirus. *Nature (London)* **341**:491.
272. Mills, D. R., C. Dobkin, and F. R. Kramer. 1978. Template-determined, variable rate of RNA chain elongation. *Cell* **15**:541–550.
273. Minor, P. D. 1990. Antigenic structure of picornaviruses. *Curr. Top. Immunol. Microbiol.* **161**:121–154.
274. Minor, P. D. 1992. The molecular biology of poliovaccines. *J. Gen. Virol.* **73**:3065–3077.
275. Minor, P. D. 1993. Attenuation and reversion of the Sabin vaccine strains of poliovirus. *Dev. Biol. Stand.* **78**:17–26.
276. Minor, P. D., and G. Dunn. 1988. The effect of sequences in the 5' non-coding region on the replication of polioviruses in the human gut. *J. Gen. Virol.* **69**:1091–1096.
277. Minor, P. D., G. Dunn, D. M. A. Evans, D. I. Magrath, A. John, J. Howlett, A. Phillips, G. Westrop, K. Wareham, J. W. Almond, and J. M. Hogle. 1989. The temperature sensitivity of the Sabin type 3 vaccine strain of poliovirus: molecular and structural effects of a mutation in the capsid protein VP3. *J. Gen. Virol.* **70**:1117–1123.
278. Minor, P. D., A. John, M. Ferguson, and J. P. Icenogle. 1986. Antigenic and molecular evolution of the vaccine strain of type 3 poliovirus during the period of excretion by a primary vaccinee. *J. Gen. Virol.* **67**:693–706.
279. Minor, P. D., G. C. Schild, J. Bootman, D. M. A. Evans, M. Ferguson, P. Reeve, M. Spitz, G. Stanway, A. J. Cann, R. Hauptmann, L. D. Clarke, R. C. Mountford, and J. W. Almond. 1983. Location and primary structure of a major antigenic site for poliovirus neutralization. *Nature (London)* **301**:674–679.
280. Mirzayan, C., and E. Wimmer. 1992. Genetic analysis of an NTP-binding motif in poliovirus polypeptide 2C. *Virology* **183**:547–555.
281. Mirzayan, C., and E. Wimmer. 1994. Biochemical studies on poliovirus polypeptide 2C: evidence for ATPase activity. *Virology* **199**:176–187.
282. Miyamura, K., M. Tanimura, N. Takeda, R. Kono, and S. Yamakazi. 1986. Evolution of enterovirus 70 in nature: all isolates were recently derived from a common ancestor. *Arch. Virol.* **89**:1–14.
283. Molla, A., K. S. Harris, A. V. Paul, S. H. Shin, J. Mugavero, and E. Wimmer. 1994. Stimulation of poliovirus proteinase 3C^{pro}-related proteolysis by the genome-linked protein VPg and its precursor 3AB. *J. Biol. Chem.* **269**:27015–27020.
284. Molla, A., S.-K. Jang, A. V. Paul, Q. Reuer, and E. Wimmer. 1992. Cardioviral internal ribosomal entry site is functional in a genetically engineered dicistronic poliovirus. *Nature (London)* **356**:255–257.
285. Molla, A., A. V. Paul, M. Schmid, S.-K. Jang, and E. Wimmer. 1993. Studies on dicistronic polioviruses implicate viral proteinase 2A^{pro} in RNA replication. *Virology* **196**:739–747.
285a. Molla, A., and E. Wimmer. Unpublished data.
286. Monroe, S. S., and S. Schlesinger. 1984. Common and distinct regions of defective-interfering RNAs of Sindbis virus. *J. Virol.* **49**:865–872.
287. Moore, M. 1982. Enteroviral disease in the United States, 1970–1979. *J. Infect. Dis.* **146**:103–108.
288. Moore, N. F., B. Reavy, and L. A. King. 1986. General characteristics, gene organization and expression of small RNA viruses of insects. *J. Gen. Virol.* **66**:647–659.
289. Moss, E. G., R. E. O'Neill, and V. R. Racaniello. 1989. Mapping of attenuating sequences of an avirulent poliovirus type 2 strain. *J. Virol.* **63**:1884–1890.
290. Moss, E. G., and V. R. Racaniello. 1991. Host range determinants located on the interior of the poliovirus capsid. *EMBO J.* **10**:1067–1074.
291. Mufson, M. A., R. Kawana, H. H. Bloom, F. Gorstein, and R. M. Chanock. 1968. Pathogenicity of coxsackie A-21 virus for suckling mice. *Proc. Soc. Exp. Biol. Med.* **128**:237–240.
292. Müller, H. J. 1964. The relation of recombination to mutational advance. *Mutat. Res.* **1**:2–9.
293. Munishkin, A. V., L. A. Voronin, and A. B. Chetverin. 1988. An *in vivo* recombinant RNA capable of autocatalytic synthesis by Qβ

replicase. *Nature* (London) **333**:473–475.
294. **Murdin, A. D., H. H. Lu, and E. Wimmer.** 1992. Poliovirus antigenic hybrids simultaneously expressing antigenic determinants from all three serotypes. *J. Gen. Virol.* **73**:607–611.
295. **Murray, M. G., J. Bradley, X. F. Yang, E. Wimmer, E. G. Moss, and V. R. Racaniello.** 1988. Poliovirus host range is determined by a short amino acid sequence in neutralization antigenic site 1. *Science* **241**:213–215.
296. **Muzychenko, A. R., G. Lipskaya, S. V. Maslova, Y. V. Svitkin, E. V. Pilipenko, B. K. Nottay, O. M. Kew, and V. I. Agol.** 1991. Coupled mutations in the 5'-untranslated region of the Sabin poliovirus strains during in vivo passages: structural and functional implications. *Virus Res.* **21**:111–122.
297. **Najita, L., and P. Sarnow.** 1990. Oxidation-reduction sensitive interaction of a cellular 50-kDa protein with an RNA hairpin in the 5'-noncoding region of the poliovirus genome. *Proc. Natl. Acad. Sci. USA* **87**:5846–5850.
298. **Nicholson, R., J. Pelletier, S.-Y. Le, and N. Sonenberg.** 1991. Structural and functional analysis of the ribosome landing pad of poliovirus type 2: in vivo translation studies. *J. Virol.* **65**:5886–5594.
299. **Nicklin, M. J. H., K. S. Harris, P. V. Pallai, and E. Wimmer.** 1988. Poliovirus proteinase 3C: large-scale expression, purification, and specific cleavage activity on natural and synthetic substrates in vitro. *J. Virol.* **62**:4586–4593.
300. **Nilsen, T. W., D. L. Wood, and C. Baglioni.** 1981. Cross-linking of viral RNA by 4'-aminomethyl-4,5',8-trimethylpsoralen in HeLa cells infected with encephalomyocarditis virus and the tsG114 mutant of vesicular stomatitis virus. *Virology* **109**:82–93.
301. **Nomoto, A., B. Detjen, R. Pozzatti, and E. Wimmer.** 1977. The location of the polio genome protein in viral RNAs and its implication for RNA synthesis. *Nature* (London) **268**:208–213.
302. **Nomoto, A., A. Jacobson, Y. F. Lee, J. Dunn, and E. Wimmer.** 1979. Defective interfering particles of poliovirus: mapping of the deletion and evidence that the deletions in the genomes of DI(1), (2) and (3) are located in the same region. *J. Mol. Biol.* **128**:179–196.
303. **Nomoto, A., S. Kajigaya, K. Suzuki, and N. Imura.** 1979. Possible point mutation sites in LSc, 2ab poliovirus RNA and a protein covalently linked to the 5' terminus. *J. Gen. Virol.* **45**:107–117.
304. **Nomoto, A., N. Kitamura, F. Golini, and E. Wimmer.** 1977. The 5'-terminal structures of poliovirion RNA and poliovirus mRNA differ only in the genome-linked protein VPg. *Proc. Natl. Acad. Sci. USA* **74**:5345–5349.
305. **Nomoto, A., T. Omata, H. Toyoda, S. Kuge, H. Horie, Y. Kataoka, Y. Genba, Y. Nakano, and N. Imura.** 1982. Complete nucleotide sequence of the attenuated poliovirus Sabin 1 strain genome. *Proc. Natl. Acad. Sci. USA* **79**:5793–5797.
306. **Nomoto, A., and E. Wimmer.** 1987. Genetic studies of the antigenicity and the attenuation phenotype of poliovirus. *Symp. Soc. Gen. Microbiol.* **35**:107–134.
306a.**Novak, J. E., and K. Kirkegaard.** 1991. Improved method for detecting poliovirus negative strands used to demonstrate specificity of positive-strand encapsidation and the ratio of positive to negative strands in infected cells. *J. Virol.* **65**:3384–3387.
307. **Novak, J. E., and K. Kirkegaard.** 1994. Coupling between genome translation and replication in an RNA virus. *Genes Dev.* **8**:1726–1737.
308. **Omata, T., M. Kohara, S. Kuge, T. Komatsu, S. Abe, B. L. Semler, A. Kameda, H. Itoh, M. Arita, E. Wimmer, and A. Nomoto.** 1986. Genetic analysis of the attenuation phenotype of poliovirus type 1. *J. Virol.* **58**:348–358.
309. **Omata, T., M. Kohara, Y. Sakai, A. Kameda, N. Imura, and A. Nomoto.** 1984. Cloned infectious complementary DNA of the poliovirus Sabin 1 genome: biochemical and biological properties of the recovered virus. *Gene* **32**:1–10.
310. **O'Neill, R. E., and V. R. Racaniello.** 1989. Inhibition of translation in cells infected with a poliovirus 2A^{pro} mutant correlates with phosphorylation of the alpha subunit of eucaryotic initiation factor 2. *J. Virol.* **63**:5069–5075.
311. **Otolea, D., S. Guillot, M. Furione, A. A. Combiescu, J. Balanant, A. Candrea, and R. Crainic.** 1993. Genomic modifications in naturally occurring neurovirulent revertants of Sabin 1 polioviruses. *Dev. Biol. Stand.* **78**:33–38.
312. **Page, G. S., A. G. Mosser, J. M. Hogle, D. J. Filman, R. R. Rueckert, and M. Chow.** 1988. Three-dimensional structure of poliovirus serotype 1 neutralizing determinants. *J. Virol.* **62**:1781–1794.
313. **Pallai, P. V., F. Burkhardt, M. Skoog, K. Schreiner, P. Bax, K. A. Cohen, G. Hansen, D. E. H. Palladino, K. S. Harris, M. J. H. Nicklin, and E. Wimmer.**

1989. Cleavage of synthetic peptides by purified poliovirus 3C proteinase. *J. Biol. Chem.* **264:**900–906.
314. **Palmenberg, A. C.** 1989. Sequence alignments of picornaviral capsids proteins, p. 221–241. *In* B. L. Semler and E. Ehrenfeld (ed.), *Molecular Aspects of Picornavirus Infection and Detection.* American Society for Microbiology, Washington, D.C.
315. **Pappenheimer, A. M., L. J. Kunz, and S. Rickardson.** 1951. Passage of coxsackievirus (Connecticut-5 strain) in adult mice with production of pancreatic disease. *J. Exp. Med.* **94:**45–65.
316. **Parvin, J. D., A. Moscona, W. T. Pan, J. M. Leider, and P. Palese.** 1986. Measurement of the mutation rates of animal viruses: influenza A virus and poliovirus type 1. *J. Virol.* **59:**377–383.
317. **Paul, A. V., A. Molla, and E. Wimmer.** 1994. Studies of a putative amphipathic helix in the N-terminus of poliovirus protein 2C. *Virology* **199:**188–199.
318. **Paul, J. R.** 1971. *A History of Poliomyelitis.* Yale University Press, New Haven, Conn.
319. **Pelletier, J., M. E. Flynn, G. Kaplan, V. R. Racaniello, and N. Sonenberg.** 1988. Mutational analysis of upstream AUG codons of poliovirus RNA. *J. Virol.* **62:**4486–4492.
320. **Pelletier, J., and N. Sonenberg.** 1988. Internal initiation of translation of eukaryotic mRNA directed by a sequence derived from poliovirus RNA. *Nature* (London) **334:**320–325.
321. **Percy, N., W. S. Barclay, M. Sullivan, and J. W. Almond.** 1992. A poliovirus replicon containing the chloramphenicol acetyltransferase gene can be used to study the replication and encapsidation of poliovirus RNA. *J. Virol.* **66:**5040–5046.
322. **Percy, N., G. J. Belsham, J. K. Brangwyn, M. Sullivan, D. M. Stone, and J. W. Almond.** 1992. Intracellular modifications induced by poliovirus reduce the requirement for structural motifs in the 5' noncoding region of the genome involved in internal initiation of protein synthesis. *J. Virol.* **66:**1695–1701.
323. **Pestova, T. V., C. U. T. Hellen, and E. Wimmer.** 1991. Translation of poliovirus RNA: the essential roles of a *cis*-acting oligopyrimidine element within the 5'-nontranslated region and a *trans*-acting 57-Da protein. *J. Virol.* **65:**6194–6204.
324. **Pestova, T. V., C. U. T. Hellen, and E. Wimmer.** 1994. A conserved AUG triplet in the 5' nontranslated region of poliovirus can function as an initiation codon *in vitro* and *in vivo*. *Virology* **204:**729–737.
325. **Pevear, D. C., C. K. Oh, L. L. Cunningham, M. Calenoff, and B. Jubelt.** 1990. Localization of genomic regions specific for the attenuated, mouse-adapted poliovirus type 2 strain W-2. *J. Gen. Virol.* **71:**43–52.
326. **Pilipenko, E. V., V. M. Blinov, B. K. Chernov, T. M. Dmitrieva, and V. I Agol.** 1989. Conservation of the secondary structure elements of the 5'-untranslated region of cardio- and aphthovirus RNAs. *Nucleic Acids Res.*
327. **Pilipenko, E. V., V. M. Blinov, L. I. Romanova, A. N. Sinyakov, S. V. Maslova, and V. I. Agol.** 1989. Conserved structural domains in the 5'-untranslated region of picornaviral genomes: an analysis of the segment controlling translation and neurovirulence. *Virology* **168:** 201–209.
328. **Pilipenko, E. V., A. P. Gmyl, S. V. Maslova, Y. V. Svitkin, A. N. Sinyakov, and V. I. Agol.** 1992. Prokaryotic-like *cis* elements in the cap-independent internal initiation of translation on picornavirus RNA. *Cell* **68:**119–131.
329. **Pilipenko, E. V., S. V. Maslova, A. N. Sinyakov, and V. I. Agol.** 1992. Towards identification of *cis*-acting elements involved in the replication of enterovirus and rhinovirus RNAs: a proposal for the existence of tRNA-like terminal structures. *Nucleic Acids Res.* **20:**1739–1745.
330. **Pincus, S., D. Diamond, E. Emini, and E. Wimmer.** 1986. Guanidine-selected mutants of poliovirus: mapping of point mutations to polypeptide 2C. *J. Virol.* **57:**638–646.
331. **Pincus, S., H. Rohl, and E. Wimmer.** 1987. Guanidine-dependent mutants of poliovirus: identification of three classes with different growth requirements. *Virology* **157:** 83–88.
332. **Pincus, S., and E. Wimmer.** 1986. Production of guanidine-resistant and -dependent poliovirus mutants from cloned cDNA: mutations in polypeptide 2C are directly responsible for altered guanidine sensitivity. *J. Virol.* **60:**793–796.
333. **Poch, O., I. Sauvaget, M. Delarue, and T. Tordo.** 1989. Identification of four conserved motifs among RNA-dependent polymerase encoding elements. *EMBO J.* **8:**3867–3874.
334. **Pollard, S. R., G. Dunn, N. Cammack, P. D. Minor, and J. W. Almond.** 1989. Nucleotide sequence of a neurovirulent variant of the type 2 oral poliovirus vaccine. *J. Virol.* **63:**4949–4951.

335. **Pöyry, T., T. Hyppia, C. Horsnell, L. Kinnunen, T. Hovi, and G. Stanway.** 1994. Molecular analysis of coxsackievirus A16 reveals a new genetic group of enteroviruses. *Virology* **202:**982–987.
336. **Pöyry, T., L. Kinnunen, and T. Hovi.** 1992. Genetic variation in vivo and proposed functional domains of the 5' noncoding region of poliovirus RNA. *J. Virol.* **66:**5313–5319.
337. **Prabhakar, B. S., M. V. Haspel, P. R. McClintock, and A. L. Notkins.** 1982. High frequency of antigenic variants among naturally occurring human coxsackievirus B4 isolates identified by monoclonal antibodies. *Nature* (London) **300:**374–376.
338. **Prabhakar, B. S., M. A. Menegus, and A. L. Notkins.** 1985. Detection of conserved and nonconserved epitopes on coxsackievirus B4: frequency of antigenic change. *Virology* **146:**302–306.
339. **Prabhakar, B. S., J. Srinivasappa, and U. Ray.** 1987. Selection of coxsackievirus B4 variants with monoclonal antibodies results in attenuation. *J. Gen. Virol.* **68:**685–689.
340. **Racaniello, V. R.** 1988. Poliovirus neurovirulence. *Adv. Virus Res.* **34:**217–246.
341. **Racaniello, V. R., and D. Baltimore.** 1981. Cloned poliovirus complementary DNA is infectious in mammalian cells. *Science* **214:**916–919.
342. **Racaniello, V. R., and D. Baltimore.** 1981. Molecular cloning of poliovirus cDNA and determination of the complete nucleotide sequence of the viral genome. *Proc. Natl. Acad. Sci. USA* **78:**4887–4891.
343. **Racaniello, V. R., and C. Meriam.** 1986. Poliovirus temperature-sensitive mutant containing a single nucleotide deletion in the 5'-noncoding region of the viral RNA. *Virology* **155:**498–507.
344. **Ramsingh, A., H. Araki, S. Bryant, and A. Hixson.** 1992. Identification of candidate sequences that determine virulence in coxsackievirus B4. *Virus Res.* **23:**281–292.
345. **Ramsingh, A., A. Hixson, B. Deuceman, and J. Slack.** 1990. Evidence suggesting that virulence maps to the P1 region of the coxsackievirus B4 genome. *J. Virol.* **64:**3078–3081.
346. **Ramsingh, A., J. Slack, J. Silkworth, and A. Hixson.** 1989. Severity of disease induced by a pancreatropic coxsackievirus B4 virus correlates with the H-2Kq locus of the major histocompatibility complex. *Virus Res.* **14:**347–358.
347. **Reagan, K. J., B. Goldberg, and R. L. Crowell.** 1984. Altered receptor specificity of coxsackievirus B3 after growth in rhabdomyosarcoma cells. *J. Virol.* **49:**635–640.
348. **Reanney, D. C.** 1984. The molecular evolution of RNA viruses. *Symp. Soc. Gen. Microbiol.* **35:**498–507.
349. **Rekosh, D.** 1972. Gene order of the poliovirus capsid proteins. *J. Virol.* **9:**479–487.
350. **Ren, R. B., F. Constantini, E. Gorgacz, J. J. Lee, and V. R. Racaniello.** 1990. Transgenic mice expressing a human poliovirus receptor: a new model for poliomyelitis. *Cell* **63:**353–362.
351. **Ren, R. B., E. G. Moss, and V. R. Racaniello.** 1991. Identification of two determinants that attenuate vaccine-related type 2 poliovirus. *J. Virol.* **65:**1377–1382.
352. **Reuer, Q., R. J. Kuhn, and E. Wimmer.** 1990. Characterization of poliovirus clones containing lethal and nonlethal mutations in the genome-linked protein VPg. *J. Virol.* **64:**2967–2975.
352a. **Rezapkin, G. Y., K. M. Chumakov, Z. Lu, Y. Ran, E. M. Dragunsky, and I. S. Levenbrook.** 1994. Microevolution of Sabin 1 strain *in vitro* and genetic stability of oral poliovirus vaccine. *Virology* **202:**370–378.
353. **Richards, O. C., S. C. Martin, H. G. Jense, and E. Ehrenfeld.** 1984. Structure of poliovirus replicative intermediate RNA. Electron microscope analysis of RNA cross-linked in vivo with psoralen derivative. *J. Mol. Biol.* **173:**325–340.
354. **Rico-Hesse, R., M. A. Pallansch, B. V. Nottay, and O. M. Kew.** 1987. Geographic distribution of wild poliovirus type 1 genotypes. *Virology* **160:**311–322.
355. **Rightsel, W., J. R. Dice, R. J. McAlpine, E. A. Timm, I. W. McLean, G. J. Dixon, and F. M. Schabel.** 1961. Antiviral effects of guanidine. *Science* **134:**558–559.
356. **Rivera, V. M., J. D. Welsh, and J. V. Maizel.** 1988. Comparative sequence analysis of the 5' noncoding region of the enteroviruses and rhinoviruses. *Virology* **165:**42–50.
357. **Rodriguez, P. L., and L. Carrasco.** 1993. Poliovirus protein 2C has ATPase and GTPase activities. *J. Biol. Chem.* **268:**8105–8110.
358. **Rohll, J. E., N. Percy, R. Ley, D. J. Evans, J. W. Almond, and W. S. Barclay.** 1994. The 5'-untranslated regions of picornavirus RNAs contain independent functional domains essential for RNA replication and translation. *J. Virol.* **68:**4384–4391.
359. **Roivainen, M., L. Piirainen, T. Hovi, I. Virtanen, T. Riikonen, J. Heino, and T. Hyppiä.** 1994. Entry of coxsackievirus A9 into host cells: specific interactions with $\alpha_v\beta_3$ integrin, the vitronectin receptor. *Virology* **203:**357–363.
360. **Romanova, L. I., V. M. Blinov, E. A.**

Tolskaya, E. G. Viktorova, M. S. Kolsenikova, E. A. Guseva, and V. I. Agol. 1986. The primary structure of crossover regions of intertypic poliovirus recombinants: a model of recombination between RNA genomes. *Virology* **155**:202–213.
361. Romanova, L. I., E. A. Tolskaya, M. S. Kolesnikova, and V. I. Agol. 1980. Biochemical evidence for intertypic genetic recombination of poliovirus. *FEBS Lett.* **118**:109–112.
362. Rossmann, M. G., E. Arnold, J. W. Erickson, E. A. Frankenberger, J. P. Griffith, H. J. Hecht, J. E. Johnson, G. Kamer, M. Luo, A. G. Mosser, R. R. Rueckert, B. Sherry, and G. Vriend. 1985. Structure of a human common cold virus and functional relationship to other picornaviruses. *Nature* (London) **317**:145–153.
363. Roux, L., A. E. Simon, and J. J. Holland. 1991. Effects of defective interfering viruses on virus replication and pathogenesis. *Adv. Virus Res.* **40**:181–211.
364. Rueckert, R. R. 1990. Picornaviridae and their replication, p. 507–548. *In* B. N. Fields, D. M. Knipe, R. M. Chanock, M. S. Hirsch, J. L. Melnick, T. P. Monath, and B. Roizman (ed.), *Virology*, 2nd ed. Raven Press, New York.
365. Rueckert, R. R., and E. Wimmer. 1984. Systematic nomenclature of picornavirus proteins. *J. Virol.* **50**:957–959.
366. Ryan, M., O. Jenkins, P. M. Hughes, A. Brown, N. J. Knowles, D. Booth, P. D. Minor, and J. W. Almond. 1990. The complete nucleotide sequence of enterovirus type 70: relationships with other members of the Picornaviridae. *J. Gen. Virol.* **71**:2291–2299.
367. Sabin, A. B. 1955. Characteristics and genetic potentialities of experimentally produced and naturally occurring variants of poliomyelitis virus. *Ann. N.Y. Acad. Sci.* **61**:924–928.
368. Sabin, A. B. 1956. Present status of attenuated live-virus poliomyelitis vaccine. *JAMA* **162**:1589–1596.
369. Sabin, A. B., and L. Boulger. 1973. History of Sabin attenuated poliovirus live vaccine strains. *J. Biol. Stand.* **1**:115–118.
370. Sabin, A. B., W. A. Hennessen, and J. Winsser. 1954. Studies on variants of poliomyelitis virus. I. Experimental segregation and properties of avirulent variants of three immunologic types. *J. Exp. Med.* **99**:551–576.
371. Sarnow, P. 1989. Role of 3'-end sequences in infectivity of poliovirus transcripts made in vitro. *J. Virol.* **63**:467–470.
372. Sarnow, P., H. D. Bernstein, and D. Baltimore. 1986. A poliovirus temperature-sensitive RNA synthesis mutant located in a noncoding region of the genome. *Proc. Natl. Acad. Sci. USA* **83**:571–575.
373. Sarnow, P., S. J. Jacobson, and L. Najita. 1990. Poliovirus genetics. *Curr. Top. Microbiol. Immunol.* **161**:155–188.
374. Schmidt, N. J., H. H. Ho, and E. H. Lennette. 1975. Propagation and isolation of group A coxsackieviruses in RD cells. *J. Clin. Microbiol.* **2**:183–185.
375. Schwerdt, C., and F. Schaffer. 1955. Some physical and chemical properties of purified poliomyelitis virus preparations. *Ann. N.Y. Acad. Sci.* **61**:740–753.
376. Schwerdt, C., and F. Schaffer. 1956. Purification of poliomyelitis viruses propagated in tissue culture. *Virology* **2**:665–678.
377. Seechurn, P., N. J. Knowles, and J. W. McCauley. 1990. The complete nucleotide sequence of a pathogenic swine vesicular disease virus. *Virus Res.* **16**:255–274.
378. Semler, B. L., C. W. Anderson, N. Kitamnura, P. G. Rothberg, W. L. Wishert, and E. Wimmer. 1981. Poliovirus replication proteins: RNA sequence encoding 1b and the sites of proteolytic processing. *Proc. Natl. Acad. Sci. USA* **78**:3464–3468.
379. Semler, B. L., A. J. Dorner, and E. Wimmer. 1984. Production of infectious poliovirus from cloned cDNA is dramatically increased by SV40 transcription and replication signals. *Nucleic Acids Res.* **12**:5123–5141.
380. Semler, B. L., R. Hanecak, C. W. Anderson, and E. Wimmer. 1981. Cleavage sites in the polypeptide precursors of poliovirus protein P2-X. *Virology* **114**:589–594.
381. Semler, B. L., V. H. Johnson, and S. Tracy. 1986. A chimeric plasmid from cDNA clones of poliovirus and coxsackievirus produces a recombinant virus that is temperature-sensitive. *Proc. Natl. Acad. Sci. USA* **83**:1777–1781.
382. Sergeev, A. G., A. V. Novoselov, A. V. Bubenschikov, and Z. N. Kondrashova. 1994. Genetic analysis of echovirus 11 variability in adsorption to human erythrocytes. *Arch. Virol.* **134**:129–139.
383. Sickles, G. M., M. Mutterer, P. Feorino, and H. Plager. 1955. Recently classified types of coxsackievirus, group A. Behaviour in tissue culture. *Proc. Soc. Exp. Biol. Med.* **90**:529–531.
384. Simoes, E. A., and P. Sarnow. 1991. An RNA hairpin at the extreme 5' end of the poliovirus RNA genome modulates viral translation in human cells. *J. Virol.* **65**:913–921.
385. Skinner, M. A., V. R. Racaniello, G. Dunn, J. Cooper, P. D. Minor, and J. W. Almond. 1989. New model for the second-

ary structure of the 5' non-coding RNA of poliovirus is supported by biochemical and genetic data that also shows that RNA secondary structure is important in neurovirulence. *J. Mol. Biol.* **207**:379–392.
386. Sommergruber, W., H. Ahorn, H. Klump, J. Seipelt, A. Zoephel, F. Fessl, E. Krystek, D. Blaas, E. Kuechler, H.-D. Liebig, and T. Skern. 1994. 2A proteinases of coxsackie- and rhinovirus cleave peptides derived from eIF-4γ via a common recognition motif. *Virology* **198**:741–745.
387. Spector, D., and D. Baltimore. 1974. Requirement of 3'-terminal poly(adenylic acid) for the infectivity of poliovirus RNA. *Proc. Natl. Acad. Sci. USA* **71**:2983–2987.
388. Sprunt, K., I. M. Mountain, W. M. Redman, and H. E. Alexander. 1955. Production of poliomyelitis virus with combined antigenic characteristics of type I and type II. *Virology* **1**:236–249.
389. Sprunt, K., W. M. Redman, and H. E. Alexander. 1955. Combination of antigenic traits of type 1 and type 2 poliovirus. *J. Immunol.* **82**:232–240.
390. Sprunt, K., W. M. Redman, and H. E. Alexander. 1959. Infectious ribonucleic acid derived from enteroviruses. *Proc. Soc. Exp. Biol. Med.* **101**:604–608.
391. Stanway, G. 1990. Structure, function and evolution of picornaviruses. *J. Gen. Virol.* **71**:2483–2501.
392. Stanway, G., A. J. Cann, R. Hauptmann, P. J. Hughes, L. D. Clarke, R. C. Mountford, P. D. Minor, G. C. Schild, and J. W. Almond. 1983. The nucleotide sequence of poliovirus type 3 Leon 12a$_1$b: comparison with poliovirus type 1. *Nucleic Acids Res.* **11**:5629–5643.
393. Stanway, G., P. J. Hughes, R. C. Mountford, P. Reeves, P. D. Minor, G. C. Schild, and J. W. Almond. 1984. Comparison of the complete nucleotide sequence of the genomes of the neurovirulent poliovirus P3/Leon/37 and its attenuated Sabin vaccine derivative P3/Leon/12 a,b. *Proc. Natl. Acad. Sci. USA* **81**:1539–1543.
394. Stanway, G., P. J. Hughes, G. D. Westrop, D. M. A. Evans, G. Dunn, P. D. Minor, G. C. Schild, and J. W. Almond. 1986. Construction of poliovirus intertypic recombinants by use of cDNA. *J. Virol.* **57**:1187–1190.
395. Stone, D. M., J. L. Almond, J. K. Brangwyn, and G. J. Belsham. 1993. *trans* complementation of cap-independent translation directed by poliovirus 5' noncoding region deletion mutants: evidence for RNA-RNA interactions. *J. Virol.* **67**:6215–6223.
396. Strauss, J. H., and E. G. Strauss. 1988. Evolution of RNA viruses. *Annu. Rev. Microbiol.* **42**:657–683.
397. Strebel, P. M., R. W. Sutter, S. L. Conchi, R. J. Biellik, E. W. Brink, O. M. Kew, M. A. Pallansch, W. A. Orenstein, and A. R. Hinman. 1992. Epidemiology of poliomyelitis in the United States one decade after the last reported case of indigenous wild virus-associated disease. *Clin. Infect. Dis.* **14**:568–579.
397a. Summers, D., and J. V. Maizel. 1971. Determination of the gene sequence of poliovirus with pactamycin. *Proc. Natl. Acad. Sci. USA* **68**:2852–2856.
398. Supanaranond, K., N. Takeda, and S. Yamakazi. 1992. The complete nucleotide sequence of a variant of coxsackievirus A24, an agent causing acute hemorrhagic conjunctivitis. *Virus Genes* **6**:149–158.
399. Svitkin, Y. V., N. Cammack, P. D. Minor, and J. W. Almond. 1990. Translation deficiency of the Sabin type 3 poliovirus genome: association with an attenuating mutation $C_{472} \rightarrow U$. *Virology* **175**:103–109.
400. Svitkin, Y. V., S. V. Maslova, and V. I. Agol. 1985. The genomes of attenuated and virulent poliovirus strains differ in their in vitro translation efficiencies. *Virology* **147**:243–252.
401. Svitkin, Y. V., T. V. Pestova, S. V. Maslova, and V. I. Agol. 1988. Point mutations modify the response of poliovirus RNA to a translation initiation factor: a comparison of neurovirulent and attenuated strains. *Virology* **166**:394–404.
402. Taber, R., D. Rekosh, and D. Baltimore. 1971. Effect of pactamycin on synthesis of poliovirus proteins: a method for genetic mapping. *J. Virol.* **8**:395–401.
403. Takeda, N. 1989. Complete nucleotide and amino acid sequences of enterovirus 70, p. 419–424. *In* K. Ishii, Y. Uchida, K. Miyamura, and S. Yamakazi (ed.), *Acute Hemorrhagic Conjunctivitis. Etiology, Epidemiology and Clinical Manifestations*. University of Tokyo Press, Tokyo.
404. Takeda, N., R. J. Kuhn, C. F. Yang, T. Takegami, and E. Wimmer. 1986. Initiation of poliovirus plus-strand RNA synthesis in a membrane complex of infected HeLa cells. *J. Virol.* **60**:43–53.
405. Takeda, N., K. Miyamura, T. Takegami, and S. Yamakazi. 1988. A temperature-sensitive defect of enterovirus 70 is located at the uridylylation of the genome-linked protein VPg in vitro. *Virus Genes* **2**:347–355.

406. Takeda, N., M. Tanimura, and K. Miyamura. 1994. Molecular evolution of the major capsid protein VP1 of enterovirus 70. *J. Virol.* **68**:854–862.
407. Takegami, T., B. L. Semler, C. W. Anderson, and E. Wimmer. 1983. Membrane fractions active in poliovirus RNA replication contain VPg precursor polypeptides. *Virology* **128**:33–47.
408. Tardy-Panit, M., B. Blondel, A. Martin, F. Tekaia, F. Horad, and F. Delpeyroux. 1993. A mutation in the RNA polymerase of poliovirus type 1 contributes to attenuation in mice. *J. Virol.* **67**:4630–4638.
409. Tatem, J. M., C. Weeks-Levy, A. Georgiu, S. J. DiMichele, E. J. Gorgacz, V. R. Racaniello, F. R. Cano, and S. J. Mento. 1992. A mutation present in the amino-terminus of Sabin 3 poliovirus VP1 protein is attenuating. *J. Virol.* **66**:3194–3197.
410. Tatem, J. M., C. Weeks-Levy, S. J. Mento, S. J. DiMichele, A. Georgiu, W. F. Waterfield, B. Scheip, C. Costalas, T. Davies, M. B. Ritchey, and F. R. Cano. 1991. Oral poliovirus vaccine in the United States: molecular characterization of Sabin type 3 after replication in the gut of vaccinees. *J. Med. Virol.* **35**:101–109.
411. Teterina, N. L., K. M. Kean, A. E. Gorbalenya, V. I. Agol, and M. Girard. 1992. Analysis of the functional significance of amino acid residues in the putative NTP-binding pattern of the poliovirus 2C protein. *J. Gen. Virol.* **73**:1977–1986.
412. Theiler, M. 1941. Studies on poliomyelitis. *Medicine* **20**:443–462.
413. Ticehurst, J., J. I. Cohen, and R. H. Purcell. 1988. Analyses of molecular sequences demonstrate that hepatitis A virus (HAV) is a unique picornavirus, p. 33–35. *In* A. Zuckerman (ed.), *Viral Hepatitis and Liver Disease*. Alan R. Liss, Inc., New York.
414. Titchener, P. A., O. Jenkins, T. M. Szopa, K. W. Taylor, and J. W. Almond. 1994. Complete nucleotide sequence of a beta-cell tropic variant of coxsackievirus B4. *J. Med. Virol.* **42**:369–373.
415. Tolskaya, E., L. Romanova, M. Kolesnikova, and V. I. Agol. 1983. Intertypic recombination in poliovirus: genetic and biochemical studies. *Virology* **124**:121–132.
416. Tolskaya, E. A., L. I. Romanova, M. S. Kolesnikova, A. P. Gmyl, A. E. Gorbalenya, and V. I. Agol. 1994. Genetic studies on the poliovirus 2C protein, and NTPase. A plausible mechanism of guanidine effect on the 2C function and evidence for the importance of 2C oligomerization. *J. Mol. Biol.* **236**:1310–1323.
417. Toyoda, H., M. Kohara, Y. Kataoka, T. Suganuma, T. Omata, N. Imura, and A. Nomoto. 1984. Complete nucleotide sequences of all three poliovirus serotype genomes. Implication for genetic relationship, gene function and antigenic determinants. *J. Mol. Biol.* **174**:561–585.
418. Toyoda, H., M. J. H. Nicklin, M. G. Murray, C. W. Anderson, J. J. Dunn, F. W. Studier, and E. Wimmer. 1986. A second virus-encoded protease involved in proteolytic processing of poliovirus polyprotein. *Cell* **45**:761–770.
419. Toyoda, H., C. F. Yang, N. Takeda, A. Nomoto, and E. Wimmer. 1987. Analysis of RNA synthesis of type 1 poliovirus by using an in vitro molecular genetic approach. *J. Virol.* **61**:2816–2822.
420. Tracy, A., N. M. Chapman, and Z. Tu. 1992. Coxsackievirus B3 from an infectious cDNA copy of the genome is cardiovirulent in mice. *Arch. Virol.* **122**:298–409.
421. Tracy, S., H.-L. Liu, and N. M. Chapman. 1985. Coxsackievirus B3: primary structure of the 5' non-coding and capsid protein-coding regions of the genome. *Virus Res.* **3**:263–270.
422. Trautman, R., and P. Sutmoller. 1971. Detection and properties of a genomic masked viral particle consisting of foot-and-mouth disease virus nucleic acid in bovine enterovirus protein capsid. *Virology* **44**:537–543.
423. Trono, D., R. Andino, and D. Baltimore. 1988. An RNA sequence of hundreds of nucleotides at the 5' end of poliovirus RNA is involved in allowing viral protein synthesis. *J. Virol.* **62**:2291–2299.
424. Trousdale, M. D., R. E. Paque, and C. J. Gauntt. 1977. Isolation of coxsackievirus B3 temperature-sensitive mutants and their assignment to complementation groups. *Biochem. Biophys. Res. Commun.* **76**:368–375.
425. Tuschall, D. M., E. Hiebert, and J. B. Flanegan. 1982. Poliovirus RNA-dependent RNA polymerase synthesizes full-length copies of poliovirion RNA, cellular mRNA, and several plant virus RNAs in vitro. *J. Virol.* **44**:209–216.
426. van der Werf, S., J. Bradley, E. Wimmer, F. W. Studier, and J. J. Dunn. 1986. Synthesis of infectious poliovirus RNA by purified T7 RNA polymerase. *Proc. Natl. Acad. Sci. USA* **83**:2330–2334.
427. van Dyke, T. A., and J. B. Flanegan. 1980. Identification of poliovirus polypeptide p63 as a soluble RNA-dependent RNA polymerase.

J. Virol. **35**:732–740.
428. **Voroshilova, M. K.** 1989. Potential use of nonpathogenic enteroviruses for control of human disease. *Prog. Med. Virol.* **36**:191–202.
429. **Ward, C. D., M. A. Stokes, and J. B. Flanegan.** 1988. Direct measurement of the poliovirus RNA polymerase error frequency in vitro. *J. Virol.* **62**:588–562.
430. **Webb, S. R., K. P. Kearse, C. L. Foulke, P. C. Hartig, and B. S. Prabhakar.** 1986. Neutralization epitope diversity of coxsackievirus B4 isolates detected by monoclonal antibodies. *J. Med. Virol.* **20**:9–15.
431. **Wecker, E., and G. Lederhilger.** 1964. Genomic masking produced by double-infection of HeLa cells with hetrotypic polioviruses. *Proc. Natl. Acad. Sci. USA* **52**:705–709.
432. **Weeks-Levy, C., J. M. Tatem, S. J. DiMichele, W. Waterfild, A. F. Georgiu, and S. J. Mento.** 1991. Identification and characterization of a new base substitution in the vaccine strain of Sabin 3 poliovirus. *Virology* **185**:934–937.
433. **Wenner, H. A., A. M. Behlebehani, and P. S. Kamitsuka.** 1965. Preparation and standardization of coxsackievirus reference antisera. II. For six group B viruses. *Am. J. Epidemiol.* **82**:27–39.
434. **Werner, G., B. Rosenwirth, E. Bauer, J.-M. Seifert, F.-J. Werner, and J. Besemer.** 1986. Molecular cloning and sequence determination of the genomic regions encoding protease and genome-linked protein of three picornaviruses. *J. Virol.* **57**:1084–1093.
435. **Westrop, G. D., K. A. Wareham, D. M. A. Evans, G. Dunn, P. D. Minor, D. I. Magrath, F. Taffs, S. Marsden, M. A. Skinner, G. C. Schild, and J. W. Almond.** 1989. Genetic basis of the attenuation of the Sabin type 3 oral poliovirus vaccine. *J. Virol.* **63**:1338–1344.
436. **Wilson, V., P. Taylor, and U. Desselberger.** 1988. Crossover regions in foot-and-mouth disease virus (FMDV) recombinants correspond to regions of high local secondary structure. *Arch. Virol.* **102**:131–139.
436a. **Wimmer, E., C. U. T. Hellen, and X. Cao.** 1993. Genetics of poliovirus. *Annu. Rev. Genet.* **27**:353–436.
437. **Yang, C.-F., L. De, S.-J. Yang, J. R. Gomez, J. R. Cruz, B. P. Holloway, M. A. Pallansch, and O. M. Kew.** 1992. Genotype-specific in vitro amplification of sequences of the wild type 3 polioviruses from Mexico and Guatemala. *Virus Res.* **24**:277–296.
438. **Yeates, T. O., D. H. Jacobson, A. Martin, C. Wychowski, M. Girard, D. J. Filman, and J. M. Hogle.** 1991. Three-dimensional structure of a mouse-adapted type 2/type 1 poliovirus chimera. *EMBO J.* **10**:2331–2341.
438a. **Yogo, Y., M. Teng, and E. Wimmer.** 1974. Poly (U) in poliovirus minus RNA is 5'-terminal. *Biochem. Biophys. Res. Commun.* **61**:1101–1109.
439. **Yogo, Y., and E. Wimmer.** 1972. Polyadenylic acid at the 3'-terminus of poliovirus RNA. *Proc. Natl. Acad. Sci. USA* **69**:1877–1882.
440. **Yogo, Y. and E. Wimmer.** 1975. Sequence studies of poliovirus RNA. III. Polyuridylic acid and polyadenylic acid as components of the purified poliovirus replicative intermediate. *J. Mol. Biol.* **92**:467–477.
441. **Yoon, J.-W., T. Onodera, and A. L. Notkins.** 1978. Virus-induced diabetes mellitus. XV. Beta cell damage and insulin-dependent hyperglycemia in mice infected with coxsackie virus B4. *J. Exp. Med.* **148**:1068–1080.
442. **Ypma-Wong, M.-F., P. G. Dewalt, V. H. Johnson, J. G. Lamb, and B. L. Semler.** 1988. Protein 3CD is the major proteinase responsible for cleavage of the P1 capsid protein precursor. *Virology* **166**:265–270.
442a. **Ypma-Wong, M.-F., D. J. Filman, J. M. Hogle, and B. L. Semler.** 1988. Structural domains of the poliovirus polyprotein are major determinants for proteolytic cleavage at Gln-Gly pairs. *J. Biol. Chem.* **263**:17846–17856.
443. **Yu, S. F., P. A. Benton, M. Bovee, J. Sessions, and R. E. Lloyd.** 1995. Defective RNA replication by poliovirus mutants deficient in 2A protease cleavage activity. *J. Virol.* **69**:247–252.
444. **Zhang, G., G. Wilsden, N. J. Knowles, and J. W. McCauley.** 1993. Complete nucleotide sequence of a coxsackievirus B5 virus and its relationship to swine vesicular disease virus. *J. Gen. Virol.* **74**:845–853.
445. **Zheng, Z., P. He, D. A. Cauefield, M. A. Newman, and S. Specter.** 1994. Enterovirus 71 (E71) isolated from China is serologically related to, but genetically different from prototype E71 BrCr strain in the 5' noncoding region. GenBank accession no. U00871.
446. **Zimmern, D.** 1988. Evolution of RNA viruses, p. 211–240. *In* D. Esteban, J. J. Holland, and P. Ahlquist (ed.), *RNA Genetics*, vol. 2. CRC Press, Inc., Boca Raton, Fla.
447. **Zoll, J., J. Galama, and W. Melchers.** 1994. Intratypic variability of the coxsackievirus B1 2A protease region. *J. Gen. Virol.* **75**:687–692.

EARLY EVENTS IN INFECTION: RECEPTOR BINDING AND CELL ENTRY

Vincent R. Racaniello

3

One of the greatest paradoxes in virology is how the virus particle, which is sufficiently stable to survive in the extracellular environment, can come apart to release its genome into a new cell and begin a productive infection. The enteroviruses in particular are remarkably stable: they are resistant to low pH, proteolytic enzymes, and detergents yet fall apart easily upon contacting a new cell. The study of virus receptors has demonstrated that these molecules do not simply bind viruses to facilitate their uptake into a cell; rather, the initial contact with a cellular receptor initiates a series of events that leads to virus disassembly. The molecular cloning of cell receptors has provided new genetic and biochemical approaches for understanding these interactions, the way they lead to uncoating of the genome, and their role in establishing viral host range and pathogenesis.

Studies of poliovirus have provided most of our understanding of the early events in enteroviral infection. Poliovirus is a particularly good model for studying virus entry into cells, because genetic manipulation of the RNA genome is possible with infectious cDNA (90),

the three-dimensional structure of the virion has been determined (33), and the poliovirus receptor (PVR), i.e., the cellular molecule to which poliovirus binds, has been molecularly cloned (76). Because knowledge of the early events in infection with enteroviruses is limited, this chapter focuses on studies with poliovirus but examines the emerging data on several other enteroviruses.

VIRAL ATTACHMENT TO CELLS

Cell Receptor for Poliovirus

Since the 1950s, it has been known that primate cells and tissues susceptible to poliovirus infection contain a membrane-associated receptor that specifically binds the virus (35). Competition and biochemical studies have demonstrated that the receptor for the three serotypes of poliovirus is distinct from those employed by the group A or B coxsackieviruses (CVA, CVB), echoviruses (ECV), and human rhinoviruses (HRV) (22, 60, 113, 114). The receptor protein was never isolated, despite solubilization of poliovirus-binding components from cell membranes (52). The first step toward identification of receptors for poliovirus came with the isolation of monoclonal antibodies (MAbs) that inhibit binding of poliovirus to cells. Two of the MAbs iso-

---

Vincent R. Racaniello, Department of Microbiology, College of Physicians and Surgeons, Columbia University, 701 West 168th Street, New York, New York 10032.

lated, 280 and 281, bind human cells and protect against infection with all three poliovirus serotypes but not with a variety of other viruses, including HRV type 1b (HRV-1b), CVA type 9 (CVA-9), CVB-5, and nine other enteroviruses (78). Antibody D171, directed against an epitope on HeLa cells, also blocked infection with all three poliovirus serotypes but not with ECV type 30 (ECV-30), CVB-5, herpes simplex virus type 1, vesicular stomatitis virus, and adenovirus type 5 (87).

To identify the poliovirus receptor, MAb D171 was used to identify mouse L cells that expressed the receptor after transformation with human DNA (75, 76). Genomic clones were isolated from libraries prepared from the susceptible mouse cell transformants, and these clones, when transformed into mouse cells, confer poliovirus susceptibility. DNA fragments from the genomic clones were used to isolate cDNA clones from a HeLa cell library. When expressed in L cells, these clones directed the synthesis of functional poliovirus receptors as assayed by susceptibility to infection with all three poliovirus serotypes.

The polypeptide encoded by these cDNA clones is a novel member of the immunoglobulin superfamily. The PVR polypeptide consists of an N-terminal signal sequence, three extracellular immunoglobulin (Ig)-like domains, a transmembrane domain, and a cytoplasmic tail. Alternative splicing results in two mRNAs that encode polypeptides of 392 and 417 amino acids (called H20A and H20B in reference 76 and PVRα and PVRδ in reference 48) that differ in the lengths of their cytoplasmic domains. Secreted PVR isoforms lacking the transmembrane domain, called PVRβ and PVRγ, are produced by translation of alternatively spliced mRNAs in different human cells and tissues, including brain, leukocytes, liver, lung, and placenta (48). The PVR gene is located on human chromosome 19 (48), the location previously identified for a gene, *pvs*, that encodes sensitivity to poliovirus in human-mouse hybrid cell lines (77).

Although the predicted molecular size of the polypeptides encoded by H20A and H20B is 43 or 45 kDa, the actual molecular sizes observed in cells are higher, owing to utilization of some of the eight predicted N-linked glycosylation sites. Expression of H20B in insect cells with baculovirus vectors produced a 67-kDa glycoprotein, and treatment of these cells with tunicamycin resulted in a polypeptide of 35 kDa (45). The 67-kDa PVR is sufficient to permit poliovirus to bind to insect cells. Western blot (immunoblot) analysis with polyclonal anti-PVR antisera was used to detect a 67-kDa protein in HeLa cells and mouse L cells that bear a PVR cosmid or express H20A cDNA by means of a vaccinia virus vector (117). In vitro translation of PVR transcripts in the presence of microsomal membranes also produced a polypeptide of 67 kDa. These two studies indicated that a PVR glycoprotein of 67 kDa is sufficient to confer poliovirus-binding ability on insect cells and susceptibility on mouse cells. A recent study employing immunoprecipitation of PVR from HeLa cells concluded that the predominant form of the protein is 80 kDa (9). Those authors show that the 67-kDa protein identified by expression in vaccinia virus is an intermediate glycoform whose further modification is blocked late in vaccinia virus infection. The 67-kDa form detected in insect cells and by in vitro translation may also have less-processed sugar chains. Both the 67- and the 80-kDa forms are observed in susceptible and nonsusceptible human tissues, as are PVR-related proteins of other sizes whose receptor activities are not known (29).

The normal cellular role of PVR is not known, although the receptor is likely to play a role in cell adhesion, as do other members of the Ig superfamily (110). Cells are likely to contain a ligand for PVR, and soluble forms of PVR may serve as ligands for other receptors. PVRα but not PVRδ is phosphorylated at a serine in the cytoplasmic tail, possibly by calcium-calmodulin kinase II at a consensus CaMK II phosphorylation site, RXXS, that is not found in the cytoplasmic domain of PVRδ (11). Phosphorylation of PVR is not required for poliovirus infection, as the cytoplasmic domain is dispensable for infection (49), but this modification may play a role in the natural function of PVR. Information on the cellular role of PVR may also come from a study of a murine PVR homolog, MPH (79), and an analysis of mice containing a targeted disruption of the MPH gene.

Role of CD44 in Poliovirus Infection

A MAb directed against an epitope on HeLa cells has the interesting property of preferentially blocking the binding of poliovirus type 2 while blocking the binding of type 1 to a lesser extent and having no effect against type 3, ECV-6, CVB-1, CVB-3, CVA-18, influenza virus, and adenovirus 2 (104). This MAb, called AF3, has been used in Western blot analysis to detect a 100-kDa protein in certain cells and tissues that are susceptible to poliovirus infection, such as HeLa cells and human neural tissue. AF3 was subsequently shown to recognize the lymphocyte homing receptor CD44, a member of the cartilage link family of proteins (103). The 100-kDa protein is the hematopoietic isoform CD44H, which has roles in lymph node homing for circulating lymphocytes, binding of hyaluronic acid, lymphocyte activation, and homotypic and heterotypic cell adhesion. CD44H has a predicted extracellular domain of 248 amino acids, a 21-amino-acid transmembrane domain, and a 72-amino-acid cytoplasmic domain (106).

Expression of CD44H cDNA in PVR-negative mouse L cells does not confer the ability to bind poliovirus, demonstrating that CD44H is not a receptor for poliovirus. The precise role of CD44H in poliovirus infection and how antibody to CD44H blocks poliovirus attachment remain unknown. PVR and CD44H may be physically associated in the membrane, and antibody to CD44H might sterically block the poliovirus-binding site on PVR. Alternatively, PVR and CD44H might be linked through signal transduction pathways, and antibody to CD44H might in some way transmit a conformational change to PVR that prevents PV binding. Several CD44-negative cell lines have been reported, and among these, the neuroblastoma line SK-N-MC and the chronic myelogenous leukemia line K562 can be infected with poliovirus, although the expression of CD44 was not determined in susceptibility studies (1, 59). If CD44H is required for infection, it might be required for binding or subsequent steps in cell entry. Because expression of PVR in mouse cells is sufficient to confer susceptibility to poliovirus infection, then if CD44H is required for infection, its role must be fulfilled by the mouse homolog of CD44H, Pgp-1 (116).

Viral Capsid Sequences That Control PVR Interaction

The three-dimensional structure of poliovirus provides clues about specific regions of the capsid that control binding of virus to PVR (33). The poliovirion is composed of 60 protomers; each protomer contains a single copy of the four capsid proteins VP1, VP2, VP3, and VP4, and the proteins are arranged with icosahedral symmetry to form a spherical particle with a diameter of 220 to 280 Å (22 to 28 nm) (Fig. 1). A 12-Å-deep, 15-Å-wide (1.2-nm-deep, 1.5-nm-wide) channel surrounds the prominent peak at the fivefold axis of symmetry. This channel, called the "canyon," is also found in rhinovirus type 14 and was proposed to be the receptor-binding site (98). A model of the interaction of HRV-16 with its soluble cell receptor, ICAM-1, constructed from cryoelectron microscopy data indicates that ICAM-1 does bind in the canyon (88). Because poliovirus and rhinovirus are structurally similar, it seems likely that the canyon of poliovirus will serve as a receptor-binding site.

The study of soluble-receptor-resistant (sn) poliovirus mutants has provided genetic evidence for the location of receptor-binding sites on the viral capsid. Detergent-solubilized PVR expressed in insect cells binds poliovirus and neutralizes its infectivity by converting native virions to 135S altered particles (45; see below for more information on altered particles). Poliovi-

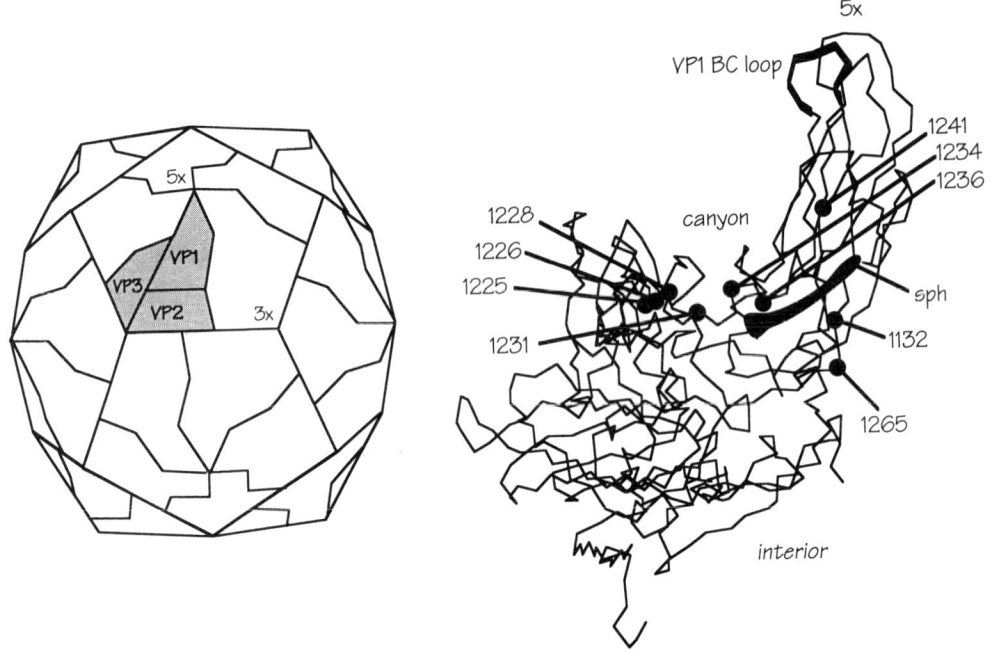

FIGURE 1 Locations of the VP1 BC loop and *srr* mutations in the poliovirus capsid. The virion is shown schematically at left, with one protomer shaded gray. At right is an α-carbon tracing of VP1 and VP2 only. The BC loop is highlighted at the fivefold axis of symmetry. Sites of amino acid changes that confer the *srr* phenotype are shown as dots, and the amino acid residues are indicated. Sphingosine in the hydrocarbon-binding pocket is shown in dark gray.

rus mutants resistant to neutralization with solubilized PVR can be readily isolated from wild-type virus stocks (46). Twenty-one *srr* mutants that still use PVR to infect cells have been isolated (19). All but one *srr* mutant contain a single amino acid change at 1 of 13 different positions in capsid protein VP1, VP2, or VP3 on the surface or in the interior of the virion. Mutations affecting any one of eight surface residues decrease the binding affinity of poliovirus for PVR on HeLa cells, indicating that multiple points in the virus-receptor interface contribute to binding. The surface mutations are located in the canyon at the interface between protomers (Fig. 1). One explanation for the mechanism of action of these mutations is that they reduce binding affinity by interfering with receptor contact. These mutations may alter the shape of the binding site or remove contact points for the receptor.

Mutations at internal capsid residues near the hydrocarbon-binding pocket of VP1 also reduce poliovirus-binding affinity. Clues about the mechanism of action of these mutations come from consideration of rhinovirus, where binding of WIN compounds in a hydrophobic pocket below the canyon results in conformational changes in the canyon floor along the protomer interface, thereby reducing binding to ICAM-1 (4, 102, 105) (see chapter 18). In poliovirus, the hydrophobic pocket is occupied by sphingosine (27), and *srr* mutations near the pocket may influence the position of this molecule, thereby modulating the receptor contact region on the virion surface.

Further information on capsid sequences that control receptor interaction comes from the analysis of viral variants that are adapted to grow on cells expressing mutant forms of PVR that cannot bind or replicate wild-type poliovirus (18). PVR mutants (see discussion below) were constructed by replacing amino acids in the first Ig-like domain with the corresponding sequence from the murine homolog of PVR, MPH (80). Stable L cell lines expressing d, g, or i receptors, three different PVR mutants, do not bind or replicate poliovirus type 1. Viral variants were selected on the mutant cell lines that restore virus binding to cells expressing mutant PVR; these variants are still able to infect cells by using wild-type PVR.

Sequence analysis and site-directed mutagenesis identified three different mutations that are responsible for the adapted viral phenotype: at positions 95 and 160 of VP1 (1095, 1160) and at position 142 of VP2 (2142). The mutation P1095S is located in the BC loop of VP1, which forms part of the prominent peak at the fivefold axis of symmetry (Fig. 1). How does this mutation permit poliovirus to use mutant receptors? One possibility is that the contact site for PVR includes both the canyon and the VP1 BC loop. These interactions must not be crucial for virus binding, because the VP1 BC loop may be deleted without a deleterious effect on virus replication (21). An alternative explanation is that the BC loop modulates the flexibility of the capsid and its ability to accommodate mutant receptors. It is interesting that other sequence changes in the VP1 BC loop permit poliovirus to utilize a receptor in mice, leading to the production of disease in that host. The expanded host range of these variants is discussed below.

Amino acid 1160, which is located at the interface between protomers near the hydrophobic binding pocket of VP1, may also facilitate the recognition of mutant receptors by changing the flexibility of the viral capsid. Both the protomer interface and the hydrophobic pocket are believed to be important for regulating structural transitions of the virus that occur during cell entry (27). Amino acid 2142 is located on the south wall of the canyon, which is probably at or near the receptor binding-site as defined by the *srr* mutations.

The nature of the amino acid at this position may influence the contact point with PVR. These results suggest that expanded receptor recognition may be mediated not only by changes at the receptor binding site but also by changes at distant sites that may influence structural transitions of the capsid.

PVR Sequences That Control Binding of Poliovirus to PVR
To complete the molecular picture of the poliovirus-PVR interaction, delineation of the precise regions of PVR that interact with poliovirus is necessary. The predicted boundaries of the Ig-like domains of PVR can be modeled after known Ig structures (domain 1, amino acids 35 to 142; domain 2, amino acids 153 to 236; domain 3, amino acids 250 to 330). Results from a number of laboratories indicate that the first Ig-like domain, a V-type Ig domain, contains the binding site for poliovirus and is sufficient for infection. Cell surface expression of domain 1 only or domain 1 linked to various other domains (CD4, ICAM-1, or MPH) leads to poliovirus binding and infection (10, 49, 79, 100, 101). However, none of these deleted or chimeric molecules are as efficient at poliovirus binding and replication as the native PVR. Domains 2 and 3 may interact with virus or with domain 1 to promote efficient binding and infection. The second domain is clearly involved in the production of altered particles, as discussed below.

The individual amino acid residues within the loops and β strands of the first Ig-like domain that are important for virus binding have been identified by site-directed mutagenesis of PVR and expression in mouse cells (2, 10, 80). The results of mutagenesis at 64 of the 114 amino acids in domain 1 by substitution or insertion of MPH or non-MPH residues indicate that three main sites are important for poliovirus binding (Fig. 2). The first is in the left-hand portion of domain 1, including the C—C' loop (positions 73 and 74 at the leading edge of the C' strand), the C' strand (position 78); the C'–C" loop (positions 80 and

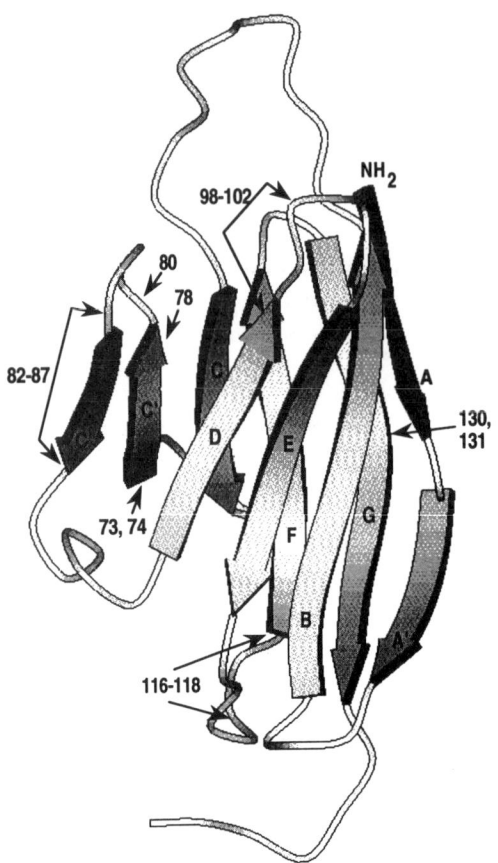

FIGURE 2 Structural model of the first Ig-like domain of PVR. The structure was predicted as described in reference 80. The β strands are lettered, and locations of mutations that affect virus binding are given as amino acid numbers, which begin with the first methionine of PVR (76). This predicted structure differs slightly from two other published versions (2, 10).

82) and the C" strand (positions 83 through 87). It is striking that all three laboratories have found that a mutation at position 82 (Q82F or Q82A) abolishes virus binding. The second region that is important for binding is the border of the D strand and the DE loop (positions 98 through 102). The third site is in the G strand, where mutations at positions 130 and 131 but not elsewhere in the strand affect virus binding. A 3-amino-acid mutation at the beginning of the F strand (positions 116 through 118) also reduces virus binding, probably by altering the domain structure (10). Extensive mutagenesis of other loops of PVR, such as the C"—D and BC loops, and parts of the β strands have not revealed other regions that are important for binding.

These studies demonstrate the clear involvement of the C'—C" ridge of PVR in binding to poliovirus. The homologous part of CD4, comprising amino acids 41 through 59, plays a major role in interaction with human immunodeficiency virus type 1 (reviewed in reference 99). In particular, the side chain of the phenylalanine at position 43 of CD4 is highly solvent accessible and appears to be extremely important for human immunodeficiency virus type 1 binding. In our model of PVR, the homologous residue is Q82, which when changed to the MPH residue, F, or A, results in abolishment of poliovirus binding. It has been suggested that the PVR equivalent of F43 of CD4 is F78; mutagenesis of this residue indicates that it is important for poliovirus binding (10). However, MPH, which does not bind poliovirus, also has a phenylalanine at this position (80).

The results of studies of PVR and poliovirus mutants suggest that the C'—C" ridge of PVR makes significant contacts with residues lining the floor of the poliovirus canyon. The DE loop of domain 1 may also contact parts of the canyon. Analysis of *srr* mutants indicates that binding determinants are distributed over a significant portion of the canyon floor and walls, a situation consistent with several contact points on PVR. It is not clear whether the G strand of PVR domain 1 is directly involved in virus binding, because it is somewhat distant from the C'—C" ridge and the DE loop. Some mutations in the G strand apparently influence domain structure, which may indirectly alter the binding site (80). Once the crystal structures of PVR and the poliovirus-PVR complex become available, the precise interactions will become apparent.

It is interesting that many of the PVR mutations that reduce virus binding have little or no effect on virus replication. In one study, mutations at positions 82, 83, and 98–99 abrogated binding and replication, but mutations at positions 80, 84, and 130 had less drastic effects on binding and permitted replication (80). In another study, few mutations (at positions 82 + 92, 83, 116, and 130) diminished binding and replication (10). In a third study, all of the binding mutants produced normal levels of poliovirus (2). Thus, it appears that the binding of poliovirus to PVR need not approach wild-type levels to achieve efficient infection. No mutations within PVR domain 1 that permit binding but not replication have been identified, suggesting that binding and the subsequent conformational alterations of PVR that lead to cell entry are tightly linked. Alternatively, postbinding events may be controlled by domains 2 and 3; in one study, a role in alteration has been assigned to domain 2 (80; see below).

PVR contains eight putative N-linked glycosylation sites, two of which are in the first Ig-like domain (76). Domain 1 of a monkey PVR homolog does not contain N-linked glycosylation sites, yet functions as a PVR (50, 118). Furthermore, removal of both N-linked glycosylation sites from PVR domain 1 has no effects on virus binding and replication (10, 118). Removal of four N-linked sites from domains 1 and 2 did not reduce virus binding and replication (10). Clearly, N-linked glycosylation of domains 1 and 2 is not required for PVR function in cell culture, although the affinity constants of the mutant receptors were not determined.

Cells expressing mutant PVR with changes at positions 80 or 85 through 88, which did not completely reduce virus binding, produced nearly normal yields of poliovirus but were not lysed by poliovirus infection (80). Similar findings have been reported for the replication of certain strains of poliovirus in L cells expressing the monkey form of PVR, which differs from human PVR at position 84 (63). It is not known how poliovirus is released from cells that do not lyse, but the results suggest that the interaction of poliovirus with its cell receptor controls the course of cell killing. Binding of poliovirus to PVR might initiate a signaling cascade that ultimately leads to cell death. A study of these mutants might provide information on the obscure mechanism of cell killing by poliovirus.

Cell Receptor for Echovirus

As discussed in chapters 10 through 13, ECVs are frequently responsible for human diseases such as febrile illness, rash, and aseptic meningitis. At least 30 viral serotypes have been distinguished by using neutralization assays (74).

To identify cell receptors for ECVs, MAbs that protect HeLa cells from ECV infection were isolated (7). Two independent MAbs, DE9 and AA10, that blocked binding and infection of ECV-1 but not other picornaviruses were identified. Each MAb immunoprecipitated from HeLa cells proteins of 125 and 145 kDa that comigrated with proteins immunoprecipitated with antibodies to the subunits of the integrin VLA-2. Immunodepletion experiments indicated that MAb DE9 recognizes the $\beta 1$ subunit, while MAb AA10 recognizes the $\alpha 2$ subunit of VLA-2. Expression of VLA-2 cDNAs was used to further understand the role of this protein in ECV infection. In one set of experiments, rhabdomyosarcoma (RD) cells, which express $\beta 1$ but low levels of $\alpha 2$, were used. RD cells bind ECV poorly and do not develop cytopathic effect after 48 h when infected at a multiplicity of infection of 2. However, when human $\alpha 2$ is expressed in RD cells, significantly more ECV-1 binds than in normal RD cells, and the cells are destroyed within 24 h by infection at a multiplicity of infection of 0.5. In a second set of experiments, CHO cells, which express hamster $\beta 1$ but not $\alpha 2$ and do not bind ECV-1, were used. Expression of human $\alpha 2$ in these cells leads to ECV-1 binding and productive infection (8). These results indicate that VLA-2 is a receptor for ECV-1 and that infection depends on the $\alpha 2$ subunit. The precise binding site of ECV-1 on VLA-2 remains to be determined.

Antibodies to $\alpha 2$ and $\beta 1$ were used in cell protection assays to determine whether other

ECV serotypes employ VLA-2 as a cell receptor (8). The results indicate that infections by ECV-1 and ECV-8 are blocked by antibodies to VLA-2, while infections with ECVs 2, 3, 5, 6, 7, 9, 11, 12, 13, 17, 18, 19, 21, 22, 25, 26, 27, 29, and 30 were not.

In contrast to PVR, the cellular function of VLA-2 is known: this molecule mediates cell attachment to collagen and laminin (38). Many integrins interact with extracellular matrix (ECM) ligands via the sequence RGD (Arg-Gly-Asp), and this sequence may therefore be present at the site of receptor contact in ECVs that bind VLA-2. However, the amino acid sequences of these ECV serotypes have not been determined. ECV-22 contains RGD in capsid protein VP1 (39), but the receptor for this serotype has not been identified (8).

There are striking differences between the binding of ECM ligands and ECV-1 to VLA-2 with respect to the epitopes involved, the cation required, the regulation of adhesion, and the role of the cytoplasmic tail (5). The interaction of ECM ligands depends on cell type-specific forms of VLA-2, while that of ECV-1 does not. Blocking studies with MAbs demonstrate that ECV-1 and ECM ligands bind different epitopes on the $\beta1$ and $\alpha2$ subunits. VLA-2 adhesion to collagen is stimulated by phorbol esters, while ECV-1 binding is not enhanced by this treatment. In addition, the cation requirements for binding of ECV-1 and collagen to VLA-2 are different. Replacement of cytoplasmic domains of $\alpha2$ with sequences from $\alpha4$ and $\alpha5$ does not affect the binding of ECM ligands but does affect postbinding events such as cell migration and collagen gel contraction. However, the different α cytoplasmic domains did not alter the course of ECV-1 binding, infection, and cell killing. These studies indicate that the interaction of ECV-1 and ECM ligands with VLA-2 is very different and that drug intervention that interferes with ECV-1 binding but not with normal VLA-2 function might be designed.

A putative cell receptor for at least six other ECV serotypes (6, 7, 11, 12, 20, and 21) was recently identified as decay-accelerating factor (DAF), or CD55 (6). To identify this receptor, a MAb that blocks attachment of ECV-7 to HeLa cells was isolated. IF7 immunoprecipitated a 70-kDa, glycosylphosphatidyl-inositol (GPI)-anchored protein from HeLa cells. Immunodepletion of cell extracts with antibodies to DAF, a 70-kDa GPI-anchored protein expressed on HeLa cells, removed all protein recognized by IF7, demonstrating that IF7 recognizes DAF. Several anti-DAF antibodies blocked attachment of ECV-7 to HeLa cells, and treatment of HeLa cells with phosphoinositol-phospholipase C prevented attachment of ECV-7. Expression of DAF cDNA in CHO cells enables binding of ECV-7 to these cells, and this binding could be blocked by anti-DAF antibodies. However, the ability of DAF to mediate infection in these cells was not determined. This experimental result is necessary to clearly demonstrate that binding of ECV-7 to DAF leads to productive infection.

DAF is a glycoprotein that protects cells from lysis by complement (62) and is predicted to consist of five extracellular domains: one serine-tyrosine-rich, membrane-proximal domain and four short consensus repeat (SCR) domains found in complement regulatory proteins. MAbs that most effectively block ECV attachment recognize epitopes in SCR2 and SCR3, suggesting that these regions are close to the virus-binding site.

There are over 30 ECV serotypes, many of which are not inhibited by antibodies to DAF or VLA-2. Therefore, at least one other receptor for this virus group remains to be identified. It has been reported that a MAb to a 44-kDa cell surface protein protects cells from infection with many ECV serotypes, including 1, 6, and 7 (69, 71). The purified 44-kDa protein blocked ECV-11 infection of KB cells, and polyclonal rabbit antibodies to this protein blocked infection of cells with ECV-7, -11, and -32 (70). The role of the 44-kDa protein in ECV infection is not clear, especially since it differs in size from the receptors for ECV-1 (VLA-2) and ECV-6, -7, and -11

(DAF). One possibility is that the 44-kDa protein is a subunit of receptors for many ECV serotypes and may be important for steps subsequent to virus binding such as entry and uncoating. Answers to these questions await molecular cloning of the 44-kDa protein.

Cell Receptor for Coxsackievirus

Coxsackieviruses are associated with a wide variety of human illnesses, such as paralytic disease, meningitis, myocarditis, pleurodynia, exanthems, and enathems (74) (chapters 10 through 14). The viruses are classified into two groups, A and B, depending on the lesions that occur after inoculation into suckling mice. CVA produces diffuse myositis, while CVB results in focal degeneration in the brain and muscle.

Competition experiments demonstrate that CVA and CVB use different receptors on HeLa cells that are distinct from the receptors used by polioviruses types 1, 2, and 3 (60). Interestingly, the CVB receptor is shared by adenovirus type 2, while the major group HRVs compete for binding with CVA-13, -18, and -21 (60). A MAb to ICAM-1, the receptor for the major group of HRVs, also blocks attachment of CVA-13, -18 and -21 (17). One MAb to HeLa cells blocks attachment of CVB -1, -5, and -6 but not of poliovirus type 3, CVA-13, or CVA-21, confirming the competition studies (14). Another MAb blocks infection by CVB-1, CVB-3, CVB-5, ECV-6, and CVA-21 but not by CVB-2, CVA-4, CVA-6, three more CVA serotypes, and four ECV serotypes (23). These results suggest a shared epitope between receptors for CVA-21, major group HRVs, ECV-6, and some CVB serotypes.

A CVB-3-binding component has been solubilized from HeLa cells; it has a molecular size of 275 kDa as determined by gel filtration (53). A nonviral polypeptide of 49.5 kDa was identified in complexes of CVB-3 and cell membranes that had been solubilized with detergent. This protein, called Rp-α, bound CVB-3 and CVB-1 but not poliovirus type 1. The authors suggest that RP-α forms part of the CVB receptor complex, but no further characterization of this protein has been reported. Recently, it was suggested that CVB-3 binds a 100-kDa protein on susceptible cells that is a member of a family of proteins with homology to nucleolin (25).

Some information is available concerning cell receptors for CVA-9, which, unlike other enteroviruses, has an insertion of 17 amino acids at the C-terminal end of VP1 that contains the RGD motif (15). RGD-containing peptides block virus attachment to cells, suggesting that the CVA-9 receptor might be an integrin (95). In support of this hypothesis, antibodies to either the α_v or the $\beta 3$ integrin subunits protect GMK cells from CVA-9 infection, and purification of cell attachment proteins with virus confirmed that the $\alpha_v\beta 3$ heterodimer, known as the vitronectin receptor, is recognized by the virus (96). However, treatment of CVA-9 with trypsin, which cleaves near the C terminus of VP1, does not alter infectivity and renders the virus resistant to the blocking effects of RGD peptides. Roivanen et al. (45) suggest that there are at least two receptor sites for CVA-9 on cells, one of which is RGD dependent and is possibly an integrin. Alteration of the receptor specificities of enteric viruses by proteolytic enzymes may have implications for the pathogenesis of infection, as these viruses normally encounter such enzymes during their passage through the gut.

VIRAL ENTRY INTO CELLS: UNCOATING OF VIRAL RNA

The ultimate goal of the early events in infection is the uncoating of the viral genome, i.e., removal of the protein shell so the viral genome can enter the cytoplasm. The events in enterovirus replication that occur immediately after receptor binding have been largely studied with poliovirus. After binding to cell surface PVR, poliovirus must then release its RNA genome into the cell. When poliovirus is bound to cells at temperatures below 33°C, the attached viruses can be released in infectious form by exposure to high salt, urea, low pH, or detergents (61). When virus-cell complexes are heated to 37°C, a large fraction of the bound virus elutes from the cell as a conformationally altered form known as the A particle (41). These A particles sediment more slowly (135S) than native viruses (160S), are noninfectious (although they contain infectious RNA), and are sensitive to detergent and proteinases. The N terminus of VP1, which is on the interior of the native particle, is exposed on the surfaces of A particles (31). At physiologic temperatures, poliovirus exists as a dynamic entity in which internal epitopes of VP4 and VP1 are reversibly exposed (57). The interaction of poliovirus with PVR results in a permanent externalization of VP4 and part of VP1.

A variety of experimental observations have been interpreted to indicate that the formation of altered particles is an essential step in the cell entry of poliovirus (31). A particles can be found within cells early after infection. The formation of altered particles is inhibited by several antiviral drugs such as arildone, which bind in an internal hydrophobic pocket in the capsid and stabilize it against structural alterations (28) (see chapter 18). Attachment of antibody-complexed poliovirus to cells via Fc receptors, which does not lead to the production of A particles, fails to lead to productive infection (68).

It has been noted that the conformational alteration that produces 135S particles has striking homologies to the receptor- or pH-induced conformational rearrangements that result in exposure of fusion peptides in many enveloped viruses (31). It has been proposed that the N terminus of VP1 forms an amphipathic helix that might insert into the cell membrane, resulting in the formation of a pore through which the viral RNA might proceed. A poliovirus mutant lacking VP1 amino acids 8 and 9 is defective in uncoating, further supporting a role for this sequence in cell entry (47). Because A particles lack VP4, it has been thought that this protein did not play a role in subsequent entry steps. However, a study of a poliovirus mutant with an amino acid change at position 28 of VP4 suggests that VP4 participates in uncoating (81). This mutant forms complete particles that bind cells and are converted to altered particles yet are noninfectious. VP4 is modified with myristate, which may target the protein to cell membranes during cell entry (16).

Analogies with the conformational transitions that are believed to occur during cell entry of plant viruses have led to the suggestion that the interfaces between protomers are important in controlling receptor-mediated conformational transitions in poliovirus (27). The protomer is a subunit of the capsid and in poliovirus consists of a single copy of each of the four virion polypeptides (Fig. 1). Upon exposure to chelators of divalent cations at alkaline pH, many icosahedral plant viruses, which are structurally similar to poliovirus, undergo an expansion in radius (40). This expansion is regulated by an interface between capsid proteins that contains a pair of divalent cation-binding sites. When divalent cations are removed, this protomer interface is destabilized. The resulting expansion of the particle also causes externalization of the amino terminus of the capsid proteins. The atomic structure of the expanded form of tomato bushy stunt virus reveals that the amino termini are extruded through a gap produced by disruption of the protomer interface. In poliovirus, the N terminus of VP1 is located directly below the analogous interface. The receptor-mediated conformational transition of poliovirus may therefore involve disruption of this interface to permit extrusion of the VP1 N terminus.

Another site that is believed to modulate receptor-mediated conformational transitions in poliovirus is the hydrocarbon-binding pocket in VP1, which is normally occupied by sphingosine (27). Antiviral drugs of the WIN class bind to the analogous pocket in HRV-14 and prevent attachment to cells. These drugs do not prevent attachment of poliovirus to cells but instead block the formation of A particles (28). The presence of drug in the pocket might make the capsid more rigid, preventing the receptor-mediated conformational rearrangements that occur during cell entry. Precisely how the drugs effect this change is not known, but one possibility is that they cause movements in residues lying directly above the hydrocarbon pocket that constitute the protomer interface. These drugs displace residues in the canyon floor and at the protomer interface in HRV-14 (4) (see chapter 18). The WIN compounds also stabilize the virion against thermal inactivation (97), further demonstrating the role of the hydrocarbon-binding pocket in controlling structural transitions. WIN-dependent mutants of poliovirus type 3 that in the absence of the thermostabilizing drug rapidly decay to noninfectious 135S particles have been isolated (84). These mutants may have a greatly reduced affinity for pocket factor sphingosine, and loss of this factor may cause them to decay in the absence of receptor unless WIN compound is present. The hydrocarbon-binding pocket may therefore be viewed as the "switch" that determines whether the virion is stable or unstable, depending on whether the pocket is occupied.

In support of the hypothesis that the protomer interface and the hydrocarbon-binding pocket regulate receptor-mediated conformational transitions of the capsid, most of the poliovirus srr mutants that are defective in binding to PVR also show a reduced ability to undergo the conversion to A particles (18). These mutants have single-amino-acid changes either on the surface of the virion, at the protomer interface, or surrounding the hydrocarbon-binding pocket. Surface srr mutations may reduce alteration by modulating the stability of the interface between protomers. Mutations at internal residues in or near the hydrocarbon-binding pocket may also reduce alteration by influencing the stability of the protomer interface. When WIN compounds bind in the pocket of a rhinovirus, several residues at the carboxyl end of the GH loop of VP1 are displaced toward the interface, allowing more extensive interactions to form between the GH loops of VP1 and VP3 and thus stabilizing the interface (4, 105). By analogy with rhinovirus, the interaction between internal srr mutations and sphingosine may result in a conformational change that leads to interactions between the GH loops of VP1 and VP3 that stabilize the interface, thereby reducing alteration.

Sequences of PVR also appear to regulate receptor-mediated conformational transitions. Replacement of the first Ig-like domain of MPH with domain 1 of PVR is sufficient to convert MPH into an active PVR (80). When stable cell lines expressing this chimeric receptor are infected with poliovirus at a low multiplicity of infection, the virus yield throughout the growth cycle is significantly lower than that in cells expressing wild-type PVR. Viral replication is normal in cells expressing a chimeric receptor in which the first two domains of MPH are replaced with those of PVR. The apparent binding affinities of poliovirus for cells expressing both chimeric receptors are identical to those for wild-type PVR. However, cells expressing the PVR domain 1 recombinant are defective in viral alteration, while cells expressing the two-domain recombinant or wild-type PVR have no alteration defect. Domain 2 of PVR may regulate the conformational transitions of the virus particle by directly interacting with poliovirus, or domain 2 may influence the structure of domain 1, thereby regulating alteration. The latter possibility is suggested by the extensive structural interactions that have been noted between the first and second Ig-like domains of CD4 (99).

A model for the early stages of poliovirus entry is presented in Fig. 3. When virus attaches to cell surface PVR, receptor sequences insert into the canyon and interact with residues of the canyon floor at the protomer interface. This interaction may displace residues at the protomer interface and residues that surround the hydrocarbon-binding pocket, located directly below the canyon floor. This displacement may lead to reduced affinity for sphingosine, causing release of the lipid, destabilization of the particle, and initiation of

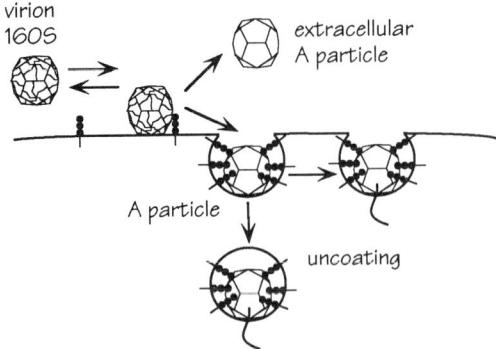

FIGURE 3 Model for poliovirus entry into cells. Binding of virus to cells is reversible when carried out at temperatures below 33°C; at higher temperatures, bound viruses are converted to A particles. These particles are found both outside and inside the cell and may be intermediates in the uncoating process. Uncoating may occur at the cell surface or from within endosomes.

conformational changes. Disruption of the interface allows extrusion of VP4 and the N terminus of VP1, forming a pore in the cell membrane through which the RNA proceeds. Precisely where in the cell the uncoating event occurs—at the cell membrane or from within an endosome—is not known. Poliovirus particles can be seen at the cell surface, in coated pits, and in endosomes early after adsorption, suggesting that entry may occur at several sites (111, 115). Consistent with the hypothesis that uncoating is receptor mediated and contrary to findings in earlier studies, poliovirus uncoating does not require low pH, although other contributions to uncoating cannot be ruled out (32, 64, 65, 89, 108, 115).

RECEPTORS AND HOST RANGE

The host range of poliovirus is limited to primates and primate cell cultures. This host range restriction is largely determined at the level of the receptor. Nonprimate cell lines are resistant to poliovirus infection because they do not bind virus (72) and do not react with anti-PVR MAbs (78, 87). This block to replication can be bypassed by transfecting the cells with viral RNA (36, 37). Expression of PVR by means of cloned human cDNA in mouse cells results in susceptibility to multicycle infection (75, 76).

Humans are the only known natural host for poliovirus, while chimpanzees and certain monkeys can be experimentally infected by a variety of routes. Most strains of poliovirus will not replicate in nonprimate hosts, although inoculation of viral RNA intracerebrally into rabbits, chicks, guinea pigs, and hamsters results in virus production without disease (36). This restriction appears to be at the level of virus binding, although in the absence of PVRs, it cannot be determined whether other factors would also limit virus replication. However, it is clear that resistance of mice to poliovirus infection is due to lack of PVRs. When the gene encoding the PVR is introduced into the germ line of mice, the resulting transgenic animals can be infected with neurovirulent strains of poliovirus, proving that the PVR is the determinant of host range in mice (51, 92).

Poliovirus has been adapted to grow in nonprimate hosts, including the mouse (3), chick embryo (94), and suckling hamster (85). Interestingly, some strains of poliovirus are naturally virulent in mice without adaptation (82). Mice inoculated with the P2/Lansing strain develop fatal poliomyelitis with the clinical, histopathologic, and age-dependent characteristics of the human disease (42, 43). In contrast to the virus that causes human disease, the virus in mice is not infectious by the oral route, and no extraneural sites of replication have been detected. In contrast, inoculation of mice with the P1/Mahoney strain does not result in disease. The Lansing strain can infect primates and primate cell cultures but not mouse cell cultures. This strain therefore has an expanded receptor recognition: it can utilize PVR in primate cells and an unidentified receptor in mice, which does not appear to be the MPH protein (79).

A host range determinant of P2/Lansing has been identified within amino acids 95 to 104 of capsid protein VP1, a sequence that forms the BC loop, an exposed sequence at the fivefold axis of symmetry (Fig. 1) that also contributes to an important antigenic site (67, 86). When the VP1 BC loop of P1/Mahoney is replaced with the sequence from P2/Lansing, the resulting recombinant virus can infect mice. Other host range determinants have been identified at the N termini of capsid proteins VP1 (positions 1022, 1040, and 1054) and VP2 (position 2031), located on the interior of the virion (20, 83). It is not clear how these host range determinants enable poliovirus strains to utilize a receptor in mice. Because the VP1 BC loop is located on the virion surface, it may enable the virus to interact with a mouse cell receptor. Comparison of the structures of P1/Mahoney and a chimeric virus containing the VP1 BC loop of P2/Lansing indicates large differences in shape, charge distribution, and solvent accessibility in a tight cluster at the apex of the fivefold peak (112). However, direct binding of the VP1 BC loop with a mouse receptor implies that there are differences in how viruses interact with mouse and primate receptors, since the BC loop can be deleted without affecting the infectivity of poliovirus on primate cells (21). Alternatively, the mouse receptor might have an expanded footprint on the virus, involving residues at the fivefold axis as well as the canyon.

Another possibility for the mechanism of host range determinants is facilitation of the structural transitions of the virus needed for binding and uncoating, which may be inefficiently induced by the mouse cell receptor. All of the host range determinants identified to date are in regions of the capsid that may regulate structural transitions of the capsid during entry (27). The VP1 BC loop might influence the structure or movement of the EF loop, which forms part of the interface between fivefold-related protomers. The EF loop is part of antigenic site I, which also consists of the DE, HI, and BC loops, and thus clearly interacts structurally with the other loops. Some of the mutations in the N termini of VP1 and VP2 that control host range are near a seven-stranded β sheet that is believed to regulate conformational transitions of the particle (27).

Some of the mutations are in regions that interact with VP4 and are part of the VP1 sequence that is extruded during the transition to A particles. By making structural transitions energetically more favorable, these mutations may enable poliovirus to utilize a mouse cell receptor to enter cells.

It is interesting that in two different experimental systems, changes in the VP1 BC loop may lead to expanded receptor recognition: utilization of a mouse cell receptor and adaptation to mutant receptors (see discussion above). Involvement of the same structure in both cases suggests a common mechanism of adaptation to different receptors. Elucidation of how the VP1 BC loop controls receptor recognition of poliovirus awaits identification of the mouse cell receptor and resolution of the structure of the virus-receptor complexes.

The relationship between host range and receptors is much less understood for coxsackieviruses and ECVs. Coxsackieviruses primarily infect primate cell cultures, primates, and suckling mice (74). Studies with CVA-9 demonstrate that the resistance of cell cultures from rabbits, cows, pigs, or mice is due to absence of receptors on these cells, which produce virus after transfection with viral RNA (73). CVB strains do not infect RD cells, because the cells do not possess CVB receptors. However, CVB variants that could grow in these cells after blind passage were obtained (91). Competition studies indicate that these viral variants recognize a new receptor on RD cells in addition to the normal CVB receptor on HeLa cells. Construction of viral recombinants between CVB-3 and the adapted variant indicates that capsid protein VP2 contains one determinant of the RD phenotype (58).

ECV multiplication is limited to primates and primate cell cultures, although certain strains can infect mice (74). Failure of ECV-1 to multiply in CHO (hamster) cells is due to the absence of the α2 subunit of VLA-2 in these cells; when human α2 is expressed in CHO cells, the cells become susceptible to infection (8). It has not been determined whether lack of receptors explains the failure of ECV to multiply in other species or in cell cultures derived from them.

RECEPTORS AND TISSUE TROPISM

Not only does poliovirus have a narrow host range, but within the infected primate, replication is limited to specific cells and tissues. Human poliovirus infections begin when virus is ingested and then replicates in the oropharyngeal and intestinal mucosa. This primary replication leads to the establishment of viremia, which enables the virus to spread to many other tissues; however, subsequent poliovirus replication is limited to a few sites: neurons of the brain and spinal cord and an undefined extraneural site. The basis for the restriction of poliovirus replication to so few sites has not been determined. Poliovirus does not replicate when inoculated directly into monkey kidney or testicular tissue (26, 44, 56). A simple explanation for this restricted tissue tropism is that it is determined by receptor distribution.

Early approaches to this question included studies of the ability of polioviruses to bind to tissue homogenates to determine whether virus binding correlated with tissue sensitivity. In one study, poliovirus bound to homogenates of susceptible but not nonsusceptible tissues (34). Occasional low levels of virus binding to kidney, liver, and lung cells were also observed. In another study, significant virus binding to some monkey and human tissues, including those that do not support virus replication, was reported (55), suggesting that some nonsusceptible tissues also express receptors. Furthermore, the binding of radiolabeled poliovirus to human regional central nervous system tissue homogenates is more widespread than the distribution of virus-induced pathologic lesions (13). There are clear difficulties in interpreting the results of binding assays conducted with tissue homogenates. For example, absence of virus-binding activity may be an experimental artifact resulting from lability of virus receptors. Nevertheless, it is often concluded that poliovirus tissue tropism is controlled at the level of receptor expression (24, 34).

The availability of PVR nucleic acid and antibody probes has made possible a reexamination of the relationship between PVR expression and poliovirus tropism. In human tissues, Northern (RNA) and Western blot analyses have demonstrated expression of PVR RNA and protein in many tissues, suggesting that PVR expression is not the primary determinant of poliovirus tropism (29, 76). However, with the exception of mononuclear cells, where PVR expression was detected on the cell surface (30), further work on the expression of poliovirus-binding sites on cell surfaces will be required. It will also be necessary to assess the permissivity of other steps in poliovirus replication. Unfortunately, most human tissues develop susceptibility to poliovirus infection when explanted into cell culture and thus cannot be used for such studies.

The establishment of transgenic mice expressing PVR (TgPVR mice) that are susceptible to poliovirus infection has provided an easily manipulatable experimental system in which to study the determinants of poliovirus tropism (51, 92, 93). When examined by Northern blot hybridization analysis and in situ hybridization, PVR RNA is expressed in virtually all TgPVR mouse tissues, including spleen, muscle, lung, heart, small intestine, liver, kidney, thymus, brain, and spinal cord, as determined by Northern blot hybridization. The results of in situ hybridization show that PVR RNA is expressed at high levels in neurons of the central and peripheral nervous systems, developing T lymphocytes in the thymus, epithelial cells of Bowman's capsule and tubules in the kidney, alveolar cells in the lung, and endocrine cells in the adrenal cortex and at low levels in intestine, spleen, skeletal muscle, and brown fat. The cell type specificity of PVR expression is striking. For example, within the central and peripheral nervous systems, PVR RNA was detected only in neurons. This restricted pattern of expression may be related to the cell function of PVR.

Despite the widespread expression of PVR

RNA in TgPVR mice, poliovirus replication was detected at only a few locations, including neurons of the brain and spinal cord, skeletal muscle, and occasionally brown adipose fat. For example, after intraperitoneal inoculation of type 1 poliovirus, infectious virus could be detected in the kidney within 24 h, but no viral replication ensued. Viral replication was also absent in a variety of other tissues from the same animals. Thus, despite expression of PVR RNA, many TgPVR tissues remain refractory to poliovirus infection.

One possible explanation for these findings is that despite expression of PVR RNA, receptor protein may not be expressed on the cell surface. Immunohistochemical analysis of TgPVR tissues with anti-PVR MAbs must be done to address this question. However, in at least some TgPVR tissues, PVR protein does reach the cell surface. Cultured thymocytes and freshly dispersed kidney cells from TgPVR mice can bind polioviruses, yet these cells are resistant to infection (93; unpublished results). In these cells, the block to poliovirus infection clearly is not at the level of binding to PVR.

If thymocytes and kidney cells can bind polioviruses, what other obstacles might prevent infection? Inability of virus to reach cells expressing PVR, such as T lymphocytes of the thymus, might preclude poliovirus infection, but this explanation cannot account for the resistance to infection of tubular epithelial cells in the kidney. Poliovirus might bind to many tissues but might not be able to deliver its RNA genome into the cell. If other factors are required for poliovirus entry and/or uncoating, these factors might be expressed only in susceptible tissues. Finally, certain cell types may be unable to support other aspects of poliovirus replication, such as translation and replication of poliovirus RNA and assembly of new virus particles. The basis for the restriction of poliovirus replication in different tissues may vary.

The tissue distribution of the 100-kDa form of CD44H recognized by MAb AF3 suggests that this protein might play a role in poliovirus tropism (104). The AF3 epitope was detected by Western blot analysis on human spinal cord, brain stem, and cortex cells, which are sites of poliovirus replication, and not on nonpermissive human kidney cells, erythrocytes, or platelets. AF3 was detected on polymorphonuclear cells, which support poliovirus infection only after stimulation with phytohemagglutinin (109). Furthermore, AF3 reacts with regions of the human brain stem that are sites of poliovirus replication, such as the reticular formation and the hypoglossal nucleus, but not with the white matter or the inferior olivary complex, which are not sites of poliovirus replication in humans (12). As discussed above, it is not yet clear whether CD44H is required for poliovirus replication in cultured cells. Furthermore, expression of PVR in mouse L cells or in transgenic mice is sufficient to confer susceptibility to poliovirus infection. If CD44H is required for poliovirus infection, then the murine CD44 homolog Pgp-1 must supply the function in certain mouse cells.

Understanding the relationship between tissue tropism of coxsackieviruses and their cellular receptors awaits identification of the cell receptors for these viruses. Studies of the ability of CVB to bind homogenates of mouse tissues suggested that susceptibility was correlated with the presence of binding sites (54). Once receptor nucleic acid and antibody probes are available, the determinants of coxsackievirus tropism will begin to be unraveled.

ECV infections are limited to humans (74). While ECV infections may result in aseptic meningitis, paralysis, encephalitis, exanthema, respiratory disease, myalgia, and myocarditis, the sites of virus replication have not been studied. The lack of an animal model has hampered studies of ECV tropism, but the recent identification of two ECV receptors should provide the impetus to carry out these studies.

SUMMARY

The early events in virus infection, from virus binding to uncoating of the viral genome, are well characterized for a number of enveloped viruses (see reference 66 for a review), but the entry of naked viruses is poorly understood. The poliovirus-receptor interaction is a particularly good model for studying virus entry because of the experimental manipulations that are possible given the known structure of the virus and our ability to mutagenize both the virus and its cellular receptor. Despite our increasing genetic and structural understanding of early events in poliovirus infection, many problems, such as the location of the uncoating event, remain unsolved. Perhaps imminent studies on the entry of ECVs and coxsackieviruses, stimulated by the identification of their receptors, will provide clues. The roles of receptors in host range and pathogenesis have been extensively studied for poliovirus, but many questions, such as the basis of tissue tropism, remain. Finally, cell receptors clearly do not exist solely for the benefit of viruses; they serve important cell functions. A study of the cell functions of virus receptors may provide information on their role in virus replication. It has been suggested that virus binding to cell receptors may lead to activation of cell events that lead to disease (107), and there is evidence that receptors may regulate virus-induced cytopathic effects (80). Studies of the interactions of cell receptors with their natural cell ligands may therefore provide clues about cell processes that are activated upon virus binding and govern the outcome of virus infections.

REFERENCES

1. **Agol, V. I., S. G. Drozdov, T. A. Ivannicova, M. S. Kolesnikova, M. B. Korolev, and E. A. Tolskaya.** 1989. Restricted growth of attenuated poliovirus strains in cultured cells of a human neuroblastoma. *J. Virol.* **63**:4035–4038.
2. **Aoki, J., S. Koike, I. Ise, Y. Sato-Yoshida, and A. Nomoto.** 1994. Amino acid residues on human poliovirus receptor involved in interaction with poliovirus. *J. Biol. Chem.* **269**:8431–8438.
3. **Armstrong, C.** 1939. Successful transfer of the Lansing strain of poliomyelitis virus from the cotton rat to the white mouse. *Public Health Rep.* **54**:2302–2305.
4. **Badger, J., I. Minor, M. J. Kremer, M. A. Oliveira, T. J. Smith, J. P. Griffith, D. M. A. Guerin, S. Krishnaswamy, M. Luo, M. G. Rossmann, M. A. McKinlay, G. D. Diana, F. J. Dutko, M. Fancher, R. R. Rueckert, and B. A. Heinz.** 1988. Structural analysis of a series of antiviral agents complexed with human rhinovirus 14. *Proc. Natl. Acad. Sci. USA* **85**:3304–3308.
5. **Bergelson, J. M., B. Chan, R. W. Finberg, and M. E. Hemler.** 1993. The integrin VLA-2 binds echovirus 1 and extracellular matrix ligands by different mechanisms. *J. Clin. Invest.* **92**:232–239.
6. **Bergelson, J. M., M. Chan, K. R. Solomon, N. F. St. John, H. Lin, and R. W. Finberg.** 1994. Decay-accelerating factor (CD55), a glycosylphosphatidylinositol-anchored complement regulatory protein, is a receptor for several echoviruses. *Proc. Natl. Acad. Sci. USA* **91**:6245–6248.
7. **Bergelson, J. M., M. P. Shepley, B. M. C. Chan, M. E. Hemler, and R. W. Finberg.** 1992. Identification of the integrin VLA-2 as a receptor for echovirus 1. *Science* **255**:1718–1720.
8. **Bergelson, J. M., N. St. John, S. Kawaguchi, M. Chan, H. Stubdal, J. Modlin, and R. W. Finberg.** 1993. Infection by echoviruses 1 and 8 depends on the alpha2 subunit of human VLA-2. *J. Virol.* **67**:6847–6852.
9. **Bernhardt, G., J. A. Bibb, J. Bradley, and E. Wimmer.** 1994. Molecular characterization of the cellular receptor for poliovirus. *Virology* **199**:105–113.
10. **Bernhardt, G., J. Harber, A. Zibert, M. deCrombrugghe, and E. Wimmer.** 1994. The poliovirus receptor: identification of domains and amino acid residues critical for virus binding. *Virology* **203**:344–356.
11. **Bibb, J. A., G. Bernhardt, and E. Wimmer.** 1994. The human poliovirus receptor alpha is a serine phosphoprotein. *J. Virol.* **68**:6111–6115.
12. **Bodian, D.** 1959. Poliomyelitis: pathogenesis and histopathology, p. 479–498. *In* T. M. Rivers and F. L. Horsfall (ed.), *Viral and Rickettsial Infections of Man*. J. B. Lippincott, Philadelphia.
13. **Brown, R. H., D. Johnson, M. Ogonowski, and H. L. Weiner.** 1987. Type 1 human poliovirus binds to human synaptosomes. *Ann. Neurol.* **21**:64–70.
14. **Campbell, B. A., and C. E. Cords.** 1983. Monoclonal antibodies that inhibit attachment of group B coxsackieviruses. *J. Virol.* **48**:561–564.

15. Chang, K. H., C. Day, J. Walker, T. Hyypiä, and G. Stanway. 1992. The nucleotide sequences of wild-type coxsackievirus A9 strains imply that an RGD motif in VP1 is functionally significant. *J. Gen. Virol.* **73:**621–626.
16. Chow, M., J. F. E. Newman, D. Filman, J. M. Hogle, D. J. Rowlands, and F. Brown. 1987. Myristylation of picornavirus capsid protein VP4 and its structural significance. *Nature* (London) **327:**482–486.
17. Colonno, R. J., P. L. Callahan, and W. L. Long. 1986. Isolation of a monoclonal antibody that blocks attachment of the major group of human rhinoviruses. *J. Virol.* **57:**7–12.
18. Colston, E., and V. R. Racaniello. Poliovirus variants selected on mutant receptor-expressing cells identify capsid residues that expand receptor recognition. Submitted for publication.
19. Colston, E., and V. R. Racaniello. Soluble receptor-resistant poliovirus mutants identify surface and internal capsid residues that control interaction with the cell receptor. *EMBO J.*, in press.
20. Couderc, T., J. Hogle, H. Le Blay, F. Horaud, and B. Blondel. 1993. Molecular characterization of mouse-virulent poliovirus type 1 Mahoney mutants: involvement of residues of polypeptides VP1 and VP2 located on the inner surface of the capsid protein shell. *J. Virol.* **67:**3808–3817.
21. Couderc, T., A. Martin, C. Wychowski, M. Girard, F. Horaud, and R. Crainic. 1991. Analysis of neutralization-escape mutants selected from a mouse virulent type 1/type 2 chimeric poliovirus: identification of a type 1 poliovirus with antigenic site 1 deleted. *J. Gen. Virol.* **72:**973–977.
22. Crowell, R. L. 1963. Specific viral interference in HeLa cell cultures chronically infected with coxsackie B5 virus. *J. Bacteriol.* **86:**517–526.
23. Crowell, R. L., A. K. Field, W. A. Schleif, W. L. Long, R. J. Colonno, J. E. Mapoles, and E. A. Emini. 1986. Monoclonal antibody that inhibits infection of HeLa and rhabdomyosarcoma cells by selected enteroviruses through receptor blockade. *J. Virol.* **57:**438–445.
24. Crowell, R. L., and B. J. Landau. 1983. Receptors in the initiation of picornavirus infections, p. 1–42. *In* H. Fraenkel-Conrat and R. R. Wagner (ed.), *Comprehensive Virology*. Academic Press, Inc., New York.
25. de Verdugo, U. R., H.-C. Selinka, M. Huber, P. H. Hofschneider, and R. Kandolf. 1994. Purification and characterization of a specific attachment protein for coxsackie B viruses, abstr. 5, p. 5. *Abstr. Europic '94*.
26. Evans, C. A., P. H. Byatt, V. C. Chambers, and W. M. Smith. 1954. Growth of neurotropic viruses in extraneural tissues. VI. Absence of in vivo multiplication of poliomyelitis virus, types I and II, after intratesticular inoculation of monkeys and other animals. *J. Immunol.* **72:**348–352.
27. Filman, D. J., R. Syed, M. Chow, A. J. Macadam, P. D. Minor, and J. M. Hogle. 1989. Structural factors that control conformational transitions and serotype specificity in type 3 poliovirus. *EMBO J.* **8:**1567–1579.
28. Fox, M. P., M. J. Otto, and M. A. McKinlay. 1986. Prevention of rhinovirus and poliovirus uncoating by WIN 51711, a new antiviral drug. *Antimicrob. Agents Chemother.* **30:**110–116.
29. Freistadt, M. F., G. Kaplan, and V. R. Racaniello. 1990. Heterogeneous expression of poliovirus receptor-related proteins in human cells and tissues. *Mol. Cell. Biol.* **10:**5700–5706.
30. Freistadt, M. S., H. B. Fleit, and E. Wimmer. 1993. Poliovirus receptor on human blood cells: a possible extraneural site of poliovirus replication. *Virology* **195:**798–803.
31. Fricks, C. E., and J. M. Hogle. 1990. The cell-induced conformational change of poliovirus: externalization of the amino terminus of VP1 is responsible for liposome binding. *J. Virol.* **64:**1934–1945.
32. Gromeier, M., and K. Wetz. 1990. Kinetics of poliovirus uncoating in HeLa cells in a nonacidic environment. *Virology* **64:**3590–3597.
33. Hogle, J. M., M. Chow, and D. J. Filman. 1985. Three-dimensional structure of poliovirus at 2.9 Å resolution. *Science* **229:**1358–1365.
34. Holland, J. J. 1961. Receptor affinities as major determinants of enterovirus tissue tropisms in humans. *Virology* **15:**312–326.
35. Holland, J. J., and B. H. Hoyer. 1962. Early stages of enterovirus infection. *Cold Spring Harbor Symp. Quant. Biol.* **27:**101–111.
36. Holland, J. J., J. C. McLaren, and J. T. Syverton. 1959. The mammalian cell virus relationship. III. Production of infectious poliovirus by non-primate cells exposed to poliovirus ribonucleic acid. *Proc. Soc. Exp. Biol. Med.* **100:**843–845.
37. Holland, J. J., J. C. McLaren, and J. T. Syverton. 1959. The mammalian cell virus relationship. IV. Infection of naturally insusceptible cells with enterovirus ribonucleic acid. *J. Exp. Med.* **110:**65–80.
38. Hynes, R. O. 1992. Integrins: versatility, modulation, and signaling in cell adhesion. *Cell*

69:11–22.
39. Hyypia, T., C. Horsnell, M. Maaronen, M. Khan, N. Kalkkinen, P. Auvinen, L. Kinnunen, and G. Stanway. 1992. A distinct picornavirus group identified by sequence analysis. *Proc. Natl. Acad. Sci. USA* **89:** 8847–8851.
40. Incardona, N. L., and P. Kaesberg. 1974. A pH-induced structural change in bromegrass mosaic virus. *Biophys. J.* **4:**11–21.
41. Joklik, W. K., and J. E. Darnell. 1961. The absorption and early fate of purified poliovirus in HeLa cells. *Virology* **13:**439–447.
42. Jubelt, B., B. Gallez-Hawkins, O. Narayan, and R. T. Johnson. 1980. Pathogenesis of human poliovirus infection in mice. I. Clinical and pathological studies. *J. Neuropathol. Exp. Neurol.* **39:**138–148.
43. Jubelt, B., O. Narayan, and R. T. Johnson. 1980. Pathogenesis of human poliovirus infection in mice. II. Age-dependency of paralysis. *J. Neuropathol. Exp. Neurol.* **39:**149–158.
44. Kaplan, A. S. 1955. Comparison of susceptible and resistant cells to infection with poliomyelitis virus. *Ann. N.Y. Acad. Sci.* **61:**830–839.
45. Kaplan, G., M. S. Freistadt, and V. R. Racaniello. 1990. Neutralization of poliovirus by cell receptors expressed in insect cells. *J. Virol.* **64:**4697–4702.
46. Kaplan, G., D. Peters, and V. R. Racaniello. 1990. Poliovirus mutants resistant to neutralization with soluble cell receptors. *Science* **250:**1596–1599.
47. Kirkegaard, K. 1990. Mutations in VP1 of poliovirus specifically affect both encapsidation and release of viral RNA. *J. Virol.* **64:**195–206.
48. Koike, S., H. Horie, I. Dise, H. Okitsu, M. Yoshida, N. Iizuka, K. Takeuthi, T. Takegami, and A. Nomoto. 1990. The poliovirus receptor protein is produced both as membrane-bound and secreted forms. *EMBO J.* **9:**3217–3224.
49. Koike, S., I. Ise, and A. Nomoto. 1991. Functional domains of the poliovirus receptor. *Proc. Natl. Acad. Sci. USA* **88:**4104–4108.
50. Koike, S., I. Ise, Y. Sato, H. Yonekawa, O. Gotoh, and A. Nomoto. 1992. A second gene for the African green monkey poliovirus receptor that has no putative N-glycosylation site in the functional N-terminal immunoglobulin-like domain. *J. Virol.* **66:**7059–7066.
51. Koike, S., C. Taya, T. Kurata, S. Abe, I. Ise, H. Yonekawa, and A. Nomoto. 1991. Transgenic mice susceptible to poliovirus. *Proc. Natl. Acad. Sci. USA.* **88:**951–955.
52. Krah, D. L., and R. L. Crowell. 1982. A solid-phase assay of solubilized HeLa cell membrane receptors for binding group B coxsackieviruses and polioviruses. *Virology* **118:** 148–156.
53. Krah, D. L., and R. L. Crowell. 1985. Properties of the deoxycholate-solubilized HeLa cell plasma membrane receptor for binding group B coxsackieviruses. *J. Virol.* **53:**867–870.
54. Kunin, C. M. 1962. Virus-tissue union and the pathogenesis of enterovirus infections. *J. Immunol.* **8:**556–559.
55. Kunin, C. M., and W. S. Jordan. 1961. In vitro adsorption of poliovirus by noncultured tissues. Effect of species, age and malignancy. *Am. J. Hyg.* **73:**245–257.
56. Ledinko, N., J. T. Riordan, and J. L. Melnick. 1951. Differences in cellular pathogenicity of two immunologically related poliomyelitis viruses as revealed in tissue culture. *Proc. Soc. Exp. Biol. Med.* **78:**83–88.
57. Li, Q., A. G. Yafal, Y. H. Lee, J. Hogle, and M. Chow. 1994. Poliovirus neutralization by antibodies to internal epitopes of VP4 and VP1 results from reversible exposure of these sequences at physiological temperature. *J. Virol.* **68:**3965–3970.
58. Lindberg, A. M., R. L. Crowell, R. Zell, R. Kandolf, and U. Pettersson. 1992. Mapping of the RD phenotype of the Nancy strain of coxsackievirus B3. *Virus Res.* **24:**187–196.
59. Lloyd, R. E., and M. Bovee. 1993. Persistent infection of human erythroblastoid cells by poliovirus. *Virology* **194:**200–209.
60. Lonberg-Holm, K., R. L. Crowell, and L. Philipson. 1976. Unrelated animal viruses share receptors. *Nature* (London) **259:**679–681.
61. Lonberg-Holm, K., and L. Philipson. 1974. Early interaction between animal viruses and cells. *Monogr. Virol.* **9:**1–148.
62. Lublin, D., and J. Atkinson. 1989. Decay-accelerating factor: biochemistry, molecular biology, and function. *Annu. Rev. Immunol.* **7:**35–57.
63. Macadam, A. J., G. Ferguson, A. Nomoto, and P. D. Minor. 1994. Sequences of the cellular receptor and viral capsid proteins influence the cytopathic effect of poliovirus, abstr. A2, p. 2. *Abstr. Europic '94.*
64. Madshus, I. H., S. Olsnes, and K. Sandvig. 1984. Mechanism of entry into the cytosol of poliovirus type 1: requirement for low pH. *J. Cell Biol.* **98:**1194–1200.
65. Madshus, I. H., S. Olsnes, and K. Sandvig. 1984. Requirements for entry of poliovirus RNA into cells at low pH. *EMBO J.* **3:**1945–1950.
66. Marsh, M., and A. Helenius. 1989. Virus entry into animal cells. *Adv. Virus Res.*

36:107–151.
67. Martin, A., C. Wychowski, T. Couderc, R. Crainic, J. Hogle, and M. Girard. 1988. Engineering a poliovirus type 2 antigenic site on a type 1 capsid results in a chimaeric virus which is neurovirulent for mice. *EMBO J.* 7:2839–2847.
68. Mason, P. W., B. Baxt, F. Brown, J. Harber, A. Murdin, and E. Wimmer. 1993. Antibody-complexed foot-and-mouth disease virus, but not poliovirus, can infect normally insusceptible cells via the Fc receptor. *Virology* 192:568–577.
69. Mbida, A. D., O. G. Gaudin, O. Sabido, B. Pozzetto, and J.-C. Le Bihan. 1992. Monoclonal antibody specific for the cellular receptor of echoviruses. *Intervirology* 33:17–22.
70. Mbida, A. D., B. Pozzetto, O. G. Gaudin, F. Grattard, J.-C. Le Bihan, Y. Akono, and A. Ros. 1992. A 44,000 glycoprotein is involved in the attachment of echovirus-11 onto susceptible cells. *Virology* 189:350–353.
71. Mbida, A. D., B. Pozzetto, O. Sabido, Y. Akono, F. Grattard, M. Habib, and O. G. Gaudin. 1991. Competition binding studies with biotinylated echovirus 11 in cytofluorimetry analysis. *J. Virol. Methods* 35:169–176.
72. McLaren, L. C., J. J. Holland, and J. T. Syverton. 1959. The mammalian cell-virus relationship. I. Attachment of poliovirus to cultivated cells of primate and non-primate origin. *J. Exp. Med.* 109:475–485.
73. McLaren, L. C., J. J. Holland, and J. T. Syverton. 1960. The mammalian cell-virus relationship. V. Susceptibility and resistance of cells in vitro to infection by coxsackie A9 virus. *J. Exp. Med.* 112:581–594.
74. Melnick, J. L. 1990. Enteroviruses: polioviruses, coxsackieviruses, echoviruses and newer enteroviruses, p. 549–605. *In* B. N. Fields, D. M. Knipe, R. M. Chanock, M. S. Hirsch, J. L. Melnick, T. P. Monath, and B. Roizman (ed.), *Virology*. Raven Press, New York.
75. Mendelsohn, C., B. Johnson, K. A. Lionetti, P. Nobis, E. Wimmer, and V. R. Racaniello. 1986. Transformation of a human poliovirus receptor gene into mouse cells. *Proc. Natl. Acad. Sci. USA* 83:7845–7849.
76. Mendelsohn, C., E. Wimmer, and V. R. Racaniello. 1989. Cellular receptor for poliovirus: molecular cloning, nucleotide sequence and expression of a new member of the immunoglobulin superfamily. *Cell* 56:855–865.
77. Miller, D. A., O. J. Miller, V. G. Dev, S. Hashmi, R. Tantravahi, L. Medrano, and H. Green. 1974. Human chromosome 19 carries a poliovirus receptor gene. *Cell* 1:167–173.
78. Minor, P. D., P. A. Pipkin, D. Hockley, G. C. Schild, and J. W. Almond. 1984. Monoclonal antibodies which block cellular receptors of poliovirus. *Virus Res.* 1:203–212.
79. Morrison, M. E., and V. R. Racaniello. 1992. Molecular cloning and expression of a murine homolog of the human poliovirus receptor gene. *J. Virol.* 66:2807–2813.
80. Morrison, M. E., H. Yuan-Jing, M. W. Wien, J. W. Hogle, and V. R. Racaniello. 1994. Homolog scanning mutagenesis reveals poliovirus receptor residues important for virus binding and replication. *J. Virol.* 68: 2578–2588.
81. Moscufo, N., A. G. Yafal, A. Rogove, J. Hogle, and M. Chow. 1993. A mutation in VP4 defines a new step in the late stages of cell entry by poliovirus. *J. Virol.* 67:5075–5078.
82. Moss, E. G., R. E. O'Neill, and V. R. Racaniello. 1989. Mapping of attenuating sequences of an avirulent poliovirus type 2 strain. *J. Virol.* 63:1884–1890.
83. Moss, E. G., and V. R. Racaniello. 1991. Host range determinants located on the interior of the poliovirus capsid. *EMBO J.* 5:1067–1074.
84. Mosser, A. G., and R. R. Rueckert. 1993. WIN 51711-dependent mutants of poliovirus type 3: evidence that virions decay after release from cells unless drug is present. *J. Virol.* 67:1246–1254.
85. Moyer, A. Q., C. Accorti, and H. R. Cox. 1952. Poliomyelitis I. Propagation of the MEF1 strain of poliomyelitis virus in the suckling hamster. *Proc. Soc. Exp. Biol. Med.* 81:513–518.
86. Murray, M. G., J. Bradley, X. F. Yang, E. Wimmer, E. G. Moss, and V. R. Racaniello. 1988. Poliovirus host range is determined by a short amino acid sequence in neutralization antigenic site I. *Science* 241: 213–215.
87. Nobis, P., R. Zibirre, G. Meyer, J. Kuhne, G. Warnecke, and G. Koch. 1985. Production of a monoclonal antibody against an epitope on HeLa cells that is the functional poliovirus binding site. *J. Gen. Virol.* 6:2563–2569.
88. Olson, N. H., P. R. Kolatkar, M. A. Oliveira, R. H. Cheng, J. M. Greve, A. McClelland, T. S. Baker, and M. G. Rossmann. 1993. Structure of a human rhinovirus complexed with its receptor molecule. *Proc. Natl. Acad. Sci. USA* 90:507–511.
89. Pérez, L., and L. Carrasco. 1993. Entry of poliovirus into cells does not require a low-pH step. *J. Virol.* 67:4543–4548.

90. **Racaniello, V. R., and D. Baltimore.** 1981. Cloned poliovirus complementary DNA is infectious in mammalian cells. *Science* **214**:916–919.
91. **Reagan, K. J., B. Goldberg, and R. L. Crowell.** 1984. Altered receptor specificity of coxsackievirus B3 after growth in rhabdomyosarcoma cells. *J. Virol.* **49**:635–640.
92. **Ren, R., F. C. Costantini, E. J. Gorgacz, J. J. Lee, and V. R. Racaniello.** 1990. Transgenic mice expressing a human poliovirus receptor: a new model for poliomyelitis. *Cell* **63**:353–362.
93. **Ren, R., and V. Racaniello.** 1992. Human poliovirus receptor gene expression and poliovirus tissue tropism in transgenic mice. *J. Virol.* **66**:296–304.
94. **Roca-Garcia, M., A. W. Moyer, and H. R. Cox.** 1952. Poliomyelitis. II. Propagation of MEF1 strain of poliomyelitis virus in developing chick embryo by yolk sac inoculation. *Proc. Soc. Exp. Biol. Med.* **81**:519–525.
95. **Roivainen, M., T. Hyypiä, L. Piirainen, N. Kalkkinen, G. Stanway, and T. Hovi.** 1991. RGD-dependent entry of coxsackievirus A9 into host cells and its bypass after cleavage of VP1 protein by intestinal proteases. *J. Virol.* **65**:4735–4740.
96. **Roivainen, M., L. Piirainen, T. Hyypiä, I. Virtanen, and T. Hovi.** 1994. Receptors for coxsackievirus A9, abstr. A7, p. 7. *Abstr. Europic '94.*
97. **Rombaut, B., P. Brioen, and A. Boeyé.** 1990. Disoxaril stabilization and immunogenicity of poliovirus procapsids. *J. Gen. Virol.* **71**:1081–1086.
98. **Rossmann, M. G., E. Arnold, J. W. Erickson, E. A. Frankenberger, J. P. Griffith, H.-J. Hecht, J. E. Johnson, and G. Kamer.** 1985. Structure of a human common cold virus and functional relationship to other picornaviruses. *Nature* (London) **317**:145–153.
99. **Ryu, S., P. D. Kwong, A. Truneh, T. G. Porter, J. Arthos, M. Rosenberg, X. Dai, N. Xuong, R. Axel, R. W. Sweet, and W. A. Hendrickson.** 1990. Crystal structure of an HIV-binding recombinant fragment of human CD4. *Nature* (London) **348**:419–426.
100. **Selinka, H.-C., A. Zibert, and E. Wimmer.** 1991. Poliovirus can enter and infect mammalian cells by way of an intercellular adhesion molecule 1 pathway. *Proc. Natl. Acad. Sci. USA* **88**:3598–3602.
101. **Selinka, H.-C., A. Zibert, and E. Wimmer.** 1992. A chimeric poliovirus/CD4 receptor confers susceptibility to poliovirus on mouse cells. *J. Virol.* **66**:2523–2526.
102. **Shepard, D. A., B. A. Heinz, and R. R. Rueckert.** 1993. WIN 52035-2 inhibits both attachment and eclipse of human rhinovirus 14. *J. Virol.* **67**:2245–2254.
103. **Shepley, M. P., and V. R. Racaniello.** 1994. A monoclonal antibody that blocks poliovirus attachment recognizes the lymphocyte homing receptor CD44. *J. Virol.* **68**:1301–1308.
104. **Shepley, M. P., B. Sherry, and H. L. Weiner.** 1988. Monoclonal antibody identification of a 100-kDa membrane protein in HeLa cells and human spinal cord involved in poliovirus attachment. *Proc. Natl. Acad. Sci. USA* **85**:7743–7747.
105. **Smith, T. J., M. J. Kremer, M. Luo, G. Vriend, E. Arnold, G. Kamer, M. G. Rossmann, M. A. McKinlay, G. D. Diana, and M. J. Otto.** 1986. The site of attachment in human rhinovirus 14 for antiviral agents that inhibit uncoating. *Science* **233**:1286–1293.
106. **Stamenkovic, I., M. Amiot, M. Pesando, and B. Seed.** 1989. A lymphocyte molecule implicated in lymph node homing is a member of the cartilage link protein family. *Cell* **56**:1057–1062.
107. **Vile, R. G., and R. A. Weiss.** 1991. Virus receptors as permeases. *Nature* (London) **352**:666–667.
108. **Wetz, K., and T. Kucinski.** 1991. Influence of different ionic and pH environments on structural alteration of poliovirus and their possible relation to virus uncoating. *J. Gen. Virol.* **72**:2541–2544.
109. **Willems, F. T. C., J. L. Melnick, and W. E. Rawls.** 1969. Replication of poliovirus in phytohemagglutinin-stimulated human lymphocytes. *J. Virol.* **3**:451–457.
110. **Williams, A. F., and A. N. Barclay.** 1988. The immunoglobulin superfamily—domains for cell surface recognition. *Annu. Rev. Immunol.* **6**:381–405.
111. **Willingmann, P., H. Barnert, H. Zeichhardt, and K. O. Habermehl.** 1989. Recovery of structurally intact and infectious poliovirus type 1 from HeLa cells during receptor-mediated endocytosis. *Virology* **168**:417–420.
112. **Yeates, T. O., D. H. Jacobson, A. Martin, C. Wychowski, M. Girard, D. J. Filman, and J. M. Hogle.** 1991. Three-dimensional structure of a mouse-adapted type 2/type 1 poliovirus chimera. *EMBO J.* **10**:2331–2341.
113. **Zajac, I., and R. Crowell.** 1965. Location and regeneration of enterovirus receptors of HeLa cells. *J. Bacteriol.* **89**:1097–1100.
114. **Zajac, I., and R. L. Crowell.** 1965. Effect

of enzymes on the interaction of enteroviruses with living HeLa cells. *J. Bacteriol.* **89:**574–582.
115. **Zeichhardt, H., K. Wetz, P. Willingmann, and K.-O. Habermehl.** 1985. Entry of poliovirus type 1 and mouse Elberfeld (ME) virus into Hep2 cells: receptor-mediated endocytosis and endosomal or lysosomal uncoating. *J. Gen. Virol.* **66:**483–492.
116. **Zhou, D. F. H., J. F. Ding, L. J. Picker, R. F. Bargatze, E. C. Butcher, and D. F. Goeddel.** 1989. Molecular cloning and expression of Pgp-1. The mouse homologue of the human H-CAM (Hermes) lymphocyte homing receptor. *J. Immunol.* **143:**3390–3395.
117. **Zibert, A., H.-C. Selinka, O. Elroy-Stern, B. Moss, and E. Wimmer.** 1991. Vaccinia virus-mediated expression and identification of the human poliovirus receptor. *Virology* **182:**250–259.
118. **Zibert, A., and E. Wimmer.** 1992. N glycosylation of the virus binding domain is not essential for function of the human poliovirus receptor. *J. Virol.* **66:**7368–7373.

VIRAL RNA SYNTHESIS

Kyle L. Johnson and Peter Sarnow

4

The entire replicative cycle of enteroviruses occurs in the cytoplasm of infected cells. Genome replication, which requires RNA-dependent RNA synthesis, demands enzymatic functions quite different from that of the host cell. It has turned out that many virus-encoded proteins in concert with a few identified host cell proteins carry out the selective amplification of the viral RNA genome in infected cells.

The life cycle of human enteroviruses is initiated by attachment of the virus to a cellular receptor. The human poliovirus receptor has been cloned, sequenced, and identified as a member of the immunoglobulin superfamily of receptors (64), which also includes the cellular receptors for human immunodeficiency virus (CD4) and the major group of human rhinoviruses (ICAM-1) (reviewed in reference 103). As described in chapter 3, the uncoated virion RNA molecule is released into the cytoplasm. The 5' end of the virion RNA is covalently attached to a small protein, VPg (3B) (38, 60), which is removed prior to

RNA translation. Viral mRNA thus bears a 5'-terminal pU nucleotide (67, 74) and lacks the 5'-terminal m^{7}GpppN cap structure normally found at the 5' end of cellular mRNAs. The viral mRNA must therefore be translated in a cap-independent manner, which occurs via an internal ribosome-binding mechanism that is mediated by sequences located in the viral 5' noncoding regions (see chapter 5). The product of poliovirus translation is an approximately 247-kDa polyprotein, which is proteolytically cleaved by three viral proteinases into individual viral proteins (reviewed in reference 59).

Figure 1 shows the genetic map of enteroviruses: the viral structural proteins are encoded in the amino-terminal (P1) part of the polyprotein, and the nonstructural proteins involved in viral genome RNA amplification are encoded in the middle (P2) and the C-terminal (P3) parts of the polyprotein. As soon as sufficient viral proteins are synthesized, the viral RNA is selectively amplified, yielding negative- and positive-strand RNA molecules. Packaging of the positive-strand RNAs results in mature, infectious progeny virus (see chapter 7).

This chapter summarizes what is known about how a single viral RNA molecule can be selectively amplified into thousands of

---

Kyle L. Johnson, Department of Biochemistry and Molecular Genetics, The University of Alabama at Birmingham, Birmingham, Alabama 35294-0005. *Peter Sarnow,* Department of Biochemistry, Biophysics and Genetics and Department of Microbiology, University of Colorado Health Sciences Center, 4200 East Ninth Avenue, Denver, Colorado 80262.

Human Enterovirus Infections, Edited by Harley A. Rotbart,
© 1995 American Society for Microbiology, Washington, DC 20005

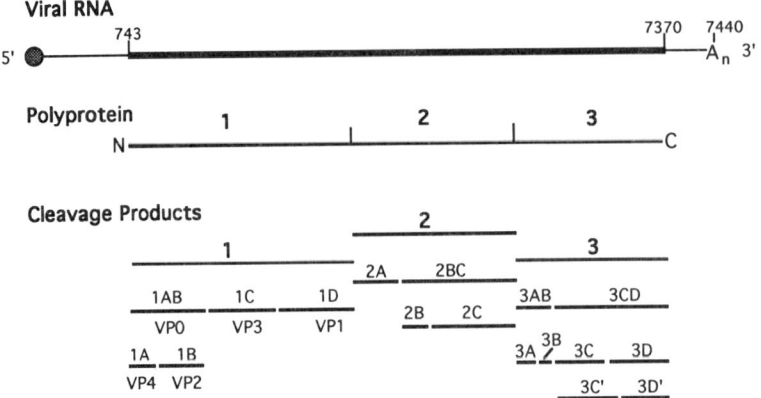

FIGURE 1 Genome organization of poliovirus. For viral RNA, the positive-strand RNA genome is shown. The presence of 3B (VPg) and polyadenosine sequences (A_n) at the 5' end and 3' ends, respectively, are indicated. The coding region is indicated by the black rectangle. For the polyprotein, the amino (N)- and carboxy (C)-terminal ends of the polyprotein are indicated. For the cleavage products, precursor proteins 1, 2, and 3 and their processed products are indicated; see the text for details.

RNA progeny in infected cells. Specifically, we (i) summarize the roles of viral proteins and RNA sequences in RNA replication, (ii) describe the kinetics and products of RNA replication in infected cells, (iii) describe the sites and compositions of viral replication complexes (RCs) in infected cells, (iv) discuss the models that have been proposed to explain how viral positive and negative RNA species are made by the viral RNA-dependent RNA polymerase, and, finally, (v) describe the coupling between translation and replication processes in infected cells. Because most of the research has been performed with poliovirus-infected cells, we use poliovirus as the prototype of an enterovirus.

POLIOVIRUS GENOME ORGANIZATION

Much has been learned about the life cycle of poliovirus and the replication of its genome since the discovery that a full-length cDNA copy of the poliovirus RNA genome produces infectious virus after being introduced into mammalian cells (80). This finding made it possible to study viral RNA genomes by using genetic approaches. Before the advent of this revolutionary tool, classic genetic approaches resulted in the generation of a genetic map of the viral genome. Cooper (25) performed chemical mutagenesis of poliovirion RNA to obtain a variety of temperature-sensitive mutants that were then used for recombination and complementation analyses (24, 26, 27). This approach allowed assignment of the structural and nonstructural regions to opposite ends of the genome (Fig. 1). However, few of the mutants could be shown to have single genetic lesions. Thus, it was not possible to use them as tools to assign functions to specific regions of the viral genome (reviewed in references 88 and 104). In addition, the viral RNA-dependent RNA polymerase, previously unknown to be the product of the 3D coding region, was identified and purified (30, 37, 39, 100). Various viral proteins suspected to be involved in RNA synthesis were localized to cytoplasmic membranous structures (13–15, 98).

With the availability of the infectious cDNA clones, however, both mapping of the gene segments encoding the various viral proteins to the viral genome and site-directed mutagenesis became possible. Cloning of the cDNA into a plasmid containing the T7ϕ-10 promoter has allowed the in vitro synthesis of infectious RNA that is 5% as infectious as virion RNA (99). Furthermore, addition of polyadenosine sequences to the 3' termini of the RNAs rendered them as infectious as virion RNA (86). By using these tools, it is possible to introduce mutations into the poliovirus cDNA, synthesize RNA transcripts from the mutated cDNA, and transfect these RNA transcripts into mammalian cells. In some but not all cases, virus with a mutant or wild-type phenotype can be recovered in this way. The genetic lesion in the resulting mutant virus can then be precisely mapped, and the phenotype can be studied. This approach in conjunction with biochemical analysis has allowed assignment of functions to most of the viral coding and noncoding regions. These functions are briefly summarized below. For a comprehensive discussion of poliovirus mutants and their phenotypes, the reader is directed to several review articles (see chapter 2 and references 52, 88, and 104).

Polioviral RNA Genome

The viral genome is a single-stranded, positive-sense RNA molecule approximately 7,500 nucleotides long, whose structure is represented schematically in Fig. 1. It contains a 743-nucleotide 5' noncoding region, a single long open reading frame encoding the viral polyprotein, a 70-nucleotide 3' noncoding region, and a genetically encoded 3'-terminal polyadenosine tail of variable length (105). The virion RNA has a 22-amino-acid protein, 3B (VPg), attached to its 5' end (38, 60) via a phosphodiester linkage between the 5'-terminal phosphate of the RNA and the O4-hydroxyl group of a unique tyrosine residue in 3B (1, 84). Other enteroviral genomes display identical organization with extensive homology within the coding sequences and only small differences in the lengths of the noncoding regions (85).

5' Noncoding Region

The poliovirus 5' noncoding region contains determinants for translation of the viral RNA by an unusual internal ribosome entry mechanism (49, 73; reviewed in reference 70), for amplification of the viral RNA (2, 3, 81), and for neurovirulence (36). This region has extensive secondary structure (83, 91), which seems to play an integral role in its functions. For example, Andino et al. (2, 3) have shown by in vitro structure analysis that a predicted cloverleaflike structure forms near the 5' end of the 5' noncoding region and that its formation is required for viral RNA synthesis (see below). Not surprisingly, there is a high degree of sequence and structure conservation among the three serotypes of poliovirus (reviewed in reference 72).

3' Noncoding Region

The 3' noncoding region is also highly conserved among the enteroviruses (46, 96). Using a combined biochemical and genetic approach, Jacobson et al. (48) have recently shown that sequences in the 3' noncoding region (in conjunction with sequences at the 3' end of the polymerase coding region) form a pseudoknot structure that is important for replication of viral RNA. This structure is also predicted to form in coxsackievirus B1, a related enterovirus. Mutations in the 3' noncoding region result in viruses defective in RNA synthesis (87).

Coding Region

Translation of virion RNA results in production of a 247-kDa polyprotein that is subsequently processed by three viral proteases, 2A (97), 3C (44), and 3CD (107), to yield the final individual polypeptides outlined in Fig. 1. A final cleavage of VP0, yielding VP2 and VP4, occurs during virion morphogenesis, possibly by autoproteolysis.

The polioviral polyprotein can be divided into three regions based on the initial products of proteolysis, P1, P2, and P3. These regions roughly correspond to the functions of the processed proteins. The proteins in the P1 region are the capsid proteins VP1, VP2, VP3, and VP4 (79). The first P2 protein, 2A, is a protease required for polyprotein processing (97), inhibition of host cell translation (10, 11), and transactivation of viral translation (43). The remaining nonstructural proteins encoded by both the P2 and P3 regions function in viral RNA amplification.

VIRAL PROTEINS INVOLVED IN VIRAL RNA SYNTHESIS

The capsid proteins encoded by the P1 region do not seem to play a major role in viral-RNA amplification. This conclusion is supported by the finding that RNAs containing large in-frame deletions within the capsid region are self-replicating after transfection into mammalian cells (23, 51). However, there is ample genetic and biochemical evidence to show that many of the poliovirus P2 and P3 nonstructural proteins (Fig. 1), with the notable exception of P2-2A, are involved in viral RNA synthesis in infected cells. That 2A does not play an essential role in RNA replication was demonstrated by the finding that a viral genome containing an in-frame deletion extending from the capsid region into the 2A coding region was self-replicating when transfected into mammalian cells (23). All remaining P2 and P3 proteins have been shown by biochemical fractionation and electron micrographic (EM) analyses to reside in the membrane-bound RCs that are the site of RNA synthesis in vivo, as discussed below (13, 14, 16, 17, 20, 42).

2B Protein

Genetic evidence has suggested that viral protein 2B is required for RNA replication (10, 50, 62). Specifically, linker insertion mutations in 2B resulted in mutant viruses that displayed specific defects in RNA synthesis. Interestingly, these 2B mutants exhibited effects that were dominant over those of wild-type viruses, suggesting a structural role of 2B or its precursor 2BC in viral RCs (50).

2C Protein

The 2C protein has been implicated in replication by genetic and cell fractionation analyses.

Mutants resistant to guanidine hydrochloride, a compound that blocks viral RNA replication, have been isolated and found to map in the coding region for 2C (76); when these mutations were reconstructed into otherwise wild-type viral cDNA, mutant viruses resistant to guanidine hydrochloride could be obtained (77). In addition, two linker insertion mutants in 2C that result in the synthesis of mutant 2C proteins are specifically defective in RNA synthesis (62). Using EM analysis, Bienz et al. (17) showed that 2C (or its precursor, 2BC) is physically present in membranous RC structures, the sites of viral RNA synthesis (see below).

3AB Protein

The 3AB protein is the precursor of 3B (VPg) and is involved in the initiation step of replication: mutants with defects in either the 3A or the 3B moiety are defective in viral RNA synthesis (10, 40, 41, 55, 56). The 3AB precursor is membrane associated and contains a hydrophobic region that could serve as a membrane anchor (90). When 3AB (32) and 2C (21) were expressed independently in the absence of other poliviral proteins, they localized to cytoplasmic membranes. Similarly, expression of 3AB in *Escherichia coli* resulted in the localization of 3AB to bacterial membranes (58). Thus, it is possible that 3AB and 2C form part of the attachment site of the viral RNA RC to membranes. It has been further suggested that cleavage of membrane-bound 3AB by the viral 3CD or 3C proteinases results in the release of 3B (58), facilitating its covalent linkage to RNA chains in the RC. The possible mechanisms by which 3B might be added to RNA are discussed in greater detail below.

Recently, it has been discovered that soluble 3AB can greatly stimulate polyuridine synthesis catalyzed by the viral 3D polymerase when polyadenosine is used as substrate (58). Lama et al. (58) concluded that 3AB has a dual function in viral RNA synthesis: to serve as primer for the initiation of new RNA chains and to function as stimulatory co-factor for the viral 3D RNA polymerase (58).

3C Protein

The role of 3C in the RC was first suspected on the basis of biochemical evidence that 3C or 3CD can cleave P2 and P3 proteins involved in RNA replication (59). Surprising genetic evidence provided support for a direct role of 3C in RNA synthesis. Specifically, a poliovirus mutant deficient in RNA replication and bearing a mutation in the cloverleaf-type structure (see above) in the viral 5' noncoding region could be suppressed by mutations in 3C (4). Subsequently, it was found that the 3CD precursor of 3C binds to the cloverleaflike structure in the viral 5' noncoding region in conjunction with a cellular protein, p36. It has been proposed that this ribonucleoprotein complex represents an initiation complex for positive-strand RNA synthesis (2, 3). Taken together, these results imply that 3C functions both as a proteinase and as an RNA-binding protein in the viral RC.

3D Protein

The 3D protein is the viral RNA-dependent RNA polymerase (30, 37, 39, 100), whose function has been studied extensively in vitro; the results of some of these studies are summarized in the discussion of in vitro replication models below. Many temperature-sensitive mutants of 3D have been constructed, and almost all of them are specifically defective in RNA synthesis at the nonpermissive temperature (18, 33).

VIRAL RNA SEQUENCES INVOLVED IN VIRAL RNA SYNTHESIS

A simple hypothesis is that the origin of negative-strand synthesis is at the 3' end of the positive strand and the origin of positive-strand synthesis is at the 3' end of the negative strand. Thus, most of the research on the putative origins of RNA replication has focused on the 3' ends of positive- and negative-strand viral RNAs. Because 3D is an RNA polymerase that is absolutely primer dependent in vitro, the search has concentrated on the identification of potential primers that can mediate RNA replication by 3D. In principle, either a *trans*-acting or a *cis*-acting primer (i.e., self-priming hairpin structures at the ends of the RNAs) could function in the initiation step. As described below, 3B-pUpU has been proposed to be a *trans*-acting primer that mediates initiation of positive strands. The genetic evidence suggests that the positioning of the replication primer for positive-strand RNA synthesis, possibly 3B-pUpU, at the 3' end of the negative-strand, is facilitated by a ribonucleoprotein complex composed of viral and cellular proteins and the RNA cloverleaf at the 5' end of the viral positive-strand RNA (see below for details). Curiously, a cloverleaf-type structure at the 5' end of the positive strand is apparently involved in the synthesis of further positive RNA strands.

Viral RNA sequences involved in the synthesis of negative-strand RNAs in vitro have been located at the very 3' end of the positive-strand RNA. Specifically, addition of uridine residues to the 3' polyadenosine sequences by a host terminal uridylyl transferase results in the formation of a snapback hairpin whereby the uridine residues pair with the adenine residues to form a primer for the initiation of negative strands (see below for details). We emphasize that most of the evidence for involvement of a snapback hairpin in the synthesis of negative strands comes from experiments performed in vitro. Thus, it is not known whether this mechanism operates in infected cells as well.

Of course, it is also conceivable that sequences located internally in the viral RNA genome may be involved in the initiation of replication at the ends of the viral RNAs. Although viral mutants that bear mutations in various parts of the viral genome and that are defective in the synthesis of RNA are available (104), it is not clear whether the primary reason for the failure to synthesize RNA is (i) the production of a mutant protein, (ii) the change in RNA structure affecting the stability of the RNA, or (iii) a mutation in a possible origin of replication.

PRODUCTS OF VIRAL RNA SYNTHESIS

During the course of replication of the viral RNA in infected cells, positive-strand virion RNA is amplified through a negative-strand intermediate. The products observed in vivo have been identified as single-stranded RNA, replicative intermediate (RI) RNA, and replicative-form (RF) RNA. Single-stranded RNA is the predominant RNA found in the infected cell. This RNA species is of positive polarity and is identical to virion RNA. Free negative-strand RNA has never been detected in vivo. RI RNA consists of a full-length RNA strand attached to six to eight nascent strands; while the predominant population of RI RNA is of positive polarity with attached nascent negative strands, negative-strand RNA with attached nascent positive strands can also be isolated. RI RNA is clearly the actively replicating species. Interestingly, all template and nascent strands in RI RNA already contain 3B (VPg) attached at their 5' termini (67, 74). RF RNA is fully double stranded and may represent a molecule no longer able to support replication or an artifact of the isolation procedures (reviewed in references 8 and 82).

SITE OF VIRAL RC

Poliovirus replication occurs on membrane-bound RCs in infected cells (13, 20, 42). During the course of poliovirus infection, smooth membrane vesicles accumulate in the cytoplasm of the infected cell (19, 29, 66), and it is on the surface of these virus-induced vesicles that the RCs reside (15) (discussed in detail in chapter 6). The RCs consist of viral nonstructural proteins (2BC, 2C, 3AB, 3C, 3D) and cellular membranes.

The structural organization of the RCs has been studied extensively. Using both EM and immunocytochemical EM, Bienz et al. (17) could examine the ultrastructural features of the RC in vivo. The RCs were found to consist of vesicular membranes containing the viral P2 proteins. In situ hybridization using positive-strand specific probes localized replicating RNAs within the RC as well (14, 98). Fractionation studies have revealed that RCs can be separated into two populations, both of which remain membrane bound (14). One population (30% sucrose fraction) contains RI RNA and can synthesize positive-strand RNA in vivo and in vitro. The second population (45% sucrose fraction) contains capsid precursors as well as free positive-strand RNA but little RI RNA (75). In vivo, no positive-strand synthesis could be detected in this population, but the complexes could be stimulated to resume positive-strand synthesis in vitro. This second fraction is proposed to represent RCs involved in encapsidation that contain a pool of viral positive strands awaiting packaging (98).

The mechanism by which the virus-induced vesicles associated with the RCs proliferate in poliovirus-infected cells is still unclear. However, several groups have shown by EM analysis that the vesicles may be derived from the endoplasmic reticulum (ER) (12, 19, 29). The proliferation of these vesicles depends on viral protein synthesis and has been correlated with the appearance of the 2BC precursor protein in infected cells (16). Indeed, the presence of 2BC in RCs has been confirmed by immunocytochemical EM (12). A model has been proposed in which 2BC combines with the membranes of the rough ER, where it induces the continuous synthesis of smooth membrane vesicles with concomitant formation of viral RCs. The vesicles detach from the rough ER, carrying the RCs on their surfaces, and accumulate in the cytoplasm (12).

However, the recent finding that poliovirus RNA amplification is inhibited by brefeldin A (BFA) suggests that the virus-induced vesicles may share properties of transport vesicles that shuttle from the ER to the *cis*-Golgi in uninfected cells (47, 63). BFA is a fungal metabolite that inhibits protein transport from the ER to the Golgi (71). BFA may therefore inhibit poliovirus replication by blocking formation of the vesicles on which the virus replicates. These findings are discussed in detail in chapter 6. Additional evidence for this model has recently been provided by Doedens et al. (34), who have shown that in two cell lines whose secretory pathways are resistant to disruption by BFA, poliovirus replication is not impaired by the drug. If indeed these vesicles are a result of subversion of transport vesicles in the cellular secretory pathway, cellular protein transport should be inhibited. Recent results from Doedens and Kirkegaard (33a) indicate that the transport of normally secreted proteins transiently expressed in poliovirus-infected cells is inhibited more than 80% by poliovirus. In addition, in the absence of viral infection, the viral proteins 2B and 3A are each sufficient to inhibit transport of the reporter protein expressed in these cells. It may be this inhibition of the protein secretory pathway that leads to the accumulation of the vesicles on which the poliovirus RCs are found in vivo. The exact role of these membranes in the process is unclear; their role may be to sequester the viral replication machinery and thus provide specificity to the reaction, or it may be to allow efficient capture of progeny RNA into virions. It is possible that host proteins that facilitate viral RNA synthesis will turn out to be components of the constitutive secretory pathways of uninfected cells.

BIPHASIC SYNTHESIS OF VIRAL RNA IN INFECTED CELLS

During the first 3 h after infection, newly synthesized viral RNA accumulates exponentially. Approximately 20% of the final RNA yield (4×10^4 RNA molecules per cell) is synthesized during this time (8). During the next hour in the infectious cycle, the remaining 80% of the viral RNA is made at a constant rate, after which RNA synthesis ceases. The time it takes to synthesize one molecule of viral RNA has been estimated to be 45 s (8). The switch from an exponential to a linear rate of RNA synthesis is not quite understood; clearly, the pool of RNA molecules destined for replication must be limited by 3 h after infection. Coincidentally, newly synthesized RNA is found in newly assembled virions at that time, suggesting that encapsidation affects the size of the RNA pool (8).

REPLICATION OF THE POLIOVIRUS RNA GENOME IS A TWO-STEP PROCESS

The first step of RNA replication involves copying the positive-strand RNA onto a negative-strand intermediate; the second step uses this negative strand as a template for further positive-strand synthesis. Both positive and negative strands are synthesized throughout the replication cycle, although positive strands are made in approximately 40-fold excess over negative strands (3, 68); the basis for this differential synthesis remains unclear (discussed in references 8 and 82).

IN VITRO RNA REPLICATION SYSTEMS

Three vitro systems have been used to study poliovirus RNA replication. A soluble system using purified proteins has been used to study the synthesis of negative strands from positive-strand templates. Also, a membranous crude RC (CRC) system has been instrumental in exploring the synthesis of further positive strands from negative-strand templates. As discussed below, neither of these models can adequately account for all of the events that occur in vivo. A new in vitro system, in which the entire replicative cycle can be reproduced in a cell-free environment, will allow further investigation of these processes. Each of these systems is considered in some detail below.

SYNTHESIS OF NEGATIVE-STRAND VIRAL RNA MOLECULES

When purified poliovirus positive strands are incubated with purified 3D polymerase in vitro, full-length negative strands can be synthesized if oligo(U) sequences are used as primers. This reaction proceeds with comparable efficiency on any 3' polyadenylated RNA, thus displaying no specificity for poliviral templates (37). A protein called host factor (HF), isolated from uninfected HeLa cells, can substitute for oligo(U) as a primer in the initiation of viral RNA synthesis (31). Andrews et al. (5, 7) discovered an explanation for this observation: purified HF preparation contains a terminal uridylyl transferase (TUTase) activity and can therefore synthesize the missing oligo(U) primer. A possible direct association between the TUTase and purified viral polymerase expressed in *E. coli* has been shown by Plotch et al. (78).

On the basis of such observations, an HF-dependent snapback model was proposed for the initiation of negative-strand RNAs (Fig. 2). The 3D-associated TUTase activity (HF) is first proposed to uridylylate the 3'-terminal polyadenosine tail of the viral RNA. Either HF or 3D promotes the annealing of the uridine residues to the 3'-terminal adenosine residues, resulting in the formation of a poly(A)-oligo(U) intramolecular duplex or a snapback structure that can function as a primer for 3D. In the presence of nucleotide triphosphates, 3D then elongates the hairpin primer, resulting in a double-stranded RI RNA molecule that is covalently closed at one end. Meanwhile, the membrane-associated precursor of 3B, 3AB, is cleaved by viral protease 3C or 3CD to release 3B (58). Protein 3B then nicks the hairpin to unlink the progeny strands while at the same time covalently attaching itself to the 5' end of the newly synthesized negative strand. Such a nicking activity for 3B has been suggested by Andrews et al. (7) and Young et al. (106) but has not yet been convincingly proven. Tobin et al. (95) presented evidence that synthetic 3B could become covalently linked to negative-strand RNA synthesized in vitro by purified 3D and HF and suggested that 3B was added by a self-catalyzed *trans*-esterification reaction in vitro (95). To return to the model (Fig. 2), newly initiated negative strands linked to 3B are then elongated by the viral 3D polymerase with the aid of the viral and hypothetical cellular factors, collectively indicated as VF and CF in Fig. 2.

This snapback model is supported by the fact that RF RNA molecules that are covalently closed at one end can be found in infected cells (106). While this model can adequately explain the synthesis of negative strands from positive-strand templates, it is somewhat less convincing as a model for the synthesis of positive strands. First, no extra uridine residues have been found on the 3' ends of the negative strands in RF RNA; the 3' ends of the negative strands in RI RNA have not been analyzed (reviewed in reference 57). Second, the suggested nicking and attaching activities for 3B would have to specifically recognize two different hairpins: one at the 3' end of the positive strand and one at the 3' end of the negative strand.

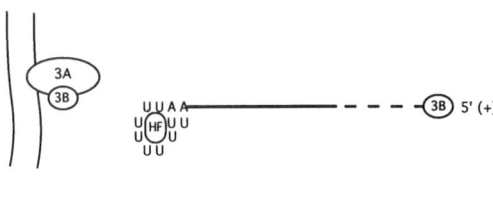

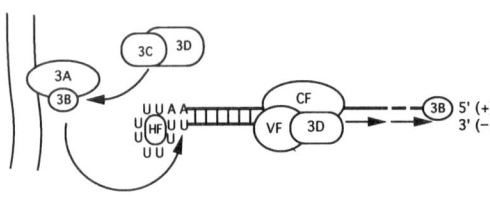

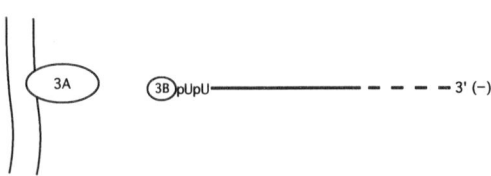

FIGURE 2 HF-dependent snapback model for the initiation of negative-strand viral RNA. Viral (VF, 3AB, 3B, 3D, and 3CD) and cellular (CF and HF) proteins and their putative actions in the replication process are shown. The direction of movement of the nascent RNA chain is indicated by two arrows. See the text for details. A hypothetical membrane is shown on the left. VF, viral factors; CF, cellular factors.

SYNTHESIS OF POSITIVE-STRAND VIRAL RNA MOLECULES

A CRC System: the 3B (VPg)-Primed Model

The synthesis of negative-strand RNA has been studied in a membrane-containing cytoplasmic extract prepared from infected cells. Fractionation of such CRC systems by discontinuous sucrose gradient centrifugation revealed that the viral 3D polymerase activity was primarily located in the smooth membrane fraction (15, 20, 94). These CRCs also contained the viral proteins 2BC, 2C, 3AB, and 3C (16). The size and polarity of the viral RNA synthesized in the CRC were monitored by performing the replication reactions in the presence of radiolabeled nucleotide triphosphates. The RNA products made in the CRC were shown to be identical to those synthesized in vivo: RI, RF, and single-stranded RNAs predominantly of positive polarity, indicating that the template was primarily negative-strand RNA (20, 92).

Several observations have led to a model, shown in Fig. 3, that describes the initiation of positive-strand RNA in the CRC system. First, it was noted that 3B (VPg) was attached not only to the 5' ends of full-length positive and negative strands but also to nascent positive strands. This suggested that 3B might act as a primer for positive-strand synthesis by 3D. Second, Takegami et al. (93) showed that 3B was uridylylated in vitro in the CRC, yielding 3B-pU and 3B-pUpU. At the same time, Crawford and Baltimore (28) reported that 3B-pUpU could be detected in infected HeLa cells. Third, 3B-pU could be chased into 3B-pUpU and, finally, in the presence of template RNA, into 3B-pUUAAAACAGp, a sequence element that represents the first nine nucleotides of positive-strand virion RNA (92). The identity of the 3B uridylylating activity remains unknown; it was shown, however, that the HF-associated TUTase activity was unable to uridylylate 3B (5). Furthermore, the synthesis of 3B-pUpU was inhibited by Nonidet P-40, a nonionic detergent, suggesting a requirement for membranes in 3B uridylylation. The fact that 3B-pUpU synthesis was most efficient in conditions in which 3D-catalyzed elongation was less efficient suggested that these were either separate activities of the same polypeptide or activities of different polypeptides (92).

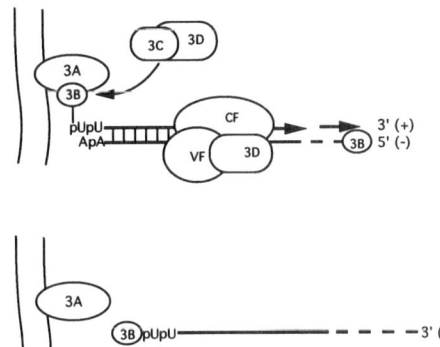

FIGURE 3 3B (VPg)-primed model for the initiation of positive-strand RNA. Viral (VF, 3AB, 3B, 3D, and 3CD) and cellular (CF and HF) proteins and their putative actions in the replication process are shown. The direction of movement of the nascent RNA chain is indicated by two arrows. See the text for details. A hypothetical membrane is shown on the left. VF, viral factors; CF, cellular factors.

The uridylylation of 3B suggested a potential mechanism for the initiation of positive-strand synthesis in which 3B-pUpU is formed in the RC and then acts as a primer for the 3D polymerase (Fig. 3). This model suggests that the membrane-bound 3AB precursor of 3B rather than 3B itself is the uridylylated species and acts as a primer for 3D. Cleavage of 3AB by 3C (or 3CD) at some point in the synthesis of the nascent strand (58) results in release of the product RNA, now attached to 3B, from the membrane. The roles in the initiation and elongation processes of viral proteins 2BC, 2B, and 2C and of hypothetical cellular proteins, collectively indicated as VF and CF in Fig. 3, are unknown.

As mentioned above, the 3B priming model for the synthesis of positive strands from negative-strand templates is supported by the detection of 3B-pUpU in vivo. Additional support for this mechanism in vivo comes from the finding that in vitro-synthesized coxsackievirus B3 (53) or poliovirus (45) RNAs missing the first two uridine nucleotides can generate infectious virus after being transfected into mammalian cells. Interestingly, the recovered viral genomes all contained two uridine nucleotides at the 5' ends of the positive-strand RNAs (45, 53). This indicated that the first two uridines were inserted template independently, consistent with the idea that 3B-pUpU functioned as primer. It is more difficult to envision how the two terminal uridines could have been regained by a snapback model. In the absence of the two adenosines at the 3' end of the negative strand, the addition of uridines by TUTase would not form a hairpin that could prime positive-strand synthesis without losing terminal nucleotides. Of course, the adenosines could always have been added by any of the abundant poly(A) polymerases in the cytoplasm of mammalian cells.

The 3B priming model describes the initiation of negative-strand RNA synthesis less adequately. First, the 5' end of the negative strand contains oligo(U) residues; to date, there has been no report stating that 3B-pUpU can be chased into 3B-oligo(U) in vitro, nor have 3B-oligo(U) molecules been detected in vivo. Second, Andrews and Baltimore (6) have shown that the attachment of 3B to nascent negative strands is the result of elongation of 3B-containing fragments of the positive-strand template rather than of de novo initiation by 3B. Thus, either 3B is not able to prime the synthesis of negative strands, or the soluble and RC in vitro systems are not adequate models for the complete replication of poliovirus RNA.

trans-Initiation Model

The *trans*-initiation model (Fig. 4) shares many aspects of the 3B priming model but incorporates the genetic and biochemical data of Andino et al. (2, 3) that describe a ribonucleoprotein complex formed between viral and cellular proteins and the 5' end of a preexisting positive-strand RNA. Mutations that disrupt the formation of this ribonucleoprotein complex cause a reduction in the synthesis of further positive-strand RNAs but not of negative-strand RNAs (2, 3). According to the *trans*-initiation model (Fig. 4), initiation of positive-strand RNA synthesis starts by formation of a functional ribonucleoprotein complex, RNP-B, at the 5'-terminal end of the positive-strand viral genome (2). RNP-B is composed of viral protein 3CD and a ribosome-associated cellular protein, p36, bound to the cloverleaf-type RNA structure formed by the 5'-terminal hundred nucleotides of the poliovirus virion RNA (2, 3). 3CD is proposed to have multiple functions in initiation. The 3C moiety of 3CD is suggested to process membrane-bound 3AB, releasing soluble 3B. The 3B can then be uridylylated by the 3D moiety of uncleaved 3CD or by processed 3D. Processing of 3CD yields the viral 3D polymerase, which can elongate 3B-pUpU, bound to the negative-strand template, to yield new positive strands. At the same time, the RC is released from the membrane, and a new RNP-B complex can form at the 5' end of either the newly synthesized or the original positive strand. Although this model is quite new and many details, such as the role of p36, are still unknown, substantial genetic and biochemical evidence (2, 3) supports the participation of the positive strand in the synthesis of additional positive-strand RNA molecules. However, this model does not describe the synthesis of negative strands, because neither the proposed cloverleaf structure nor the binding of 3CD and p36 has been observed at the 5' end of the negative strand. Overall, these data tend to suggest that there are separate mechanisms for the synthesis of positive- and negative-strand viral RNA molecules.

CELL-FREE SYSTEM SUPPORTS DE NOVO SYNTHESIS OF POLIOVIRUS

Recently, Molla et al. (65) established a cell-free system in which both viral protein synthesis and RNA replication can occur, resulting in the production of infectious poliovirus de novo. This is the first demonstration of the cell-free morphogenesis of an animal RNA virus. To do this, Molla and coworkers prepared a translation-competent extract from human HeLa cells; following addition of only poliovirion RNA, this extract was capable of translating poliovirus RNA and producing

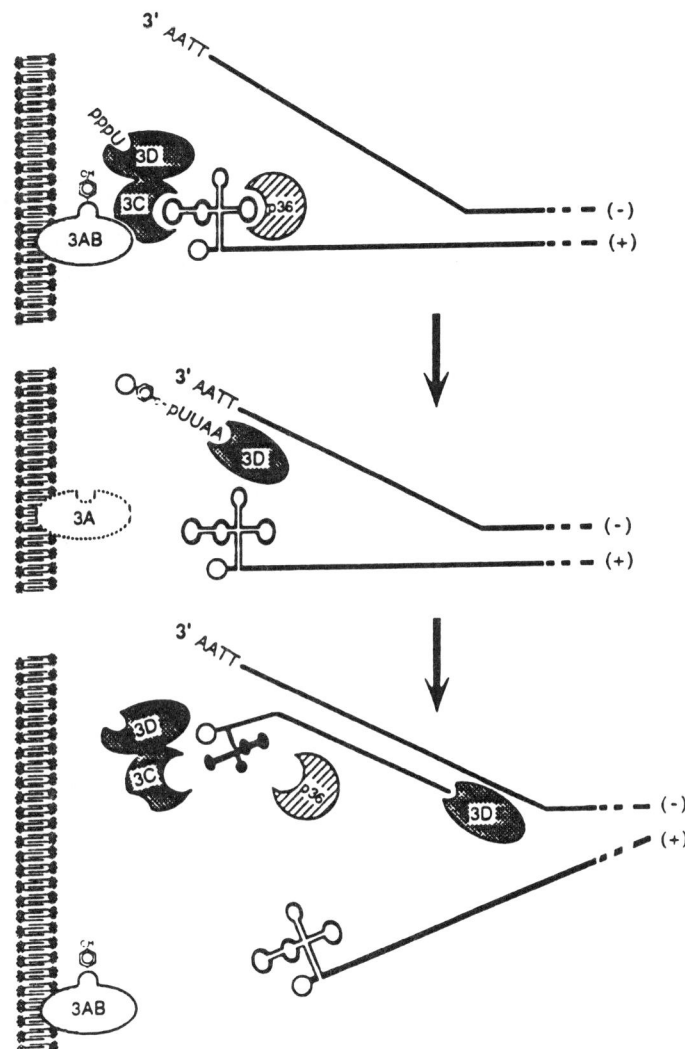

FIGURE 4 *trans*-Initiation model for the initiation of positive-strand RNAs. Viral (3AB, 3D, and 3CD) and cellular (p36) proteins and their putative actions in the replication process are shown. The cloverleaf-type RNA structure at the 5' end of the positive-strand RNA is indicated. 3B (open circle) is shown attached to the 5' ends of the positive strands and positioned as primer in the RC. See the text for details. A hypothetical membrane is shown on the left. This figure is reprinted from Andino et al. (2) by permission of Oxford University Press.

correctly processed viral proteins. Even after RNase treatment, addition of these extracts to monolayers of human cells resulted in the recovery of infectious poliovirus. Molla et al. demonstrated in several ways that virus production was dependent on the new synthesis of viral RNA in the translation extract. First, synthesis of viral negative-strand RNA in the translation was demonstrated by PCR assays designed to amplify any newly synthesized negative-strand RNA molecules. Second, treatment of the translation extract with guanidine hydrochloride, an inhibitor of viral RNA synthesis, abolished virus production. However, when translation was initiated with viral RNA from a guanidine-resistant viral mutant, guanidine treatment did not inhibit virus production. In addition, Barton and Flanegan (9) demonstrated that the kinetics of viral RNA translation, the activity of 3D polymerase, and the production of infectious virions were all comparable to the time course of events in infected cells (9).

These systems in which cell-free translation

of poliovirus RNA results in the production of infectious viruses will be powerful new tools with which to examine viral RNA translation, RNA synthesis, and morphogenesis. The cell-free system may obviate the often cumbersome task of isolating and propagating mutant viruses. Instead, it may be possible to examine interactions between the 3D polymerase and different RNA templates as well as interactions between 3D and other viral and cellular proteins involved in replication of the viral RNA in an in vitro system known to mimic the entire intracellular replicative cycle.

IN VIVO SPECIFICITY OF THE VIRAL RC

Purified viral polymerase 3D can copy any RNA in the presence of a primer in a soluble in vitro system (31, 39). Thus, neither the 3B priming model nor the snapback model explains why the 3D polymerase exclusively replicates poliovirus RNA in infected cells. It has been speculated that the in vivo specificity of 3D for viral RNAs results from (i) host cell or viral factors absent from the in vitro replication systems, (ii) particular structures in the viral RNA that are formed only in the infected-cell environment, or (iii) compartmentalization and sequestration of the viral RC in infected cells (52).

In this respect, it was observed that an RNA pseudoknot can form in the 3' noncoding region of the viral positive strand (48). Mutations that disrupted the pseudoknot structure resulted in a mutant virus that displayed temperature-dependent synthesis of viral RNA molecules in infected cells (48). Revertant viruses that were able to synthesize RNA at the restrictive temperature restored the pseudoknot structure. Thus, this structural element is a good candidate for modulating the efficiency with which negative-strand RNAs are made in infected cells. This is supported by the observation that a similar pseudoknot structure has been predicted to form in the 3' noncoding region of coxsackievirus (48). Similarly, the RNP-B complex, consisting of the RNA cloverleafs at the 5'

ends of positive-strand RNAs and its associated viral and cellular factors (see above), may confer in vivo specificity on the viral RC during the initiation of positive-strand RNA synthesis. In addition, the sequestration of the viral RC in the *trans*-initiation model may aid in the establishment of a sequestered RC. Finally, new roles for viral or cellular proteins in establishing template specificity may be discovered.

COUPLING BETWEEN VIRAL RNA TRANSLATION AND REPLICATION

Translation in *cis* through Internal Region (CTR) of Viral RNA Genome Is Required for Viral RNA Replication

It has been known for a long time that naturally occurring defective interfering (DI) particles of poliovirus, which contain large deletions in the capsid-encoding region of the viral RNA, can accumulate in infected cells (22, 54). Since these DI RNAs can be replicated in infected cells in the presence of a wild-type helper virus, the helper virus must provide the missing capsid proteins in *trans*. However, not all mutant genomes with deletions in the capsid region can be replicated, even in the presence of helper viral RNA genomes. The sequence determination of several DI genomes has revealed that DI RNAs that can be replicated contain deletions that do not disrupt the translation of the remainder of the viral genome (54). DI RNAs that cannot be replicated contain P1 deletions that change the open reading frame in the RNA, resulting in the production of truncated P1 proteins and none of the downstream P2 and P3 proteins. Because such out-of-frame DI RNAs could not be replicated in the presence of a helper virus, it was suggested that each viral RNA needs to be translated in order to be replicated (23, 54). This hypothesis could not easily be tested, however, because changes in RNA structures or dominant negative effects of truncated P1 proteins could have explained these findings.

Very recently, Novak and Kirkegaard (69) rigorously demonstrated that a region of the poliovirus RNA genome from P2-2A to the first 81 nucleotides of P3-3D (Fig. 1) needs to be translated for the RNA to be replicated (69). This demonstration was performed by constructing mutated RNAs containing nonsense codons in the 2A or 3D coding region. Mutant virus stocks could be obtained after transfection of the mutant RNAs into a cell line expressing nonsense-suppressing tRNA molecules (89), indicating that the mutant RNAs did not harbor any defects deleterious to viral growth. Neither mutant virus could grow on nonsuppressing cell lines. While the 3D-nonsense mutant virus could be complemented in nonsuppressing cell lines by wild-type virus, the 2A-nonsense mutant virus could not. Because the stabilities of the two nonsense mutant RNA genomes were similar in infected cells, it could be concluded that the viral RNA genome needs to be translated at least into the P3-3D coding region (Fig. 1) to be replicated (69), even when the P2 and P3 proteins are produced in *trans* from a helper virus. Novak and Kirkegaard speculated that the coupling of translation and replication could provide a proofreading mechanism whereby RNA genomes bearing deleterious mutations are prevented from being amplified (69). This is an attractive hypothesis considering that the viral 3D polymerase does not possess a proofreading activity and has an error rate of approximately 4×10^{-3} (101, 102).

Viral RNA Replication Does Not Require Continuous Translation

The observed in vivo specificity of the viral RC for viral RNA (see above) could be explained if the RNA can be replicated only by proteins translated from the same RNA molecule. If this is the case, this function must be required only early in infection. By the middle of the infectious cycle, RNA replication can continue, albeit at a reduced rate, after translation is blocked by inhibitors of protein biosynthesis (35, 61). Recently, Novak and Kirkegaard (69) showed that positive-strand RNA synthesis continued for at least 30 min after the addition of the protein synthesis inhibitor puromycin; similarly, negative-strand synthesis did not cease until 1 h after the addition of puromycin (69). Because it takes only approximately 45 s to complete the synthesis of one RNA strand, it could be concluded that RNA replication can continue in the absence of translation. Thus, ongoing translation is not required for the RNA to be replicated at the same time. However, as described above, ribosomes need to passage through the viral CTR (*cis* translation required) region at least once to allow the RNAs to be competent for later use as replication templates. The mechanism by which replication competence is gained is unclear. It is conceivable that scanning ribosomes modulate the stabilization or destabilization of RNA structures that are involved in the initiation of RNA synthesis. Another reason that this finding is of interest is that how ribosomes engaged in translation and an RC synthesizing new RNA molecules can move in opposite directions on the same positive-strand RNA molecule is still an enigma.

CONCLUDING REMARKS

To accomplish the unique task of RNA-dependent RNA polymerization in infected cells, enteroviruses encode several proteins required for viral RNA synthesis. In addition, evidence is accumulating that both proteins and membranous structures from the host cell are recruited for RNA synthesis, although their precise roles have yet to be established. Open questions about the mechanism of viral synthesis include the nature of the RNA primers for positive- and negative-strand RNA synthesis, the source of specificity for the viral template RNA, and the relationship between translation and RNA synthesis, which may occur simultaneously in the infected host cell cytoplasm. Some of these questions may be studied with the recently discovered cell-free system that is able to direct the de novo synthesis of poliovirus, thus mimicking events that take place in the infected host.

ACKNOWLEDGMENTS

We thank Karla Kirkegaard for critical reading of the manuscript. We are grateful to Valerie Ray Vaden for the artwork.

Work in the authors' laboratory was supported by grants from the U.S. Public Health Service (AI-25105 and AG-07347). P.S. acknowledges the receipt of a Faculty Research Award from the American Cancer Society.

REFERENCES

1. Ambros, V., and D. Baltimore. 1978. Protein is linked to the 5' end of poliovirus RNA by a phosphodiester linkage to tyrosine. *J. Biol. Chem.* **60:**5263–5266.
2. Andino, R., G. E. Rieckhof, P. L. Achacosco, and D. Baltimore. 1993. Poliovirus RNA synthesis utilizes an RNP complex formed around the 5'-end of viral RNA. *EMBO J.* **12:**3587–3598.
3. Andino, R., G. E. Rieckhof, and D. Baltimore. 1990. A functional ribonucleoprotein complex forms around the 5' end of poliovirus RNA. *Cell* **63:**369–380.
4. Andino, R., G. E. Rieckhof, D. Trono, and D. Baltimore. 1990. Substitutions in the protease 3C gene of poliovirus can suppress a mutation in the 5' noncoding region. *J. Virol.* **64:**607–612.
5. Andrews, N., and D. Baltimore. 1986. Purification of a terminal uridylyltransferase that acts as host factor in the *in vitro* poliovirus replicase reaction. *Proc. Natl. Acad. Sci. USA* **83:**221–225.
6. Andrews, N. C., and D. Baltimore. 1986. Lack of evidence for VpG priming of poliovirus RNA synthesis in the HF-dependent in vitro replicase reaction. *J. Virol.* **58:**212–215.
7. Andrews, N. C., D. Levin, and D. Baltimore. 1985. Poliovirus replicase stimulation by TUTase. *J. Biol. Chem.* **260:**7628–7635.
8. Baltimore, D. 1969. *The Replication of Picornaviruses.* Marcel Dekker, Inc., New York.
9. Barton, D., and J. B. Flanegan. 1993. Coupled translation and replication of poliovirus RNA in vitro: synthesis of functional 3D polymerase and infectious virus. *J. Virol.* **67:**822–831.
10. Bernstein, H. D., P. Sarnow, and D. Baltimore. 1986. Genetic complementation among poliovirus mutants derived from an infectious cDNA clone. *J. Virol.* **60:**1040–1049.
11. Bernstein, H. D., N. Sonenberg, and D. Baltimore. 1985. Poliovirus mutant that does not selectively inhibit host cell protein synthesis. *Mol. Cell. Biol.* **5:**2913–2923.
12. Bienz, K., D. Egger, and L. Pasamontes. 1987. Association of poliviral proteins of the P2 genomic region with the viral replication complex and virus-induced membrane synthesis as visualized by electron microscopic immunocytochemistry and autoradiography. *Virology* **160:**220–226.
13. Bienz, K., D. Egger, and T. Pfister. 1994. Characteristics of the poliovirus replication complex, p. 147–157. *In* M. A. Brinton, C. H. Calisher, and R. Rueckert (ed.), *Positive-Strand RNA Viruses.* Springer-Verlag, Vienna.
14. Bienz, K., D. Egger, T. Pfister, and M. Troxler. 1992. Structural and functional characterization of the poliovirus replication complex. *J. Virol.* **66:**2740–2747.
15. Bienz, K., D. Egger, Y. Rasser, and W. Bossart. 1980. Kinetics and location of poliovirus macromolecular synthesis in correlation to virus-induced cytopathology. *Virology* **100:**390–399.
16. Bienz, K., D. Egger, Y. Rasser, and W. Bossart. 1983. Intracellular distribution of poliovirus proteins and the induction of virus-specific cytoplasmic structures. *Virology* **131:**39–48.
17. Bienz, K., D. Egger, M. Troxler, and L. Pasamontes. 1990. Structural organization of poliovirus RNA replication is mediated by viral proteins of the P2 genomic region. *J. Virol.* **64:**1156–1163.
18. Burns, C. C., O. C. Richards, and E. Ehrenfeld. 1992. Temperature-sensitive poliovirus containing mutations in RNA polymerase. *Virology* **189:**568–582.
19. Butterworth, B. E., E. J. Shimshick, and F. H. Yin. 1976. Association of the poliviral RNA polymerase complex with phospholipid membranes. *J. Virol.* **19:**457–466.
20. Caliguiri, L. A., and I. Tamm. 1970. Characterization of poliovirus-specific structures associated with cytoplasmic membranes. *Virology* **42:**112–122.
21. Cho, M. W., N. Teterina, D. Egger, K. Bienz, and E. Ehrenfeld. 1994. Membrane rearrangement and vesicle induction by recombinant poliovirus 2C and 2BC in human cells. *Virology* **202:**129–145.
22. Cole, C. N., D. Wimmer, and D. Baltimore. 1971. Defective interfering particles of poliovirus. I. Isolation and physical properties. *J. Virol.* **7:**478–485.
23. Collis, P. S., J. B. O'Donnell, D. J. Barton, J. A. Rogers, and J. B. Flanegan. 1992. Replication of poliovirus RNA and subgenomic RNA transcripts in transfected cells. *J. Virol.*

66:6480–6488.
24. Cooper, P. 1968. A genetic map of poliovirus temperature-sensitive mutants. *Virology* 35:584–596.
25. Cooper, P. D. 1964. An improved agar cell-suspension plaque assay for poliovirus: some factors affecting efficiency of plating. *Virology* 13:153–157.
26. Cooper, P. D. 1965. Rescue of one phenotype in mixed infections with heat-defective mutants of type 1 poliovirus. *Virology* 25:431–438.
27. Cooper, P. D. 1977. Genetics of picornaviruses. *Comp. Virol.* 9:133–207.
28. Crawford, N. M., and D. Baltimore. 1983. Genome-linked protein VPg of poliovirus is present as free VPg and VPg-pUpU in poliovirus-infected cells. *Proc. Natl. Acad. Sci. USA* 80:7452–7455.
29. Dales, S., H. J. Eggers, I. Tamm, and G. E. Palade. 1965. Electron microscopic study of the formation of poliovirus. *Virology* 26:379–389.
30. Dasgupta, A., M. H. Baron, and D. Baltimore. 1979. Poliovirus replicase: a soluble enzyme able to initiate copying of poliovirus RNA. *Proc. Natl. Acad. Sci. USA* 76:2679–2683.
31. **Dasgupta, A., P. Zabel, and D. Baltimore.** 1980. Dependence of the activity of the poliovirus replicase on a host cell protein. *Cell* 19:423–429.
32. Datta, U., and A. Dasgupta. 1994. Expression and subcellular localization of poliovirus VPg-precursor protein 3AB in eukaryotic cells: evidence for glycosylation in vitro. *J. Virol.* 68:4468–4477.
33. Diamond, S. E., and K. Kirkegaard. 1994. Clustered charged-to-alanine mutagenesis of poliovirus RNA-dependent RNA polymerase yields multiple temperature-sensitive mutants defective in RNA synthesis. *J. Virol.* 68:863–876.
33a. Doedens, J., and K. Kirkegaard. Inhibition of protein secretion by poliovirus proteins 2B and 3A. *EMBO J.*, in press.
34. Doedens, J., L. A. Maynell, M. W. Klymkowski, and K. Kirkegaard. 1994. Secretory pathway function, but not cytoskeletal integrity, is required in poliovirus infection, p. 159–172. *In* M. A. Brinton, C. H. Calisher, and R. Rueckert (ed.), *Positive-Strand RNA Viruses*. Springer-Verlag, Vienna.
35. Ehrenfeld, E., J. V. Maizel, and D. F. Summers. 1970. Soluble RNA polymerase complex from poliovirus-infected HeLa cells. *Virology* 40:840–846.
36. Evans, D. M., G. Dunn, P. D. Minor, G. C. Schild, A. J. Cann, G. Stanway, J. W. Almond, K. Currey, and J. V. Maizel. 1985. Increased neurovirulence associated with a single nucleotide change in a noncoding region of the Sabin type 3 poliovaccine genome. *Nature* (London) 314:548–550.
37. Flanegan, J. B., and D. Baltimore. 1977. Poliovirus-specific primer-dependent RNA polymerase able to copy poly(A). *Proc. Natl. Acad. Sci. USA* 74:3677–3680.
38. **Flanegan, J. B., R. F. Pettersson, V. Ambros, M. J. Hewlett, and D. Baltimore.** 1977. Covalent linkage of a protein to a defined nucleotide sequence at the 5'-terminus of virion and replicative intermediate RNAs of poliovirus. *Proc. Natl. Acad. Sci. USA* 74:961–965.
39. Flanegan, J. B., and T. A. van Dyke. 1979. Isolation of a soluble and template-dependent poliovirus RNA polymerase that copies virion RNA *in vitro*. *J. Virol.* 32:155–161.
40. Giachetti, C., S. S. Hwang, and B. L. Semler. 1992. *cis*-Acting lesions targeted to the hydrophobic domain of a poliovirus membrane protein involved in RNA replication. *J. Virol.* 66:6045–6057.
41. Giachetti, C., and B. L. Semler. 1991. Role of a viral membrane polypeptide in strand-specific initiation of poliovirus RNA synthesis. *J. Virol.* 65:2647–2654.
42. **Girard, M., D. Baltimore, and J. E. Darnell.** 1967. The poliovirus replication complex: sites for synthesis of poliovirus RNA. *J. Mol. Biol.* 24:59–74.
43. **Hambidge, S. J., and P. Sarnow.** 1992. Translation enhancement of the poliovirus 5' noncoding region mediated by virus-encoded polypeptide 2A. *Proc. Natl. Acad. Sci. USA* 89:10272–10276.
44. **Hanecak, R., B. L. Semler, C. W. Anderson, and E. Wimmer.** 1982. Proteolytic processing of poliovirus polypeptides: antibodies to polypeptide P3-7c inhibit cleavage of glutamine-glycine pairs. *Proc. Natl. Acad. Sci. USA* 79:3973–3977.
45. **Harmon, S. A., O. C. Richards, D. F. Summers, and E. Ehrenfeld.** 1991. The 5'-terminal nucleotides of hepatitis A virus RNA, but not poliovirus RNA, are required for infectivity. *J. Virol.* 65:2757–2760.
46. Iizuka, N., S. Kuge, and A. Nomoto. 1987. Complete nucleotide sequence of the genome of coxsackievirus B1. *Virology* 156:64–73.
47. Irurzun, A., L. Perez, and L. Carrasco. 1992. Involvement of membrane traffic in the replication of poliovirus genomes: effect of brefeldin A. *Virology* 191:166–175.
48. **Jacobson, S. J., D. A. M. Konings, and P.**

Sarnow. 1993. Biochemical and genetic evidence for a pseudoknot structure at the 3' terminus of the poliovirus RNA genome and its role in viral RNA amplification. *J. Virol.* **67**:2961-2971.

49. Jang, S. K., H. G. Krausslich, M. J. H. Nicklin, G. M. Duke, A. C. Palmenberg, and E. Wimmer. 1988. A segment of the 5' nontranslated region of encephalomyocarditis virus RNA directs internal entry of ribosomes during in vitro translation. *J. Virol.* **62**:2636-2643.

50. Johnson, K. L., and P. Sarnow. 1991. Three poliovirus 2B mutants exhibit noncomplementable defects in viral RNA amplification and display dosage-dependent dominance over wild-type poliovirus. *J. Virol.* **65**:4341-4349.

51. Kaplan, G., and V. R. Racaniello. 1988. Construction and characterization of poliovirus subgenomic replicons. *J. Virol.* **62**:1687-1696.

52. Kirkegaard, K. 1992. Genetic analysis of picornaviruses. *Curr. Opin. Genet. Dev.* **2**:64-70.

53. Klump, W. M., I. Bergmann, B. C. Müller, D. Ameis, and R. Kandolf. 1990. Complete nucleotide sequence of infectious coxsackievirus B3 cDNA: two initial 5' uridine residues are regained during plus-strand synthesis. *J. Virol.* **64**:1573-1583.

54. Kuge, S., I. Saito, and A. Nomoto. 1986. Primary structure of poliovirus defective-interfering particle genomes and possible generation mechanisms of the particles. *J. Mol. Biol.* **192**:473-487.

55. Kuhn, R. J., H. Tada, M. F. Ypma-Wong, J. J. Dunn, B. L. Semler, and E. Wimmer. 1988. Construction of a "mutagenesis cartridge" for poliovirus genome-linked viral protein: isolation and characterization of viable and nonviable mutants. *Proc. Natl. Acad. Sci. USA* **85**:519-523.

56. Kuhn, R. J., H. Tada, M. F. Ypma-Wong, B. L. Semler, and E. Wimmer. 1988. Mutational analysis of the genome-linked protein VPg of poliovirus. *J. Virol.* **62**:4207-4215.

57. Kuhn, R. J., and E. Wimmer. 1987. The replication of piconaviruses, p. 17-51. *In* D. J. Rowlands, M. A. Mayo, and B. W. J. Mahy (ed.), *The Molecular Biology of Positive Strand RNA Viruses.* Academic Press, London.

58. Lama, J., A. V. Paul, K. V. Harris, and E. Wimmer. 1994. Properties of purified recombinant poliovirus 3AB as substrate for viral proteinases and as co-factor for RNA polymerase 3D$^{pol.}$ *J. Biol. Chem.* **269**:66-70.

59. Lawson, M. A., and B. L. Semler. 1990. Picornavirus protein processing: enzymes, substrates and genetic regulation. *Curr. Top. Microbiol. Immunol.* **161**:49-88.

60. Lee, Y. F., A. Nomoto, B. M. Detjen, and E. Wimmer. 1977. A protein covalently linked to poliovirus genome RNA. *Proc. Natl. Acad. Sci. USA* **74**:59-63.

61. Levintow, L., M. M. Thoren, J. E. Darnell, and J. L. Hooper. 1962. Effect of p-fluorophenylalanine and puromycin on the replication of poliovirus. *Virology* **16**:220-229.

62. Li, J.-P., and D. Baltimore. 1988. Isolation of poliovirus 2C mutants defective in viral RNA synthesis. *J. Virol.* **62**:4016-4021.

63. Maynell, L. A., K. Kirkegaard, and M. W. Kymkowsky. 1992. Inhibition of poliovirus RNA synthesis by brefeldin A. *J. Virol.* **66**:1985-1994.

64. Mendelsohn, C. L., E. Wimmer, and V. R. Racaniello. 1989. Cellular receptor for poliovirus: molecular cloning, nucleotide sequence, and expression of a new member of the immunoglobulin superfamily. *Cell* **56**:855-865.

65. Molla, A., A. V. Paul, and E. Wimmer. 1991. Cell-free, de novo synthesis of poliovirus. *Science* **254**:1647-1651.

66. Mosser, A. G., L. A. Caliguiri, and I. Tamm. 1972. Incorporation of lipid precursors into cytoplasmic membranes of poliovirus-infected HeLa cells. *Virology* **47**:39-47.

67. Nomoto, A., N. Kitamura, F. Golini, and E. Wimmer. 1977. The 5'-terminal structures of poliovirion RNA and poliovirus mRNA differ only in the genome-linked protein VPg. *Proc. Natl. Acad. Sci. USA* **74**:5345-5349.

68. Novak, J. E., and K. Kirkegaard. 1991. Improved method for detecting poliovirus negative strands used to demonstrate specificity of positive-strand encapsidation and the ratio of positive to negative strands in infected cells. *J. Virol.* **65**:3384-3387.

69. Novak, J. E., and K. Kirkegaard. 1994. Coupling between translation and replication in an RNA virus. *Genes Dev.* **8**:1726-1737.

70. Oh, S. K., and P. Sarnow. 1993. Gene regulation: translational initiation by internal ribosome binding. *Curr. Opin. Genet. Dev.* **3**:295-300.

71. Orci, L., M. Tagaya, M. Amherdt, A. Perrelet, J. G. Donaldson, J. Lippincott-Schwartz, R. D. Klausner, and J. E. Rothman. 1991. Brefeldin A, a drug that blocks secretion, prevents the assembly of non-clathrin-coated buds on Golgi cisternae. *Cell* **64**:1183-1195.

72. Palmenberg, A. C. 1987. Comparative organization and genome structure in picornaviruses. *UCLA Symp. Mol. Cell. Biol.* **54**:25-34.

73. Pelletier, J., and N. Sonenberg. 1988. In-

ternal initiation of translation of eukaryotic mRNA directed by a sequence derived from poliovirus RNA. *Nature* (London) **334:**320–325.
74. Pettersson, R. F., J. B. Flanegan, J. K. Rose, and D. Baltimore. 1977. 5'-Terminal nucleotide sequence of poliovirus polyribosomal RNA and virion RNA are identical. *Nature* (London) **268:**270–272.
75. Pfister, T., L. Pasamontes, M. Toxler, D. Egger, and K. Bienz. 1992. Immunocytochemical localization of capsid-related proteins in subcellular fractions of poliovirus-infected cells. *Virology* **188:**676–684.
76. Pincus, S. E., D. C. Diamond, E. A. Emini, and E. Wimmer. 1986. Guanidine-selected mutants of poliovirus: mapping of point mutations to polypeptide 2C. *J. Virol.* **57:**638–646.
77. Pincus, S. E., H. Rohl, and E. Wimmer. 1987. Guanidine-dependent mutants of poliovirus: identification of three classes with different growth requirements. *Virology* **157:**83–88.
78. Plotch, S. J., O. Palant, and Y. Gluzman. 1989. Purification and properties of poliovirus RNA polymerase expressed in *Escherichia coli*. *J. Virol.* **63:**216–225.
79. Putnak, J. R., and B. A. Phillips. 1981. Picornaviral structure and assembly. *Microbiology* **45:**287–315.
80. Racaniello, V. R., and D. Baltimore. 1981. Cloned poliovirus complementary DNA is infectious in mammalian cells. *Science* **214:**916–919.
81. Racaniello, V. R., and C. Meriam. 1986. Poliovirus temperature-sensitive mutant containing a single nucleotide deletion in the 5'-noncoding region of the viral RNA. *Virology* **155:**498–507.
82. Richards, O. C., and E. Ehrenfeld. 1990. Poliovirus RNA replication. *Curr. Top. Microbiol. Immunol.* **161:**89–120.
83. Rivera, V. M., J. D. Welsh, and J. V. Maizel. 1988. Comparative sequence analysis of the 5' noncoding region of the enteroviruses and rhinoviruses. *Virology* **165:**42–50.
84. Rothberg, P. G., T. J. R. Harris, A. Nomoto, and E. Wimmer. 1978. The genome-linked protein of picornaviruses. V. O4-(5'uridylyl)-tyrosine is the bond between the genome-linked protein and the RNA of poliovirus. *Proc. Natl. Acad. Sci. USA* **75:**4868–4872.
85. Rueckert, R. R. 1990. Piconaviridae and their replication, p. 507–548. *In* B. N. Fields et al. (ed.), *Virology*, 2nd ed., vol. 1. Raven Press, New York.
86. Sarnow, P. 1989. Role of 3'-end sequences in infectivity of poliovirus transcripts made in vitro. *J. Virol.* **63:**467–470.
87. Sarnow, P., H. D. Bernstein, and D. Baltimore. 1986. A poliovirus temperature-sensitive RNA synthesis mutant located in a noncoding region of the genome. *Proc. Natl. Acad. Sci. USA* **83:**571–575.
88. Sarnow, P., S. J. Jacobson, and L. Najita. 1990. Poliovirus genetics. *Curr. Top. Microbiol. Immunol.* **161:**155–188.
89. Sedivy, J. M., J. P. Capone, U. L. RajBhandary, and P. A. Sharp. 1987. An inducible mammalian amber suppressor: propagation of a poliovirus mutant. *Cell* **50:**379–389.
90. Semler, B. L., C. W. Anderson, R. Hanecak, L. Dorner, and E. Wimmer. 1982. A membrane-associated precursor to poliovirus VPg identified by immunoprecipitation with antibodies directed against a synthesis heptapeptide. *Cell* **28:**405–412.
91. Skinner, M. A., V. R. Racaniello, G. Dunn, J. R. Cooper, P. D. Minor, and J. W. Almond. 1989. New model for the secondary structure of the 5' non-coding RNA of poliovirus is supported by biochemical and genetic data that also shows that RNA secondary structure is important in neurovirulence. *J. Mol. Biol.* **207:**379–392.
92. Takeda, N., R. J. Kuhn, C. F. Yang, T. Takegami, and E. Wimmer. 1986. Initiation of poliovirus plus-strand RNA synthesis in a membrane complex of infected HeLa cells. *J. Virol.* **60:**43–53.
93. Takegami, T., R. J. Kuhn, C. W. Anderson, and E. Wimmer. 1983. Membrane-dependent uridylylation of the genome-linked protein VPg of poliovirus. *Proc. Natl. Acad. Sci. USA* **80:**7447–7451.
94. Takegami, T., B. L. Semler, C. W. Anderson, and E. Wimmer. 1983. Membrane fractions active in poliovirus RNA replication contain VPg precursor polypeptides. *Virology* **128:**33–47.
95. Tobin, G. J., D. C. Young, and J. B. Flanegan. 1989. Self-catalyzed linkage of poliovirus terminal protein VPg to poliovirus RNA. *Cell* **59:**511–519.
96. Toyoda, H., M. Kohara, Y. Kataoka, T. Suganuma, T. Omata, N. Imura, and A. Nomoto. 1984. Complete nucleotide sequences of all three poliovirus serotype genomes: implication for genetic relationship, gene function and antigenic determinants. *J. Mol. Biol.* **174:**561–585.
97. Toyoda, H., M. J. H. Nicklin, M. G. Murray, C. W. Anderson, J. J. Dunn, F. W. Studier, and E. Wimmer. 1986. A second virus-encoded proteinase involved in proteolytic

processing of poliovirus polyprotein. *Cell* **45:**761–770.

98. **Troxler, M., D. Egger, T. Pfister, and K. Bienz.** 1992. Intracellular localization of poliovirus RNA by in situ hybridization at the ultrastructural level using single-stranded riboprobes. *Virology* **191:**687–697.

99. **van der Werf, S., J. Bradley, E. Wimmer, F. W. Studier, and J. J. Dunn.** 1986. Synthesis of infectious poliovirus RNA by purified T7 RNA polymerase. *Proc. Natl. Acad. Sci. USA* **83:**2330–2334.

100. **van Dyke, T. A., and J. B. Flanegan.** 1980. Identification of poliovirus polypeptide p63 as a soluble RNA-dependent RNA polymerase. *J. Virol.* **35:**732–740.

101. **Ward, C. D., and J. B. Flanegan.** 1992. Determination of the poliovirus RNA polymerase error frequency at eight sites in the viral genome. *J. Virol.* **66:**3784–3793.

102. **Ward, C. D., M. A. Stokes, and J. B. Flanegan.** 1988. Direct measurement of the poliovirus RNA polymerase error frequency in vitro. *J. Virol.* **62:**558–562.

103. **White, J. M., and D. R. Littman.** 1989. Viral receptors of the immunoglobulin superfamily. *Cell* **56:**725–728.

104. **Wimmer, E., C. U. T. Hellen, and X. Cao.** 1993. Genetics of poliovirus. *Annu. Rev. Genet.* **27:**353–436.

105. **Yogo, Y., and E. Wimmer.** 1975. Sequence studies of poliovirus RNA. III. Polyuridylic acid and polyadenylic acid as components of the purified poliovirus replicative intermediate. *J. Mol. Biol.* **92:**467–477.

106. **Young, D. C., D. M. Tuschall, and J. B. Flanegan.** 1985. Poliovirus RNA-dependent RNA polymerase and host cell protein synthesize product RNA twice the size of poliovirion RNA in vitro. *J. Virol.* **54:**256–264.

107. **Ypma-Wong, M. F., P. G. Dewalt, V. H. Johnson, J. G. Lamb, and B. L. Semler.** 1988. Protein 3CD is the major poliovirus proteinase responsible for cleavage of the P1 capsid precursor. *Virology* **166:**265–270.

TRANSLATION AND HOST CELL SHUTOFF

Aurelia A. Haller and Bert L. Semler

5

Poliovirus represents the prototypic enterovirus, and thus, much of the information available on the mechanism of protein synthesis of enteroviruses has been derived from its study. The other members of the genus *Enterovirus*, such as coxsackieviruses A and B and enteric cytopathic human orphan (ECHO) virus, presumably display similar modes of translation initiation. Enteroviruses, like all members of the *Picornaviridae* family, have a positive-sense (i.e., message-sense), single-stranded RNA genome that is translated in the cellular cytoplasm immediately after the virions have been uncoated. Enteroviral RNAs resemble cellular mRNAs to such an extent that the viral mRNAs are translated efficiently by the host cell translation machinery, although, as discussed below, the mechanism for initiation of protein synthesis appears to be distinct from that employed for most eukaryotic mRNAs. As described in previous chapters, the prototypic enteroviral RNA is composed of approximately 7,500 nucleotides (nt), and its polyprotein coding region is preceded by a long 5' noncoding region (NCR) (~750 nt) that is characteristic of picornaviruses (51, 92).

A much shorter untranslated region (~60 to 70 nt), implicated in RNA replication (44, 99), is located at the 3' terminus of the viral genome, and this stretch of noncoding sequence is followed by a poly(A) tail 40 to 100 nt long. A virus-encoded protein, VPg (a 22-amino acid polypeptide), is covalently linked via an O^4-(5'-uridylyl)-tyrosine to the 5' terminal moiety of genomic poliovirus RNA (1, 96) instead of the 7-methyl-guanosine cap structure normally present at the 5' ends of cellular mRNAs. The cap structure at the 5' ends of eukaryotic cellular mRNAs is essential for efficient translation initiation in a cap-dependent manner. Eukaryotic translation initiation factors (eIF-4A, eIF-4B, and eIF-4F) initially recognize the 7-methyl-guanosine cap structure, and the ensuing macromolecular interactions result in binding of the 40S ribosomal subunit at the 5' end of the mRNA (75). In contrast, enteroviruses employ an alternative mechanism of translation initiation. It is of interest that poliovirus mRNA that is associated with polyribosomes does not contain VPg at its 5' terminus (79). Either as a prerequisite for association with ribosomes or as a consequence of that association, VPg is removed from the viral RNA by a cellular unlinking enzyme that still awaits identification. The presence of VPg at the 5' ends of

---

Aurelia A. Haller and Bert L. Semler, Department of Microbiology and Molecular Genetics, College of Medicine, University of California, Irvine, California 92717.

viral RNAs does not interfere with ribosome binding in vitro, nor does VPg interfere with in vitro translation of poliovirus RNA (30). Perhaps enteroviruses use the unlinking activity to regulate which progeny RNAs are destined to be mRNAs and which RNAs are to be packaged into virion particles.

Enteroviruses initiate viral protein synthesis via a cap-independent mechanism. The determinants directing internal ribosome entry are located in the unusually long 5' NCR that precedes the enteroviral single, long open reading frame. This region of RNA exhibits several features that will not accommodate the RNA-protein dynamics implicated in the ribosome scanning model predicted for translation initiation on eukaryotic mRNAs (54). The 5' NCRs of enteroviruses display an extensive computer-predicted RNA secondary structure that has been verified in part by chemical and RNase probing experiments (61, 90, 94, 101). A model of the secondary structure of the 5' NCR of enteroviral RNA is shown in Fig. 1. Ribosomes initiating at the 5' end of the viral RNA appear to be unable to melt and open up the extensive secondary structure of the 5' NCR for scanning. A highly conserved polypyrimidine tract (from nt 559 to 577) and an 8-base consensus sequence, CTTATGGT (from nt 583 to 590), are located in the 5' NCR of enteroviral RNA. The numbering refers to the nucleotide sequence of poliovirus type 1. Both of these conserved sequence elements appear to be crucial for viral protein synthesis, and their roles in cap-independent translation initiation are discussed below.

An interesting characteristic of enteroviruses is the presence of multiple AUG codons in the 5' NCR of the viral RNA (six to eight AUG codons in poliovirus depending on the serotype) that are followed by in-frame termination codons. The positions of three of these AUGs are conserved among the three poliovirus serotypes (Sabin and wild-type strains). The upstream AUGs are not believed to be utilized for initiation of translation, since expression of proteins from this region in vivo or in vitro has not been observed (20). In addition, they lack the preferred consensus sequence context displayed by the initiator AUG codon of cellular mRNAs (54). Pelletier et al. (84) individually mutated all seven upstream AUG codons in the 5' NCR of poliovirus type 2 to UUG. Mutation of the first six AUG codons had no effect on viral functions, but the seventh AUG mutation (nt 588) generated a virus with a small-plaque phenotype. Upon fusion of the 5' NCR containing the mutated AUG7 to a chloramphenicol acetyltransferase (CAT) reporter gene, decreased translation efficiency in vitro was detected. When mutant virus containing the AUG7 mutation was used to infect HeLa cells in culture, a defect in virus-specific RNA synthesis was observed, presumably as a result of decreased levels of viral protein synthesis. Thus, a disruption of the adenosine of AUG7 alters a motif that plays a positive role in poliovirus translation. This same nucleotide, nt 588, is located within a conserved octamer region. The other six upstream AUGs apparently do not inhibit ribosome migration, since none of the mutated AUGs increased the translation efficiency when placed upstream of a reporter gene.

Sequence analysis of the 5' NCR showed it to be highly conserved among the three poliovirus serotypes. More than 90% nucleotide sequence identity occurs from nt 1 to 650, and this region is followed by a highly variable region showing little nucleotide sequence homology (105). The computer-predicted secondary structures of the 5' NCRs of genomic RNA from all three poliovirus serotypes are nearly identical (94). Interestingly, the 5' NCR of a related enterovirus, coxsackievirus B3, displays a 70% nucleotide sequence identity with poliovirus and shares many structural features with the 5' NCR of poliovirus genomic RNA (61, 90, 94). These observations suggested that the determinants responsible for translation initiation by internal ribosome entry may be the RNA secondary structures of the 5' NCR per se in concert with conserved nucleotide

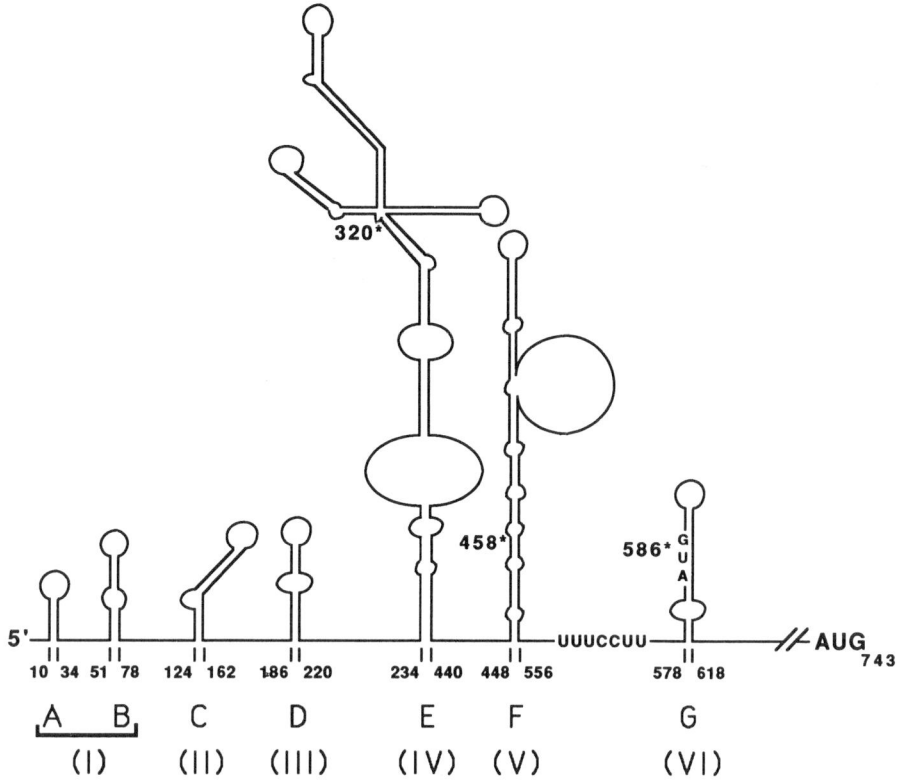

FIGURE 1 Diagram of computer-predicted secondary structure of the 5' NCR of poliovirus RNA. This structure has been confirmed, in part, by RNase and chemical probing experiments. Numbers refer to the poliovirus type 1 RNA genome. The seven stem-loop structures are labeled A through G. An alternative nomenclature employing roman numerals for the stem-loop structures is indicated in parentheses (36). In addition, Andino et al. (2) suggested that stem-loops A and B form a cloverleaf structure. This structure would compose the I stem-loop region shown in the figure. The asterisks indicate AUGs conserved among the enteroviruses and rhinoviruses. The conserved polypyrimidine tract (UUUCCUU) is located at nt 558 to 577; the conserved AUG at position 586 is indicated. The AUG at nt 743 represent the authentic translation start codon. The figure is modified from that of Dildine and Semler (18).

sequence elements, both of which may be recognized by host cellular and possibly viral factors providing a nucleation point for ribosome-viral RNA interactions. The region of the 5' NCR of enteroviral RNA where the ribosome-RNA contact takes place has been termed the internal ribosome entry site (IRES) (45) or the ribosome landing pad (85).

TRANSLATION INITIATION BY INTERNAL RIBOSOME ENTRY ON ENTEROVIRAL RNAs

Investigators observed early on that enteroviral RNAs are very inefficient mRNAs in an in vitro cell-free translation system such as rabbit reticulocyte lysate or wheat germ extract. Indeed, in addition to some of the predicted viral polypeptides observed in vivo, some unexpected translation products were generated in these translation systems in vitro. The proteins were subsequently identified by using poliovirus antibodies as aberrant internal translation initiation products originating from the P2 and P3 regions of the poliovirus genome (21). The addition of cytoplasmic extracts derived from HeLa cells to the cell-free translation reactions corrected the pattern of proteins produced, indicating that aberrant translation initiation could be suppressed. Further, the overall level of viral protein synthesis was stimulated to a great extent (9). These experiments suggested that present in the cytoplasmic extracts prepared from uninfected human cells are factors capable of both suppressing aberrant internal translation initiation on enteroviral RNAs and stimulating the levels of viral protein synthesis.

Enteroviruses were long suspected of using an alternative mechanism of translation initiation, since the viral RNAs were translated in the host cell at times when most of the cellular cap-dependent protein synthesis had ceased. In 1988, Pelletier and Sonenberg (85) demonstrated that poliovirus mRNAs are translated in a cap-independent manner that employs internal ribosome entry (Fig. 2). In this elegant experiment, the cDNA encoding the poliovirus 5' NCR was cloned into an artificially created bicistronic mRNA construct between an upstream herpes simplex virus thymidine kinase (TK) gene and a downstream CAT gene. By translating the mRNA from this construct in poliovirus-infected cells, which are unable to support cap-dependent translation, and still obtaining CAT protein at normal levels, Pelletier and Sonenberg (85) demonstrated that translation initiation had occurred by internal binding of ribosomes. To further substantiate these results, three XbaI linkers that form a stable hairpin structure were separately inserted into the cDNA encoding the poliovirus 5' NCR at nt 70 and at nt 631 of the bicistronic mRNA. The linker insertion at nt 70 had no effect on CAT expression, but the linker insertion at nt 631 caused a severe decrease in CAT expression.

These results suggested that prior to initiation of translation at the AUG for the CAT protein, ribosomes bound to the poliovirus 5' NCR downstream of nt 70 but upstream of nt 631. Another multiple linker insertion at the 5' end of the TK gene resulted in the loss of cap-dependent translation of the TK mRNA. Apparently, ribosomes initiating at the 5' end of an mRNA cannot efficiently melt a stable secondary structure to continue scanning (55). Thus, the ribosomes translating the CAT mRNA must initiate internally to circumvent the majority of the secondary structure of the 5' NCR, which precludes ribosome scanning. These experiments were extended to show that cap-independent translation is supported in an extract from uninfected HeLa cells that implicates cellular rather than viral factors in mediating cap-independent translation (86). Concurrently, a bicistronic construct containing the 5' NCR of encephalomyocarditis virus (EMCV), a related picornavirus, in the intercistronic region was used to demonstrate translation initiation by internal ribosome entry on EMCV RNAs (45). Recently, Macejak and Sarnow (70) discovered a cellular mRNA encoding the GRP78/Bip protein that can direct internal ribosome entry, although Bip encodes a capped mRNA. Additionally, *Drosophila melanogaster* mRNAs of the antennapedia gene were shown to harbor IRES elements (80). Thus, translation initiation by internal ribosome entry is not a mechanism employed by only a small subset of RNA viruses but appears to represent an alternative mode used by eukaryotic cellular mRNAs for protein synthesis.

The question of how ribosomes initiate internally in the 5' NCRs of enteroviral mRNAs remains to be elucidated. The site of ribosome entry most likely consists of single-stranded RNA devoid of secondary structure. This requirement implies an involvement of eukaryotic translation initiation factors 4A and 4B in their function as RNA helicases (97). However, a direct interaction of these two initiation factors with picornavirus RNAs has not yet been demonstrated. The IRES element

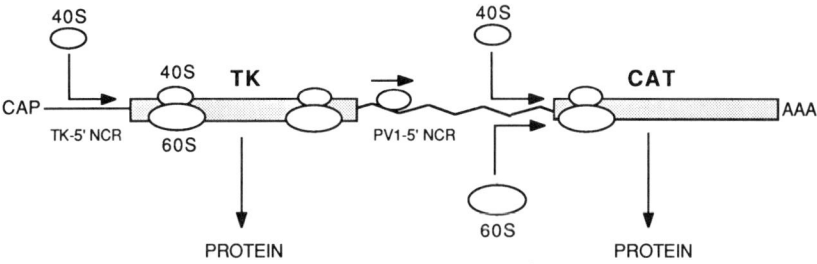

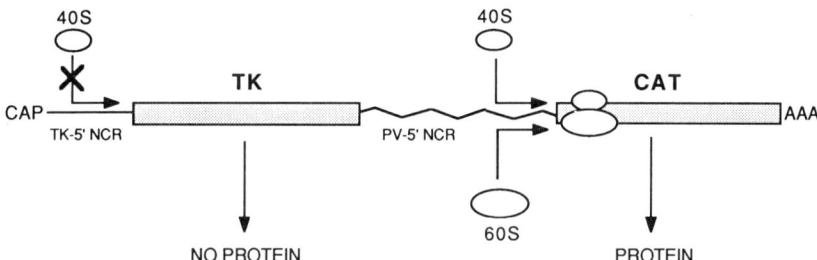

FIGURE 2 Diagram of bicistronic mRNAs directing cap-independent translation initiation in uninfected and poliovirus-infected cells. The bicistronic RNA consists of a capped mRNA encoding TK that is fused to the poliovirus 5' NCR linked to the second cistron encoding CAT. In uninfected cells, the capped mRNA encoding TK is translated in a cap-dependent manner. Translation of the second cistron encoding CAT could occur in two ways: by ribosomal readthrough and reinitiation of ribosomes that bound at the 5' end of the bicistronic mRNA or by internal ribosome entry in the 5' NCR of poliovirus. In poliovirus-infected cells, cap-dependent translation initiation is inhibited by the proteolytic processing of translation initiation factor eIF-4F. Thus, no TK protein is observed. However, the CAT mRNA is still translated, presumably by ribosomes binding internally at the IRES element within the 5' NCR of poliovirus RNA. Reprinted with permission from *Nature* (85). © 1988 Macmillan Magazines Limited.

may have to first bind other cellular factors that subsequently support interactions with eIF-4A and eIF-4B to eliminate secondary structures present in the 5' NCR of the viral RNA genome. The factor eIF-4F may also be part of this model, since eIF-4F stimulates internal ribosome entry on poliovirus RNAs in a cell-free translation system (3). In poliovirus-infected cells, eIF-4F is targeted for proteolysis, thereby causing a shutoff of host cell translation (discussed in detail below), but the processed form of eIF-4F is still capable of stimulating poliovirus protein synthesis (10). Finally, the 40S ribosomal subunit binds to the IRES element and, in the case of enteroviruses, may scan the RNA until it encounters the authentic translation AUG. Alternatively, the 40S ribosomal subunit may translocate from its entry site in the 5' NCR directly to the translation start site without scanning of the viral RNA, perhaps by RNA looping.

Evidence for scanning by the ribosomal subunit of poliovirus mRNAs was provided by inserting a 70-nt segment containing an AUG codon in the highly variable region of poliovirus RNA between nt 630 and 742 (57). The resulting virus displayed a small-plaque phenotype, and revertants that retained the inserted sequence but had deleted or altered the inserted AUG sequence were isolated. As mentioned above, other data in support of scanning of poliovirus RNA after ribosome entry were produced by Pelletier and Sonenberg (85), who introduced stable secondary structures downstream of the IRES element in a bicistronic mRNA that dramatically reduced protein synthesis in vitro. In contrast, other picornaviruses such as EMCV do not display a selection of the translation initiation site by scanning of the viral RNA. Rather, the ribosome appears to enter directly at the site of the translation start codon (49). The 5' NCR of rhinovirus, another member of the *Picornaviridae* family, lacks the variable region, and thus, the selection of the initiation site of protein synthesis is not predicted to occur by scanning of the viral RNA. Once the start site of protein synthesis is located, the 60S ribosomal subunit interacts with the 40S subunit to form a translation-competent 80S ribosome complex, and viral protein synthesis ensues (for reviews, see references 43 and 102).

VIRAL IRES ELEMENTS

The IRES elements of picornaviruses can be separated along the lines of the phylogenetic division of the virus family. The genera *Enterovirus* and *Rhinovirus*, composed of the coxsackieviruses, polioviruses, echoviruses, and rhinoviruses, display one kind of IRES element (type 2). The viruses belonging to the genus *Cardiovirus*, such as EMCV, Theiler's murine encephalomyelitis virus, and aphthovirus (foot-and-mouth disease virus [FMDV]), harbor a different type of IRES (type 1). The IRES element of hepatitis A viruses resembles that of the cardioviruses. Members of these different virus genera employ slightly different mechanisms of internal ribosome binding, as alluded to in the previous section. However, the two types of IRES elements contain common characteristics that

may be essential for the translation initiation mechanisms used by picornaviruses (Fig. 3). A polypyrimidine tract, highly conserved among all members of the picornaviruses, is located approximately 20 to 25 nt from a conserved AUG triplet. For the enteroviruses, the initiator AUG is the next AUG, located 150 nt downstream. Interestingly, a region from nt 567 to 627 (containing a large part of the polypyrimidine tract) was described previously as an essential element for efficient translation initiation of poliovirus mRNAs in vitro (5). A mutational analysis of the pyrimidine-rich sequences from nt 556 to 585 in poliovirus type 2 revealed that a sequence from nt 560 to 564 (UUUCC) is important for translation initiation by internal ribosome entry in vitro and in vivo (72, 78, 89). The experiments carried out by Pelletier and colleagues (83) in which the upstream AUG codons located in the 5' NCR were altered (described above), indicated a special function of AUG7 in po-

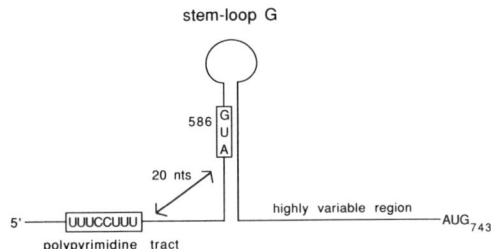

FIGURE 3 Diagram of conserved sequence elements in the IRES of enteroviral RNAs. The conserved sequence elements, i.e., the polypyrimidine tract and the upstream AUG codon (at nt 586 in poliovirus type 1), are boxed. The AUG codon is present in stem-loop G of the 5' NCR of enterovirus RNA. The nucleotide sequences of the AUG codon are predicted to be base paired in a stem structure. A distance of 20 nt between the pyrimidine-rich region and the AUG at nt 586 is required for efficient translation initiation by internal ribosome entry on viral RNAs. Stem-loop G sequences are followed by a region of viral RNA that is not well conserved among the enteroviruses (the variable region). The authentic translation start codon is located at nt 743 and is thus ~150 nt downstream of the polypyrimidine tract. This AUG codon may be located by ribosome scanning of the viral RNA.

liovirus replication. A change of the conserved AUG7 sequences also resulted in a decrease in translation initiation, and these data suggested a role for this AUG codon, not as an initiator AUG but as an element involved in the formation of a functional IRES structure. The distance between the two conserved RNA nucleotide sequences appears to be critical as well. If the spacing of 20 to 25 nt between the polypyrimidine tract and the downstream AUG is decreased or increased, translation initiation is affected in a negative manner (29, 91).

Further information about the spacing requirements of the above-described conserved sequences (the polypyrimidine tract and the downstream AUG triplet) was obtained by isolating poliovirus revertants displaying gross rearrangements of the RNA genome. A poliovirus revertant which contained a large deletion of ~150 nt in the 5' NCR of poliovirus RNA that removed stem-loop G and most of the upstream variable region was isolated (33). The originally introduced mutated RNA contained a linker sequence substitution in the 5' NCR that altered the conserved AUG located in stem-loop G. The mutation of this conserved AUG perturbed the ~20-nt distance normally present in wild-type RNAs between the polypyrimidine tract and an AUG codon. In the isolated poliovirus revertant bearing the stem-loop G deletion, the wild-type spacing of ~20 nt between the two conserved sequence elements, the polypyrimidine tract and an AUG codon (in this case the authentic translation start codon), was restored. Surprisingly, this revertant behaved similarly to wild-type poliovirus in tissue culture experiments despite the loss of one-fifth of the 5' NCR sequences. Other than these two short conserved sequences, no additional significant RNA sequence identity or similar predicted RNA secondary structures exist between the two viral IRES types (for a review, see reference 46). Although most of the described studies employed polioviruses, an experiment carried out by Johnson and Semler (48) suggested that coxsackieviruses employ a similar mechanism for viral protein synthesis. Those authors generated a chimeric enterovirus containing nearly the entire coxsackievirus 5' NCR fused to the poliovirus single, long open reading frame. The resulting recombinant virus displayed a wild-type-like phenotype for growth in tissue culture. Further, a region encompassing the polypyrimidine tract of coxsackievirus B1 strain from nt 546 to 566 was determined by deletion analysis to play an important role in directing the levels of translation initiation (42). These data show that the determinants located in the 5' NCRs of coxsackieviruses that direct internal ribosome entry are very similar, if not functionally analogous, to those present in the 5' NCRs of polioviruses.

What are the boundaries of the IRES element located in the 5' NCRs of enterovirus RNAs? For poliovirus, a long RNA sequence from nt 130 to 630 (containing predicted stem-loops C, D, E, F, and G; Fig. 1) affects efficient translation initiation (106). However, two of the predicted stem-loop structures (D and G) of the 5' NCR may not be essential for translation initiation by internal ribosome entry in cell culture. A poliovirus revertant that displayed a deletion of sequences corresponding to stem-loop D (from nt 184 to 228) was isolated. The phenotype of this revertant was very similar yet not identical to that of the wild type (17). Haller and Semler (33) isolated a poliovirus pseudorevertant that contained a gross deletion of 151 nt (from nt 564 to 715) that removed stem-loop G and most of the upstream variable region. Two other mutant viruses containing deletions with very similar boundaries were constructed by site-specific deletion mutagenesis of cDNAs corresponding to the type 1 (Mahoney) strain of poliovirus and Sabin type 1 vaccine strain (41, 91). Surprisingly, all of these mutant polioviruses displayed a wild-type-like phenotype despite the missing stem-loop G sequences. The mutant poliovirus type 1 (Mahoney) bearing the stem-loop G deletion exhibited a reduced lesion score in monkey neurovirulence tests (41, 91). A genetically engineered poliovirus RNA lacking stem-loops D and G of the 5' NCR proved to be infectious, although this mutant virus displayed a decreased level of translation efficiency in vitro (~30% of the levels directed by wild-type RNAs) and reduced protein synthesis in virus-infected cells (32). Similar results were obtained when 5' NCRs containing various stem-loop deletions were placed between two open reading frames expressed as a single transcription unit. Stem-loops D and G are not absolutely essential for translation initiation by internal ribosome entry in these assay systems (78, 87, 103). Nevertheless, they are probably required in vivo for a fully functional IRES element or perhaps in functions related to viral pathogenesis during proliferation in primate tissues.

Experimental evidence generated to date suggests that stem-loops E and F compose the essential core structures of the IRES element. Mutated poliovirus RNAs bearing deletions of stem-loop F did not yield virus upon transfection of HeLa cells. Further, deletion of stem-loop F of the 5' NCR of poliovirus RNA is highly detrimental to viral translation initiation in vitro (33). In addition, it was shown by electrophoretic mobility shift analysis that stem-loop E sequences were required for the formation of specific RNA-protein complexes within the 5' NCR of poliovirus RNA (18). The structural requirements for internal ribosome entry on viral RNAs may change during the early and late phases of poliovirus infection. The virus infection may modify the cellular translation apparatus so that shortened forms of the 5' NCR are sufficient for cap-independent translation late in the infectious cycle. Transient assays suggest that in poliovirus-infected cells, a decreased requirement for stem-loop F exists during the late phases of infection (87). The 5' NCR containing a deletion of stem-loop F is complemented in some unknown fashion by full-length poliovirus RNA molecules, perhaps by serving as a "sink" for cellular factors that are able to act in *trans* to facilitate internal ribosome binding of the mutated RNAs (103).

CELLULAR AND VIRAL FACTORS INTERACTING WITH THE IRES ELEMENTS OF ENTEROVIRAL RNAs

The observation that factors present in uninfected cells mediate internal ribosome entry on enteroviral RNAs resulted in a search for proteins binding to RNAs harboring IRES elements. Two approaches were employed to identify *trans*-acting factors: electrophoretic mobility shift analysis and UV cross-linking assays (95). In electrophoretic mobility shift assays, radiolabeled RNAs containing the sequence of interest are incubated with cellular extracts in binding buffer. Before the radiolabeled RNAs are added to the binding reaction mixtures, the extracts are saturated with a nonspecific riboheteropolymer, poly[I-C], to remove nonspecific RNA binding proteins present in eukaryotic cells. After complexes have formed, the bound and free radiolabeled RNAs are separated on a nondenaturing polyacrylamide gel. The gel migration of the RNAs bound to cellular factors is retarded owing to its increased molecular mass compared to that of the unbound RNA molecules. To determine whether the observed RNA-protein interactions are specific for enteroviral RNAs, competitions for binding of these factors are carried out by adding a large molar excess of specific or nonspecific RNAs to the binding reaction mixtures. If RNA-protein complex formation can be prevented in the presence of heterologous, nonspecific RNA, then the protein(s) does not bind to the viral RNA in a specific fashion. However, if complex formation can be inhibited by homologous competitor RNAs, then the RNA-protein interaction is specific. Thus, electrophoretic mobility shift assays determine whether polypeptides interact specifically with the RNA segment of interest. Electrophoretic mobility shift assays do not provide information regarding the number or sizes of the cellular proteins composing the retarded complex.

In contrast to electrophoretic mobility shift assays, RNA UV cross-linking assays indicate how many polypeptides bind directly to the

RNA and their approximate molecular weights. The disadvantage of this technique lies in the fact that only proteins that contact the RNA directly can be studied. In cross-linking assays, the cellular extracts are first incubated with a large excess of nonspecific poly[I-C] in binding buffer, and then the radiolabeled RNAs are added to the binding reaction. After complexes have formed, the reactions are exposed to UV irradiation (254 nm). An RNase cocktail is then added to the binding reactions such that RNA fragments not protected by proteins are degraded. Finally, the reactions are analyzed on a sodium dodecyl sulfate-polyacrylamide gel. The proteins that are bound to radiolabeled RNA fragments are detected after autoradiography.

By electrophoretic mobility shift analysis and UV cross-linking assays, a 50-kDa HeLa cell protein was shown to interact with stem-loop D of poliovirus RNA (nt 178 to 224) (Fig. 1). The protein appears to interact directly via a transient covalent adduct with the single-stranded loop, since an alteration of the loop sequence abolishes p50 binding. The nucleotide sequence context of the lower base-paired stem does not appear to be important, but the stem structure itself is required for binding (18, 77). The importance of this RNA-protein interaction with respect to internal ribosome entry is not known, since the sequences containing stem-loop D can be removed without significantly affecting internal ribosome binding (17, 103). However, this RNA-protein interaction is conserved among members of the enteroviruses, rhinoviruses, and cardioviruses (18). This observation suggests that the RNA-p50 interaction may play a role in the poliovirus life cycle in vivo that is not essential in a tissue culture system.

Additional RNA-protein interactions were revealed by electrophoretic mobility shift assays with labeled, subgenomic poliovirus RNAs. These experiments demonstrated that proteins present in HeLa cells interacted with poliovirus RNA sequences encompassing stem-loop E (nt 220 to 445) (Fig. 1). This observation is especially interesting, since stem-loop E of poliovirus is thought to be an integral part of the IRES element. The cellular factors binding to stem-loop E sequences may play an essential role in directing internal ribosome entry. Like the one described for stem-loop D, this RNA-protein interaction appears to be conserved among the *Enterovirus, Rhinovirus*, and *Cardiovirus* genera (18). Further studies showed that HeLa cell proteins binding to stem-loop E RNA have molecular masses of 38 and 48 kDa (27). The functions of p38 and p48 in the poliovirus life cycle and their roles in the uninfected cell are currently under investigation.

By using both electrophoretic mobility shift analysis and UV cross-linking assays, a 52-kDa protein present in HeLa cells was shown to interact with poliovirus RNA sequences from nt 559 to 624 (encompassing stem-loop G; Fig. 1). The binding site for p52 contains part of the conserved polypyrimidine tract. The factor, p52, is most abundant in HeLa cells and is present to a lesser extent in rabbit reticulocyte lysate and wheat germ extracts. No amino acid sequence homologies of p52 to known eukaryotic translation initiation factors were found (73). The 52-kDa protein was purified from HeLa cells, and subsequent protein sequencing identified this factor as the human La antigen. Interestingly, the La protein, predominantly a nuclear factor, is recognized by antibodies from patients with autoimmune disorders such as systemic lupus erythematosus and Sjögren's syndrome. In the uninfected cell, the La protein plays a role as an RNA polymerase III transcription termination factor. Scatchard analysis of a saturation binding curve yielded a dissociation constant for p52 binding to poliovirus RNA (nt 559 to 624) of 4×10^{-9} M. Poliovirus RNA translation was stimulated in a cell-free system upon the addition of purified p52. Attempts to reconstitute a HeLa cell cytoplasmic extract depleted of p52 (using antibodies directed against p52) by adding the recombinant La protein back to it failed to stimulate poliovirus RNA translation (74). These data suggest that the antibodies to p52 may fortuitously remove other cellular factors that are closely associated with p52 and that, alone or in concert with p52, mediate internal ribosome binding. The role of the La protein may indeed be to stimulate internal ribosome entry at the authentic start codon and to suppress the aberrant internal translation initiation in the P2-P3 regions of poliovirus RNA that has been observed when a cell-free translation system (rabbit reticulocyte lysate) was programmed with poliovirus RNA (21).

Three putative binding sites in the 5' NCR of poliovirus RNA (nt 70 to 288, 443 to 539, and 630 to 730) for a 57-kDa polypeptide present in partially purified fractions from HeLa cells were identified by UV cross-linking analysis (38). Studies using electrophoretic mobility shift assays demonstrated a binding site for recombinant p57 that was composed in part of the pyrimidine-rich sequences and the adjacent stem-loop structures, F and G (34). A mutated RNA bearing sequence alterations in the conserved polypyrimidine tract was not capable of interacting with recombinant p57 in vitro. However, a poliovirus harboring the same lesions in the polypyrimidine tract displayed a wild-type phenotype for growth in tissue culture (34). Thus, p57 binding to this region of the poliovirus 5' NCR may occur in a functionally nonspecific manner in vitro.

The factor p57 was initially identified in rabbit reticulocyte lysate as a polypeptide that interacted with EMCV RNAs containing the IRES element (46). Further characterization of p57 revealed that it is a member of a family of polypyrimidine tract-binding proteins (PTB) involved in pre-mRNA splicing (26, 76, 82). Immunoprecipitation experiments using antibodies directed against purified recombinant PTB suggested an antigenic relationship between p57 and PTB. In addition, binding studies using UV cross-linking assays with both proteins and the cyanogen bromide and V8 protease cleavage patterns strongly suggest that p57 and PTB are the same polypeptide (39). However, Witherell et al. (107) demonstrated that the recombinant p57 and the PTB present in cytoplasmic extracts derived from HeLa cells display different binding characteristics. Thus, p57 may obtain binding specificity for the IRES element from direct or indirect association with other polypeptides present in the cytoplasm of human cells.

PTB displays a dissociation constant of 20 nM in binding to subgenomic RNAs corresponding to EMCV IRES sequences and, although it is a nuclear factor, is associated with ribosomes (39). PTB contains four repeated RNA binding motifs, each 80 amino acids long, that can conceivably make multiple contacts with the 5' NCR of viral RNA (28, 50). The addition of antibodies to p57 to a cell-free translation system (rabbit reticulocyte lysate) inhibited translation of EMCV RNA as well as of poliovirus RNA, while the synthesis of globin was not affected. This experiment suggests a role for p57 in the process of mediating internal ribosome binding. However, a p57-immunodepleted HeLa cell extract could not support EMCV RNA translation upon addition of either purified or recombinant p57, implying that the p57 antibodies removed another factor closely associated with PTB that is essential for either p57 interaction with the 5' NCR or ribosome binding per se. Recently, evidence suggesting that p57 may not play an essential role in translation initiation by internal ribosome entry on viral RNAs harboring a type 2 IRES element was presented (8). A cytoplasmic extract prepared from HeLa cells was fractionated, and the individual fractions were tested for their abilities to stimulate cap-independent translation on rhinovirus RNAs. The results showed that p57 (or PTB) is part of a complex containing the stimulatory activity. However, within this complex, the translation stimulatory activity copurified with a 97-kDa protein that cross-linked to the rhinovirus 5' NCR but not to that of EMCV RNA. Collectively, these data demonstrate the presence in eukaryotic cells of specific *trans*-acting factors that can interact with the putative IRES elements of enteroviruses.

Additional studies that investigated the role

of the secondary structures formed by the 5' NCR of poliovirus RNA in the binding of cellular factors were initiated. In UV cross-linking assays, a 39-kDa protein present in extracts from HeLa and neuronal cells bound to stem-loop G sequences of poliovirus RNA. The question arose of whether additional cellular polypeptides bind to RNAs containing not only stem-loop G sequences but also the upstream sequences encompassing stem-loop F. While specific RNA-protein interactions were not observed with RNAs bearing stem-loop F sequences alone, an additional 36-kDa protein bound to an RNA encompassing stem-loops F and G of poliovirus RNA. The 36-kDa polypeptide is present in HeLa cells and neuronal cells (34). These data suggest that some cellular polypeptides require a synergistic interaction of neighboring stem-loop structures, perhaps at the level of RNA-RNA interactions, prior to binding. Presumably, the RNA-RNA interactions result in a protein-binding site within a tertiary structure context. The functional significance of these interactions and their importance for translation initiation by internal ribosome entry remain to be determined.

Stem-loop G sequences of poliovirus RNA also interact specifically with a 60-kDa protein found in neuronal cells but not detected in HeLa cells (32, 34). It is tempting to speculate that this 60-kDa polypeptide plays a functional role in the neurovirulence-attenuation phenotype displayed by polioviruses. Polioviruses are neurovirulent agents causing human poliomyelitis, a paralytic disease. Previous studies have demonstrated a correlation between the attenuation phenotype displayed by polioviruses, a point mutation in the 5' NCR of genomic RNA, and decreased levels of virus-specific protein synthesis in neuronal cells (58).

How do ribosomes bind internally on the viral RNAs of enteroviruses, and what are the possible roles of the above-described proteins? Some of the cellular polypeptides may interact with the IRES element directly, functioning as scaffolding proteins necessary to result in an active IRES configuration. These RNA-binding proteins may have not just one but multiple binding sites within the 5' NCRs of enterovirus RNAs. The multiple RNA-protein interactions may initiate the formation of a higher-order structure of the IRES element. The existence of a higher-order structure of the 5' NCR of poliovirus RNA is supported by the observation that point mutations and single nucleotide insertions or deletions in the 5' NCR are nearly always detrimental for viral functions (19, 84, 93, 100, 106). These data also suggest that some of the tertiary interactions are accomplished via RNA-RNA contacts, although no direct experimental evidence in support of this theory has been provided. Alternatively, the RNA-binding proteins may interact with the IRES to facilitate the binding of the 40S ribosomal subunit directly or, by recruiting other proteins involved in this complex process, indirectly. After binding of the 40S ribosomal subunit at the IRES, the ribosome either scans the viral RNA until the authentic translation initiation codon is located, or the 40S subunit is translocated in a nonlinear fashion to the start site of protein synthesis. When the 60S subunit joins the 40S subunit, synthesis of the viral proteins begins.

To date, no direct interactions of viral IRES sequences and virally encoded proteins have been reported. Intriguing results, however, suggest that polypeptide 2A, a viral proteinase, stimulates cap-independent translation initiation of mRNAs bearing the poliovirus 5' NCR during the early phases of infection of mammalian cells. For the first 2 h of infection, poliovirus mRNAs compete for the translation machinery with cellular mRNAs. This is a time during the virus life cycle when the virus has not completely effected the shutoff of cellular, cap-dependent translation. In addition to its role in host cell shutoff (see below), protein 2A appears to be a stimulatory *trans*-activator for the internal ribosome entry required for translation initiation of poliovirus mRNAs (35). If 2A interacts directly with the IRES element of poliovirus RNA, stem-loop F may harbor the 2A binding site, as Percy et al. (87) have shown a reduced requirement for these RNA sequences when they are used to direct translation of a reporter gene in cells coinfected with wild-type poliovirus. However, more recent results have allowed reinterpretation of these data to suggest that the IRES function can, in part, be complemented in *trans* by the presence of wild-type 5' NCR sequences (in the absence of any poliovirus coding region), possibly by RNA-RNA interactions (103). Genetic evidence supporting a direct interaction between stem-loop F of the 5' NCR of poliovirus RNA and the viral 2A proteinase was provided by Macadam et al. (69). In that study, non-temperature-sensitive revertants of temperature-sensitive polioviruses bearing nucleotide sequence alterations located in stem-loop F of the 5' NCR were isolated. An analysis of the revertant viral RNA genomes identified mutations in the coding region of the 2A proteinase. The revertant viruses containing mutated 2A proteinases had increased levels of viral protein synthesis during infection compared to the levels seen in cells infected by the *ts* mutants or parental Sabin virus. These data suggest a role for the viral 2A proteinase in cap-independent translation initiation. However, 2A may carry out the stimulation of internal ribosome binding of poliovirus mRNAs by other mechanisms, e.g., protein-protein-mediated activation, that remain to be elucidated.

HOST CELL SHUTOFF

Enteroviruses are virulent viruses that lyse the host cell upon release of the viral progeny. Prior to cell lysis, the global macromolecular synthesis of the host cell (RNA transcription, DNA replication, and protein synthesis), the membrane structures of the cell, and the cytoskeletal-microtubule-associated proteins are perturbed by poliovirus infection (6, 11, 12, 15, 23, 47, 53, 67) (see chapter 6). In poliovirus-infected cells, an inhibition of host cell protein synthesis is followed by a stimulation of viral protein synthesis (22) (Fig. 4). The inhibition of cap-dependent translation initia-

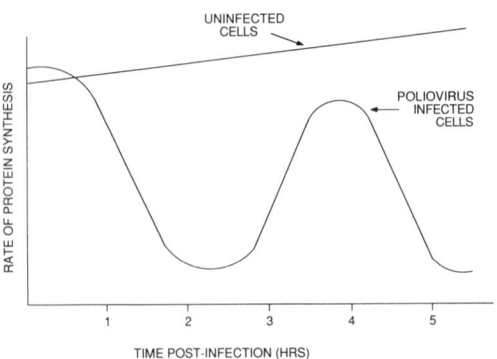

FIGURE 4 Kinetics of protein synthesis in poliovirus-infected cells compared to the rate of protein synthesis in uninfected cells. By approximately 2 h postinfection, cap-dependent cellular protein synthesis has ceased in infected cells. By 3.5 to 4 h postinfection, cap-independent virus-specific protein synthesis occurs at high levels. In uninfected cells, continuous cellular protein synthesis is observed. (Adapted from reference 22 with permission.)

tion is quite rapid, and within 2 h postinfection, cell protein synthesis is severely impaired. This inhibition results in the preferential translation of virus-specific uncapped mRNAs over cellular capped mRNAs.

The defect in host cell protein synthesis is thought to involve the inactivation of polypeptides associated with a cap-binding protein complex (CBP or eIF-4F). The translation initiation factor eIF-4F is also referred to as eIF-4 by an alternative nomenclature. An antiserum against eIF-3 detected a protein with a molecular weight of 220,000 (p220) in lysates from uninfected HeLa cells that was not present in lysates from infected cells. Cytoplasmic extracts from poliovirus-infected cells contained antigenically related polypeptides of 100,000 to 130,000 Da, presumably proteolytic degradation products (23). p220 was shown to be part of the multiprotein complex eIF-4F, but its function in cap-dependent translation initiation is not known. p220 may provide an electrostatic interaction with RNA and the major protein contacts necessary for interaction with eIF-3 and the 40S ribosomal subunit (75).

The gene for human p220 was recently cloned and shown to encode a 154-kDa polypeptide that contains numerous potential glycosylation and phosphorylation sites and a high PEST score (the latter property indicating a predisposition toward proteolytic degradation; 110). eIF-4F is composed of p220 and eIF-4E, the cap recognition protein. Two other cellular factors, namely, eIF-4A (an ATP-dependent bidirectional RNA helicase and a member of the D-E-A-D box protein family) and eIF-4B (a polypeptide that stimulates the activities of eIF-4F and eIF-4A) are closely associated with eIF-4F (65, 97). In a time course experiment, the degradation of p220 correlated well with that observed for the inhibition of cellular protein synthesis in vivo (23). The results suggested that p220 can associate with eIF-3, although p220 constitutes an integral component of eIF-4F. The degradation of p220 may be responsible for the shutoff of host cell protein synthesis in virus-infected cells (23). Further support for this idea is provided by the observation that the inhibition of translation initiation of capped mRNAs in extracts from virus-infected cells can be alleviated by the addition of intact eIF-4F (63).

The proteolysis of p220 prompted a search for either viral or cellular proteases directing this cleavage. A natural candidate was the poliovirus proteinase 3C. Data derived from partial purification of an activity from poliovirus-infected cells that cleaves the p220 component of eIF-4F suggested that viral proteinase 3C is not involved in the shutoff of cap-dependent cellular translation. In the presence of 3C antibodies, the protease activity of 3C was inhibited, although p220 cleavage still occurred (62, 66). A similar approach was applied to test the involvement of the second viral proteinase, 2A, in host cell shutoff. Lloyd et al. (68) demonstrated that the activity that cleaves p220 and the viral 2A proteinase do not copurify, that partially purified fractions containing the p220 cleavage activity do not react with 2A antibodies, and that 2A antibodies cannot inhibit p220 cleavage in vitro.

However, a functionally active 2A proteinase appears to be required for efficient cleavage of p220 in poliovirus-infected cells. Perhaps a functional 2A^{pro} is necessary to activate a latent cellular protease in a cascade of molecular events (67). Mutated poliovirus cDNAs that harbored lesions (insertions or deletions) disrupting the 2A coding sequence resulted in an inactive 2A^{pro} enzyme. The 2A activity was assayed by the ability of 2A to autocatalyze the *cis* cleavage between its own amino terminus and the P1 capsid precursor. An inactive 2A proteinase of poliovirus did not mediate the cleavage of p220 (56). An 18-amino-acid segment in the carboxy terminus of 2A is highly conserved among the enteroviruses and rhinoviruses. The conserved 2A sequence is homologous with essential elements of the active site of the 3C proteinase of poliovirus. The picornaviruses that cleave p220, such as the enteroviruses and rhinoviruses, bear this amino acid sequence of 2A. In contrast, the picornaviruses that do not cleave p220 in vivo, i.e., the cardioviruses, do not encode the equivalent proteinase sequence in the 2A region (67). Further mutational analyses of the 2A proteinase of poliovirus indicated that 2A is a trypsinlike serine proteinase. These data also suggested that the cellular factor that is responsible for p220 degradation may be activated by 2A-catalyzed proteolytic cleavage itself (37).

The role of other cellular proteins in the virus-induced host cell shutoff of protein synthesis was further investigated. A cell-free assay was developed to identify the components involved in this process. In this assay, a partially purified p220 substrate was incubated with an extract from *Escherichia coli* expressing the viral 2A proteinase. As expected, p220 was not efficiently cleaved, suggesting that 2A alone is not sufficient for p220 cleavage. Fractions of a cytoplasmic extract from HeLa cells containing translation initiation factors were added to the in vitro assay to define the cellular factors catalyzing p220 cleavage. Proteolysis of p220 was observed in the presence of the 2A proteinase and a fraction enriched in eIF-3 (108). These data allowed the formation of various models. In one model, an eIF-3–eIF-4F complex presents p220 in the proper conformation to be a substrate for cleavage by the viral 2A proteinase or by the cellular protease activated by 2A (Fig. 5). In the other model, eIF-3 is the cellular protease that cleaves p220 after activation by 2A. To date, eIF-3 has not been reported to be a protease, and this activity appears to be disadvantageous for a factor involved in protein synthesis. It was further demonstrated that eIF-3 was functional in extracts derived from uninfected as well as from virus-infected cells (24). The p220 cleavage activity present in eukaryotic cells and eIF-3 do not copurify. However, eIF-3 is composed of seven subunits, and it is possible that one of these subunits is modified during poliovirus infection and mediates the p220 cleavage.

Further research resolved the p220 cleavage activity from eIF-3-containing fractions by gel filtration and anion-exchange chromatography. The cellular protease activity was partially purified, and it was shown to be a protein of 55 to 60 kDa. Alkylating agents and metals inhibit the p220 protease, indicating the presence of reactive thiol groups. Upon incubation of this partially purified cellular protease with p220, cleavage occurred, but only in the presence of eIF-3. Thus, eIF-3 plays an essential role in p220 proteolysis after the latent cellular protease is already activated by the viral 2A proteinase (109). The precise function of eIF-3 in the shutoff of cap-dependent protein synthesis is still not known.

Recently, the 2A proteinases of coxsackievirus type B4 and a closely related picornavirus, human rhinovirus type 2, were expressed in *E. coli* in soluble form and purified. In contrast to the reported activity of the 2A proteinase of poliovirus, both enzymes cleaved the p220 subunit of eIF-4F directly at a single site in vitro. A drastic reduction in the translation efficiencies of capped mRNAs was observed in HeLa cell cytoplasmic extracts preincubated with 2A proteinase. The addition of purified eIF-4F restored the translation of capped mRNAs to the initial level. Interestingly, in the presence of the human rhinovirus 2A proteinase, the levels of synthesis of a reporter gene driven by the 5' NCR of human rhinovirus were stimulated two- to threefold (64). This observation correlates well with the data obtained by Hambidge and Sarnow (35), who reported that the 2A proteinase of poliovirus could act as a stimulatory *trans*-activator of mRNAs employing internal ribosome entry for translation initiation. The presence of eIF-3 did not affect the cleavage activity of the 2A proteinases (59). These observations suggest that the 2A proteinases of poliovirus, coxsackievirus, and rhinovirus may employ different mechanisms to cleave eIF-4F, ultimately resulting in the inhibition of host cell protein synthesis (Fig. 5).

Picornavirus strategies for achieving a pref-

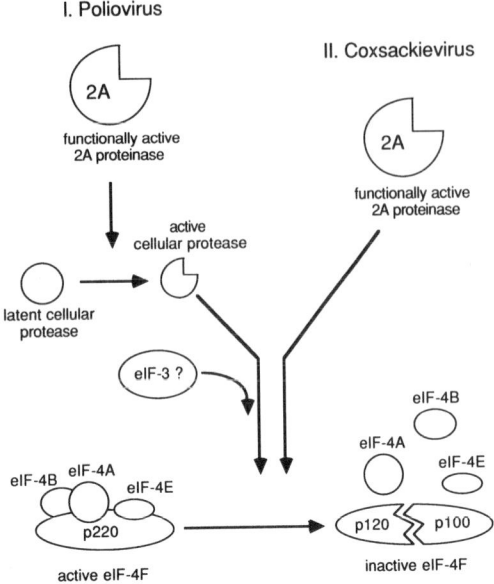

FIGURE 5 Models of shutoff of host cell protein synthesis for poliovirus and coxsackievirus. In poliovirus-infected cells, a latent cellular protease is activated by the viral 2A^{pro}, perhaps by proteolysis. The cellular protease carries out the cleavage of p220, a component of eIF-4F, in the presence of eIF-3, resulting in inactive eIF-4F and an inhibition of cap-dependent translation initiation. In contrast, the coxsackievirus 2A^{pro} can carry out p220 cleavage itself without a requirement for eIF-3.

erential translation of viral mRNAs utilizing the host cell translation machinery have evolved in many different directions. As described above, enteroviruses and rhinoviruses require the 2A proteinase activity to mediate p220 cleavage directly or indirectly. FMDV, an aphthovirus, contains only 16 amino acids reminiscent of the picornavirus 2A proteinase. However, a small leader protein that is translated from two open reading frames, since initiation of protein synthesis on FMDV RNA occurs at two sites, functions as a protease that directs the p220 cleavage (16, 71). The L protein cleaves itself autocatalytically from the structural protein precursor, P1 (104). It is not known whether the L protein cleaves p220 directly or whether it activates a latent cellular protease that carries out the p220 cleavage. The L protein has been predicted by amino acid sequence alignment to be a thiol protease related to the papain family of proteases (31). An inhibitor of papain proteases [L-*trans*-epoxysuccinyl-leucylamido(4-guanidino)butane, or E-64] was tested as an inhibitor of the L protein of FMDV. The results demonstrated an interference in virus assembly, a reduction in virus yield, a decrease in viral protein and RNA synthesis, and a delay in cleavage of p220 (52). The cleavage products of p220 in FMDV-infected cells differ from those found in poliovirus-infected cells. This observation may imply a different mechanism or may simply underscore the differences between the trypsinlike serine proteinases (like 2A) and the papain proteases (like the L protein) (52). Interestingly, EMCV, a member of the genus *Cardiovirus*, possesses both a functional cleavage activity encoded in a position comparable to enterovirus 2A sequences and a leader protein. The leader protein does not appear to have a protease activity, and the 3C proteinase carries out its cleavage from the P1 precursor (81). Cardioviruses do not cause a shutoff of host cell protein synthesis by p220 cleavage. Rather, EMCV competes for the cellular translation machinery by means of a strong ribosome-binding element (60).

Other investigators reported that p220 cleavage is not the sole event that brings about the shutoff of host cell translation observed in poliovirus-infected cells. Experiments were carried out in the presence of viral replication inhibitors to show that at a time during infection when the majority of p220 was cleaved, cellular translation still occurred at significant levels (88). A careful look at the genetic experiments of Bernstein et al. (4) suggests additional complexities in the pathway leading to shutoff of cap-dependent translation by enteroviruses. Those authors described a mutant poliovirus, bearing a lesion in the 2A proteinase-coding sequence, that was unable to catalyze p220 cleavage. However, at late times during infection by this mutant, a global shutoff of viral and cellular protein synthesis was observed (4). In addition, upon transient expression of 2A as part of a dicistronic construct in COS-1 monkey kidney cells, only a threefold reduction of translation of the capped reporter mRNA (globin mRNA) was observed (15). Finally, Bonneau and Sonenberg (7) demonstrated that proteolysis of p220 results in only partial inhibition of host cell shutoff of protein synthesis 3.5 h after poliovirus infection (about 55 to 77% of host protein synthesis is suppressed). These observations allow speculation that it may not be the cleavage of the p220 component of eIF-4F that is responsible for the inhibition of host cell protein synthesis but rather a viral protein that promotes or stimulates this process. Alternatively, more than one pathway to inhibit cellular protein synthesis upon enteroviral infection may have evolved.

It has long been recognized that enteroviral infections of primate cells lead to inhibition of cellular RNA synthesis (40). The inhibition of RNA synthesis could result from an alteration of the cellular RNA polymerases (I, II, and III) or from the modification of transcription-associated cellular proteins. Observations that support the latter hypothesis have been made. In vitro transcription assays with crude and fractionated extracts demonstrated that poliovirus infection inactivates one or more transcription factors associated with RNA polymerase I (98), II (14), or III (25). Indeed, a loss of the phosphorylated form of transcription factor CREB/ATF, a factor involved in RNA polymerase II-mediated transcription, was detected in poliovirus-infected cells (53).

The viral proteins that mediate the inhibition of cellular RNA synthesis include the 2A and 3C proteinases. Davies et al. (15) observed that the expression of the 2A proteinase of poliovirus had a dramatic effect on RNA polymerase II transcription and, to a lesser extent, on cellular DNA replication. In addition, Clark et al. (12) demonstrated that proteinase 3C converted an active form of transcription factor IIIC, required for RNA polymerase III-mediated transcription, to an inactive form via proteolytic cleavage, thereby inhibiting host cell RNA polymerase III activity. More recently, the human TATA-binding protein was shown to be susceptible to direct cleavage by poliovirus 3C proteinase in vivo and in vitro. The cleavage of the TATA-binding protein resulted in an inhibition of host cell RNA polymerase II-mediated transcription (13). Further studies are required to determine the precise roles of different viral proteins in the inhibition of cellular RNA synthesis during an enteroviral infection of cultured cells.

The results given above describe a synergistic interplay between the levels of translation initiation on viral RNAs by internal ribosome entry and the shutoff of host cell macromolecular synthesis observed in enterovirus-infected cells. The rate of cap-independent translation initiation of viral RNAs directs the viral 2A proteinase concentrations in the virus-infected host cell. Apparently, low levels of 2A enzyme are sufficient for p220 cleavage mediated directly or indirectly. The 2A enzyme must be proteolytically active to initiate the cellular cascade that culminates in p220 cleavage, thereby inactivating eIF-4F and presumably inhibiting host cell protein synthesis. The processed form of eIF-4F was shown to positively influence translation initiation by internal ribosome binding. Additionally, the viral 2A^{pro} enzyme itself stimulates cap-independent translation initiation during the early phases of the virus infection. These results implicate the viral 2A proteinase as a key factor involved not only in the shutoff of host cell protein synthesis, which in itself stimulates cap-independent translation initiation, but also in the stimulation of internal ribosome entry of viral RNAs during infection.

REFERENCES

1. **Ambros, V., and D. Baltimore.** 1978. Protein is linked to the 5' end of poliovirus RNA by phosphodiester linkage to tyrosine. *J. Biol. Chem.* **253:**5263–5266.
2. **Andino, R., G. E. Rieckhof, and D. Baltimore.** 1990. A functional ribonucleoprotein complex forms around the 5' end of poliovirus RNA. *Cell* **63:**369–380.
3. **Anthony, D. D., and W. C. Merrick.** 1991. Eukaryotic initiation factor (eIF)-4F: implications for a role in internal initiation of translation. *J. Biol. Chem.* **266:**10218–10226.
4. **Bernstein, H. D., N. Sonenberg, and D. Baltimore.** 1985. Poliovirus mutant that does not selectively inhibit host cell protein synthesis. *Mol. Cell. Biol.* **5:**2913–2923.
5. **Bienkowska-Szewczyk, K., and E. Ehrenfeld.** 1988. An internal 5'-noncoding region required for translation of poliovirus RNA in vitro. *J. Virol.* **62:**3068–3072.
6. **Bienz, K., D. Egger, Y. Rasser, and W. Bossart.** 1983. Intracellular distribution of poliovirus proteins and the induction of virus-specific cytoplasmic structures. *Virology* **131:**39–48.
7. **Bonneau, A.-M., and N. Sonenberg.** 1987. Proteolysis of the p220 component of the cap-binding protein complex is not sufficient for complete inhibition of host cell protein synthesis after poliovirus infection. *J. Virol.* **61:**986–991.
8. **Borman, A., M. T. Howell, J. G. Patton, and R. J. Jackson.** 1993. The involvement of a spliceosome component in internal initiation of human rhinovirus RNA translation. *J. Gen. Virol.* **74:**1775–1788.
9. **Brown, B. A., and E. Ehrenfeld.** 1979. Translation of poliovirus RNA in vitro: changes in cleavage pattern and initiation sites by ribosomal salt wash. *Virology* **97:**396–405.
10. **Buckley, B., and E. Ehrenfeld.** 1987. The cap-binding protein complex in uninfected and poliovirus-infected HeLa cells. *J. Biol. Chem.*

262:13599–13606.
11. **Clark, M., and A. Dasgupta.** 1990. A transcriptionally active form of TFIIIC is modified in poliovirus-infected HeLa cells. *Mol. Cell. Biol.* **10:**5106–5113.
12. **Clark, M., T. Haemmerle, E. Wimmer, and A. Dasgupta.** 1991. Poliovirus proteinase 3C converts an active form of transcription factor IIIC to an inactive form: a mechanism for inhibition of host cell polymerase III transcription by poliovirus. *EMBO J.* **10:**2941–2947.
13. **Clark, M. E., P. M. Lieberman, A. J. Berk, and A. Dasgupta.** 1993. Direct cleavage of human TATA-binding protein by poliovirus protease 3C in vivo and in vitro. *Mol. Cell. Biol.* **13:**1232–1237.
14. **Crawford, N., A. Fire, M. Samuels, P. A. Sharp, and D. Baltimore.** 1981. Inhibition of transcription factor activity by poliovirus. *Cell* **27:**555–561.
15. **Davies, M. V., J. Pelletier, K. Meerovitch, N. Sonenberg, and R. J. Kaufman.** 1991. The effect of poliovirus proteinase 2A^{pro} expression on cellular metabolism. *J. Biol. Chem.* **266:**14714–14720.
16. **Devaney, M. A., V. N. Vakharia, R. E. Lloyd, E. Ehrenfeld, and M. J. Grubman.** 1988. Leader protein of foot-and-mouth disease virus is required for cleavage of the p220 component of the cap-binding protein complex. *J. Virol.* **62:**4407–4409.
17. **Dildine, S. L., and B. L. Semler.** 1989. The deletion of 41 proximal nucleotides reverts a poliovirus mutant containing a temperature-sensitive lesion in the 5' noncoding region of genomic RNA. *J. Virol.* **63:**847–862.
18. **Dildine, S. L., and B. L. Semler.** 1992. Conservation of RNA-protein interactions among picornaviruses. *J. Virol.* **66:**4364–4376.
19. **Dildine, S. L., K. R. Stark, A. A. Haller, and B. L. Semler.** 1991. Poliovirus translation initiation: differential effects of directed and selected mutations in the 5' noncoding region of viral RNAs. *Virology* **182:**742–752.
20. **Dorner, A. J., L. F. Dorner, G. R. Larsen, E. Wimmer, and C. W. Anderson.** 1982. Identification of the initiation site of poliovirus polyprotein synthesis. *J. Virol.* **42:**1017–1028.
21. **Dorner, A. J., B. L. Semler, R. J. Jackson, R. Hanecak, E. Duprey, and E. Wimmer.** 1984. In vitro translation of poliovirus RNA: utilization of internal initiation sites in reticulocyte lysate. *J. Virol.* **50:**507–514.
22. **Ehrenfeld, E.** 1984. Picornavirus inhibition of host cell protein synthesis, p. 177–221. *In* H. Fraenkel-Conrat and R. R. Wagner (ed.), *Comprehensive Virology*, vol. 19. Plenum Press, New York.
23. **Etchison, D., S. Milburn, I. Edery, N. Sonenberg, and J. W. B. Hershey.** 1982. Inhibition of HeLa cell protein synthesis following poliovirus infection correlates with the proteolysis of a 220,000 dalton polypeptide associated with eucaryotic initiation factor 3 and a cap binding protein complex. *J. Biol. Chem.* **257:**14806–14810.
24. **Etchison, D. S., J. Hansen, E. Ehrenfeld, I. Edery, N. Sonenberg, S. Milburn, and J. W. B. Hershey.** 1984. Demonstration in vitro that eucaryotic initiation factor 3 is active but that a cap-binding protein complex is inactive in poliovirus-infected cells. *J. Virol.* **51:**832–837.
25. **Fradkin, L. G., S. K. Yoshinaga, A. J. Berk, and A. Dasgupta.** 1987. Inhibition of host cell RNA polymerase III-mediated transcription by poliovirus: inactivation of specific transcription factors. *Mol. Cell Biol.* **7:**3880–3887.
26. **Garcia-Blanco, M. A., S. F. Jamison, and P. A. Sharp.** 1989. Identification and purification of a 62,000-dalton protein that binds specifically to the polypyrimidine tract of introns. *Genes Dev.* **3:**1874–1886.
27. **Gebhard, J. R., and E. Ehrenfeld.** 1992. Specific interactions of HeLa cell proteins with proposed translation domains of the poliovirus 5' noncoding region. *J. Virol.* **66:**3101–3109.
28. **Ghetti, A., S. Piol-Roma, W. M. Michael, C. Morandi, and G. Dreyfuss.** 1992. hnRNP I, the polypyrimidine tract-binding protein: distinct nuclear localization and association with hn RNAs. *Nucleic Acids Res.* **20:**3671–3678.
29. **Gmyl, A. P., E. V. Pilipenko, S. V. Maslova, G. A. Belov, and V. I. Agol.** 1993. Functional and genetic plasticities of the poliovirus genome: quasi-infectious RNAs modified in the 5'-untranslated region yield a variety of pseudorevertants. *J. Virol.* **67:**6309–6316.
30. **Golini, F., B. L. Semler, A. J. Dorner, and E. Wimmer.** 1980. Protein-linked RNA of poliovirus is competent to form an initiation complex of translation *in vitro*. *Nature* (London) **287:**600–603.
31. **Gorbalenya, A. E., E. V. Koonin, and M. M.-C. Lai.** 1991. Putative papain-related thiol proteases of positive-strand RNA viruses: identification of rubi- and aphthovirus proteases and delineation of a novel conserved domain associated with proteases of rubi-, alpha-, and coronaviruses. *FEBS Lett.* **288:**201–205.
32. **Haller, A. A., J. H. C. Nguyen, and B. L. Semler.** 1993. Minimum internal ribosome entry site required for poliovirus infectivity. *J. Virol.* **67:**7461–7471.
33. **Haller, A. A., and B. L. Semler.** 1992.

Linker scanning mutagenesis of the internal ribosome entry site of poliovirus RNA. *J. Virol.* **66:**5075–5086.

34. **Haller, A. A., and B. L. Semler.** Stem-loop structure synergy in binding cellular proteins to the 5' noncoding region of poliovirus RNA. *Virology,* in press.

35. **Hambidge, S. J., and P. Sarnow.** 1992. Translational enhancement of the poliovirus 5' noncoding region mediated by virus-encoded polypeptide 2A. *Proc. Natl. Acad. Sci. USA* **89:**10272–10276.

36. **Harber, J., and E. Wimmer.** 1993. Aspects of the molecular biology of picornaviruses, p. 189–224. *In* L. Carrasco, N. Sonenberg, and E. Wimmer (ed.), *Regulation of Gene Expression in Animal Viruses.* Plenum Press, New York.

37. **Hellen, C. U. T., M. Faecke, H.-G. Kraeusslich, C.-K. Lee, and E. Wimmer.** 1991. Characterization of poliovirus 2A proteinase by mutational analysis: residues required for autocatalytic activity are essential for induction of cleavage of eukaryotic initiation factor 4F polypeptide p220. *J. Virol.* **65:**4226–4231.

38. **Hellen, C. U. T., T. V. Pestova, M. Litterst, and E. Wimmer.** 1994. The cellular polypeptide p57 (pyrimidine tract-binding protein) binds to multiple sites in the poliovirus 5' nontranslated region. *J. Virol.* **68:**941–950.

39. **Hellen, C. U. T., G. W. Witherell, M. Schmid, S. H. Shin, T. V. Pestova, A. Gil, and E. Wimmer.** 1993. A cytoplasmic 57 kDa protein (p57) that is required for translation of picornavirus RNA by internal ribosome entry is identical to the nuclear polypyrimidine tract-binding protein. *Proc. Natl. Acad. Sci. USA* **90:**7642–7646.

40. **Holland, J. J.** 1962. Inhibition of DNA-primed RNA synthesis during poliovirus infection of human cells. *Biochem. Biophys. Res. Commun.* **9:**556–573.

41. **Iizuka, N., M. Kohara, K. Hagino-Yamagishi, S. Abe, T. Komatsu, K. Tago, M. Arita, and A. Nomoto.** 1989. Construction of less neurovirulent polioviruses by introducing deletions into the 5' noncoding sequence of the genome. *J. Virol.* **63:**5354–5363.

42. **Iizuka, N., H. Yonekawa, and A. Nomoto.** 1991. Nucleotide sequences important for translation initiation of enterovirus RNA. *J. Virol.* **65:**4867–4873.

43. **Jackson, R. J., M. T. Howell, and A. Kaminski.** 1990. The novel mechanism of initiation of picornavirus RNA translation. *Trends Biochem. Sci.* **15:**477–483.

44. **Jacobson, S. J., D. A. M. Konings, and P. Sarnow.** 1993. Biochemical and genetic evidence for a pseudoknot structure at the 3' terminus of the poliovirus RNA genome and its role in viral RNA amplification. *J. Virol.* **67:**2961–2971.

45. **Jang, S. K., H. G. Kräusslich, M. J. H. Nicklin, G. M. Duke, A. C. Palmenberg, and E. Wimmer.** 1988. A segment of the 5' untranslated region of encephalomyelitis virus RNA directs internal entry of ribosomes during in vitro translation. *J. Virol.* **62:**2636–2643.

46. **Jang, S. K., T. V. Pestova, C. U. T. Hellen, G. W. Witherell, and E. Wimmer.** 1990. Cap-independent translation of picornavirus RNAs: structure and function of the internal ribosomal entry site. *Enzyme* **44:**292–309.

47. **Joachims, M., and D. Etchison.** 1992. Poliovirus infection results in structural alteration of a microtubule-associated protein. *J. Virol.* **66:**5797–5804.

48. **Johnson, V. H., and B. L. Semler.** 1988. Defined recombinants of poliovirus and coxsackievirus: sequence-specific deletions and functional substitutions in the 5'-noncoding regions of viral RNAs. *Virology* **162:**47–57.

49. **Kaminski, A., T. Howell, and R. J. Jackson.** 1990. Initiation of encephalomyocarditis virus RNA translation: the authentic initiation site is not selected by a scanning mechanism. *EMBO J.* **9:**3753–3759.

50. **Kenan, D. J., C. C. Query, and J. D. Keene.** 1991. RNA recognition: towards identifying determinants of specificity. *Trends Biochem. Sci.* **16:**214–220.

51. **Kitamura, N., B. L. Semler, P. G. Rothberg, G. R. Larsen, C. J. Adler, A. J. Dorner, E. A. Emini, R. Hanecak, J. J. Lee, S. van der Werf, C. W. Anderson, and E. Wimmer.** 1981. Primary structure, gene organization, and polypeptide expression of poliovirus RNA. *Nature* (London) **291:**547–553.

52. **Kleina, L. G., and M. J. Grubman.** 1992. Antiviral effects of a thiol protease inhibitor on foot-and-mouth disease virus. *J. Virol.* **66:**7168–7175.

53. **Kliewer, S., C. Muchardt, R. Gaynor, and A. Dasgupta.** 1990. Loss of a phosphorylated form of transcription factor CREB/ATF in poliovirus-infected cells. *J. Virol.* **64:**4507–4515.

54. **Kozak, M.** 1989. The scanning model for translation: an update. *J. Cell Biol.* **108:**229–241.

55. **Kozak, M.** 1991. Structural features in eukaryotic mRNAs that modulate the initiation of translation. *J. Biol. Chem.* **266:**19867–19870.

56. **Kraeusslich, H. G., M. J. H. Nicklin, H. Toyoda, D. Etchison, and E. Wimmer.** 1987. Poliovirus proteinase 2A induces cleav-

age of eukaryotic initiation factor 4F polypeptide p220. *J. Virol.* **61:**2711–2718.
57. Kuge, S., N. Kawamura, and A. Nomoto. 1989. Genetic variation occurring in the genome of an in vitro insertion mutant of poliovirus type 1. *J. Virol.* **63:**1069–1075.
58. La Monica, N., and V. R. Racaniello. 1989. Differences in replication of attenuated and neurovirulent polioviruses in human neuroblastoma cell line SH-SY5Y. *J. Virol.* **63:**2357–2360.
59. Lampheart, B. J., R. Yan, F. Yang, D. Waters, H.-D. Liebig, H. Klump, E. Kuechler, T. Skern, and R. E. Rhoads. 1993. Mapping the cleavage site in protein synthesis initiation factor eIF-4 gamma of the 2A proteases from human coxsackievirus and rhinovirus. *J. Biol. Chem.* **268:**19200–19203.
60. Lawrence, C., and R. E. Thatch. 1974. Encephalomyocarditis virus infection of mouse plasmacytoma cells. *J. Virol.* **14:**598–610.
61. Le, S.-Y., and M. Zuker. 1990. Common structures of the 5' non-coding RNA in enteroviruses and rhinoviruses. *J. Mol. Biol.* **216:**729–741.
62. Lee, K. A. W., I. Edery, R. Hanecak, E. Wimmer, and N. Sonenberg. 1985. Poliovirus protease 3C (P3-7c) does not cleave p220 of the eukaryotic mRNA cap-binding protein complex. *J. Virol.* **55:**489–493.
63. Lee, K. A. W., and N. Sonenberg. 1982. Inactivation of cap-binding proteins accompanies the shut-off of host protein synthesis by poliovirus. *Proc. Natl. Acad. Sci. USA* **79:**3447–3451.
64. Liebig, H.-D., E. Ziegler, R. Yan, K. Hartmuth, H. Klump, H. Kowalski, D. Blaas, W. Sommergruber, L. Frasel, B. J. Lampheart, R. E. Rhoads, E. Kuechler, and T. Skern. 1993. Purification of two picornaviral 2A proteinases: interaction with eIF-4 gamma and influence on in vitro translation. *Biochemistry* **32:**7581–7588.
65. Linder, P., P. F. Lasko, P. Leroy, M. Ashburner, P. Nielsen, K. Nishi, J. Schnier, and P. P. Slonimski. 1989. Birth of the D-E-A-D box. *Nature* (London) **337:**121–122.
66. Lloyd, R. E., D. Etchison, and E. Ehrenfeld. 1985. Poliovirus protease does not mediate cleavage of the 220,000-Da component of the cap binding protein complex. *Proc. Natl. Acad. Sci. USA* **82:**2723–2727.
67. Lloyd, R. E., M. Grubman, and E. Ehrenfeld. 1988. Relationship of p220 cleavage during picornavirus infection to 2A proteinase sequences. *J. Virol.* **62:**4216–4223.
68. Lloyd, R. E., H. Toyoda, D. Etchison, E. Wimmer, and E. Ehrenfeld. 1986. Cleavage of the cap binding protein complex polypeptide p220 is not effected by the second poliovirus protease 2A. *Virology* **150:**299–303.
69. Macadam, A. J., G. Ferguson, T. Fleming, D. M. Stone, J. W. Almond, and P. D. Minor. 1994. Role for poliovirus protease 2A in cap independent translation. *EMBO J.* **13:**924–927.
70. Macejak, D. G., and P. Sarnow. 1991. Internal initiation of translation mediated by the 5' leader of a cellular mRNA. *Nature* (London) **353:**90–94.
71. Medina, M., E. Domingo, J. K. Brangwyn, and G. J. Belsham. 1993. The two species of the foot-and-mouth disease virus leader protein, expressed individually, exhibit the same activities. *Virology* **194:**355–359.
72. Meerovitch, K., R. Nicholson, and N. Sonenberg. 1991. In vitro mutational analysis of cis-acting RNA translational elements within the poliovirus type 2 5' untranslated region. *J. Virol.* **65:**5895–5901.
73. Meerovitch, K., J. Pelletier, and N. Sonenberg. 1989. A cellular protein that binds to the 5'-noncoding region of poliovirus RNA: implications for internal translation initiation. *Genes Dev.* **3:**1026–1034.
74. Meerovitch, K., Y. U. Svitkin, H. S. Lee, F. Lejbkowicz, D. J. Kenan, E. K. L. Chan, V. I. Agol, J. D. Keene, and N. Sonenberg. 1993. La autoantigen enhances and corrects aberrant translation of poliovirus RNA in reticulocyte lysate. *J. Virol.* **67:**3798–3807.
75. Merrick, W. C. 1990. Overview: mechanism of translation initiation in eukaryotes. *Enzyme* **44:**7–16.
76. Morris, D. R., T. Kakegawa, R. L. Kaspar, and M. W. White. 1993. Polypyrimidine tracts and their binding proteins: regulatory sites for posttranscriptional modulation of gene expression. *Biochemistry* **32:**2931–2937.
77. Najita, L., and P. Sarnow. 1990. Oxidation-reduction sensitive interaction of a cellular 50-kD protein with an RNA hairpin in the 5' noncoding region of the poliovirus genome. *Proc. Natl. Acad. Sci. USA* **87:**5846–5850.
78. Nicholson, R., J. Pelletier, S. Le, and N. Sonenberg. 1991. Structural and functional analysis of the ribosome landing pad of poliovirus type 2: in vivo translational studies. *J. Virol.* **65:**5886–5894.
79. Nomoto, A., Y. F. Lee, and E. Wimmer. 1976. The 5'-end of poliovirus mRNA is not capped with m7G(5')ppp(5')Np. *Proc. Natl. Acad. Sci. USA* **73:**375–380.
80. OH, S.-K., M. P. Scott, and P. Sarnow. 1992. Homeotic gene Antennapedia mRNA

contains 5'-noncoding sequences that confer translational initiation by internal ribosome binding. *Genes Dev.* **6:**1643–1653.
81. **Parks, G. D., G. M. Duke, and A. C. Palmenberg.** 1986. Encephalomyocarditis virus 3C protease: efficient cell-free expression from clones which link viral 5' noncoding sequences to the P3 region. *J. Virol.* **60:**376–384.
82. **Patton, J. G., S. A. Mayer, P. Tempst, and B. Nadal-Ginard.** 1991. Characterization and molecular cloning of polypyrimidine tract-binding protein: a component of a complex necessary for pre-mRNA splicing. *Genes Dev.* **5:**1237–1251.
83. **Pelletier, J., M. E. Flynn, G. Kaplan, V. Racaniello, and N. Sonenberg.** 1988. Mutational analysis of upstream AUG codons of poliovirus RNA. *J. Virol.* **62:**4486–4492.
84. **Pelletier, J., G. Kaplan, V. R. Racaniello, and N. Sonenberg.** 1988. Cap-independent translation of poliovirus mRNA is conferred by sequence elements within the 5' noncoding region. *Mol. Cell. Biol.* **8:**1103–1112.
85. **Pelletier, J., and N. Sonenberg.** 1988. Internal initiation of translation of eukaryotic mRNA directed by a sequence derived from poliovirus RNA. *Nature* (London) **334:**320–325.
86. **Pelletier, J., and N. Sonenberg.** 1989. Internal binding of eukaryotic ribosomes on poliovirus RNA: translation in HeLa cell extracts. *J. Virol.* **63:**441–444.
87. **Percy, N., G. J. Belsham, J. K. Brangwyn, M. Sullivan, D. M. Stone, and J. W. Almond.** 1992. Intracellular modifications induced by poliovirus reduce the requirement for structural motifs in the 5' noncoding region of the genome involved in internal initiation of protein synthesis. *J. Virol.* **66:**1695–1701.
88. **Perez, L., and L. Carrasco.** 1992. Lack of direct correlation between p220 cleavage and the shut-off of host translation after poliovirus infection. *Virology* **189:**178–186.
89. **Pestova, T. V., C. U. T. Hellen, and E. Wimmer.** 1991. Translation of poliovirus RNA: role of an essential *cis*-acting oligopyrimidine element within the 5' nontranslated region and involvement of a cellular 57-kilodalton protein. *J. Virol.* **65:**6194–6204.
90. **Pilipenko, E. V., V. M. Blinov, L. I. Romanova, A. N. Sinyakov, S. V. Maslova, and V. I. Agol.** 1989. Conserved structural domains in the 5' untranslated region of picornaviral genomes: an analysis of the segment controlling translation and neurovirulence. *Virology* **168:**201–209.
91. **Pilipenko, E. V., A. P. Gmyl, S. V. Maslova, Y. V. Svitkin, A. N. Sinyakov, and V. I. Agol.** 1992. Prokaryotic-like cis-elements in the cap-independent internal initiation of translation on picornavirus RNA. *Cell* **68:**119–131.
92. **Racaniello, V. R., and D. Baltimore.** 1981. Molecular cloning of poliovirus cDNA and determination of the complete nucleotide sequence of the viral genome. *Proc. Natl. Acad. Sci. USA* **78:**4887–4891.
93. **Racaniello, V. R., and C. Meriam.** 1986. Poliovirus temperature-sensitive mutant containing a single nucleotide deletion in the 5'-noncoding region of the viral RNA. *Virology* **155:**498–507.
94. **Rivera, V. M., J. D. Welsh, and J. V. Maizel.** 1988. Comparative sequence analysis of the 5' noncoding region of the enteroviruses and rhinoviruses. *Virology* **165:**42–50.
95. **Roehl, H. H., and B. L. Semler.** 1994. In vitro biochemical methods for investigating RNA-protein interactions in picornaviruses. *Methods Mol. Genet.* **4:**160–182.
96. **Rothberg, P. G., T. J. R. Harris, A. Nomoto, and E. Wimmer.** 1978. O4-(5'-uridylyl)tyrosine is the bond between the genome-linked protein and the RNA of poliovirus. *Proc. Natl. Acad. Sci. USA* **75:**4868–4872.
97. **Rozen, F., I. Edery, K. Meerovitch, T. E. Dever, W. C. Merrick, and N. Sonenberg.** 1990. Bidirectional RNA helicase activity of eukaryotic translation initiation factors 4A and 4F. *Mol. Cell. Biol.* **10:**1134–1144.
98. **Rubinstein, S. J., and A. Dasgupta.** 1989. Inhibition of rRNA synthesis by poliovirus: specific inactivation of transcription factors. *J. Virol.* **63:**4689–4696.
99. **Sarnow, P., H. S. Bernstein, and D. Baltimore.** 1986. A poliovirus temperature-sensitive mutant located in a non-coding region of the genome. *Proc. Natl. Acad. Sci. USA* **83:**571–575.
100. **Simoes, E. A. F., and P. Sarnow.** 1991. An RNA hairpin at the extreme 5' end of the poliovirus RNA genome modulates viral translation in human cells. *J. Virol.* **65:**913–921.
101. **Skinner, M. A., V. R. Racaniello, G. Dunn, J. Cooper, P. D. Minor, and J. W. Almond.** 1989. New model for the secondary structure of the 5' non-coding RNA of poliovirus is supported by biochemical and genetic data that also show that RNA secondary structure is important in neurovirulence. *J. Mol. Biol.* **207:**379–392.
102. **Sonenberg, N., and K. Meerovitch.** 1990.

Translation of poliovirus mRNA. *Enzyme* **44:**278–291.
103. **Stone, D. M., J. W. Almond, J. K. Brangwyn, and G. J. Belsham.** 1993. *trans* complementation of cap-independent translation directed by poliovirus 5' noncoding region deletion mutants: evidence for RNA-RNA interactions. *J. Virol.* **67:**6215–6223.
104. **Strebel, K., and E. Beck.** 1986. A second protease of foot-and-mouth disease virus. *J. Virol.* **58:**893–899.
105. **Toyoda, H., M. Kohara, Y. Kataoka, T. Suganuma, T. Omata, N. Imura, and A. Nomoto.** 1984. Complete nucleotide sequences of all three poliovirus serotype genomes: implication for genetic relationship, gene function, and antigenic determinants. *J. Mol. Biol.* **174:**561–585.
106. **Trono, D., R. Andino, and D. Baltimore.** 1988. An RNA sequence of hundreds of nucleotides at the 5' end of poliovirus RNA is involved in allowing viral protein synthesis. *J. Virol.* **62:**2291–2299.
107. **Witherell, G. W., A. Gil, and E. Wimmer.** 1993. Interaction of polypyrimidine tract binding protein with the encephalomyocarditis virus mRNA internal ribosome entry site. *Biochemistry* **32:**8268–8275.
108. **Wyckoff, E. E., J. W. B. Hershey, and E. Ehrenfeld.** 1990. Eukaryotic initiation factor 3 is required for poliovirus 2A protease-induced cleavage of the p220 component of eukaryotic initiation factor 4F. *Proc. Natl. Acad. Sci. USA* **87:**9529–9533.
109. **Wyckoff, E. E., R. E. Lloyd, and E. Ehrenfeld.** 1992. Relationship of eukaryotic initiation factor 3 to poliovirus-induced p220 cleavage activity. *J. Virol.* **66:**2943–2951.
110. **Yan, R., W. Rychlik, D. Etchison, and R. E. Rhoads.** 1992. Amino acid sequence of the human protein synthesis initiation factor eIF-4 gamma. *J. Biol. Chem.* **267:**23226–23231.

CELL BIOLOGY OF ENTEROVIRUS INFECTION

Andreas Schlegel and Karla Kirkegaard

6

When most cells in culture are infected with enteroviruses, profound alterations in cellular morphology and metabolism ensue. Poliovirus, coxsackievirus, and echoviruses are cytopathic in most cell types, and the cytopathic effect (CPE) of enteroviral infection has been frequently described (reviewed in references 54 and 81). By light microscopy, the most easily observed changes are the rounding and detachment from the tissue culture dish of adherent cells (Fig. 1). Immunofluorescence microscopy can also reveal alterations in nuclear shape and cytoskeletal organization during the course of enteroviral infection. Electron microscopy of enterovirus-infected cells has shown several changes characteristic of enteroviral infection. First, the nucleus gradually alters in morphology until it acquires a characteristic crescent shape late in infection. This is accompanied by margination of the chromatin, in which chromosomal DNA is found in increasingly smaller regions of the nucleus, often associated with the nuclear membrane. Second, in the cytoplasm, ribosomes appear to aggregate, and third and most strikingly, clusters of membranous vesicles form in great numbers (Fig. 2). Eventually, the rounded, detached cells lyse.

Many biochemical and physiologic changes accompany the morphologic ones. In most enteroviral infections, host translation and transcription become inhibited (37, 57) and the plasma membrane becomes more permeable (68, 81). Recently, poliovirus has been shown to inhibit the protein secretory apparatus; this inhibition was shown not to be a consequence of the inhibition of host cell translation (29). Which of these biochemical alterations cause the morphologic ones? Which changes are required to facilitate growth or spread of the virus during infection? What is it that eventually kills the cells?

There is no real agreement in the literature as to the definition of the CPE caused by cytocidal enteroviruses. Many different techniques that measure different aspects have been employed to monitor the development of CPE in infected cells. Classically, the rounding of adherent cells (2, 3) or observations of intracellular changes observable by light or electron microscopy (9, 44) have been used to monitor cytopathology. Two useful biochemical assays are the release of lysosomal enzymes into the cytoplasm (44) and the increase in penetration of dyes such as erthrosin B (1) that

---

Andreas Schlegel and Karla Kirkegaard, Department of Molecular, Cellular and Developmental Biology, Howard Hughes Medical Institute, University of Colorado, Boulder, Colorado 80309.

Human Enterovirus Infections, Edited by Harley A. Rotbart,
© 1995 American Society for Microbiology, Washington, DC 20005

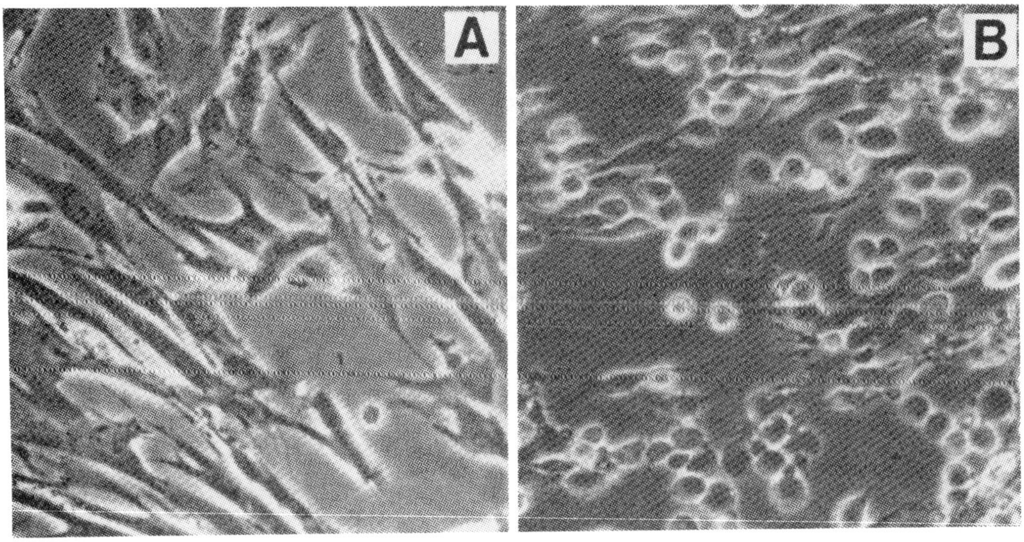

FIGURE 1 Morphologic changes in human embryonic lung cells upon poliovirus infection. Phase contrast photomicrographs are of uninfected (A) and infected (B) cells. Reprinted from reference 2 with permission.

accompany the increase in membrane permeability late in infection. Clearly, different assays monitor distinct cellular events that may or may not have the same biochemical cause.

Early studies of the CPE in poliovirus infection were aimed at differentiating among three theories of the cause of the morphologic alterations: (i) early inhibition of host nucleic acid and protein synthesis, (ii) release of lysosomal enzymes, and (iii) synthesis or accumulation of viral proteins late in infection. The first hypothesis was discarded because treatment of uninfected cells with actinomycin D to inhibit cellular transcription and DNA synthesis (37) or with puromycin to inhibit cellular translation (3) did not cause changes reminiscent of virally induced CPE. Although a correlation between the development of CPE and the release of lysosomal enzymes was documented in some cells (9, 44, 78), HEp-2 cells that were experimentally enucleated before infection did not release lysosomal enzymes but did develop the morphologic changes characteristic of CPE, thus causing the second hypothesis to be discarded (10). When cells infected with poliovirus were treated with puromycin to inhibit both viral and cellular protein synthesis at 3.5 h postinfection, no CPE ensued. However, when the cells were treated at the same time with guanidine, which specifically inhibits viral RNA synthesis but allows continued viral protein synthesis, CPE developed at the same time as in the absence of guanidine treatment (2, 3). Thus, it appeared that the late accumulation of viral proteins is necessary for development of the characteristic CPE.

Which viral proteins cause different aspects of the CPE, and which aspects are useful for the viruses? The well-studied inhibition of cellular translation and its role in virus-specific translation are discussed by Haller and Semler in chapter 5. Here, we discuss alterations in chromatin structure and transcription, rearrangement of cytoskeleton, accumulation of membranous vesicles, inhibition of protein secretion, and eventual lysis of cells infected with cytopathic enteroviruses. Wherever possible, the known or suspected viral proteins involved in these processes are identified (Table 1), and the evidence for their involvement is presented.

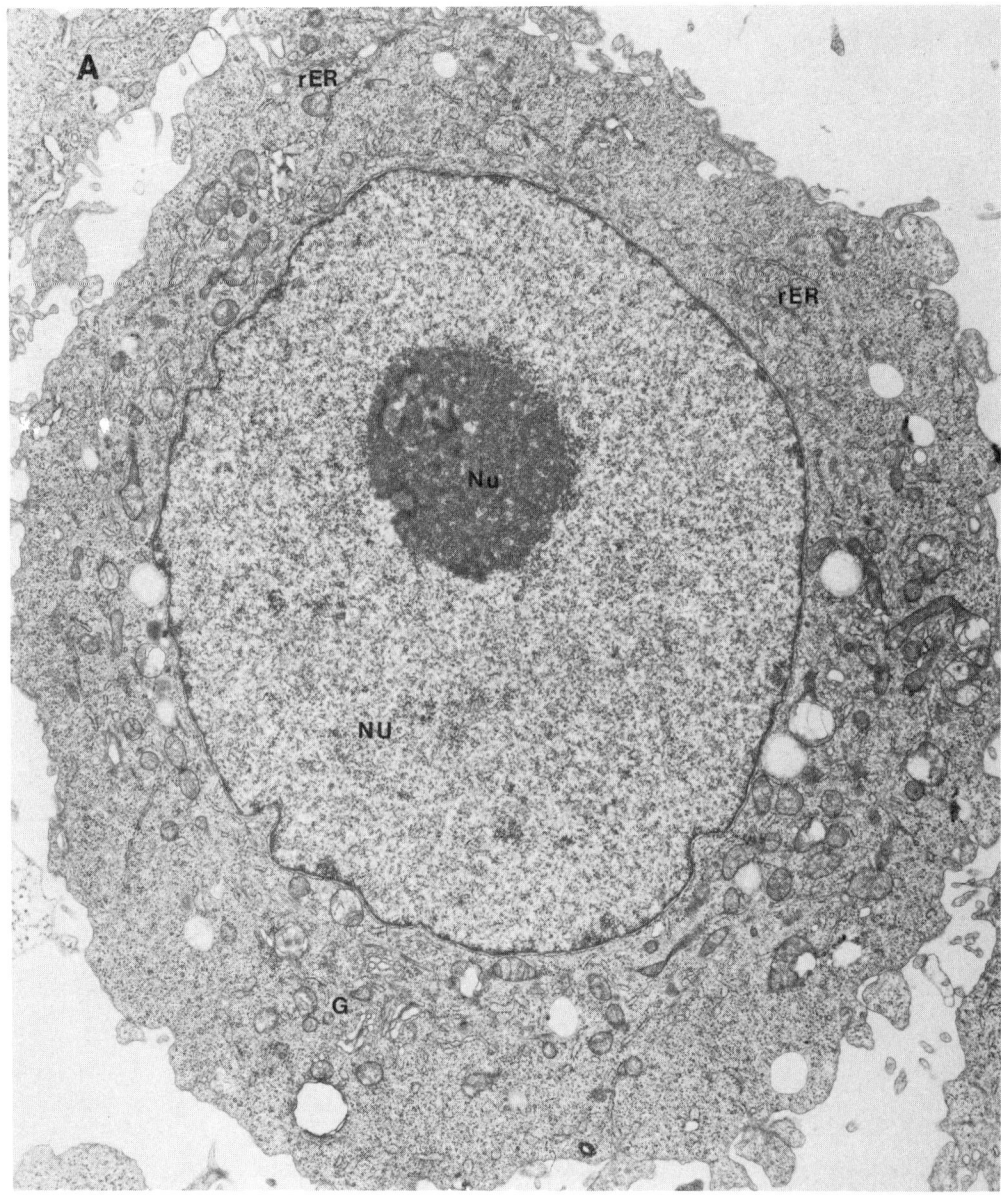

FIGURE 2 Electron micrographs of HEp-2 cells: (A) uninfected; (B) infected with poliovirus for 3 h; (C) infected with poliovirus for 4 h. NU, nucleus; Nu, nucleolus; rER, rough endoplasmic reticulum; G, Golgi apparatus; V, virus-induced vesicles. Images courtesy of K. Bienz and D. Egger, University of Basel.

NUCLEAR EFFECTS OF ENTEROVIRAL INFECTION

Although enteroviral RNA translation, positive- and negative-strand RNA synthesis, and virion assembly all occur in the cytoplasm, numerous changes occur in the nuclei of infected cells as well. Within 2 to 3 h of infection with poliovirus, transcription by polymerase

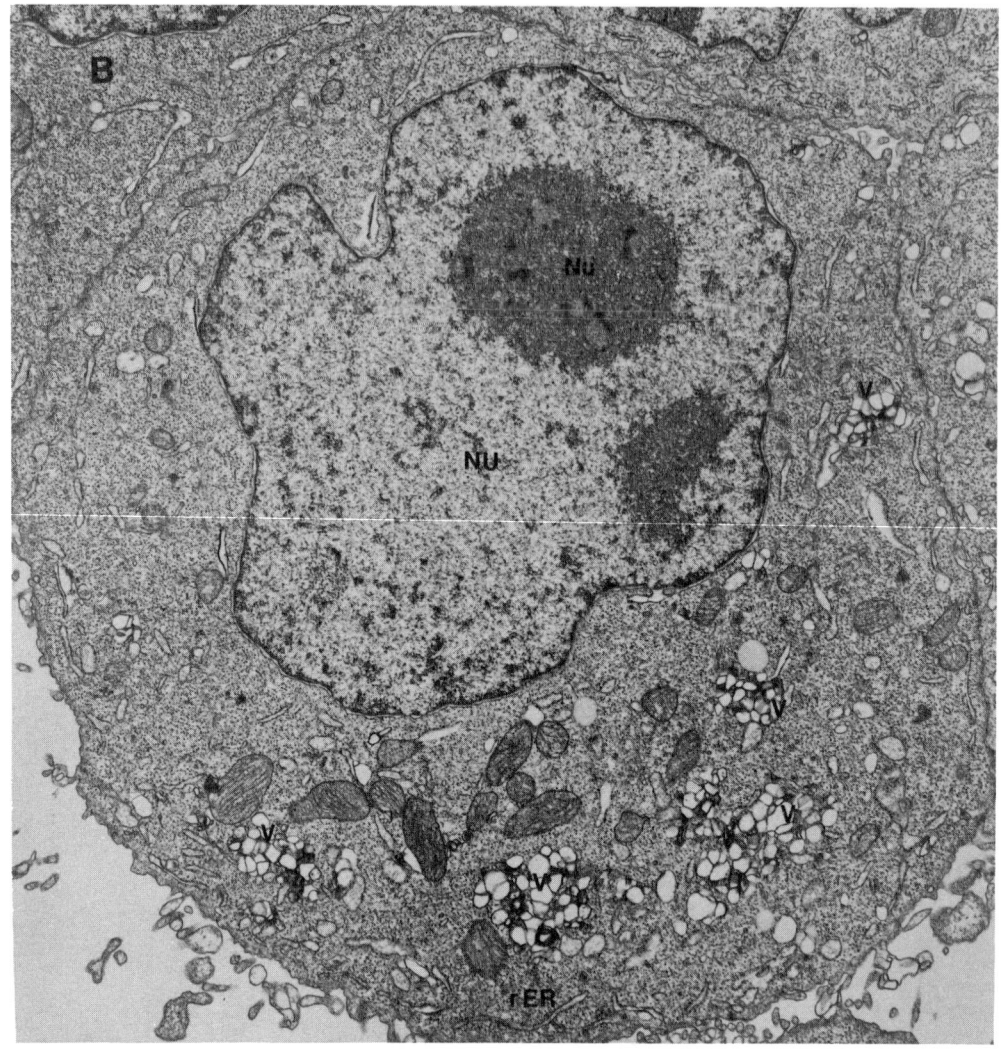

FIGURE 2 *Continued.*

I (Pol I) is inhibited; by 4 h postinfection, Pol II transcription is inhibited; and by 4 to 5 h postinfection, Pol III transcription also declines dramatically (18; reviewed in reference 81). Four hours into the usual 6- to 7-h infectious cycle of poliovirus, cellular DNA synthesis ceases, and the chromatin condenses to occupy only a small part of the nucleus (Fig. 2C; 37).

Since host translation is inhibited by about 2 h postinfection (chapter 5), it is often suggested that many of these nuclear effects are secondary to the inhibition of new host protein synthesis. In some cases, this hypothesis has been tested by examining the effects of protein synthesis inhibitors on nuclear function. For example, in some human and murine tissue culture cell lines, inhibition of protein synthesis greatly reduces the fraction of cells in mitosis within a few hours (76). Thus, the effects of poliovirus infection on DNA synthesis in any particular cell line could be a secondary consequence of inhibition of protein synthesis. Treatment of human lymphosarcoma cells with cycloheximide was shown to

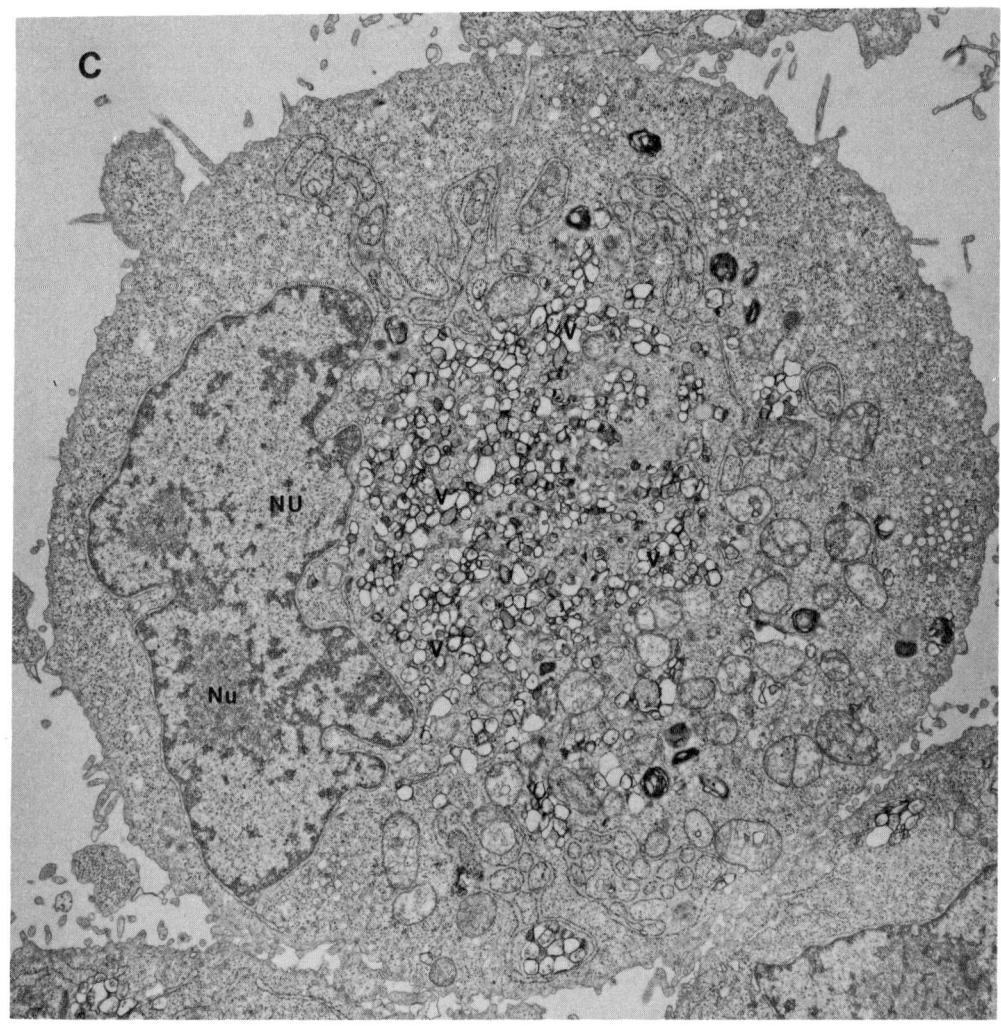

FIGURE 2 *Continued.*

inhibit Pol I and Pol III transcription by about 50% within 2 h, while no effect on Pol II transcription was seen for hours after treatment (40).

While many changes in the cell biology of infected cells may result directly from the inhibition of cellular translation, it is also true that several preexisting proteins in the infected cell are specifically degraded during infection by poliovirus. HeLa cell proteins were labeled with [^{35}S]methionine and then either infected or mock infected with poliovirus. Two-dimensional gel electrophoresis of the labeled cellular proteins revealed that although most proteins were unaffected during the course of poliovirus infection, 10 to 14 different cellular proteins were missing from the infected samples (95).

Inhibition of Pol II Transcription Is Caused by TBP Cleavage

A clear example of inhibition of host transcription by direct cleavage of a transcription factor by a poliovirus protease has been docu-

TABLE 1 Known effects of individual viral proteins on host functions or proteins

Virus	Protein(s)	Effect	Altered host target	Reference
Poliovirus	2A	Inhibition of cap-dependent protein synthesis	p220	33
Coxsackievirus B4 and rhinovirus[a]	2A	Inhibition of cap-dependent protein synthesis by direct proteolysis of p220	p220	60
Poliovirus	2B	Inhibition of ER-to-Golgi protein traffic	?	29
Poliovirus	2C, 2BC	Membranous vesicle accumulation	?	15
Poliovirus	3A	Inhibition of ER-to-Golgi protein traffic	?	29
Poliovirus	3C	1. Alteration of Pol I promoter-specific protein DNA complex	?	80
		2. Inhibition of Pol II transcription; direct cleavage of TBP	TBP	18
		3. Inhibition of Pol III transcription; proteolytic alteration of TFIIIC complex	TFIIIC complex	17
Foot-and-mouth disease virus[a]	3C	Direct proteolytic cleavage of histone H3	Histone H3	34, 89
Poliovirus	?	Alteration of MAP 4 by unknown mechanism	MAP 4	50

[a]Known effects of homologous nonenteroviral picornaviral proteins are included.

mented for Pol II transcription. When the Pol II transcription activities of extracts from infected and uninfected cells were compared in vitro, a particular fraction from poliovirus-infected cells did not function (23). This fraction was later identified as TFIID, a general transcription factor complex required for preinitiation complex formation (53). The TATA-binding protein (TBP), a component of the TFIID fraction, is directly cleaved in vitro by poliovirus protease 3C (18) near the N terminus of the protein, probably after residue 18 (26). Cleavage of TBP abolishes Pol II transcription activity in vitro, and presumably in vivo as well (18).

Pol I Inhibition Correlates with Altered DNA-Binding Proteins

The inhibition of Pol I transcription by poliovirus can also be observed in vitro; extracts of cells infected with poliovirus for 4 h displayed lower Pol I transcription activity than did extracts of uninfected cells (80). Interestingly, extracts from cells treated with cycloheximide for 1.5 h showed even lower transcription activity than did extracts from poliovirus-infected cells. However, in the infected-cell extracts, this inhibition correlated with the disappearance of a protein-DNA complex with a characteristic electrophoretic mobility formed upon incubation of uninfected extracts with Pol I promoter DNA. When infected-cell extracts were incubated with promoter DNA, a protein-DNA complex with greatly increased mobility was formed. This change in the protein-DNA complexes was not observed in the cycloheximide-treated extracts. Therefore, although inhibition of protein synthesis was sufficient to explain the observed inhibition of Pol I transcription, it could not explain the apparent alteration in the Pol I transcription factors (80). However, the recent findings that TBP is cleaved during poliovirus infection might explain the altered Pol I transcription factor complexes. TBP is required not only for Pol II transcription but also for Pol I and III transcription (21, 22, 77, 83, 100) and is now known to be a component of specific Pol I transcription factor SL1 (21). Thus, the observed alterations in Pol I promoter-specific complexes from poliovirus-infected extracts could result from the altered TBP-containing SL1 fraction. It has been argued that since inhibition of Pol I transcription in poliovirus-infected cells occurs earlier in the infectious cycle than the cleavage of TBP, depletion of TBP cannot be solely responsible for the inhibition of Pol I transcription (18). However, the combined effects of protein synthesis inhibition and TBP cleavage are sufficient to explain the effects of poliovirus infection on Pol I transcription, although a third virus-specific effect is also possible (26).

Inhibition of Pol III Transcription by Protease 3C

Poliovirus inhibition of Pol III transcription by poliovirus has also been observed by comparing extracts prepared from uninfected and poliovirus-infected cells. Two transcription factor fractions, TFIIIB and TFIIIC, were defective in extracts from cells infected with poliovirus for 4 to 5 h (36). The inhibition of transcription correlated with a change in the electrophoretic mobilities of the protein-DNA complexes formed between a Pol III promoter and proteins from infected extracts, and the change in the TFIIIC could be mimicked by incubating it with purified poliovirus protein 3C (17). This change is probably not a result of TBP cleavage by protease 3C. TBP is known to fractionate with a different Pol III transcription factor, TFIIIB (62), which probably explains the effect of poliovirus infection on the TFIIIB fraction. Cycloheximide treatment for 2 h was not sufficient to explain the magnitude of the inhibition of Pol III transcription in vitro (36). Thus, it is likely that in addition to the effects of poliovirus-induced cleavage of TBP and inhibition of protein synthesis, the action of protease 3C on Pol III transcription, specifically on the TFIIIC fraction, also contributes to the inhibition of Pol III transcription during poliovirus infection (17).

Other Nuclear Effects

What causes the effect of enteroviral infection on chromatin morphology? The only documented effect of any picornavirus on a known component of chromatin structure is the direct cleavage by the 3C protease of foot-and-mouth disease virus of histone H3, removing the N-terminal 20 amino acids (34, 89). Proteolytic removal of these N-terminal residues is not expected to affect DNA binding or the assembly of individual nucleosomes. However, this region is proposed to mediate interactions with DNA and nonnucleosomal proteins and contains several highly conserved lysine residues whose posttranslational acetylation has been correlated with activation of transcription and unfolding of chromatin (reviewed in reference 43). Mutations in this region of *Saccharomyces cerevisiae* histone H3 cause defects in transcriptional silencing (90). Effects similar to the cleavage of histone H3 by foot-and-mouth disease virus 3C protease have not yet been observed during infection for any enterovirus.

What is the role of these nuclear events in enteroviral infection? Enucleated mouse L cells transfected with single-stranded poliovirion RNA allowed the replication of poliovirus to titers comparable to that in cells with nuclei (28). Thus, it is clear that nuclear presence and function are not required for poliovirus infection. Instead, it might be the case that when the nucleus is physically present, inhibition of its function is needed to prevent an inhibitory effect on viral replication. Alternatively, it is possible that nuclear effects such as the inhibition of cellular transcription serve functions that optimize but are not absolutely required for viral replication, such as increasing the pools of ribonucleotides available for viral RNA synthesis.

ENTEROVIRAL INFECTION AND THE CYTOSKELETON

Alteration of the Cytoskeletal Framework in Virus-Infected Cells

The cell cytoskeleton is composed of three distinct but interconnected filament systems: actin microfilaments, microtubules, and intermediate filaments. The cytoskeleton functions to maintain cell shape and mobility and may also provide anchoring points for other intracellular structures. The cytoskeleton is extensively remodeled during enteroviral infection.

The data summarized below are from experiments using poliovirus-infected cells; there is evidence, however, that the described effects are similar in other enteroviral infections and possibly in a wide variety of animal and plant virus infections as well (64).

The most obvious alteration of the host cell cytoskeleton in poliovirus-infected cells is the increased concentration of intermediate filaments around the nucleus, which was revealed by electron microscopy (58) and immunofluorescence (30). Neither the mechanism of this alteration in intermediate filament organization nor the viral products involved have been identified. Two observations, however, suggest that the rearranged intermediate filaments serve as sites for viral RNA replication. First, a considerable amount of viral RNA remains associated with the framework when cytoskeletal fractions are prepared from infected cells (58). Second, the cytoskeleton becomes associated with electron-dense particles with diameters of 40 to 70 nm during infection (96); these particles are postulated to be viral RNA replication complexes composed of the viral RNA polymerase, template, and nascent RNA.

The suggestion that the cytoskeleton provides the site of viral RNA synthesis, however, contrasts with the model that viral RNA replication occurs on the outer surfaces of membranous vesicles that accumulate in infected cells (5, 6, 93). The apparent conflict between these models may be due to the different experimental approaches used to visualize morphologic changes in infected cells. In the cytoskeleton studies, nonionic detergents were used to remove cytosolic components from the cells while keeping the cytoskeletal framework intact, and thus the involvement of any membranes in forming the viral replication complex would not have been detected. The membranous vesicles, on the other hand, were isolated from infected cells following mechanical disruption to release intracellular structures. Cytoskeletal elements would have been removed in the subsequent fractionation, and their possible role in RNA replication would not have been detected. Thus, it is possible that the viral replication complexes associate with both membranes and cytoskeletal structures. Molecular aspects and the significance of these associations are still under investigation.

Another alteration of the cytoskeleton in poliovirus-infected HeLa cells is the proteolytic degradation of a microtubule-associated protein 4 to 5 h postinfection (50). This proteolytic alteration was found by screening an antibody library designed to detect differences in antigenic patterns in infected and uninfected cells. The altered antigen was cloned, sequenced, and identified as microtubule-associated protein 4 (MAP 4). The function of MAP 4 in uninfected cells, the role of its cleavage during infection, and the identity of the responsible protease are unknown.

Is a Rearranged Cytoskeleton Required for Enteroviral Infection?

Rearrangement of the intermediate filament framework, association of viral RNA with the cytoskeleton, and proteolytic degradation of a microtubule-associated protein in infected cells have been shown to accompany poliovirus infection. Those studies, however, did not test whether the cytoskeletal alterations are required for virus replication. The significance of these alterations in poliovirus-infected cells was tested recently: when host cells were treated from the beginning of the infection with chemicals that disrupt all three filament systems, the characteristic virus-induced rearrangements of the intermediate filament network were not detected. Virus accumulation during a single cycle of infection, however, was not affected by drug treatment (30). These results suggested that neither the virus-induced cytoskeletal rearrangements nor the integrity of the host cell cytoskeleton is required for poliovirus replication.

Further work needs to be done to test the importance of the cytoskeleton for virus replication in tissue culture and in animal models to identify the steps in infection, if any, that require the modified cytoskeletal structures and proteins observed in infected cells. An attractive role for cytoskeletal alterations is in cell lysis or in cell-cell contact within the infected animal, both steps in the virus replicative cycle that were not addressed by previous studies.

MEMBRANE REARRANGEMENT IN ENTEROVIRUS-INFECTED CELLS

Formation of Specific Class of Vesicles in Infected Cells

Enteroviral infection is accompanied by a striking alteration in the organization of the host cell's cytoplasmic membranes. In the middle of the infectious cycle, membranous vesicles begin to form. By the end of the infection, the cell is virtually filled with virus-induced vesicles. A variety of enteroviruses, including echovirus 9 (38, 39), echovirus 12 (84), poliovirus (25), and coxsackievirus B4 (49), induce vesicle accumulation in their host cells. The most intensively studied example, however, is poliovirus, and the following discussion is restricted to poliovirus-host cell interactions.

Electron microscopy and autoradiography of newly synthesized polioviral macromolecules revealed that synthesis of viral proteins occurs before virus-induced cytoplasmic membranes are formed. Viral RNA synthesis, however, begins concomitantly with the accumulation of membranous vesicles and is associated with these membranes (6). From these results it was concluded that viral proteins induce formation of the vesicles and that these membranes are required for viral RNA synthesis.

A variety of findings support the hypothesis that the synthesis of viral RNA is membrane associated. First, subcellular fractions of poliovirus-infected cells that contain virus-induced membranes are able to synthesize viral RNA (12, 13). Second, a complex of proteins containing the RNA-dependent RNA polymerase was shown to be membrane associated: when such complexes were isolated from poliovirus-infected cells under conditions that disrupted the membranes, many proteins, including the RNA polymerase, associated spontaneously with liposomes in vitro (11). Third, membranous complexes isolated from poliovirus-infected cells contain all of the viral proteins thought to be involved in RNA replication (85, 86, 92). Finally, hybridization studies using single-stranded RNA probes followed by electron microscopy localized polioviral RNA molecules in close vicinity to virus-induced membranous vesicles (93). The composition and known functions of viral RNA replication complexes are discussed in chapter 4.

Electron microscopy revealed that at least some of the virus-induced vesicles bud from the rough endoplasmic reticulum (rER) of infected cells and that poliovirus protein 2C or 2C-containing precursors are associated with the growing buds. Furthermore, protein 2C and 2C-containing precursors seem to migrate with the budding vesicles into the host cell cytoplasm and remain associated with the vesicles (4). This finding is supported by biochemical data from subcellular fractions containing virus-induced vesicles: viral proteins 2C, 2BC, and 3AB are tightly bound to the vesicular membrane and cannot be removed from the lipid bilayer with high-ionic-strength buffers or 4 M urea (88). Electron microscopic immunocytochemistry of subcellular fractions containing virus-induced vesicles further confirmed that poliovirus protein 2C and 2C-containing precursors were asssociated with the outer surfaces of the membranes (5, 8). 2B, 2BC, 3A, and 3AB, independently expressed in HeLa cells by using vaccinia virus vectors, all localized to structures proposed to be ER and Golgi membranes (15, 27).

Using $ZnCl_2$ as a partial inhibitor of poliovirus polyprotein cleavage, electron microscopic analysis showed that the timing of vesicle formation was most coincident with the accumulation of poliovirus protein 2BC; thus, it was proposed that polypeptide 2BC may be the vesicle-inducing protein (7). The expression of recombinant poliovirus proteins 2C and 2BC in human cells by using vaccinia vectors recently confirmed and refined this finding (15). Both 2C and 2BC, when expressed in the absence of other poliovirus proteins, associated with cytoplasmic membranes and induced the formation of membranous vesicles. Some of these vesicles displayed morphology similar to that of vesicles in poliovirus-infected cells. Protein 2C but not 2BC also induced the formation of myelinlike spiral membrane structures enclosed in the lumen of the rER. The spirals, which have not been seen in poliovirus-infected cells, were continuous with the parental rER membrane and were composed of quadruple rather than double layers of lipids. Together, these results suggest that poliovirus protein 2BC is involved in vesicle formation in infected cells and that protein 2C alone may not be able to induce correct and efficient membrane vesiculation.

At the moment, the molecular basis of the interaction of poliovirus proteins 2C and 2BC with host cell membranes is not clear. That the interaction of 2BC and 2C with the membrane might be mediated by other poliovirus proteins was ruled out by the clear association of the two proteins with intracellular membranes when the proteins are expressed in the absence of other poliovirus proteins (15). However, the possibility that proteins 2BC and 2C interact indirectly with the lipid bilayer via an association with host cell proteins remains to be investigated. At the moment, the degree to which cellular polypeptides are involved in vesicle formation is unknown. Therefore, it is possible that a cellular mechanism slightly diverted by viral proteins might be used to form and accumulate virus-induced membranes.

Comparison of Membranous Vesicle Formation in Uninfected and Infected Cells

The formation of transport vesicles along the secretory pathways of uninfected cells (reviewed in references 79 and 82) shows some similarities to the formation of membranous vesicles in poliovirus-infected cells. First, uninfected cells constantly release transport vesicles from the ER and other organelles by forming protein-coated buds that grow into coated vesicles (75). Second, as in virus-infected cells, specific proteins are required for efficient release of transport vesicles from the donor organelles. Third, the released transport vesicles found in uninfected cells contain the same coat proteins as the growing buds (74). In uninfected cells, coat proteins are released only when the transport vesicles prepare to fuse with the next organelle along the secretory pathway (87). The flow of membranous transport vesicles along the secretory pathway, termed forward or anterograde transport, is accompanied by a constant backflow of membranous material. This latter process, termed retrograde transport, is thought to occur via tubular membrane extensions rather than via the coated vesicles that mediate forward transport (reviewed in reference 55).

There are also several differences between poliovirus-induced vesicles and the coated transport vesicles found in uninfected cells. First, there is a difference in size and morphology: virus-induced vesicles vary in diameter from 50 to 400 nm (15), whereas coated transport vesicles have quite homogenous diameters of approximately 75 nm. A transport vesicle is composed of a spherical membrane compartment that is completely coated with a protein shell, whereas poliovirus-induced vesicles appear smooth, with some protein bound to the outer surfaces. However, because the morphologic characterization of virus-induced membranes was based on partially purified vesicles subjected to several isolation steps, it is not clear whether all the substituents present in the cell remained associated. Observation of these partially purified virus-induced membranes also revealed that they form rosettelike aggregates (8). A second, more compact membrane system was detected at the center of the rosettes; the viral RNA replication complexes seemed to localize to this inner membrane system (5).

A second difference between intracellular transport vesicles and virus-induced vesicles is their function: transport vesicles are carriers of secretory material being transported along the anterograde transport pathway. After budding from the donor organelle (vesicle generation), transport vesicles attach to a target membrane and fuse with this compartment (vesicle consumption). Small GTP-binding proteins, which are part of the transport vesicle coat and are specific for different vesicular transport steps, are thought to regulate vesicle generation and consumption (reviewed in references 35 and 102). Vesicle generation at a donor compartment, vesicle consumption at a target membrane, and retrograde transport of membranes back to the donor compartment keep the balance between forward and backward membrane flow and are responsible for the maintenance of organelle integrity in uninfected cells. This balance in membrane flow seems not to be the case in poliovirus-infected cells, which generate vesicles that constantly increase in number, apparently without being recycled (4). Recent findings, in fact, provide evidence for a disruption of intracellular membrane organization in poliovirus-infected cells: at later stages of the infection, no material corresponding to the Golgi apparatus could be identified (15). A loss of Golgi stacks was also reported when poliovirus proteins 2BC and 2C were expressed in the absence of other poliovirus proteins (15), suggesting that protein 2C or its precursors directly or indirectly alter the integrity of the Golgi apparatus.

What is the function of virus-induced vesicles in enteroviral infection, and why is the intracellular membrane so profoundly rearranged? The finding that viral RNA synthesis occurs in close association with virus-induced vesicles (5, 6, 93) and the observation that inhibitors of intracellular vesicle generation (see below) inhibit viral RNA synthesis in poliovirus-infected cells (48, 66) suggest that the main function of virus-induced vesicles is to support or assemble the viral RNA replication complex. Continuous accumulation of these membranes during the infectious cycle may contribute to the efficiency of virus production at the expense of intracellular membrane organization.

Effects of Inhibitors on Intracellular Transport and Poliovirus Infection

The secretory pathways of uninfected cells, several steps of which have been faithfully reconstituted in vitro, can be modulated by several chemicals and drugs (reviewed in references 35, 67, 79, and 98). For example, in both intact cells and in vitro extracts, brefeldin A (BFA), a fungal metabolite, inhibits the formation of coated buds and coated transport vesicles. BFA affects a small GTP-binding protein termed ADP ribosylation factor (ARF), which is found on Golgi membranes. The drug blocks the binding of GTP to ARF and thereby prevents ARF from becoming membrane associated (31, 45). Binding of ARF to the membrane is required to induce vesicle budding in vitro (74). Because retrograde transport in BFA-treated cells is not inhibited (55), the overall effect of BFA in living cells is the collapse of the Golgi apparatus into the ER (reviewed in reference 35).

Interestingly, BFA is a potent inhibitor of poliovirus replication, specifically inhibiting poliovirus RNA synthesis (48, 66). Maynell and coworkers (66) linked the antiviral activity of BFA with its known effects on vesicle formation in uninfected cells. They proposed that BFA might inhibit the formation of virus-induced vesicles by a mechanism similar to that described for uninfected cells. Blocking the generation of these specific membranes might directly inhibit membrane-dependent viral RNA replication. Furthermore, they postulated that the accumulation of virus-induced membranes in infected cells may be due to a viral product that directly or indirectly inhibits further transport and consumption of these vesicles (66). The finding that poliovirus growth is not affected by BFA in cell lines that have a BFA-resistant secretory pathway (30) further supported this model and ruled out a trivial interaction of the inhibitor with a viral product. An alternative model was proposed by Irurzun and coworkers (48), who took into account the inhibitory effects of BFA on intra-Golgi transport. They postulated that the replication complexes assemble on secretory membranes that are shuttled through the Golgi apparatus. Virus-induced membranes containing mature replication complexes would then, according to this model, bud from the trans-Golgi network. BFA was proposed to interfere with the assembly of viral replication complexes on Golgi membranes (48).

Several newer findings argue against the latter model. First, the typical stacks of the Golgi apparatus seem to disappear in infected cells (15). Second, the model proposed by Irurzun and coworkers (48) predicts that the Golgi apparatus remains functionally active, allowing transport and posttranslational modifications of secreted proteins. However, glycosylation studies with transiently expressed secretory proteins have revealed that the Golgi apparatus is functionally disrupted during poliovirus infection (29). Third, immunoisolation of virus-induced vesicles revealed that these membranes contain marker proteins of the early secretory pathway that in normally secreting cells would not reach the trans-Golgi network (81a).

Inhibition of Protein Secretion in Poliovirus-Infected Cells

How are membrane-mediated housekeeping functions of the host cell affected by the profound virus-induced rearrangement of intracellular membranes described above? Recent data have shown that the ability of the host cell to transport secretory proteins from the rER to the cell periphery is severely impaired in poliovirus-infected cells. Specifically, it was shown that poliovirus infection leads to an arrest of secretory proteins in the ER, the trans-ER network (TEN), or the cis-Golgi network (29). A similar inhibition of the secretory pathway was observed when each of the poliovirus nonstructural proteins 2B, 2BC, and 3A was expressed in animal cells in the absence of other viral proteins. Finally, by using double immunofluorescence microscopy, it was shown that protein 3A induced the retention of a secretory protein in an organelle that also contained an ER-resident cellular protein, suggesting that poliovirus infection leads to an arrest of secretory proteins in the ER or an ER-like compartment (29).

Enterovirus-Induced Rearrangement of Intracellular Membranes: a Model

Taken together, these data support the model that the virus-induced vesicles that accumulate in the cytoplasm of infected cells derive from the secretory pathway of the host cell (66). Specifically, we propose (Fig. 3) that the poliovirus-induced vesicles bud from the ER or the TEN by a mechanism involving viral protein 2BC or 3A or both and probably cellular proteins of the vesicle generation apparatus as well. One of the cellular vesicle-inducing proteins may be the target of BFA inhibition. Subsequently, one of the viral products may, directly or indirectly, inhibit the consumption of virus-induced vesicles with a target membrane. Blocking membrane flow at this step of intracellular secretion would explain both the accumulation of membranous vesicles and the inhibition of host cell secretion in poliovirus-infected cells. In addition, by specifically inhibiting anterograde membrane transport, viral infection would reduce the amount of membrane that fuses with the Golgi complex. Thus, the disappearance of the Golgi apparatus during infection could be explained by retrograde membrane flow (Fig. 3B). Alternatively, if retrograde membrane flow is also inhibited in infected cells, the Golgi stacks could disappear because of anterograde flow downstream of the Golgi (Fig. 3C).

It is interesting that nonenveloped viruses such as enteroviruses, which do not need the protein secretion apparatus for transport of any viral products, may make efficient use of the constituents of this apparatus to assemble RNA replication complexes during infection. Other direct advantages to enteroviruses of dismantling the protein secretion apparatus early in infection may include the inhibition of antigen presentation in the context of major histocompatibility complex molecules and the inhibition of interferon secretion.

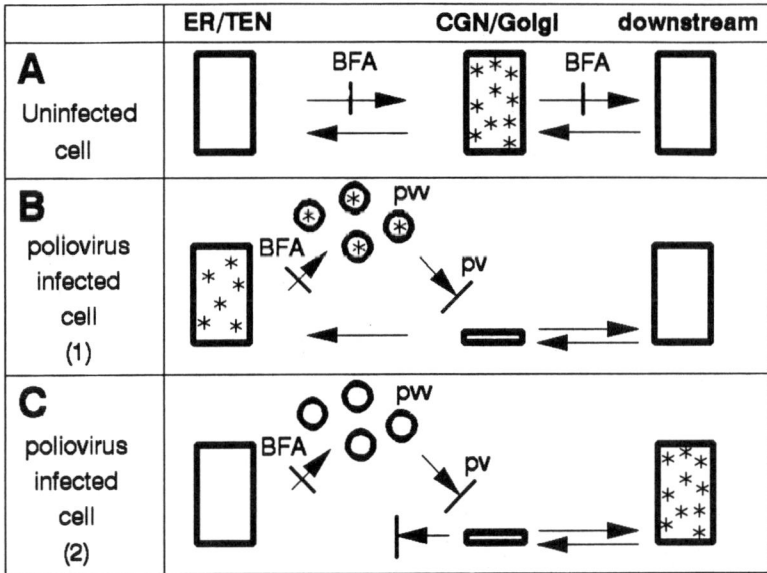

FIGURE 3 Model for vesicle accumulation and inhibition of vesicular transport in poliovirus (pv)-infected cells. In uninfected cells (A), secretory material is transported from the ER and the TEN to the cis-Golgi-network and via the Golgi apparatus further down the secretory pathway. Transport in this direction (anterograde transport) is inhibited by BFA, whereas backward (retrograde) transport remains unaffected by BFA. Infection (B and C) leads to the accumulation of poliovirus-induced vesicles (pvv). The inhibitory effect of BFA on poliovirus replication may be because the generation of poliovirus-induced vesicles is inhibited. A viral product may inhibit further transport of virus-induced vesicles and therefore cause vesicle accumulation and secretion inhibition. This virus-induced block of membrane traffic may lead to the disintegration of the Golgi apparatus, which may be consumed by upstream (B) or downstream (C) compartments as schematically depicted for a Golgi resident protein (✱). For details, see the text.

VIRAL EXIT FROM INFECTED CELLS AND CELL LYSIS

Exit of Assembled Viruses from Infected Cells

Although the eventual lysis of cells by cytopathic enterovirus provides an efficient route for viral exit, there is clear evidence that viruses can be released prior to the lysis of their cellular host. For example, during infection with a noncytopathic variant of hepatitis A virus, 50% of the infectious virus was released into the medium at times when no cell lysis was observed (24). These and similar findings with enteroviruses (20, 94) can always be dismissed by the argument that a small subset of cells is responsible for producing most of the virus and that the lysis of this small number of cells is not detected. However, other data argue that enteroviruses can be released without cell lysis. When human blood cell lines representing various stages of differentiation were compared for their abilities to support poliovirus infection and their susceptibilities to lysis by poliovirus, these two variables were found to be separable (73). Specifically, a differentiated granulocytic cell line supported high levels of poliovirus replication and was killed by lysis within 3 days. Another cell line, similar to an undifferentiated stem cell, supported equally high levels of poliovirus replication, as assayed by measuring both cell-associated virus titers and virus titers in the medium for up to 3 days postinfection. However, the stem cell line showed no detectable CPE or lysis for 14 days (73). Taken together, these data argue that there is a mechanism for viral release from infected cells in the absence of overt cellular lysis and that different cell lines are differentially susceptible to the killing effects of enteroviral infection. Nonlytic spread of viruses could clearly play a role during persistent infection. However, the mechanism of this nonlytic release is not yet understood.

The epithelial lining of the gastrointestinal tract is both the portal of entry for most enteroviruses and a means for virus spread. In tissue culture, polarized epithelial cell lines can be propagated, and virus adsorption and exit from their apical and basolateral surfaces can be monitored. When such experiments were performed with a human intestinal epithelial cell line (Caco-2), poliovirus was released almost exclusively from the apical surface (94). This finding places some restrictions on the possible mechanisms of virus release from this polarized cell line (Fig. 4). If lysis of the infected cell within the epithelial sheet is the mechanism of cell exit, this lysis can be only partial, on the apical surfaces of the infected cells (Fig. 4A). Alternatively, the infected cell could be expelled from the monolayer sheet before lysis (Fig. 4B), or a nonlytic mechanism could allow the vectorial release of virus (Fig. 4C; 94). Such a nonlytic mechanism is not likely to be secretion via the normal secretory pathway, which releases the internal components of membranous vesicles, because the secretion of reporter proteins is blocked in poliovirus-infected cells (29). Nonlytic release of virus by some other mechanism could be restricted to the apical surfaces of cells, or preferential release from the apical surface could reflect a polarized intracellular concentration of poliovirus membrane-associated replication complexes and mature viruses.

Cell Lysis and Death
Infection of most cell lines with most enteroviruses eventually leads to cell lysis and death.

What causes the cells to die? Persistent infections, in which host cells are not killed by the infecting viruses, have been used as model systems for studying the mechanism of cell killing. Combinations of viral (14) and cellular (51, 61, 63, 73) variants that can lead to nonlytic infections have been reported; in most cases, however, the reduced cytopathology also correlates with reduced amounts of viral growth, making it difficult to separate these two variables. Cell type-dependent restrictions to viral growth at the levels of receptor expression (52) and viral translation (63) have been documented for cell lines that allow persistent infection by wild-type poliovirus, again making it difficult to distinguish between effects on viral growth and viral persistence. However, in the case of the human blood cell lines discussed above, it is clear that different cell lines are differentially susceptible to killing by poliovirus infection independently of their abilities to support viral growth (73). Therefore, there must be cellular targets for the killing functions of poliovirus that are differentially susceptible in different cell lines.

What are the functions of enteroviruses that promote cell killing and lysis? Two lines of evidence trace the lytic function to the capsid proteins. When a neuroblastoma cell line was infected with neurovirulent type 1 poliovirus in the presence of antibodies against the viral capsid, many cells were not killed. When these cells were maintained in culture in the presence of the antiserum, they displayed the properties of persistent infection. Although the cells did not lyse, the intracellular viral titer was not diminished by the presence of the antiserum. Cell lysis could be inhibited either by the extracellular antiserum or by some fraction of the antiserum that was internalized; in either case, a role for the capsid proteins in cell lysis was suggested (91). A region from nucleotides 1148 to 3481 of a nonlytic poliovirus variant containing mutations only in VP1 and VP2 was sufficient to confer on a lytic poliovirus strain the ability to infect cells persistently (14). However, since these mutations conferred both slower growth of the virus and the ability to

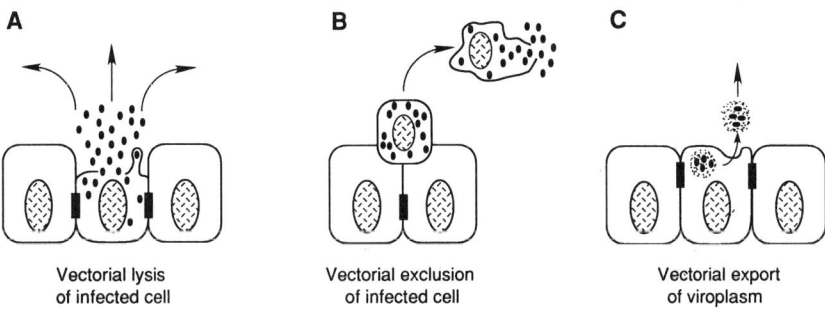

FIGURE 4 Models for release of poliovirus from polarized Caco-2 cells, redrawn from reference 94. (A) Cell membrane of infected cell within an epithelial sheet lyses on its apical surface only. (B) An infected cell is expelled from an epithelial sheet before lysis. (C) A portion of the cytoplasm of an infected cell that contains a high concentration of virus, termed viroplasm, is released from the infected cell without cell lysis.

maintain persistent infection, it is difficult to conclude that the lytic function lies solely in the mutations in VP1 and VP2 within these sequences. Another study suggested that protein 3A might play a role in cell lysis. Comparison of cytopathic and noncytopathic strains of hepatitis A (a hepatovirus, formerly classified as enterovirus 72) reveals many mutations, the most consistent of which map to the coding region for viral protein 3A (70). However, none of the mutations found in cytopathic strains has been independently cloned into a nonlytic hepatitis A genome to test for the ability to confer cytopathology.

By what mechanism do enteroviruses kill cells? For poliovirus, the known effects of protein 2A in inhibiting cap-dependent translation, of 3C in inhibiting cellular transcription, and of 2B and 3A in inhibiting protein secretion are not sufficient to explain the rapid demise of infected cells. It is possible that one or more viral proteins lyse cells directly. Possible mechanisms for such direct killing include disruption of the cellular membranes (56) or alteration of microtubule structure (50).

Another possible reason for cell death during enteroviral infection is that a viral product induces apoptosis, the cell death program wired into the cells themselves. In uninfected organisms, programmed cell death is triggered by cell-cell interactions and removes superfluous cells. Cells undergoing apoptosis shrink, their nuclei condense, and the DNA typically becomes fragmented; phagocytosis soon follows. In the free-living nematode *Caenorhabditis elegans*, several steps in the apoptotic pathway have been identified genetically; the later steps of DNA fragmentation and phagocytosis require new protein synthesis and are not required for execution of the cell death program. Expression of the first identified gene in the pathway, *ced-9*, prevents apoptosis. Its mammalian homolog, *bcl-2*, previously identified as a cellular oncogene, can also prevent apoptosis in mammalian cells in response to extracellular signals such as hormone addition, cytokine withdrawal, or exposure to toxins (reviewed in references 46 and 101). Expression of two genes, *ced-3* and *ced-4*, from *C. elegans* (32) and one, *reaper*, from the fruit fly *Drosophila melanogaster* (99) induces apoptosis. A mammalian homolog of the *ced-3* product, ICE (interleukin-1β converting enzyme), has been identified. ICE is a cysteine protease that, when overexpressed, can induce apoptosis in rat fibroblasts (69).

Recently, viral functions analogous to those of the proteins involved in the cellular apoptotic pathway have been discovered. Like the cellular *bcl-2* protein, gene products from Epstein-Barr virus, adenovirus, herpes simplex virus, and baculovirus are all capable of preventing apoptosis, presumably to prolong cell viability during infection by these viruses (16, 19, 42, 97). On the other hand, cell killing by several lytic viruses, including human immunodeficiency, Sindbis, and influenza viruses, can be blocked by *bcl-2* overexpression (41, 47, 59, 71), suggesting that these viruses normally kill cells by triggering apoptosis. Experiments to test a possible role for the cellular apoptotic pathway in enteroviral infection or the ability of any enteroviral proteins to induce programmed cell death have not yet been reported.

Given their small genomes, enteroviruses cause a remarkable number of alterations in cellular physiology and morphology. In some cases, it might be more efficient for viruses to harness preexisting mechanisms within host cells than to invent new ones. For example, as discussed in chapter 5, translation by internal ribosome binding was originally thought to be a uniquely viral process. However, internal ribosome binding now appears to have a normal function in uninfected cells (65, 72). Perhaps other aspects of the interactions between enteroviruses and their host cells, such as the accumulation of membranous vesicles and the death of infected cells, also represent viral subversions of normal cellular programs.

ACKNOWLEDGMENTS

We thank Kurt Bienz and Denise Egger for the micrographs shown in Fig. 2. We are grateful to John Doedens and Peter Sarnow for ongoing discussions of the topics discussed here and for thoughtful comments on the manuscript.

The work described from this laboratory was supported in part by grant AI-25166 from the Public Health Service. A.S. is a recipient of fellowships from the Swiss National Science Foundation and the Howard Hughes Medical Institute. K.K. is an Assistant Investigator of the Howard Hughes Medical Institute.

REFERENCES

1. **Amako, K., and S. Dales.** 1967. Cytopathology of mengovirus infection. II. Proliferation of membranous cisternae. *Virology* **32:**201–215.
2. **Bablanian, R., H. J. Eggers, and I. Tamm.** 1965. Studies on the mechanism of poliovirus-induced cell damage. I. *Virology* **26:**100–113.
3. **Bablanian, R., H. J. Eggers, and I. Tamm.** 1965. Studies on the mechanism of poliovirus-induced cell damage. II. *Virology* **26:**114–121.
4. **Bienz, K., D. Egger, and L. Pasamontes.** 1987. Association of polioviral proteins of the P2 genomic region with the viral replication complex and virus-induced membrane synthesis as visualized by electron microscopic immunocytochemistry and autoradiography. *Virology* **160:**220–226.
5. **Bienz, K., D. Egger, T. Pfister, and M. Troxler.** 1992. Structural and functional characterization of the poliovirus replication complex. *J. Virol.* **66:**2740–2747.
6. **Bienz, K., D. Egger, Y. Rasser, and W. Bossart.** 1980. Kinetics and location of poliovirus macromolecular synthesis in correlation to virus-induced cytopathology. *Virology* **100:**390–399.
7. **Bienz, K., D. Egger, Y. Rasser, and W. Bossart.** 1983. Intracellular distribution of poliovirus proteins and the induction of virus-specific cytoplasmic structures. *Virology* **131:**39–48.
8. **Bienz, K., D. Egger, M. Troxler, and L. Pasamontes.** 1990. Structural organization of poliovirus RNA replication is mediated by viral proteins of the P2 genomic region. *J. Virol.* **64:**1156–1163.
9. **Bienz, K., D. Egger, and D. A. Wolff.** 1973. Virus replication, cytopathology, and lysosomal enzyme response of mitotic and interphase Hep-2 cells infected with poliovirus. *J. Virol.* **11:**565–574.
10. **Bossart, W., and K. Bienz.** 1979. Virus replication, cytopathology, and lysosomal enzyme release in enucleated HEp-2 cells infected with poliovirus. *Virology* **92:**331–339.
11. **Butterworth, B. E., E. J. Shimshick, and F. H. Yin.** 1976. Association of the poliovirial RNA polymerase complex with phospholipid membranes. *J. Virol.* **19:**457–466.
12. **Caliguiri, L. A., and I. Tamm.** 1970. The role of cytoplasmic membranes in poliovirus biosynthesis. *Virology* **42:**100–111.
13. **Caliguiri, L. A., and I. Tamm.** 1970. Characterization of poliovirus-specific structures associated with cytoplasmic membranes. *Virology* **42:**112–122.
14. **Calvez, V., I. Pelletier, S. Borzakian, and F. Colbére-Garapin.** 1993. Identification of a region of the poliovirus genome involved in persistent infection of HEp-2 cells. *J. Virol.* **67:**4432–4435.

15. Cho, M. W., N. Teterina, D. Egger, K. Bienz, and E. Ehrenfeld. 1994. Membrane rearrangement and vesicle induction by recombinant poliovirus 2C and 2BC in human cells. *Virology* **202**:129–145.
16. Chou, J., and B. Roizman. 1992. The d134.5 gene of herpes simplex virus 1 precludes neuroblastoma cells from triggering total shutoff of protein synthesis characteristic of programmed cell death in neuronal cells. *Proc. Natl. Acad. Sci. USA* **89**:3266–3270.
17. Clark, M. E., T. Hammerle, E. Wimmer, and A. Dasgupta. 1991. Poliovirus proteinase 3C converts an active form of trancription factor IIIC to an inactive form: a mechanism for inhibition of host cell polymerase III transcription by poliovirus. *EMBO J.* **10**:2941–2947.
18. Clark, M. E., P. M. Lieberman, A. J. Berk, and A. Dasgupta. 1993. Direct cleavage of human TATA-binding protein by poliovirus protease 3C in vivo and in vitro. *Mol. Cell. Biol.* **13**:1232–1237.
19. Clem, R. J., M. Fechheimer, and L. K. Miller. 1991. Prevention of apoptosis by a baculovirus gene during infection of insect cells. *Science* **254**:1388–1390.
20. Colbére-Garapin, F., C. Christodoulou, R. Crainic, and I. Pelletier. 1989. Persistent poliovirus infection of human neuroblastoma cells. *Proc. Natl. Acad. Sci. USA* **86**:7590–7594.
21. Comai, L., N. Tanese, and R. Tjian. 1992. The TATA-binding protein and associated factors are integral components of the RNA polymerase I transcription factor, SL1. *Cell* **68**:965–976.
22. Cormack, B. P., and K. Struhl. 1992. The TATA-binding protein is required for transcription by all three nuclear RNA polymerases in yeast cells. *Cell* **69**:685–696.
23. Crawford, N., A. Fire, M. Samuels, P. A. Sharp, and D. Baltimore. 1981. Inhibition of transcription factor activity by poliovirus. *Cell* **27**:555–561.
24. Cromeans, T., M. D. Sobsey, and H. A. Fields. 1987. Development of a plaque assay for a cytopathic, rapidly replicating isolate of hepatitis A virus. *J. Med. Virol.* **22**:45–56.
25. Dales, S., H. J. Eggers, I. Tamm, and G. E. Palade. 1965. Electron microscopic study of the formation of poliovirus. *Virology* **26**:379–389.
26. Das, S., and A. Dasgupta. 1993. Identification of the cleavage site and determinants required for poliovirus 3CPro-catalyzed cleavage of human TATA-binding transcription factor TBP. *J. Virol.* **67**:3326–3331.
27. Datta, U., and A. Dasgupta. 1994. Expression and subcellular localization of poliovirus VPg-precursor protein 3AB in eukaryotic cells: evidence for glycosylation in vitro. *J. Virol.* **68**:4468–4477.
28. Detjen, B. M., J. Lucas, and E. Wimmer. 1978. Poliovirus single-stranded RNA and double-stranded RNA: differential infectivity in enucleate cells. *J. Virol.* **27**:582–586.
29. Doedens, J., and K. Kirkegaard. Inhibition of cellular protein secretion by poliovirus proteins 2B and 3A. *EMBO J.*, in press.
30. Doedens, J., L. A. Maynell, M. W. Klymkowsky, and K. Kirkegaard. 1994. Secretory pathway function, but not cytoskeletal integrity, is required in poliovirus infection. *Arch. Virol.* **9**(Suppl.):159–172.
31. Donaldson, J. G., D. Finazzi, and R. D. Klausner. 1992. Brefeldin A inhibits Golgi membrane-catalysed exchange of guanine nucleotide onto ARF protein. *Nature* (London) **360**:350–352.
32. Ellis, H. M., and H. R. Horvitz. 1986. Genetic control of programmed cell death in the nematode *C. elegans*. *Cell* **47**:817–829.
33. Etchison, D., S. C. Milburn, I. Edery, N. Sonenberg, and J. W. B. Hershey. 1982. Inhibition of HeLa cell protein synthesis following poliovirus infection correlates with the proteolysis of a 220,000-dalton polypeptide associate with eukaryotic initiation factor 3 and a cap binding protein complex. *J. Biol. Chem.* **257**:14806–14810.
34. Falk, M. M., P. R. Grigera, I. E. Bergmann, A. Zibert, G. Multhaup, and E. Beck. 1990. Foot-and-mouth disease virus protease 3C induces specific proteolytic cleavage of host cell histone H3. *J. Virol.* **64**:748–756.
35. Ferro-Novick, S., and P. Novick. 1993. The role of GTP-binding proteins in transport along the exocytic pathway. *Annu. Rev. Cell Biol.* **9**:575–599.
36. Fradkin, L. G., S. K. Yoshinaga, A. J. Berk, and A. Dasgupta. 1987. Inhibition of host cell RNA polymerase III-mediated transcription by poliovirus: inactivation of specific transcription factors. *Mol. Cell. Biol.* **7**:3880–3887.
37. Franklin, R. M., and D. Baltimore. 1962. Patterns of macromolecular synthesis in normal and virus-infected mammalian cells. *Cold Spring Harbor Symp. Quant. Biol.* **27**:175–194.
38. Godman, G. C., R. A. Rifkind, C. Howe, and H. M. Rose. 1964. A description of ECHO 9 virus infection in cultured cells. I. The cytopathic effect. *Am. J. Pathol.* **44**:1–27.
39. Godman, G. C., R. A. Rifkind, R. B. Page, C. Howe, and H. M. Rose. 1964. A

description of ECHO 9 virus infection in cultured cells. II. Cytochemical observations. *Am. J. Pathol.* **44**:215–245.
40. **Gokal, P. K., A. H. Cavanaugh, and E. A. Thompson, Jr.** 1986. The effects of cycloheximide upon transcription of rRNA, 5S RNA and tRNA genes. *J. Biol. Chem.* **261**:2536–2541.
41. **Gougeon, M., and L. Montagnier.** 1993. Apoptosis in AIDS. *Science* **260**:1269–1270.
42. **Gregory, C. D., C. Dive, S. Henderson, C. A. Smith, G. T. Williams, F. Gordon, and A. B. Rickenson.** 1991. Activation of Epstein-Barr virus latent genes protects human B cells from death by apoptosis. *Nature* (London) **349**:612–614.
43. **Grunstein, M.** 1990. Histone function in transcription. *Annu. Rev. Cell Biol.* **6**:643–678.
44. **Guskey, L. E., P. C. Smith, and D. A. Wolff.** 1970. Patterns of cytopathology and lysosomal enzyme release in poliovirus-infected HEp-2 cells. *J. Gen. Virol.* **6**:151–161.
45. **Helms, J. B., and J. E. Rothman.** 1992. Inhibition by brefeldin A of a Golgi membrane enzyme that catalyses exchange of guanine nucleotide bound to ARF. *Nature* (London) **360**:352–354.
46. **Hengartner, M. O., and H. R. Horvitz.** 1994. *C. elegans* cell survival gene *ced-9* encodes a functional homolog of the mammalian protooncogene *bcl-2*. *Cell* **76**:665–676.
47. **Hinshaw, V. S., C. W. Olsen, N. Dybdahl-Sissoko, and D. Evans.** 1994. Apoptosis: a mechanism of cell killing by influenza A and B viruses. *J. Virol.* **68**:3667–3673.
48. **Irurzun, A., L. Perez, and L. Carrasco.** 1992. Involvement of membrane traffic in the replication of poliovirus genomes: effects of brefeldin A. *Virology* **191**:166–175.
49. **Jezequel, A. M., and J. W. Steiner.** 1966. Some ultrastructural and histochemical aspects of Coxsackie virus-cell interactions. *Lab. Invest.* **15**:1055–1083.
50. **Joachims, M., and D. Etchison.** 1992. Poliovirus infection results in structural alteration of a microtubule-associated protein. *J. Virol.* **66**:5797–5804.
51. **Kaplan, G., A. Levy, and V. R. Racaniello.** 1989. Isolation and characterization of HeLa cell lines blocked at different steps in the poliovirus life cycle. *J. Virol.* **63**:43–51.
52. **Kaplan, G., and V. R. Racaniello.** 1991. Down regulation of poliovirus receptor RNA in HeLa cells resistant to poliovirus infection. *J. Virol.* **65**:1829–1835.
53. **Kliewer, S., and A. Dasgupta.** 1988. An RNA polymerase II transcription factor inactivated in poliovirus-infected cells copurifies with transcription factor TFIID. *Mol. Cell. Biol.* **8**:3175–3182.
54. **Koch, F., and G. Koch.** 1985. *The Molecular Biology of Poliovirus.* Springer-Verlag, Vienna.
55. **Kreis, T. E.** 1992. Regulation of vesicular and tubular membrane traffic of the Golgi complex by coat proteins. *Curr. Opin. Cell Biol.* **4**:609–615.
56. **Lama, J., and L. Carrasco.** 1992. Expression of poliovirus nonstructural proteins in *Escherichia coli* cells. Modification of membrane permeability induced by 2B and 3A. *J. Biol. Chem.* **267**:15932–15937.
57. **Leibowitz, R., and S. Penman.** 1971. Regulation of protein synthesis in HeLa cells. III. Inhibition during poliovirus infection. *J. Virol.* **8**:661–668.
58. **Lenk, R., and S. Penman.** 1979. The cytoskeletal framework and poliovirus metabolism. *Cell* **16**:289–301.
59. **Levine, B., Q. Huang, J. T. Isaacs, J. C. G. Reed, D. E. Griffin, and J. M. Hardwick.** 1993. Conversion of lytic to persistent alphavirus infection by the *bcl-2* cellular oncogene. *Nature* (London) **361**:739–742.
60. **Liebig, H. D., E. Ziegler, R. Yan, K. Hartmuth, H. Klump, H. Kowalski, D. Blaas, W. Sommergruber, L. Frasel, B. J. Lamphear, R. E. Rhoads, E. Kuechler, and T. Skern.** 1993. Purification of two picornaviral proteases: interaction with eIF-4 gamma and influence on in vitro translation. *Biochemistry* **32**:7581–7588.
61. **Lloyd, R. E., and M. Bovee.** 1993. Persistent infection of human erythroblastoid cells by poliovirus. *Virology* **194**:200–209.
62. **Lobo, S. M., M. Tanaka, M. L. Sullivan, and N. Hernandez.** 1992. A TBP complex essential for transcription from TATA-less but not TATA-containing RNA polymerase III promoters is part of the TFIIIB fraction. *Cell* **71**:1029–1040.
63. **Lopez-Guerrero, J. A., L. Carrasco, F. Martinez-Abarca, M. Fresno, and M. A. Alonso.** 1989. Restriction of poliovirus RNA translation in a human monocytic cell line. *Eur. J. Biochem.* **186**:577–582.
64. **Luftig, R. B.** 1982. Does the cytoskeleton play a significant role in animal virus replication? *J. Theor. Biol.* **99**:173–191.
65. **Macejak, D. G., and P. Sarnow.** 1991. Internal initiation of translation mediated by the 5' leader of a cellular mRNA. *Nature* (London) **353**:90–94.
66. **Maynell, L. A., K. Kirkegaard, and M. W. Klymkowsky.** 1992. Inhibition of poliovirus

RNA synthesis by brefeldin A. *J. Virol.* **66**:1985–1994.
67. Melançon, P. 1993. G whizz. *Curr. Biol.* **3**:230–233.
68. Melnick, J. L. 1990. Enteroviruses: polioviruses, coxsackieviruses, echoviruses and newer enteroviruses, p. 549–606. *In* B. M. Fields and D. M. Knipe (ed.), *Virology.* Raven Press, New York.
69. Miura, M., H. Zhu, R. Rotello, and E. A. Y. Hartweig. 1993. Induction of apoptosis in fibroblasts by IL-1b-converting enzyme, a mammalian homology of the *C. elegans* cell death gene *ced-3. Cell* **75**:653–660.
70. Morace, G., G. Pisani, F. Beneduce, M. Divizia, and A. Pana. 1993. Mutations in the 3A genomic region of two cytopathic strains of hepatitis A virus isolated in Italy. *Virus Res.* **28**:187–194.
71. Noteborn, M. H. M., D. Todd, A. J. Vershueren, H. W. F. M. de Gauw, W. L. Curran, S. Verdkamp, A. J. Douglas, M. S. McNulty, A. J. van der Eb, and G. Koch. 1994. A single chicken anemia virus protein induces apoptosis. *J. Virol.* **68**:346–351.
72. Oh, S.-K., M. P. Scott, and P. Sarnow. 1992. Homeotic gene Antennapedia mRNA contains 5'-noncoding sequences that confer translational initiation by internal ribosome binding. *Genes Dev.* **6**:1643–1653.
73. Okada, Y., G. Toda, H. Oda, A. Nomoto, and H. Yoshikura. 1987. Poliovirus infection of established human blood cell lines: relationship between the differentiation stage and susceptibility or cell killing. *Virology* **156**:238–245.
74. Ostermann, J., L. Orci, K. Tani, M. Amherdt, M. Ravazzola, Z. Elazar, and J. E. Rothman. 1993. Stepwise assembly of functionally active transport vesicles. *Cell* **75**:1015–1025.
75. Peter, F., H. Plutner, H. Zhu, T. E. Kreis, and W. E. Balch. 1993. β-COP is essential for transport of protein from the endoplasmic reticulum to the Golgi *in vitro. J. Cell Biol.* **122**:1155–1167.
76. Phillips, S. G., and J. B. Rattner. 1976. Dependence of centriole formation on protein synthesis. *J. Cell Biol.* **70**:9–19.
77. Pugh, B. F., and R. Tjian. 1991. Transcription from a TATA-less promoter requires a multisubunit TFIID complex. *Genes Dev.* **5**:1935–1945.
78. Rice, J. M., and D. A. Woff. 1975. Phospholipase in the lysosomes of HEp-2 cells and its release during poliovirus infection. *Biochim. Biophys. Acta* **381**:17–21.
79. Rothman, J. E., and L. Orci. 1992. Molecular dissection of the secretory pathway. *Nature* (London) **355**:409–415.
80. Rubinstein, S. J., T. Hammerle, E. Wimmer, and A. Dasgupta. 1992. Infection of HeLa cells with poliovirus results in modification of a complex that binds to the rRNA promoter. *J. Virol.* **66**:3062–3068.
81. Rueckert, R. R. 1990. Picornaviridae and their replication, p. 507–548. *In* B. M. Fields and D. M. Knipe (ed.), *Virology.* Raven Press, New York.
81a. Schlegel, A., K. Bienz, D. Egger, and K. Kirkegaard. Unpublished data.
82. Schmid, S. L. 1993. Biochemical requirements for the formation of clathrin- and COP-coated transport vesicles. *Curr. Opin. Cell Biol.* **5**:621–627.
83. Schultz, M. C., R. H. Reeder, and S. Hahnm. 1992. Variants of the TATA-binding protein can distinguish subsets of RNA polymerase I, II and III promoters. *Cell* **69**:697–702.
84. Skinner, M. S., S. Halperen, and J. C. Harkin. 1968. Cytoplasmic membrane-bound vesicles in echovirus 12-infected cells. *Virology* **36**:241–253.
85. Takeda, N., R. J. Kuhn, C.-F. Yang, T. Takegami, and E. Wimmer. 1986. Initiation of poliovirus plus-strand RNA synthesis in a membrane complex of infected HeLa cells. *J. Virol.* **60**:43–53.
86. Takegami, T., B. L. Semler, C. W. Anderson, and E. Wimmer. 1983. Membrane fractions active in poliovirus RNA replication contain VPg precursor polypeptides. *Virology* **128**:33–47.
87. Tanigawa, G., L. Orci, M. Amherdt, M. Ravazzola, J. B. Helms, and J. E. Rothman. 1993. Hydrolysis of bound GTP by ARF protein triggers uncoating of Golgi-derived COP-coated vesicles. *J. Cell Biol.* **123**:1365–1371.
88. Tershak, D. R. 1984. Association of poliovirus proteins with the endoplasmic reticulum. *J. Virol.* **52**:777–783.
89. Tesar, M., and O. Marquardt. 1990. Foot-and-mouth disease virus protease 3C inhibits cellular transcription and mediates cleavage of histone H3. *Virology* **174**:364–374.
90. Thompson, J. S., X. Ling, and M. Grunstein. 1994. Histone H3 amino terminus is required for telomeric and silent mating locus repression in yeast. *Nature* (London) **369**:245–247.
91. Tolskaya, E. A., T. A. Ivannikova, M. S. Kolesnikova, S. G. Drozdov, and V. I. Agol. 1992. Postinfection treatment with antiviral serum results in survival of neural cells produc-

tively infected with virulent poliovirus. *J. Virol.* **66:**5152–5156.
92. **Toyoda, H., C.-F. Yang, N. Takeda, A. Nomoto, and E. Wimmer.** 1987. Analysis of RNA synthesis of type 1 poliovirus by using an in vitro molecular genetic approach. *J. Virol.* **61:**2816–2822.
93. **Troxler, M., D. Egger, T. Pfister, and K. Bienz.** 1992. Intracellular localization of poliovirus RNA by in situ hybridization at the ultrastructural level using single-stranded riboprobes. *Virology* **191:**687–697.
94. **Tucker, S. P., C. L. Thornton, E. Wimmer, and R. W. Compans.** 1993. Vectorial release of poliovirus from polarized human intestinal epithelial cells. *J. Virol.* **67:**4274–4282.
95. **Urzainqui, A., and L. Carrasco.** 1989. Degradation of cellular proteins during poliovirus infection: studies by two-dimensional gel electrophoresis. *J. Virol.* **63:**4729–4735.
96. **Weed, H. G., G. Krochmalnic, and S. Penman.** 1985. Poliovirus metabolism and the cytoskeletal framework: detergent extraction and resinless section electron microscopy. *J. Virol.* **56:**549–557.
97. **White, E. P., P. Sabbatini, M. Debbas, W. S. M. Wold, D. I. Dusher, and L. R. Gooding.** 1992. The 19-kilodalton adenovirus E1B transforming protein inhibits programmed cell death and prevents cytolysis by tumor necrosis factor a. *Mol. Cell. Biol.* **12:**2570–2580.
98. **White, J. M.** 1992. Membrane fusion. *Science* **258:**917–924.
99. **White, K., M. E. Grether, J. M. Abrams, L. Young, K. Farrell, and H. Steller.** 1994. Genetic control of programmed cell death in *Drosophila*. *Science* **264:**677–683.
100. **White, R. J., S. P. Jackson, and P. W. J. Rigby.** 1992. A role for the TATA-box binding protein component of the transcription factor IID complex as a general RNA polymerase III transcription factor. *Proc. Natl. Acad. Sci. USA* **89:**1949–1953.
101. **Williams, G. T., and C. A. Smith.** 1993. Molecular regulation of apoptosis: genetic controls on cell death. *Cell* **74:**777–779.
102. **Zerial, M., and H. Stenmark.** 1993. Rab GTPases in vesicular transport. *Curr. Opin. Cell Biol.* **5:**613–620.

ENTEROVIRUS STRUCTURE AND ASSEMBLY

Christopher U. T. Hellen and Eckard Wimmer

7

Enterovirus particles protect the encapsidated RNA genome from degradation and serve a number of more specialized functions, such as interacting with processing enzymes, selectively packaging newly synthesized genomes, and binding to specific cellular receptors on susceptible host cells in a manner that results in internalization of the genome. The structural information that specifies these different interactions must be conserved, yet the virion surface must also be sufficiently mutable to avoid immune surveillance by the host. Viruses undergo a number of structural rearrangements during assembly and disassembly to accommodate these different biological functions. In this chapter, we describe the structures of enterovirus capsid proteins and virions and the process by which virions are assembled and the genome is encapsidated.

PHYSICAL PROPERTIES OF VIRIONS

Enterovirus particles are small (about 30 nm in diameter), roughly spherical, and relatively simple, consisting of an outer protein shell and an inner RNA core (19, 60, 105). There is no lipid envelope, and virus infectivity is therefore insensitive to organic solvents (110). Enteroviruses are also acid stable, surviving pH 3 or lower, although several group A coxsackieviruses are thermolabile in low-ionic-strength solutions at neutral pH (35). Genomic RNA constitutes about 30% of the virion mass, which is about 8.5×10^6 kDa. All enteroviruses have a buoyant density of about 1.34 g/cm^3 in CsCl and a sedimentation coefficient of about 156S (Table 1). Density gradient centrifugation reveals that virus preparations contain a second, more slowly sedimenting top component (107); these empty capsids do not contain RNA (148, 168) and have a sedimentation coefficient of 70S to 80S (60, 74, 79, 112, 130, 133, 148, 157). Empty capsids are less stable than virions, and denaturation occurs readily, causing antigenic changes (145, 146, 157). Cytoplasmic extracts of enterovirus-infected cells contain a number of additional protein complexes that are antigenically related to virions and probably correspond to assembly precursors and intermediates (66, 139, 153, 169). These structures are discussed in greater detail below.

A number of enteroviruses have been crystallized, and X-ray diffraction analysis and electron microscopic studies have revealed that

Christopher U. T. Hellen, Department of Microbiology and Immunology, State University of New York Health Sciences Center at Brooklyn, 450 Clarkson Avenue, Box 44, Brooklyn, New York 11203-2098.   *Eckard Wimmer,* Department of Microbiology, State University of New York at Stony Brook, Stony Brook, New York 11794-8621.

Human Enterovirus Infections, Edited by Harley A. Rotbart,
© 1995 American Society for Microbiology, Washington, DC 20005

TABLE 1 Physical properties of enterovirus virions

Virus[a]	Sedimentation coefficient (S)[b]	Buoyant density[b]	Molecular size of capsid protein (kDa)[c]				References
			VP4	VP2	VP3	VP1	
Poliovirus 1 (M)[d]	160	1.34	7.4 (68)	30.0 (271)	26.4 (238)	33.5 (302)	78, 105, 120, 154–156
Poliovirus 2 (S)[d]	160	1.34	7.4 (69)	30.0 (271)	26.4 (238)	33.1 (301)	138, 154
Coxsackievirus A2[d]			7.4 (68)	28.1 (255)	26.3 (240)	32.6 (294)	
Coxsackievirus A9[d]		1.34	7.0 (69)	28.9 (261)	26.3 (238)	34.2 (303)	105
Coxsackievirus A10	153	1.34					
Coxsackievirus A16[d]			7.4 (68)	27.6 (254)	26.6 (242)	32.9 (297)	105
Coxsackievirus A21							105
Coxsackievirus A24[d]			7.3 (69)	29.8 (271)	26.6 (240)	34.4 (305)	
Coxsackievirus B1[d]			7.4 (68)	29.1 (263)	26.6 (240)	33.4 (298)	
Coxsackievirus B2							78
Coxsackievirus B3[d]			7.4 (68)	28.8 (263)	26.1 (238)	31.3 (281)	
Coxsackievirus B4[d]			7.4 (68)	28.5 (261)	26.4 (238)	32.0 (284)	
Coxsackievirus B5[d]	160	1.35	7.4 (68)	28.6 (261)	26.0 (238)	31.6 (283)	62
ECBO virus SA1	156	1.34					137
Echovirus 4		1.35					78
Echovirus 7	160	1.33					63, 154
Echovirus 9	156		7	28	30	33	148
Echovirus 11		1.33					38
Echovirus 12		1.33	7	31	24	33	60, 148, 149
Echovirus 16		1.32					78
Echovirus 19		1.34					78
SVDV[d]	160	1.34	7.3 (69)	28.6 (261)	26.0 (238)	31.5 (283)	62, 75, 112
EV70[d]	150	1.34	7.3 (69)	27.5 (250)	26.4 (242)	34.3 (310)	47, 173
EV71[d]	165	1.35	9.0	27.0	25.8	37.2	29, 176
BEV[d]	165	1.34	6.9 (64)	27.2 (248)	26.6 (242)	31.1 (281)	104, 120
PEV	150	1.34					119
CrPV	167	1.34	(8)	34	30	35	113
DCV	153	1.34	8.5	30	28	31	113

[a]ECBO, enteric cytopathogenic bovine orphan; SVDV, swine vesicular disease virus; EV70, enterovirus type 70; BEV, bovine enterovirus; PEV, porcine enterovirus; CrPV, cricket paralysis virus; DCV, *Drosophila* C virus.
[b]Values are from the indicated references.
[c]Values in parentheses are numbers of amino acids.
[d]Numbers of amino acids and molecular sizes of most capsid proteins are derived from published nucleotide sequences (see Table 1 in chapter 2).

virions have icosahedral symmetry owing to the regular organization of identical protein subunits arranged in axes of two-, three-, and fivefold symmetry within the protein shell (39, 51, 72). The surface lattice of icosahedral viruses necessarily has 60 equivalent subdivisions, which can consist of single or multiple subunits (40). In picornaviruses, this subdivision is the protomer, which consists of a single copy of each of four distinct capsid proteins, termed VP4, VP3, VP2, and VP1. The basic virion assembly unit is the protomer, which consists of one copy each of VP0, VP1, and VP3. The protomeric unit illustrated in Fig. 1 is suggested by the intertwining of the N and C termini of these proteins in the virion and is energetically the most favorable configuration according to calculation of the "buried" surface area between pairwise combinations of human rhinovirus type 14 capsid protein (7). All enteroviruses contain equimolar amounts of these four capsid proteins (26, 41, 148, 149, 164); traces of a fifth polypeptide (VP0, which is the precursor of VP2 and VP4) can be de-

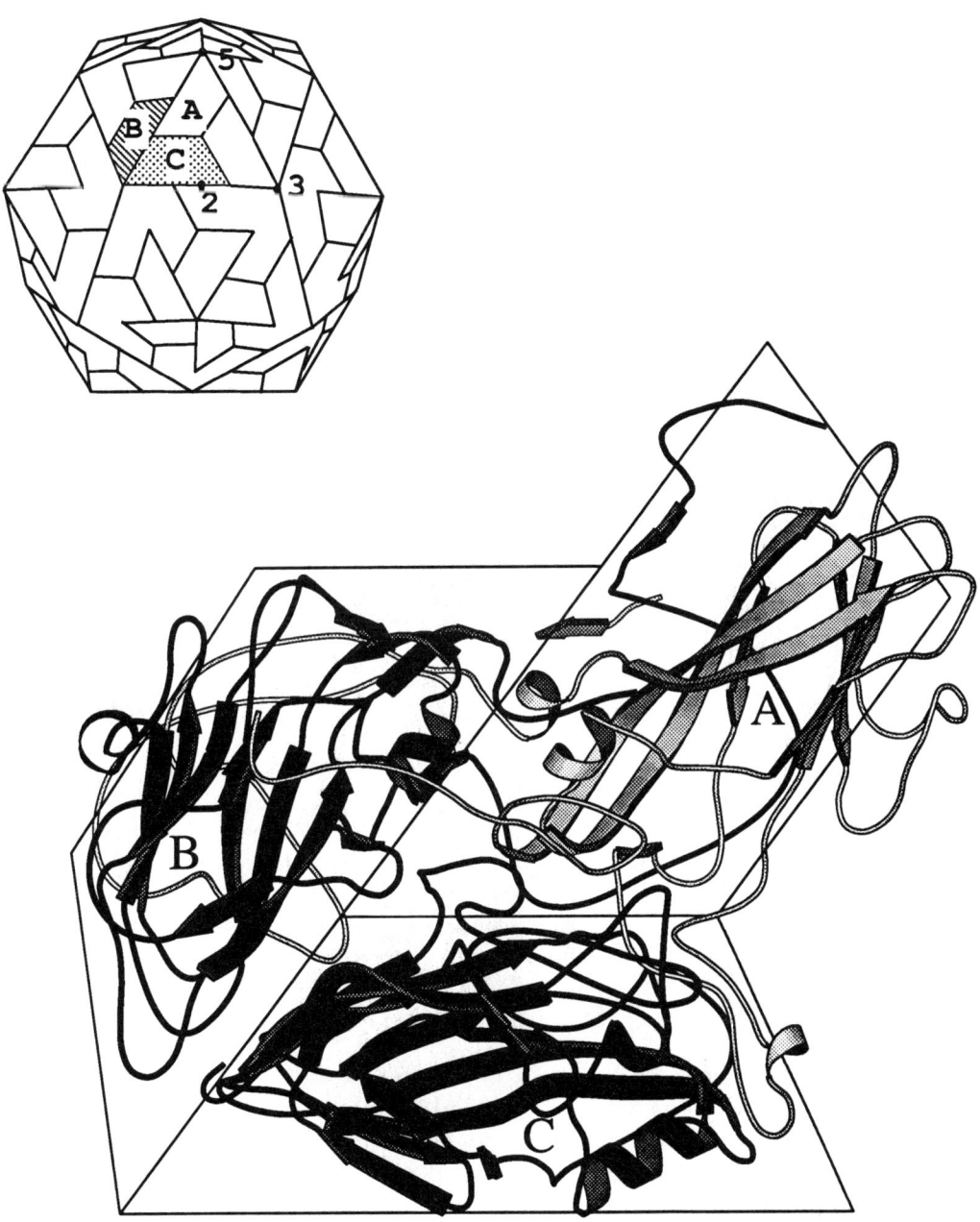

Poliovirus Protomer

FIGURE 1 Quaternary organization of poliovirus capsid proteins VP2, VP3, and VP1 within the protomer. The ribbon drawing represents the arrangement of the three β barrels within the virus quaternary structure. The heavy outline in the capsid model represents the biological protomer, which is not identical to the triangular asymmetric unit. The shading matches the β barrel units found in each trapezoid. Quasi-twofold, fivefold, and quasi-sixfold axes of symmetry are indicated by solid diamonds, pentagons, and triangles, respectively.

tected in highly purified virus preparations. Bovine enteroviruses contain submolar amounts of VP4 (79). This polypeptide is also readily lost from some group A coxsackieviruses at neutral pH (35), and from enteroviruses such as poliovirus and group B coxsackieviruses following heat or alkaline treatment (20, 41, 97). Empty capsids lack VP4 and VP2 but contain equimolar amounts of VP0, VP3, and VP1 (77, 148, 149).

ENTEROVIRUS CAPSID PROTEINS

Enterovirus capsid proteins are translated in the order VP4-VP2-VP3-VP1 as part of a large polyprotein and are separated by proteolytic cleavage (Fig. 2). Cleavage sites in the poliovirus P1 capsid protein precursor have been determined experimentally (46, 87), and those in other enteroviruses have been deduced by sequence alignment (Table 2). They fall into three groups (N, K/S; Q, A, N/G; and Y, F, T/G) that correspond to the three distinct cleavage activities that process the capsid proteins (see below). The four poliovirus capsid proteins and their precursors have been mapped onto the genome by alignment of its nucleotide sequence (84, 140) with partial amino acid sequences derived from the amino and carboxy termini of these polypeptides. The amino termini of VP4 and its precursors VP0 and P1 are blocked (44) by amide linkage of a myristic acid moiety to the amino terminus of VP4 (28, 129), and the initiation codon of the viral polyprotein was instead identified by analysis of tryptic peptides derived from VP4 (44).

The number of amino acid residues in the capsid proteins VP3 and VP4 is similar in all enteroviruses, whereas the lengths of VP1 and VP2 species differ by up to 10% (Table 1). The sequences of these polypeptides appear to be very variable, but in fact, much of this variation represents limited divergence from a conserved sequence (Table 3). VP1 capsid proteins show the least degree of similarity, a fact that may be related to their involvement in interactions with a variety of cell surface receptors and in antibody binding; the greater similarity of structural elements in VP2 could be related to functions (such as assembly and disassembly) that are common to all enteroviruses (7). Consideration of other picornavirus sequences indicates that rhinoviruses are the most similar to enteroviruses (Table 3) and could be considered part of the same virus group; the sequences of equivalent entero- and rhinovirus capsid proteins are sufficiently closely related to be aligned (128). Structural superimposition of individual capsid proteins also permits alignment of VP1, VP2, and VP3 with each other, although sequence and structural similarities between the three capsid proteins in any single virus isolate are less than those between equivalent picornavirus capsid proteins (95). This suggests that capsid proteins diverged from a single primordial ancestor before the polyproteins of present-day viruses diverged from one another.

PROTEOLYTIC PROCESSING OF CAPSID PROTEIN PRECURSORS

The RNA genomes of poliovirus and other enteroviruses are translated into single large polyproteins that are subsequently proteolytically processed to yield diverse structural and nonstructural proteins (71, 77, 82, 98, 163; reviewed in reference 65). The initial event in this proteolytic cascade is the primary cleavage by which the P1 structural protein precursor is separated from the nascent P2-P3 precursor in a reaction catalyzed by 2A proteinase, which hydrolyzes a Tyr-Gly bond at its own amino terminus (166) (Fig. 2). The activity of 2A^{pro} is not dependent on its excision from the P2 precursor (64), but the initial cleavage that it catalyzes must occur before the P1 precursor can be processed further to yield capsid proteins (121).

Secondary cleavage of Gln-Gly dipeptides between nonstructural proteins of the P2-P3 region can be catalyzed by 3C proteinase alone (179), although it is more likely that they are normally catalyzed by 3C precursors (86, 88). The structure of the related 3C^{pro} of hepatitis A virus indicates that it is unlikely that cleavage releasing the enzyme from the polyprotein is intramolecular (2). However, 3C^{pro} is unable

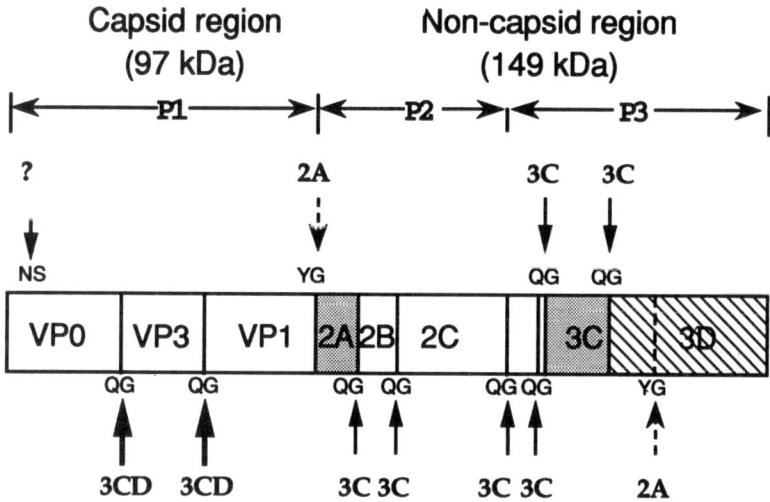

FIGURE 2 Gene organization, processing scheme, and cleavage sites of the P1 poliovirus capsid protein precursor. Proteolytic cleavages occur between amino acid pairs, indicated by standard single-letter code. Arrows above and below the P1 partial polyprotein indicate sites that are cleaved in inter- and intramolecular reactions, respectively, by proteinases as indicated. The question mark indicates that the mechanism of cleavage at this site is not known.

to catalyze efficient cleavage between VP0-VP3 and VP3-VP1, even though these capsid proteins are separated by Gln-Gly dipeptides. These reactions are instead catalyzed by 3CD^{pro}, which contains the sequence of the polymerase 3D in addition to 3C^{pro} (80, 177). The efficiency and fidelity of P1 cleavage depend both on recognition of an extended cleavage site by 3C^{pro} (in which residues flanking the scissile bond and at the -4 position are primary determinants of cleavage [4, 16, 17, 122, 126]) and on specific interactions between 3CD^{pro} and the P1 polyprotein (88). The importance of the integrity of the ordered structure of the P1 precursor for cleavage has been demonstrated by making specific truncations, deletions, and insertions within or at the termini of P1 (106, 121, 178). Cleavage of the P1 precursor appears to be a requirement for entry of capsid proteins into the virion assembly pathway (6, 127), so these stringent requirements for P1 processing may enhance the fidelity of assembly by excluding incorrectly folded precursors.

The final processing step is cleavage of VP0 to VP4 and VP2, which occurs at an Asn-Ser dipeptide in poliovirus (87), and at similar dipeptides in other enteroviruses (Table 3). This maturation cleavage occurs late in capsid assembly, after assembly of pentamers and probably concomitantly with encapsidation of RNA. The termini generated by VP0 cleavage are close to one another in the interior of mature virions, and the scissile bond therefore appears to be inaccessible to exogenous viral or cellular proteinases. It has been suggested that cleavage is catalyzed by some aspect of the virion structure itself, but the mechanism by which it occurs is not known. The proximity of a conserved serine residue in VP2 to one of the cleaved termini of VP0 led Arnold et al. (6) to suggest a novel RNA-aided serine proteinase-like mechanism for this cleavage, but participation of Ser-10 in this reaction had been ruled out, since this residue can be replaced without impairment of VP0 cleavage (61a). Although ordered purine nucleotides have been identified in the vicinity of the amino terminus of VP2 (7, 50), the identification of a *ts* poliovirus mutant that failed to

TABLE 2 Proteolytic cleavage sites within P1 structural protein precursor of enteroviruses

Virus[a]	Cleavage site[b]			
	VP4/VP2	VP2/VP3	VP3/VP1	VP1/2A
Poliovirus 1 (M)	N-S	Q-G	Q-G	Y-G
Coxsackievirus A2	Q-S	Q-G	Q-G	T-G
Coxsackievirus A9	N-S	Q-G	Q-G	F-G
Coxsackievirus A16	K-S	Q-G	Q-G	L-G
Coxsackievirus A21	N-S	Q-G	Q-G	F-G
Coxsackievirus A24	N-S	Q-G	Q-G	Y-G
Coxsackievirus B1	N-S	Q-G	Q-G	Y-G
Coxsackievirus B3	N-S	Q-G	Q-G	T-G
Coxsackievirus B4	N-S	Q-G	Q-G	Y-G
Coxsackievirus B5	N-S	Q-G	Q-G	T-G
Echovirus 11	ND	ND	ND	Y-G
Echovirus 12	N-S	Q-G	Q-G	T-G
SVDV	N-S	Q-G	Q-G	T-G
EV70	K-S	Q-G	Q-A	Y-G
BEV	K-S	Q-G	Q-N	Y-G
CrPV	ND	ND	ND	Y-G

[a] Abbreviations: SVDV, swine vesicular disease virus; EV70, enterovirus type 70; BEV, bovine enterovirus; CrPV, cricket paralysis virus.
[b] Amino acids are indicated by the single-letter code.

cleave VP0 and instead accumulated provirions at the nonpermissive temperature indicates that RNA packaging can be uncoupled from VP0 cleavage (32). Cleavage of VP0 does not occur at 30°C, a temperature at which 14S pentamers accumulate in vivo (145). Thus, although conformational changes induced by pentamer-pentamer interactions and by encapsidation of RNA may be necessary to trigger cleavage of VP0, neither process is in itself sufficient. Nevertheless, the dependence of VP0 cleavage on RNA encapsidation may serve to make this step in viral assembly irreversible.

A functionally similar autocatalytic maturation cleavage occurs in nodaviruses, and it has been suggested that capsid assembly initiates cleavage by raising the pK_a of an Asp residue, which then acts as the proton donor in an acid-catalyzed hydrolysis reaction (172). This proposal may be relevant to enterovirus maturation, since Asp residues probably occur in the vicinity of the VP4-VP2 bond (61a).

STRUCTURAL INTERMEDIATES IN ENTEROVIRUS ASSEMBLY

A number of potential intermediates in picornavirus assembly have been identified (139, 153); their positions in the enterovirus assembly pathway are shown in Fig. 3. The earliest assembly precursor is the 5S immature protomer, which consists of one copy each of VP0, VP3, and VP1 and results from cleavage of the P1 capsid protein precursor. It is likely that the individual VP2, VP3, and VP1 β bar-

TABLE 3 Amino acid sequence similarity between capsid proteins of poliovirus type 1 (Mahoney) and other enteroviruses and rhinoviruses

Virus[a]	Amino acid sequence similarity (%) with poliovirus type 1 (Mahoney) protein			
	VP4	VP2	VP3	VP1
PV3/23127	93	83	83	71
CA21	75	72	74	56
CB3	65	56	53	41
CB4	70	56	56	47
CB5	65	55	56	48
SVDV	65	50	53	43
BEV	60	55	41	33
EV70	62	53	43	36
HRV2	58	45	49	17

[a] The sources of virus sequences are as in Table 1 except for that of human rhinovirus type 2 (HRV2) (158). Abbreviations: CA21, coxsackievirus type A21; CB3, CB4, and CB5, coxsackievirus types B3, B4, and B5, respectively. Other abbreviations are defined in Table 2, footnote a.

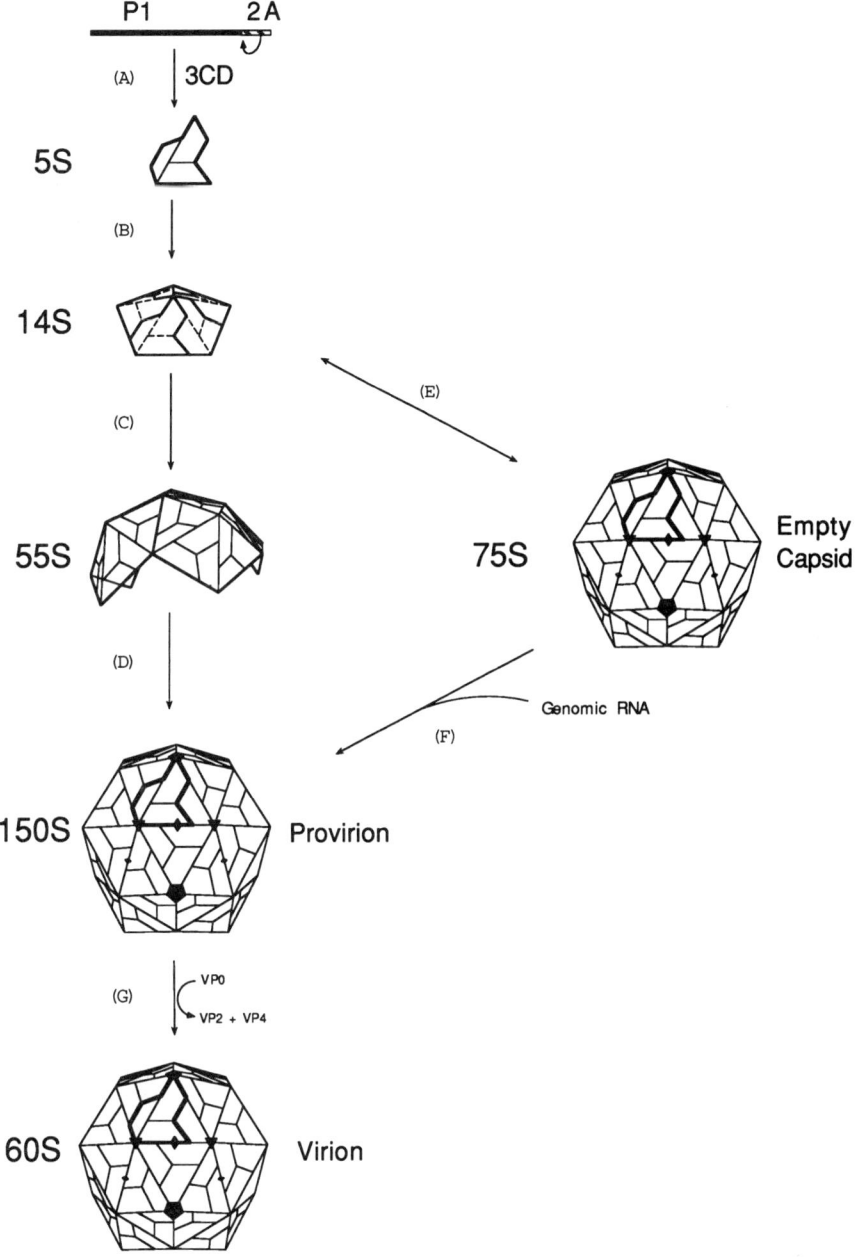

FIGURE 3 Enterovirus morphogenesis. (A) The P1 capsid protein precursor is released from the nascent polyprotein following autocatalytic cleavage by 2A^{pro} at its own amino terminus and is then cleaved twice by 3CD^{pro}. The cleaved termini of all three capsid proteins undergo considerable rearrangement after P1 cleavage, and cleavage is a prerequisite for assembly (B) of five 5S monomers into 14S pentamers. Twelve 14S pentamers either may associate directly with genomic RNA to form provirions, possibly by way of 55S half-shell intermediates (C and D), or may assemble to form empty capsids (E) into which genomic RNA is subsequently inserted (F). Maturation cleavage (G) of VP0 to yield VP4 and VP2 results in conversion of 150S provirions into 160S virions.

rels are formed as the P1 capsid protein precursor is being synthesized, and consideration of probable changes in free energy strongly suggests that these domains fold and organize themselves within the P1 precursor prior to proteolytic cleavage by 3CD^{pro} (7, 55). Cleavage sites occur in structurally flexible regions between β barrels (6) and after cleavage, the free ends could reposition themselves into the orientations observed in the mature virus without disrupting the contacts between β barrels. The 5S protomer is the precursor of the 14S pentamer, which has the composition (VP0-VP3-VP1)$_5$ (56, 131, 136, 162, 170). By analogy with cardioviruses, cleavage of P1 may be a prerequisite for assembly of immature protomers into stable pentamers and would provide spatial and temporal control over the initiation of assembly (127). This possibility is strongly supported by structural analysis of mature virions: the β cylinder at the fivefold axis of symmetry is formed by the amino termini of adjacent VP3 molecules and is surrounded by a concentric bundle formed from the amino termini of VP0 and VP1 (see below). These interactions are obviously dependent on proteolytic cleavage to free the amino termini of capsid proteins.

Pentamers are key assembly intermediates common to all picornaviruses (18, 145). Poliovirus 14S pentamers are capable of self-association to form 75S procapsids in vivo and in vitro (131, 134–136, 144), and radioactively labeled pentamers can be chased into mature virions in vivo (145). Moreover, cardiovirions can be dissociated under mild conditions into 13.4S pentameric structures with the composition (VP2-VP3-VP1)$_5$ (45). Pentamers are thus stabilized by strong interactions between protomers, which are likely to include the interactions of the amino termini of VP1, VP0, and VP3 at the fivefold axis of symmetry described above. Particles of 45S to 55S that may correspond to half-shell assembly intermediates have been identified; they are composed of the polypeptides VP0, VP3, and VP1, and some reports indicate that they can be converted into procapsids in vitro (36, 112, 114, 147, 162).

Procapsids correspond to the empty capsids that were first detected by density gradient centrifugation (60, 74, 107, 157). They contain 12 pentamers and have the composition (VP0-VP3-VP1)$_{60}$. The term "procapsid" was coined to reflect their proposed role as virion precursors in a model for assembly in which newly synthesized virion RNA is inserted into the central cavity of the procapsid to form provirions (76) (Fig. 4). Stable procapsids were reported to accumulate in the presence of guanidine and could be chased into mature virions after alleviation of guanidine inhibition (76). However, poliovirus procapsids are known to readily undergo irreversible antigenic and structural alterations, so purification of stable procapsids may be artifactual (153). Other reports indicate that natural empty capsids purified at low temperature can dissociate reversibly into 14S pentamers (50, 102). This observation would be consistent with an alternative morphogenesis pathway in which 14S pentamers assemble directly with virion RNA to form provirions and procapsids act as nothing more than storage forms of 14S pentamers.

150S provirions have the same protein composition as procapsids [i.e., (VP0-VP3-VP1)$_{60}$] and are the final assembly intermediate; they contain 35S virion RNA but are not infectious even though they are able to bind to HeLa cells and to elute in a conformationally altered 125S to 130S form (32, 48, 49, 58). Provirions have also been isolated from bovine enterovirus-infected cells (68); their precursor role in virion formation is supported by analysis of the kinetics of VP0 cleavage and of associated changes in particle infectivity and structure, using *wt* hepatitis A virus and genetically engineered mutants of poliovirus and human rhinovirus (15, 32, 90).

POLIOVIRUS ARCHITECTURE

The mature picornavirus particle consists of a single copy of the genome packaged in an icosahedrally symmetric protein shell composed of 60 protomers, each consisting of a single copy of the capsid proteins VP1 through

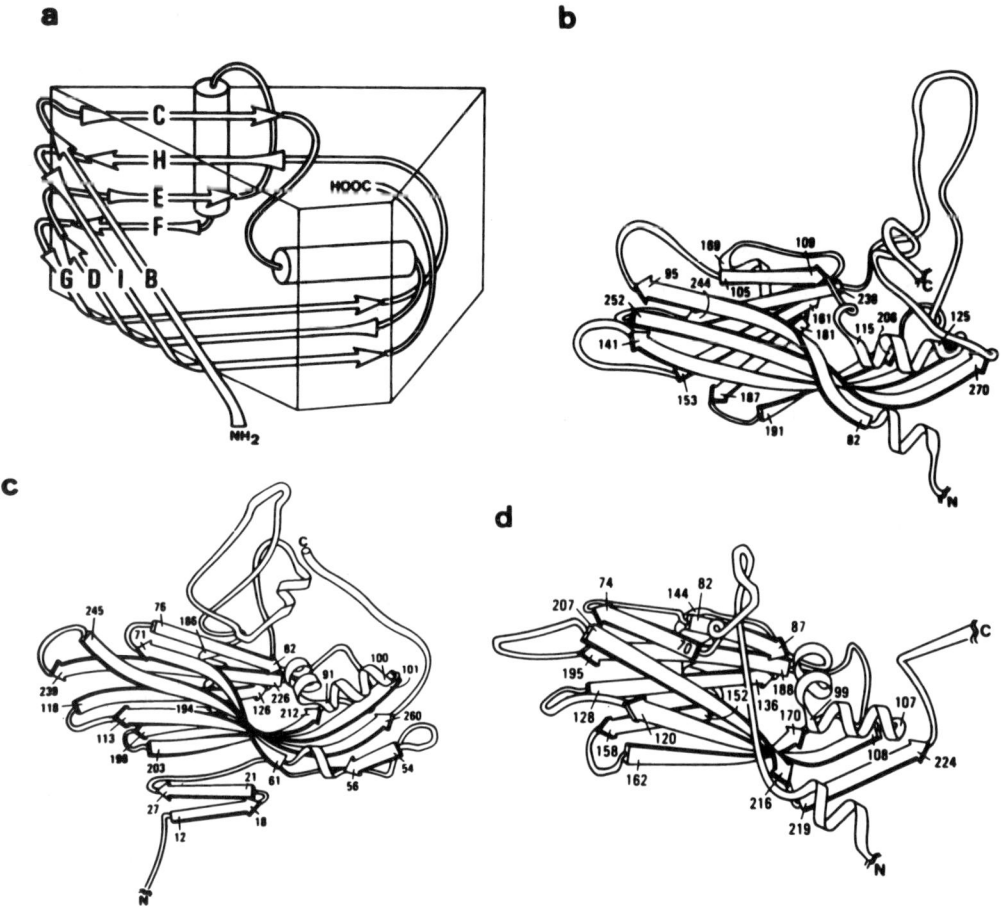

FIGURE 4 Structures of the three major capsid proteins of poliovirus. (a) Schematic representation of the wedgelike eight-stranded antiparallel β barrel protein fold shared by VP1, VP2, and VP3. Individual β strands are shown as arrows and labeled with letters. Flanking helices are shown as cylinders. (b to d) Ribbon diagrams of VP1 (b), VP2 (c), and VP3 (d). The numbers indicate amino acid residues; extensions at the amino and carboxy termini of VP1 and VP3 have been truncated for clarity.

VP4, which are the subunits of the protomers. The structures of two serotypes of poliovirus (50, 69) and of representatives of three other genera of picornaviruses have been determined by X-ray crystallography (see reference 89 and references therein).

The three major picornavirus capsid proteins, VP1, VP2, and VP3, each contain about 250 amino acids and have a relatively compact structure. VP4 is much smaller (ca. 70 amino acids) and can be regarded as a (detached) N-terminal extension of VP2 by virtue of its extended conformation and its internal position in the mature virion. The core structures of the three large proteins are topologically identical; each consists of an eight-stranded antiparallel β barrel with two flanking helices (Fig. 4b, c, and d). This folding pattern is conserved in the capsid proteins of icosahedral eukaryotic RNA viruses (152). The β strands are conventionally designated alphabetically (151): one antiparallel β sheet is made up of strands B, I, D, and G, and the other is made up of strands C, H, E, and F (Fig. 4a). These two β sheets form the front and back surfaces of the barrel and enclose a hydrophobic pocket that is empty in VP2 and VP3 but may be occupied by a lipid substituent in VP1 (50, 174). The β strands are joined at one end by four short loops, and as a result, the β barrel is wedge-shaped. The greatest differences between capsid proteins are in the size and conformation of the loops that connect the outer strands of the β barrels and in the extensions at their N and C termini. These loops decorate the surface of the virion and mostly determine the antigenic sites of the virus, whereas the flexible N-terminal extensions (including VP4) form an intertwined network within the virion that contributes significantly to its stability. The carboxy termini are located on the outer surface of the virion and are spatially distant from the amino termini, indicating that significant local rearrangement must occur within structural precursors of the virion following proteolytic cleavage of the P1 capsid protein precursor.

The triangular shapes of the three major capsid proteins allow them to pack tightly around the symmetry axes of the virion. The narrow ends of the VP1 β barrels are canted up from the plane of the virion surface, exposing the uppermost three loops of the barrel and forming a peak at the fivefold axis that extends to a 165-Å (16.5-nm) radius. The exposed BC loop of VP1 constitutes a major portion of neutralizing antigenic site 1; it is the site of the greatest conformational difference between poliovirus serotypes and has a pronounced effect on poliovirus host range (50, 103, 118). The peak at the fivefold axis of symmetry is surrounded by a deep canyon that is inaccessible to antibodies because of steric hindrance and is the putative site of receptor binding (150). A hydrophobic pocket within the β barrel of VP1 lies just beneath the floor of the canyon and is normally occupied by a lipid pocket factor that must be displaced by interaction with the receptor before the conformational changes within the capsid that lead to uncoating and release of incoming RNA can occur (50, 125, 174). The pocket can be filled by lipophilic antiviral WIN compounds, which stabilize the capsid against thermal denaturation and prevent conformational rearrangements associated with uncoating (108) (see chapter 18). Interestingly, the presence of WIN 51711 promotes self-assembly of 14S subunits into native procapsids (144), which raises the possibility that this pocket also plays a role in virus assembly. The narrow ends of VP2 and VP3 alternate around the quasi-sixfold axes, and their outward tilt is less pronounced; only the outermost two loops are exposed, and they form part of a broad plateau.

The N termini of five VP3 molecules form an unusual cylindrically parallel β sheet at the fivefold axis of symmetry, and this sheet is in turn surrounded by five three-stranded β sheets formed by the N termini of VP4 and VP1. Interaction between these two structures is mediated by the myristate moiety that is attached to the N terminus of VP4 (28, 129; see also below). Adjacent pentamers form an interlocking seven-stranded β sheet; four strands of the VP3 β barrel and one strand comprising residues close to the N terminus of VP1 flank a two-stranded β sheet formed by the N terminal residues of VP2 from a neighboring pentamer (50).

Peptide-scanning analyses indicate that the poliovirus virion is conformationally flexible and that VP4 and an immunodominant region from the amino terminus of VP1 can be reversibly exposed in solution at physiologic temperatures (93, 142, 143). The irreversible exposure of these residues following interaction with the cellular poliovirus receptor has been implicated in early events in infection (37, 54, 83, 116, 117) (see chapter 3).

STRUCTURAL AND CONFORMATIONAL CHANGES DURING MORPHOGENESIS

Proteolytic cleavage of enterovirus capsid proteins from the P1 precursor, assembly, and eventual maturation of the virion are regulated, sequential processes that appear to be intimately connected. Structural rearrangement of the capsid domains (and particularly their N-terminal extensions) consequent to successive cleavage events regulates and directs the association and assembly of capsid subunits.

The initial modification of the P1 capsid protein precursor is the cotranslational removal of the initiating fMet moiety and subsequent linkage of myristic acid to the exposed amino-terminal glycine residue of VP4 (and its precursors VP0 and P1) (28, 44, 129). The myristate moieties participate in a network of intersubunit interactions that is formed on assembly of protomers into pentamers; the moieties cluster around the fivefold axis of symmetry and stabilize the β cylinder formed by the amino termini of five VP3 molecules (28, 50). Systematic mutational analysis indicates that myristoylation is dependent on residues at the N terminus of VP4 that match the eukaryotic consensus sequence (57); analysis of defective mutants has confirmed a role for the myristate moiety in stabilizing pentamers and consequently virions (5, 99, 100, 101, 114, 115). Substitutions that reduced the level of myristoylation resulted in the formation of some mature virions, but these either had greatly reduced specific activities or were completely unable to initiate a second round of infection (100, 101, 115). This indicates that VP4 plays a role in at least one of the early steps in viral infection.

Enterovirus capsid proteins probably adopt the β-barrel folding pattern as the capsid protein precursor is being synthesized, but considerable rearrangement of the amino and carboxy termini of capsid proteins after proteolytic cleavage is apparent from structural analysis (69). The carboxy termini of VP1, VP2, and VP3 are located on the outer surface of the capsid, whereas the amino termini of these three proteins participate in an extensive interior network of interactions between protomers on the inner surface of the virion. The formation of this network depends on proteolytic cleavage of P1, which accounts for the coupling of proteolytic processing with events early in assembly. Cleavage of VP0 to VP4 and VP2 is associated with the acquisition of infectivity and an increase in particle stability. The latter is due in part to the formation of an interlocking seven-stranded β sheet by residues from adjacent pentamers (50). Four strands of the VP3 β barrel and one strand consisting of residues from VP1 flank a two-stranded β sheet formed by the amino-terminal residues from a neighboring pentamer. Formation of this structure results from rearrangement of the innermost three strands during the assembly of pentamers into capsids. This structure does not occur in empty capsids (53), an observation suggesting that its formation is correlated either with cleavage of VP0 or with encapsidation of RNA. The residues forming the interdigitating fifth and sixth strands of this β sheet are part of the VP2 domain of a neighboring pentamer and are disordered in empty capsids. This suggests that cleavage of VP0 could dictate their positioning and thus regulate the adhesion of pentamers into a growing capsid.

The temperature-sensitive growth of the attenuated Sabin strain of poliovirus type 3 is attributable to a Ser3091Phe substitution in VP3 (111). This residue is located at a protomer-protomer interface at the base of the canyon (50), and the ts defect is thought to take effect during the assembly of protomers into pentamers and presumably to result from an altered equilibrium between assembly intermediates (96). A number of non-ts revertants contain second-site suppressor mutations that may stabilize interfaces between capsid proteins that are altered during thermally induced conformational changes, thus accelerating steps in assembly after pentamer formation. Most occur close to Phe-3091, but the remainder mapped either to the assembly-dependent β sheet that stabilizes the association of adjacent pentamers or to the lipid-binding pocket that lies below the canyon floor (96, 111). This genetic analysis supports the identification by structural means of locations that are thought to regulate or stabilize conformational changes that occur during assembly.

MECHANISM OF RNA ENCAPSIDATION

Enteroviral infection of cells involves the formation of smooth cytoplasmic vesicles that are the sites of virus-specific RNA synthesis (24, 25, 42, 159). The viral proteins 2C, 2BC, and 3D are closely associated with these vesicles (13, 21, 25, 165) and can be visualized by electron microscopic immunocytochemistry in membrane-associated structures that probably correspond to the viral replication complex (12, 56a). 3D is the viral RNA polymerase (9, 52). The function of 2BC, if any, is unknown, but poliovirus 2C appears to be involved in viral RNA synthesis (91); it can be cross-linked to viral RNA by UV radiation in situ and may attach viral RNA to the surfaces of vesicles (14). Mutations within 2C also confer an uncoating defect on virions that can be complemented by wt 2C and can be suppressed by an additional substitution within 2C (92). These observations imply that 2C plays a role in determining virion structure. 2C is a nucleoside triphosphatase whose activity is stimulated by RNA (141), and one can speculate that it might act as an ATP-dependent RNA translocase. There is some evidence that 2C is involved in the release of completed viral RNA from the replication complex (73). Poliovirus capsid proteins are found in smooth membrane fractions containing the viral RNA replication complex (22, 23, 175). They have been detected in the form of pentamers and pentamer assemblies by using electron microscopic immunocytochemistry and monoclonal antibodies specific for assembly intermediates (132).

Two models have been proposed for virion formation (Fig. 3). The first involves encapsidation into procapsids and is supported by the reported association of procapsids with the viral replication complex (22, 175) and the conversion of procapsids into virions in pulse-chase experiments (76). However, it has been suggested that purification of stable procapsids may be irrelevant to morphogenesis or may even be artifactual (153) and that the procapsids may result from detergent-mediated destruction of intracellular membranes (132). The second model involves the association of pentamers or pentamer assemblies around virion RNA. It is supported by electron microscopic investigations (see above), the kinetics of assembly of mutant protomers (4), and reports that pentamers accumulated in the presence of a guanidine or a low-temperature block could be chased directly into virions without the appearance of a procapsid intermediate when the block was removed (56, 145).

The pool of capsid proteins is probably large, since RNA synthesis and encapsidation normally continue for 25 min after inhibition of viral translation by cycloheximide (10). Kinetic studies have shown that the pool of viral RNA available for encapsidation is much smaller, since newly synthesized RNA can be detected in complete virions within 5 min, whereas incorporation of capsid proteins into virus particles requires at least 20 min (8, 10, 130). Unencapsidated viral RNA accumulated in the presence of an inhibitor of virion formation (p-fluorophenylalanine) does not serve as a precursor of virions after removal of the inhibitor (61). These observations suggest that RNA encapsidation is coupled to RNA synthesis. The reverse is not true, since defective interfering RNA genomes that lack capsid protein coding sequences are replication competent (30, 31, 59, 81).

Encapsidation of enterovirus RNA is specific, since purified polio virions contain only positive-sense genomic viral RNA and exclude positive-sense viral mRNA, negative-sense viral RNA, rRNA, tRNA, and other cytoplasmic mRNAs (123, 124). Viral mRNA lacks the 5'-terminal VPg that is covalently linked to genomic RNA, but there is no evidence that this oligopeptide constitutes a packaging signal; VPg-linked negative-sense viral RNA is excluded from virions, and extensive mutagenesis of VPg has not revealed packaging mutants (172a). A more likely explanation for the exclusion of viral mRNA is the apparent coupling of encapsidation to RNA synthesis. Specific cis-acting encapsidation signals ranging in size from 30 to >1,200 nucleotides have been identified in a variety of retroviruses and some positive-sense RNA viruses (67, 180). Similar signals have not been identified in enterovirus genomes, and indeed the internal ribosome entry site and much of the P1 region of poliovirus can be deleted without influencing encapsidation (1, 85).

Analysis of dicistronic polioviruses indicates that poliovirus capsids have an upper packaging limit of about 9,000 nucleotides (1), and the failure of some replication-competent defective interfering genomes to be encapsidated suggests that capsid stability may also require that a minimum length of RNA be encapsidated (59). The possibility that enterovirus capsids are stabilized by internal interaction with viral RNA is supported by structural and biophysical analyses of the bean pod mottle virus, which is genetically and structurally related to picornaviruses. It contains ordered domains of viral RNA at the threefold vertices of the capsid and packaging of viral RNA stabilizes subunit-subunit interactions (27, 43, 94). Although little is known about picornavirus capsid protein-RNA interactions, nucleotides have tentatively been identified in a similar location in PV3(S) and human rhinovirus type 14 (7, 50).

Infection of single cells with antigenically unrelated enteroviruses frequently results in the formation of pseudotypes in which the RNA genome of one virus is enclosed within the capsid of a heterologous enterovirus. For example, pseudotypic enteroviruses have been generated by coinfection of monkey kidney cells with echovirus type 7 and coxsackievirus A9 (75a) and by coinfection of HeLa cells with poliovirus type 1 and either poliovirus type 2, coxsackievirus B1, coxsackievirus B5, or echovirus type 1 (11, 33, 34, 70, 74a, 109, 160, 161, 171). One report even indicates that bovine enterovirus coat proteins can encapsidate the genome of the aphthovirus foot-and-mouth disease virus (167). It is not yet apparent whether the formation of such a variety of pseudotypes indicates that enteroviruses contain conserved determinants of encapsidation. Specific residues within the poliovirus capsid, including those at the amino terminus of VP1 and three relatively conserved arginine residues in VP1, VP3, and VP4, are known to be required for encapsidation (3, 4, 83).

ACKNOWLEDGMENTS

We thank M. de Crombrugghe for assistance in preparing figures.

This work was supported in part by Public Health Service grants AI 32100 and AI 15122 from the National Institute of Allergy and Infectious Diseases to E.W.

REFERENCES

1. **Alexander, L., H. H. Lu, and E. Wimmer.** 1994. Polioviruses containing picornavirus type 1 and/or type 2 internal ribosomal entry site elements: genetic hybrids and the expression of a foreign gene. *Proc. Natl. Acad. Sci. USA* **91:**1406–1410.
2. **Allaire, M., M. M. Chermaia, B. A. Malcolm, and M. N. G. James.** 1994. Picornaviral 3C cysteine proteinases have a fold similar to the chymotrypsin-like serine proteinases. *Nature* (London) **369:**72–76.
3. **Ansardi, D. C., M. Luo, and C. D. Morrow.** 1994. Mutations in the poliovirus P1 capsid precursor at arginine residues VP4-ARG34, VP3-ARG223, and VP1-ARG129 affect virus assembly and encapsidation of genomic RNA. *Virology* **188:**20–34.
4. **Ansardi, D. C., and C. D. Morrow.** 1993. Poliovirus capsid proteins derived from P1 precursors with glutamine-valine cleavage sites have defects in assembly and RNA encapsidation. *J. Virol.* **67:**7284–7297.
5. **Ansardi, D. C., D. C. Porter, and C. D. Morrow.** 1992. Myristylation of poliovirus capsid precursor P1 is required for assembly of subviral particles. *J. Virol.* **66:**4556–4563.
6. **Arnold, E., M. Luo, G. Vriend, M. G. Rossmann, A. C. Palmenberg, G. D. Parks, M. J. H. Nicklin, and E. Wimmer.** 1987. Implications of the picornavirus capsid structure for processing. *Proc. Natl. Acad. Sci. USA* **84:**21–25.
7. **Arnold, E., and M. G. Rossman.** 1990. Analysis of the structure of a common cold virus, human rhinovirus 14, refined at a resolution of 3.0 Å. *J. Mol. Biol.* **211:**763–801.
8. **Baltimore, D.** 1969. The replication of picor-

naviruses, p. 101–176. *In* H. B. Levy (ed.), *The Biochemistry of Viruses*. Marcel Dekker, New York.
9. **Baltimore, D., H. J. Eggers, R. M. Franklin, and I. Tamm.** 1963. Poliovirus-induced RNA polymerase and the effects of virus-specific inhibitors on its production. *Proc. Natl. Acad. Sci. USA* **49**:843–849.
10. **Baltimore, D., M. Girard, and J. E. Darnell.** 1966. Aspects of the synthesis of poliovirus RNA and the formation of virus particles. *Virology* **29**:179–189.
11. **Benyesh, M., H. Itoh, G. D. Hsiung, and J. L. Melnick.** 1957. Mixed infections between ECHO and polioviruses. *Fed. Proc.* **16**:365.
12. **Bienz, K., D. Egger, and L. Pasamontes.** 1987. Association of polioviral proteins of the P2 genomic region with the viral replication complex and virus-induced membrane synthesis as visualized by electron microscopic immunocytochemistry and autoradiography. *Virology* **160**:220–226.
13. **Bienz, K., D. Egger, T. Pfister, and M. Troxler.** 1992. Structural and functional characterization of the poliovirus replication complex. *J. Virol.* **66**:2740–2747.
14. **Bienz, K., D. Egger, M. Troxler, and L. Pasamontes.** 1990. Structural organization of poliovirus RNA replication is mediated by viral proteins of the P2 genomic region. *J. Virol.* **64**:1156–1163.
15. **Bishop, N. E., and D. A. Anderson.** 1993. RNA-dependent cleavage of VP0 capsid protein in provirions of hepatitis A virus. *Virology* **197**:616–623.
16. **Blair, W. S., S.-S. Huang, M. F. Ypma-Wong, and B. L. Semler.** 1990. A mutant poliovirus containing a novel proteolytic cleavage site in VP3 is altered in viral maturation. *J. Virol.* **64**:1784–1793.
17. **Blair, W. S., and B. L. Semler.** 1991. A role for the P4 amino acid residue in substrate utilization by the poliovirus 3CD proteinase. *J. Virol.* **65**:6111–6123.
18. **Boege, U., D. S. W. Ko, and D. G. Scraba.** 1986. Toward an in vitro system for picornavirus assembly: purification of mengovirus 14S capsid precursor particles. *J. Virol.* **57**:275–284.
19. **Boublik, M., and R. Drzeniek.** 1976. Demonstration of a core in poliovirus particles by electron microscopy. *J. Virol.* **31**:447–449.
20. **Breindl, M.** 1971. The structure of heated poliovirus particles. *J. Gen. Virol.* **11**:147–166.
21. **Butterworth, B. E., E. J. Shimschick, and F. H. Yin.** 1976. Association of the polioviral replication complex with phospholipid membranes. *J. Virol.* **19**:457–466.
22. **Caliguiri, L. A., and R. W. Compans.** 1973. The formation of poliovirus particles in association with the RNA replication complexes. *J. Gen. Virol.* **21**:99–108.
23. **Caliguiri, L. A., and A. G. Mosser.** 1971. Proteins associated with the poliovirus RNA replication complex. *Virology* **46**:375–386.
24. **Caliguiri, L. A., and I. Tamm.** 1969. Membranous structures associated with translation and transcription of poliovirus RNA. *Science* **166**:885–886.
25. **Caliguiri, L. A., and I. Tamm.** 1970. The role of cytoplasmic membranes in poliovirus biosynthesis. *Virology* **42**:100–111.
26. **Chatterjee, N. K., and C. Tuchowski.** 1981. Comparison of capsid polypeptides of group B coxsackieviruses and polypeptide synthesis in infected cells. *Arch. Virol.* **70**:255–269.
27. **Chen, Z., C. Stauffacher, Y. Li, T. Schmidt, B. Wu., G. Kamer, M. Shanks, G. Lomonossoff, and J. E. Johnson.** 1989. Protein-RNA interactions in an icosahedral virus at 3.0 Å resolution. *Science* **245**:154–159.
28. **Chow, M., J. F. E. Newman, D. Filman, J. M. Hogle, D. J. Rowlands, and F. Brown.** 1987. Myristylation of picornavirus capsid protein VP4 and its structural significance. *Nature* (London) **327**:482–486.
29. **Chumakov, K. M., I. K. Lavrova, L. I. Martianova, M. B. Korolev, V. N. Bashkirtsev, and M. K. Voroshilova.** 1979. Investigation of physicochemical properties of Bulgarian strain 258 of enterovirus type 71. *Arch. Virol.* **60**:359–362.
30. **Cole, C. N., and D. Baltimore.** 1973. Defective interfering particles of poliovirus. II. Nature of the defect. *J. Mol. Biol.* **76**:325–343.
31. **Collis, P. S., B. J. O'Donnell, D. J. Barton, J. A. Rogers, and J. B. Flanegan.** 1992. Replication of poliovirus RNA and subgenomic RNA transcripts in transfected cells. *J. Virol.* **66**:6480–6488.
32. **Compton, S. R., B. Nelsen, and K. Kirkegaard.** 1990. Temperature-sensitive poliovirus mutant fails to cleave VP0 and accumulates provirions. *J. Virol.* **64**:4067–4075.
33. **Cords, C. E., and J. J. Holland.** 1964. Replication of poliovirus RNA induced by heterologous virus. *Proc. Natl. Acad. Sci. USA* **51**:1080–1082.
34. **Cords, C. E., and J. J. Holland.** 1964. Alteration of the species and tissue specificity of poliovirus by enclosure of its RNA within the protein capsid of coxsackie B1 virus. *Virology* **24**:492–495.
35. **Cords, C. E., C. G. James, and L. C. McLaren.** 1975. Alteration of capsid proteins

of coxsackievirus A13 by low ionic concentrations. *J. Virol.* **15**:244–252.
36. **Corrias, M. V., O. Flore, E. Broi, M. E. Marongiu, A. Pani, S. Torelli, and P. La Colla.** 1987. Characterization and role in morphogenesis of a new subviral particle (55S) isolated from poliovirus-infected cells. *J. Virol.* **61**:561–569.
37. **Couderc, T., J. Hogle, H. Le Bleu, F. Horaud, and B. Blondel.** 1993. Molecular characterization of mouse-virulent poliovirus type 1 Mahoney mutants: involvement of residues of polypeptides VP1 and VP2 located on the inner surface of the capsid protein shell. *J. Virol.* **67**:3808–3817.
38. **Cova, L., and M. Aymard.** 1980. Isolation and characterization of non-haemagglutinating echovirus 11. *J. Gen. Virol.* **51**:219–222.
39. **Crick, F. H. K., and J. D. Watson.** 1956. Structure of small viruses. *Nature* (London) **177**:473–475.
40. **Crick, F. H. K., and J. D. Watson.** 1957. Virus structure: general principles. *Ciba Found. Symp.* **12**:5–13.
41. **Crowell, R. L., and L. Phillipson.** 1971. Specific alterations of coxsackievirus B3 eluted from HeLa cells. *J. Virol.* **8**:509–515.
42. **Dales, S., H. J. Eggers, I. Tamm, and G. E. Palade.** 1965. Electron microscopic study of the formation of poliovirus. *Virology* **26**:379–389.
43. **Da Poian, A. T., J. E. Johnson, and J. L. Silva.** 1994. Differences in pressure stability of the three components of cowpea mosaic virus: implications for virus assembly and disassembly. *Biochemistry* **33**:8339–8346.
44. **Dorner, A. J., L. F. Dorner, G. R. Larsen, E. Wimmer, and C. W. Anderson.** 1982. Identification of the initiation site of poliovirus polyprotein synthesis. *J. Virol.* **42**:1017–1028.
45. **Dunker, A. K., and R. R. Rueckert.** 1971. Fragments generated by pH dissociation of ME-virus and their relation to the structure of the virion. *J. Mol. Biol.* **58**:217–235.
46. **Emini, E. A., M. Elzinga, and E. Wimmer.** 1982. Carboxy-terminal analysis of poliovirus proteins: the termination of poliovirus RNA translation and the location of unique poliovirus polyprotein cleavage sites. *J. Virol.* **42**:194–199.
47. **Esposito, J. J., and J. F. Obijeski.** 1976. Enterovirus type 70 virion and intracellular proteins. *J. Virol.* **18**:1160–1162.
48. **Fernandez-Tomas, C. B., and D. Baltimore.** 1973. Morphogenesis of poliovirus. II. Demonstration of a new intermediate, the provirion. *J. Virol.* **12**:1122–1130.
49. **Fernandez-Tomas, C. B., N. Guttman, and D. Baltimore.** 1973. Morphogenesis of poliovirus. III. Formation of provirion in cell-free extracts. *J. Virol.* **12**:1181–1183.
50. **Filman, D. J., R. Syed, M. Chow, A. J. Macadam, P. D. Minor, and J. M. Hogle.** 1989. Structural factors that control conformational transitions and serotype specificity in type 3 poliovirus. *EMBO J.* **8**:1567–1579.
51. **Finch, J. T., and A. Klug.** 1959. Structure of poliomyelitis virus. *Nature* (London) **183**:1709–1714.
52. **Flanegan, J. B., and T. Van Dyke.** 1979. Isolation of a soluble and template dependent poliovirus RNA polymerase that copies virion RNA in vitro. *J. Virol.* **32**:155–161.
53. **Flore, O., C. E. Fricks, D. J. Filman, and J. M. Hogle.** 1990. Conformational changes in poliovirus assembly and cell entry. *Semin. Virol.* **1**:429–438.
54. **Fricks, C. E., and J. M. Hogle.** 1990. Cell-induced conformational changes in poliovirus: externalization of the amino terminus of VP1 is responsible for liposome binding. *J. Virol.* **64**:1934–1945.
55. **Fry, E., D. Logan, R. Acharya, G. Fox, D. Rowlands, F. Brown, and D. Stuart.** 1990. Architecture and topography of an aphthovirus. *Semin. Virol.* **1**:439–452.
56. **Ghendon, Y., E. Yakobson, and A. Mikhejeva.** 1972. Study of some stages of poliovirus morphogenesis in MiO cells. *J. Virol.* **10**:261–266.
56a. **Girard, M., D. Baltimore, and J. E. Darnell.** 1967. The poliovirus replication complex: site for synthesis of poliovirus RNA. *J. Mol. Biol.* **24**:59–74.
57. **Gordon, J. L., R. J. Duronio, D. A. Rudnick, S. P. Adams, and G. W. Gokel.** 1991. Protein N-myristoylation. *J. Biol. Chem.* **266**:8647–8650.
58. **Guttman, N., and D. Baltimore.** 1977. Morphogenesis of poliovirus. IV. Existence of particles sedimenting at 150S and having the properties of provirion. *J. Virol.* **23**:363–367.
59. **Hagino-Yamagishi, K., and A. Nomoto.** 1989. In vitro construction of poliovirus defective interfering particles. *J. Virol.* **63**:5386–5392.
60. **Halperen, S., H. J. Eggers, and I. Tamm.** 1964. Complete and coreless hemagglutinating particles produced in echovirus 12 virus-infected cells. *Virology* **23**:81–89.
61. **Halperen, S., H. J. Eggers, and I. Tamm.** 1964. Evidence for uncoupled synthesis of viral RNA and viral capsids. *Virology* **24**:36–46.
61a. **Harber, J. J., J. Bradley, C. W. Anderson, and E. Wimmer.** 1991. Catalysis of poliovi-

rus VP0 maturation is not mediated by serine 10 of VP2. *J. Virol.* **65**:326-334.
62. **Harris, T. J. R., and F. Brown.** 1975. Correlation of polypeptide composition with antigenic variation in the swine vesicular disease and coxsackievirus B5 viruses. *Nature* (London) **258**:758-760.
63. **Hasegawa, A., and S. Inouye.** 1979. Antigenicity and polypeptide composition of native and heated echovirus type 7 procapsids. *J. Gen. Virol.* **42**:119-125.
64. **Hellen, C. U. T., M. Fäcke, H. G. Kräusslich, C.-K. Lee, and E. Wimmer.** 1991. Characterization of poliovirus 2A proteinase by mutational analysis: residues required for autocatalytic activity are essential for induction of cleavage of eukaryotic initiation factor 4F polypeptide p220. *J. Virol.* **65**:4226-4231.
65. **Hellen, C. U. T., H. G. Kräusslich, and E. Wimmer.** 1989. Proteolytic processing of polyproteins in the replication of RNA viruses. *Biochemistry* **28**:9881-9890.
66. **Hellen, C. U. T., and E. Wimmer.** 1992. Maturation of poliovirus capsid proteins. *Virology* **187**:391-397.
67. **Hirsch, R. C., D. L. Loeb, J. R. Pollack, and D. Ganem.** 1992. cis-Acting sequences required for encapsidation of duck hepatitis B virus pregenomic RNA. *J. Virol.* **65**:3309-3316.
68. **Hoey, E. M., and S. J. Martin.** 1974. A possible precursor containing RNA of a bovine enterovirus: the provirion 11. *J. Gen. Virol.* **24**:515-524.
69. **Hogle, J. M., M. Chow, and D. J. Filman.** 1985. Three-dimensional structure of poliovirus at 2.9 Å resolution. *Science* **229**:1358-1365.
70. **Holland, J. J., and C. E. Cords.** 1964. Maturation of poliovirus RNA with capsid protein coded by heterologous enteroviruses. *Proc. Natl. Acad. Sci. USA* **51**:1082-1085.
71. **Holland, J. J., and E. D. Kiehn.** 1968. Specific cleavage of viral proteins as steps in the synthesis and maturation of enteroviruses. *Proc. Natl. Acad. Sci. USA* **60**:1015-1022.
72. **Horne, R. W., and J. Nagington.** 1959. Electron microscope studies of the development and structure of poliomyelitis virus. *J. Mol. Biol.* **1**:333-338.
73. **Huang, A. S., and D. Baltimore.** 1970. Initiation of polysome formation in poliovirus-infected cells. *J. Mol. Biol.* **47**:275-291.
74. **Hummeler, K., T. F. Anderson, and R. A. Brown.** 1962. Identification of poliovirus particles of different antigenicity by specific agglutination as seen in the electron microscope. *Virology* **16**:84-90.
74a. **Ikegami, N., H. J. Eggers, and I. Tamm.** 1964. Rescure of drug-requiring and drug-inhibited enteroviruses. *Proc. Natl. Acad. Sci. USA* **52**:1419-1426.
75. **Inoue, T., T. Suzuki, and K. Sekiguchi.** 1989. The complete nucleotide sequence of swine vesicular disease virus. *J. Gen. Virol.* **70**:919-934.
75a. **Itoh, H., and J. D. Melnick.** 1959. Double infections of single cells with ECHO 7 and coxsackie A9 viruses. *J. Exp. Med.* **109**:393-406.
76. **Jacobson, M. F., and D. Baltimore.** 1968. Morphogenesis of poliovirus. I. Association of the viral RNA with coat proteins. *J. Mol. Biol.* **33**:369-378.
77. **Jacobson, M. F., and D. Baltimore.** 1968. Polypeptide cleavages in the formation of poliovirus proteins. *Proc. Natl. Acad. Sci. USA* **61**:77-84.
78. **Jamison, R. M., and H. D. Mayor.** 1966. Comparative study of seven picornaviruses of man. *J. Bacteriol.* **91**:1971-1976.
79. **Johnston, M. D., and S. J. Martin.** 1971. Capsid and procapsid proteins of a bovine enterovirus. *J. Gen. Virol.* **11**:71-79.
80. **Jore, J., B. de Geus, R. J. Jackson, P. H. Pouwels, and B. E. Enger-Valk.** 1988. Poliovirus protein 3CD is the active protease for processing of the precursor protein P1 in vitro. *J. Gen. Virol.* **69**:1627-1636.
81. **Kaplan, G., and V. R. Racaniello.** 1988. Construction and characterization of poliovirus subgenomic replicons. *J. Virol.* **62**:1687-1696.
82. **Kiehn, E. D., and J. J. Holland.** 1968. Synthesis and cleavage of enterovirus polypeptides in mammalian cells. *J. Virol.* **5**:358-367.
83. **Kirkegaard, K.** 1990. Mutations in VP1 of poliovirus specifically affect both encapsidation and release of viral RNA. *J. Virol.* **64**:195-206.
84. **Kitamura, N., B. L. Semler, P. G. Rothberg, G. R. Larsen, C. J. Adler, A. J. Dorner, E. A. Emini, R. Hanecak, J. Lee, S. van der Werf, C. W. Anderson, and E. Wimmer.** 1981. Primary structure, gene organization and polypeptide expression of poliovirus RNA. *Nature* (London) **291**:547-553.
85. **Kuge, S., I. Saito, and A. Nomoto.** 1986. Primary structure of poliovirus defective-interfering particle genomes and possible generation mechanisms of the particles. *J. Mol. Biol.* **192**:473-487.
86. **Kuhn, R. J., H. Tada, M. F. Ypma-Wong, B. L. Semler, and E. Wimmer.** 1988. Mutational analysis of the genome-linked protein VPg of poliovirus. *J. Virol.* **62**:4207-4215.
87. **Larsen, G. R., C. W. Anderson, A. J. Dorner, B.L. Semler, and E. Wimmer.** 1982. Cleavage sites within the poliovirus

capsid protein precursors. *J. Virol.* **41:**340–344.
88. **Lawson, M. A., and B. L. Semler.** 1990. Picornavirus protein processing: enzymes, substrates and genetic regulation. *Curr. Top. Microbiol. Immunol.* **161:**49–88.
89. **Lea, S., J. Hernandez, W. Blakemore, E. Brocchi, S. Curry, E. Domingo, E. Fry, R. Abu-Ghazaleh, A. King, J. Newman, D. Stuart, and M. G. Mateu.** 1994. The structure and antigenicity of a type C foot-and-mouth disease virus. *Structure* **2:**123–139.
90. **Lee, W.-M., S. S. Monroe, and R. R. Rueckert.** 1993. Role of maturation cleavage in infectivity of picornaviruses: activation of an infectosome. *J. Virol.* **67:**2110–2122.
91. **Li, J. P., and D. Baltimore.** 1988. Isolation of poliovirus 2C mutants defective in viral RNA synthesis. *J. Virol.* **62:**4016–4021.
92. **Li, J. P., and D. Baltimore.** 1990. An intragenic revertant of a poliovirus 2C mutant has an uncoating defect. *J. Virol.* **64:**1102–1107.
93. **Li, Q., A. G. Yafal, Y. M.-H. Lee, J. Hogle, and M. Chow.** 1994. Poliovirus neutralization by antibodies to internal epitopes of VP4 and VP1 results from reversible exposure of these sequences at physiological temperature. *J. Virol.* **68:**3965–3970.
94. **Li, T., Z. Chen, J. E. Johnson, and G. J. Thomas.** 1992. Conformations, interactions, and thermostabilities of RNA and proteins in bean pod mottle virus: investigation of solution and crystal structures by laser Raman spectroscopy. *Biochemistry* **31:**6673–6682.
95. **Luo, M., G. Vriend, G. Kamer, I. Minor, E. Arnold, M. G. Rossmann, U. Boege, D. G. Scraba, G. M. Duke, and A. C. Palmenberg.** 1987. The atomic structure of mengo virus at 3.0 Å resolution. *Science* **235:**182–191.
96. **Macadam, A. J., G. Ferguson, C. Arnold, and P. D. Minor.** 1991. An assembly defect as a result of an attenuating mutation in the capsid proteins of the poliovirus type 3 vaccine strain. *J. Virol.* **65:**5225–5231.
97. **Maizel, J. V., B. A. Phillips, and D. F. Summers.** 1967. Composition of artificially produced and naturally occurring empty capsids of poliovirus type 1. *Virology* **32:**692–699.
98. **Maizel, J. V., and D. F. Summers.** 1968. Evidence for differences in size and composition of the poliovirus-specific polypeptides in infected HeLa cells. *Virology* **36:**48–54.
99. **Marc, D., G. Drugeon, A.-L. Haenni, M. Girard, and S. van der Werf.** 1989. Role of myristoylation of poliovirus capsid protein VP4 as determined by site-directed mutagenesis of its N-terminal sequence. *EMBO J.* **8:**2661–2668.
100. **Marc, D., M. Girad, and S. van der Werf.** 1991. A Gly^1 to Ala substitution in poliovirus capsid protein VP0 blocks its myristoylation and prevents viral assembly. *J. Gen. Virol.* **72:**1151–1157.
101. **Marc, D., G. Masson, M. Girard, and S. van der Werf.** 1990. Lack of myristoylation of poliovirus capsid polypeptide VP0 prevents the formation of virions or results in the assembly of noninfectious virus particles. *J. Virol.* **64:**4099–4107.
102. **Marongiu, M. E., A. Pani, M. V. Corrias, M. Sau, and P. LaColla.** 1981. Poliovirus morphogenesis. I. Identification of 80S dissociable particles and evidence for the artefactual production of procapsids. *J. Virol.* **39:**341–347.
103. **Martin, A., C. Wychowski, T. Couderc, R. Crainic, J. Hogle, and M. Girard.** 1988. Engineering a poliovirus type 2 antigenic site on a type 1 capsid results in a chimaeric virus which is neurovirulent for mice. *EMBO J.* **7:**2839–2847.
104. **Martin, S. J., M. D. Johnston, and J. B. Clements.** 1970. Purification and characterization of bovine enteroviruses. *J. Gen. Virol.* **7:**103–113.
105. **Mattern, C. F. T.** 1962. Some physical and chemical properties of Coxsackieviruses A9 and A10. *Virology* **17:**520–532.
106. **Mattion, N. M., P. A. Reilly, S. J. DiMichele, J. C. Crowley, and C. Weeks-Levy.** 1994. Attenuated poliovirus strain as a live vector: expression of regions of rotavirus outer capsid protein VP7 by using recombinant Sabin 3 viruses. *J. Virol.* **68:**3925–3933.
107. **Mayer, M. M., H. J. Rapp, B. Roizman, S. W. Klein, K. M. Cowan, D. Lukens, C. E. Schwerdt, F. L. Schaffer, and J. Charney.** 1957. The purification of poliomyelitis virus as studied by complement fixation. *J. Immunol.* **78:**435–455.
108. **McKinley, M. A., D. C. Pevear, and M. G. Rossmann.** 1992. Treatment of the picornavirus common cold by inhibitors of viral uncoating and attachment. *Annu. Rev. Microbiol.* **46:**635–654.
109. **Melnick, J. L.** 1957. ECHO viruses. *Spec. Publ. N.Y. Acad. Sci.* **5:**365.
110. **Melnick, J. L., G. Dalldorf, J. F. Enders, H. M. Gelfaud, W. M. Hammond, A. B. Sabin, J. T. Syverton, and H. A. Wenner.** 1962. Classification of human enteroviruses. *Virology* **16:**501–504.
111. **Minor, P. D., G. Dunn, D. M. A. Evans,**

D. I. Magrath, A. John, J. Howlett, A. Phillips, G. Westrop, K. Wareham, J. W. Almond, and J. M. Hogle. 1989. The temperature sensitivity of the Sabin type 3 vaccine strain of poliovirus: molecular and structural effects of a mutation in the capsid protein VP3. *J. Gen. Virol.* **70:**1117–1123.
112. Moore, D. M. 1977. Characterization of three antigenic particles of swine vesicular disease virus. *J. Gen. Virol.* **34:**431–445.
113. Moore, N. F., B. Reavy, and L. King. 1985. General characteristics, gene organization and expression of small RNA viruses of insects. *J. Gen. Virol.* **66:**647–659.
114. Moscufo, N., and M. Chow. 1992. Myristate-protein interactions in poliovirus: interactions of VP4 threonine 28 contribute to the structural conformation of assembly intermediates and the stability of assembled virions. *J. Virol.* **66:**6849–6857.
115. Moscufo, N., J. Simons, and M. Chow. 1991. Myristoylation is important at multiple stages in poliovirus assembly. *J. Virol.* **65:**2372–2380.
116. Moscufo, N., A. G. Yafal, A. Rogrove, J. M. Hogle, and M. Chow. 1993. A mutation in VP4 defines a new step in the late stages of cell entry by poliovirus. *J. Virol.* **67:**5075–5078.
117. Moss, E. G., and V. R. Racaniello. 1991. Host range determinants located on the interior of the poliovirus capsid. *EMBO J.* **10:**1067–1074.
118. Murray, M. G., J. Bradley, X.-F. Yang, E. Wimmer, E. G. Moss, and V. R. Racaniello. 1988. Poliovirus host range is determined by a short amino acid sequence in neutralizing antigenic site 1. *Science* **241:**213–215.
119. Nardelli, L., E. Lodetti, G. L. Gualandi, R. Burros, D. Goodridge, F. Brown, and B. Cartwright. 1968. A foot and mouth disease syndrome in pigs caused by an enterovirus. *Nature* (London) **219:**1275–1276.
120. Newman, J. F. E., D. J. Rowlands, and F. Brown. 1973. A physico-chemical sub-grouping of the mammalian picornaviruses. *J. Gen. Virol.* **18:**171–180.
121. Nicklin, M. J. H., H.-G. Kräusslich, H. Toyoda, J. J. Dunn, and E. Wimmer. 1987. Poliovirus polypeptide precursors: expression *in vitro* and processing by exogenous 3C and 2A proteinases. *Proc. Natl. Acad. Sci. USA* **84:**4002–4006.
122. Nicklin, M. J. H., H. Toyoda, M. G. Murray, and E. Wimmer. 1986. Proteolytic processing in the replication of polio and related viruses. *Bio/Technology* **4:**33–42.
123. Nomoto, A., N. Kitamura, F. Golini, and E. Wimmer. 1977. The 5'-terminal structures of poliovirion RNA and poliovirus mRNA differ only in the genome-linked protein VPg. *Proc. Natl. Acad. Sci. USA* **74:**5345–5349.
124. Novak, J. E. K., and K. Kirkegaard. 1991. Improved method for detecting poliovirus negative strands used to demonstrate specificity of positive-strand encapsidation and the ratio of positive to negative strands in infected cells. *J. Virol.* **65:**3384–3387.
125. Oliviera, M. A., R. Zhao, W.-M. Lee, M. J. Kremer, I. Minor, R. R. Rueckert, G. D. Diana, D. C. Pevear, F. J. Dutko, M. A. McKinlay, and M. G. Rossmann. 1993. The structure of human rhinovirus 16. *Structure* **1:**51–68.
126. Pallai, P. V., F. Burkhardt, M. Skoog, K. Schreiner, P. Bax, K. A. Cohen, G. Hansen, D. E. H. Palladino, K. S. Harris, M. J. Nicklin, and E. Wimmer. 1989. Cleavage of synthetic peptides by purified 3C proteinase. *J. Biol. Chem.* **264:**9738–9741.
127. Palmenberg, A. C. 1982. In vitro synthesis and assembly of picornaviral capsid intermediate structures. *J. Virol.* **44:**900–906.
128. Palmenberg, A. C. 1989. Sequence alignments of picornaviral capsid proteins, p. 211–241. *In* E. Ehrenfeld and B. Semler (ed.), *Molecular Aspects of Picornavirus Infection and Detection.* American Society for Microbiology, Washington, D.C.
129. Paul, A. V., A. Schultz, S. E. Pincus, S. Oroszalan, and E. Wimmer. 1987. Capsid protein VP4 of poliovirus is N-myristoylated. *Proc. Natl. Acad. Sci. USA* **84:**7827–7831.
130. Penman, S., Y. Becker, and J. Darnell. 1964. A cytoplasmic structure involved in the synthesis and assembly of poliovirus components. *J. Mol. Biol.* **8:**541–555.
131. Perlin, M., and B. A. Phillips. 1973. In vitro assembly of polioviruses. III. Assembly of 14S particles into empty capsids by poliovirus-infected HeLa cell membranes. *Virology* **53:**107–114.
132. Pfister, T., L. Pasamontes, M. Troxler, D. Egger, and K. Bienz. 1992. Immunocytochemical localization of capsid-related particles in subcellular fractions of poliovirus-infected cells. *Virology* **188:**676–684.
133. Philipson, L., S. T. Beatrice, and R. I. Crowell. 1973. A structural model of picornaviruses as suggested from analysis of urea-degraded virions and procapsids of coxsackievirus B3. *Virology* **54:**69–79.
134. Phillips, B. A. 1969. In vitro assembly of

polioviruses. I. Kinetics of the assembly of empty capsids and the role of extracts from infected cells. *Virology* **39:**811–821.
135. **Phillips, B. A.** 1971. In vitro assembly of poliovirus. II. Evidence for the self-assembly of 14S particles into empty capsids. *Virology* **44:**307–316.
136. **Phillips, B. A., D. F. Summers, and J. V. Maizel.** 1968. In vitro assembly of poliovirus-related particles. *Virology* **35:**216–226.
137. **Polson, A., and A. Kipps.** 1965. Physicochemical investigation of an enteric cytopathogenic bovine orphan virus, ECBO SA.1. *Arch. Gesamte Virusforsch.* **17:**488–494.
138. **Polson, A., and J. Levitt.** 1963. Density determination in a preformed gradient of caesium chloride. *Biochim. Biophys. Acta* **75:**88–95.
139. **Putnak, J. R., and B. A. Phillips.** 1981. Picornaviral structure and assembly. *Microbiol. Rev.* **45:**287–315.
140. **Racaniello, V. R., and D. Baltimore.** 1981. Molecular cloning of poliovirus cDNA and determination of the complete nucleotide sequence of the viral genome. *Proc. Natl. Acad. Sci. USA* **78:**4887–4901.
141. **Rodriguez, P. L., and L. Carrasco.** 1993. Poliovirus protein 2C has ATPase and GTPase activities. *J. Biol. Chem.* **268:**8105–8110.
142. **Roivainen, M., A. Närvänen, M. Korkolainen, M.-L. Huhtala, and T. Hovi.** 1991. Antigenic regions of poliovirus type 3/Sabin capsid proteins recognized by human sera in the peptide scanning technique. *Virology* **180:**99–107.
143. **Roivainen, M., L. Piirainen, T. Rysä, A. Närvänen, and T. Hovi.** 1993. An immunodominant N-terminal region of VP1 protein of poliovirion that is buried in crystal structure can be exposed in solution. *Virology* **195:**762–765.
144. **Rombaut, B., and A. Boeye.** 1991. In vitro assembly of poliovirus 14S subunits: disoxaril stabilization as a model for the antigenicity-conferring activity of infected cell extracts. *Virology* **180:**788–792.
145. **Rombaut, B., R. Vrijsen, and A. Boeye.** 1990. New evidence for the precursor role of 14S subunits in poliovirus morphogenesis. *Virology* **117:**411–414.
146. **Rombaut, B., R. Vrijsen, P. Brioen, and A. Boeye.** 1982. A pH-dependent antigenic conversion of empty capsids of poliovirus studied with the aid of monoclonal antibodies to N and H antigen. *Virology* **122:**215–218.
147. **Rombaut, B., R. Vrijsen, A. Delgadillo, D. vanden Berghe, and A. Boeye.** 1985. Characterization and assembly of poliovirus-related 45S particles. *Virology* **146:**111–119.
148. **Rosenwirth, B., and H. J. Eggers.** 1978. Structure and replication of echovirus type 12. I. Analysis of the polypeptides and RNA of echovirus 12 particles. *Eur. J. Biochem.* **92:**53–60.
149. **Rosenwirth, B., and H. J. Eggers.** 1982. Biochemistry and pathogenicity of echovirus 9. I. Characterization of the virus particles of strains Barty and Hill. *Virology* **123:**102–112.
150. **Rossmann, M. G.** 1989. The canyon hypothesis. *J. Biol. Chem.* **264:**14587–14590.
151. **Rossman, M. G., C. Abad-Zapatero, M. A. Hermodson, and J. W. Erickson.** 1983. Subunit interactions in southern bean mosaic virus. *J. Mol. Biol.* **166:**37–83.
152. **Rossman, M. G., and J. E. Johnson.** 1989. Icosahedral RNA virus structure. *Annu. Rev. Biochem.* **58:**533–573.
153. **Rueckert, R. R.** 1990. Picornaviridae and their replication, p. 507–548. *In* B. N. Fields, D. M. Knipe, R. M. Chanock, M. S. Hirsch, J. L. Melnick, R. T. P. Morath, and B. Roizman (ed.), *Virology*. Raven Press, New York.
154. **Schaffer, C. E., and L. H. Frommhagen.** 1965. Similarities of biophysical properties of several human enteroviruses as shown by density gradient ultracentrifugation of mixtures of the viruses. *Virology* **25:**662–664.
155. **Schaffer, C. E., and F. L. Schwerdt.** 1955. Some physical and chemical properties of purified poliomyelitis virus preparations. *Ann. N.Y. Acad. Sci.* **61:**740–750.
156. **Schaffer, C. E., and F. L. Schwerdt.** 1959. Purification and properties of poliovirus. *Adv. Virus Res.* **6:**159–204.
157. **Scharff, M. D., and L. Levintow.** 1963. Quantitative study of the formation of poliovirus antigens in infected HeLa cells. *Virology* **17:**491–500.
158. **Skern, T., W. Sommergruber, D. Blaas, P. Gruendler, F. Fraundorfer, C. Pieler, I. Fogy, and E. Kuechler.** 1985. Human rhinovirus 2: complete nucleotide sequence and proteolytic processing signals in the capsid protein region. *Nucleic Acids Res.* **13:**2111–2126.
159. **Skinner, M. S., S. Halperen, and J. C. Harkin.** 1968. Cytoplasmic membrane–bound vesicles in echovirus 12-infected cells. *Virology* **36:**241–253.
160. **Sprunt, K., I. M. Mountain, W. M. Redman, and H. E. Alexander.** 1955. Production of poliomyelitis virus with combined antigenic characteristics of type I and type II. *Virology* **1:**236–249.
161. **Sprunt, K., W. M. Redman, and H. E.**

Alexander. 1958. Combination of antigenic traits of type 1 and type 2 poliovirus. *J. Immunol.* **82**:232–240.
162. Su, R. T., and M. W. Taylor. 1976. Morphogenesis of picornaviruses: characterization and assembly of bovine enterovirus subviral particles. *J. Gen. Virol.* **30**:317–328.
163. Summers, D. F., and J. V. Maizel. 1968. Evidence for large precursor proteins in poliovirus synthesis. *Proc. Natl. Acad. Sci. USA* **59**:966–971.
164. Summers, D. F., J. V. Maizel, and J. E. Darnell. 1965. Evidence for virus-specific non-capsid proteins in poliovirus-infected HeLa cells. *Proc. Natl. Acad. Sci. USA* **54**:505–513.
165. Takegami, T., B. L. Semler, C. W. Anderson, and E. Wimmer. 1983. Membrane fractions active in poliovirus RNA replication contain VPg precursor polypeptides. *Virology* **126**:33–47.
166. Toyoda, H., M. J. H. Nicklin, M. G. Murray, C. W. Anderson, J. J. Dunn, F. W. Sudier, and E. Wimmer. 1986. A second virus-encoded proteinase involved in proteolytic processing of poliovirus polyprotein. *Cell* **45**:761–770.
167. Trautman, R., and P. Sutmoller. 1971. Detection and properties of a genomic masked viral particle consisting of foot-and-mouth disease virus nucleic acid in bovine enterovirus protein capsid. *Virology* **44**:537–545.
168. Van Elsen, A., and A. Boeye. 1966. Disruption of type 1 poliovirus under alkaline conditions: role of pH, temperature and sodium dodecyl sulphate (SDS). *Virology* **28**:481–483.
169. Vrijsen, R., P. Brioen, and A. Boeye. 1980. Identification of poliovirus precursor proteins by immunoprecipitation. *Virology* **107**:567–569.
170. Watanabe, Y., K. Watanabe, and Y. Hinuma. 1962. Synthesis of poliovirus specific proteins in HeLa cells. *Biochim. Biophys. Acta* **61**:976–977.
171. Wecker, E., and G. Lederhilger. 1964. Genomic masking produced by double infection of HeLa cells with heterotypic polioviruses. *Proc. Natl. Acad. Sci. USA* **52**:705–709.
172. Wery, J.-P., V. S. Reddy, M. V. Hosur, and J. E. Johnson. 1994. The refined three dimensional structure of an insect virus at 2.8A resolution. *J. Mol. Biol.* **235**:565–586.
172a. Wimmer, E., C. U. T. Hellen, and X. Cao. 1993. Poliovirus genetics. *Annu. Rev. Genet.* **27**:353–436.
173. Yamazaki, S., K. Natori, and R. Kono. 1974. Purification and biophysical properties of acute haemorrhagic conjunctivitis virus. *J. Virol.* **14**:1357–1360.
174. Yeates, T. O., D. H. Jacobson, A. Martin, C. Wychowski, M. Girard, D. J. Filman, and J. M. Hogle. 1991. Three-dimensional structure of a mouse-adapted type 2/type 1 poliovirus chimera. *EMBO J.* **10**:2331–2341.
175. Yin, F. H. 1977. Involvement of viral procapsid in the RNA synthesis and maturation of poliovirus. *Virology* **82**:299–307.
176. Yoneyama, T., A. Hagiwara, and I. Tagaya. 1980. Structural proteins of hand, foot and mouth disease viruses. *Intervirology* **13**:130–132.
177. Ypma-Wong, M.-F., P. G. Dewalt, V. H. Johnson, J. G. Lamb, and B. L. Semler. 1988. Protein 3CD is the major proteinase responsible for cleavage of the P1 capsid precursor. *Virology* **166**:265–270.
178. Ypma-Wong, M. F., D. J. Filman, J. M. Hogle, and B. L. Semler. 1988. Structural domains of the poliovirus polyprotein are major determinants for proteolytic cleavage at Gln-Gly pairs. *J. Biol. Chem.* **263**:17846–17856.
179. Ypma-Wong, M.-F., and B. L. Semler. 1987. In vitro molecular genetics as a tool for determining the differential cleavage specificities of the poliovirus 3C proteinase. *Nucleic Acids Res.* **15**:2069–2088.
180. Zhong, W., R. Dasgupta, and R. Rueckert. 1992. Evidence that the packaging signal for nodaviral RNA2 is a bulged stem-loop. *Proc. Natl. Acad. Sci. USA* **89**:11146–11150.

HOST IMMUNE RESPONSES TO ENTEROVIRUS INFECTIONS

Steven Tracy, Nora M. Chapman, Ronald J. Rubocki, and Melinda A. Beck

8

Enteroviral infections in vertebrates induce both cell-mediated and humoral immune responses. Enteroviruses cause a wide array of human diseases (79), a common feature of which is often acute inflammation: of central nervous system tissue (poliomyelitis, encephalitis, meningitis), of cardiac muscle (myocarditis), and of skeletal muscle (myositis, polymyositis). It is widely accepted that neutralizing-antibody titers against enteroviruses, such as those gained following vaccination with poliovirus (PV) vaccines, provide lifelong protection against enterovirus-induced disease. Enteroviruses are also etiologically linked to chronic inflammatory diseases such as those of the heart (117, 119, 127) and skeletal muscle (22, 114); among the immunologic mechanisms proposed are epitope mimicry (25, 123) and autoimmunity (38, 52, 92, 110) (see chapters 14 and 16).

At present, the best readily available experimental small-animal model for studying host immune responses to enterovirus infection is coxsackievirus, particularly coxsackievirus B3 (CVB3), replication in mice. Three infectious cDNA copies of CVB3 genomes have been reported; two of them induce severe inflammatory heart disease (myocarditis) in most mice (59, 118), and one is noncardiovirulent (18). The viral genetic site that controls the expression of the cardiovirulence phenotype in mice has been mapped and identified for the two strains of CVB3 characterized in our laboratory (17a, 18). In addition to being completely characterized viral tools, cardiovirulent CVB3 strains induce severe acute inflammatory heart disease in many murine strains (117, 119, 127) and can induce a chronic murine disease similar to dilated cardiomyopathy in humans (70, 78, 102, 126). Complementing the normal murine strains are a number of strains that have various immunologic defects. A host of studies since seminal work by Woodruff in the 1970s (127, 128) have defined many of the parameters in the system of CVB3-induced acute and chronic inflammatory heart diseases.

Other murine-enterovirus-induced disease models exist. A useful model of CVB1-induced polymyositis (114) (see chapter 16) and an actively studied model of CVB4-induced pancreatic disease, which mimics diabetes (95, 122) (see chapter 15), are available. Important

---

Steven Tracy, Nora M. Chapman, and Ronald J. Rubocki, Department of Pathology and Microbiology, University of Nebraska Medical Center, 600 South 42nd Street, Omaha, Nebraska 68198-6495. *Melinda A. Beck,* FPG Child Development Center, Department of Pediatrics, University of North Carolina at Chapel Hill, 105 Smith Level Road, Chapel Hill, North Carolina 27599-8180.

for these models, the genomes of CVB1 and CVB4 have also been cloned as infectious cDNAs (55, 57). PVs do not naturally replicate in mice, and so until recently, studies of murine immune reactions to replicating PVs and subsequent virus-induced tissue damage have been limited. The advent of transgenic mice expressing the human PV receptor (64, 97) should change this situation rapidly.

Humoral immunity is antibody mediated and plays a key role in neutralizing the infectivity of extracellular virus during viremia. Cell-mediated immunity (T cells) is involved in clearing intracellular viral infection and providing help to the humoral response. Characteristics of acquired immune responses against viral infections include specificity, diversity, and memory. Specificity involves the selection of antigen-specific B and T cells prior to antigenic stimulation (14, 58). The diversity of antibody and T-cell·receptor specificities is extraordinarily large: for B- and T-cell repertoires, it is approximately 10^{11} and 10^{16} to 10^{18}, respectively (27). A unique component of acquired immunity is the capacity of the immune response to mount a memory (or secondary) response to antigen (virus) reexposure; this memory response is more rapid and higher in titer than the primary response and it may differ qualitatively.

Antigenic determinants, or epitopes, can be divided into those recognized by B cells and those recognized by T cells (hereafter, B- and T-cell epitopes). Antibodies can recognize epitopes that can be combinatorial (composed of residues from more than one protein strand) or linear and are conformational in nature. The T-cell epitope is a linear oligopeptide sequence of a protein antigen that binds in the peptide-binding pocket, or groove, of major histocompatibility complex (MHC) class I or II molecules (12). Viral epitopes recognized by the immune system can be encoded for by either surface or internal viral proteins (116).

In the early 1970s, it was observed that the immune system recognized only antigen-associated target cells that shared cell surface molecules with the effector cells (104, 131). The self components that are critical in this restricted recognition of self plus nonself antigen are encoded by the MHC (26), which in humans is called the human leukocyte antigen complex and in mice is called the *H-2* complex. Two types of MHC-encoded molecules are the class I and II alleles, which are codominantly expressed but differ in distribution: MHC class I molecules are found on nearly all nucleated cells, while class II molecules are limited to certain lineages (20). Murine and human class I and II gene products are highly polymorphic in number of alleles and loci. Both class I and class II MHC-encoded molecules function as receptors for binding and presenting peptides to the immune system. Naturally processed peptides eluted from MHC molecules suggest that thousands of different peptides can be associated with a particular MHC molecule (53). Different MHC alleles tend to bind different peptide motifs owing to the polymorphic amino acid residues lining the peptide-binding groove within these MHC molecules (20, 53, 108).

Class I molecules are trimolecular structures composed of a heavy chain (α), β-2 microglobulin, and a peptide (usually 8- to 9-mers; 12, 20). They function as restriction elements for presenting MHC-bound peptides to CD8$^+$ T lymphocytes. Class II molecules are composed of α/β MHC-encoded chains in association with a peptide; they function as restriction elements for CD4$^+$ T cells (13). The class II MHC-binding peptides are generally 13 to 17 amino acids long (20, 108). The variation in the lengths of the peptides bound to class II in contrast to those bound to class I is due to the open ends of the MHC peptide-binding groove (13). Class II reactive CD4$^+$ T cells can be divided into at least two groups, T helper 1 (Th1) and Th2, based on the cytokines synthesized by these cells (86). Th1 cells, defined as producers of interleukin-2 (IL-2) and gamma interferon, are involved to a greater degree in cellular and delayed-type hypersensitivity reactions, while Th2 cells are defined as producers of IL-4 and IL-10 and stimulate B-cell activity.

HUMORAL IMMUNE RESPONSES

Normal humoral immune responses to enteroviral infections result in the rapid production of antiviral immunoglobulin (IgM) and then IgG and IgA. Antienteroviral IgM normally persists for less than 6 months, but IgA and IgG to enteroviruses can persist for years (11). IgM titers have been used to predict recent or ongoing infection with enteroviruses (40, 99). IgM titers against CVBs are present more frequently in patients with acute or chronic diseases in which CVB infection has been implicated (87). However, subclinical enteroviral infections are common: in one study, 5 to 10% of healthy people had detectable IgM to the CVB group (62). The importance of a functional humoral immune response in overcoming enteroviral infection is demonstrated by the chronic and life-threatening enteroviral infections that can occur in agammaglobulinemic patients (77) (see chapter 13) and the propensity of neonates for severe and fulminant enteroviral illness (19) (see chapter 10). Treatment of agammaglobulinemic patients with intravenous immunoglobulin has made the occurrence of chronic enteroviral meningoencephalitis in these patients relatively rare (85). Transfer of enterovirus immunity (in the form of IgA) via breast milk protects humans (130) and mice (80) against infection.

Vaccination has provided extensive data on protective immunity associated with inactivated and live attenuated PV vaccines (see chapter 9). While inactivated PV vaccines can generate higher neutralizing serum antibody to PVs, live attenuated viruses reduce the incidence of fecal PV excretion upon challenge (93), presumably as a result of superior mucosal immunity. Secretory IgA to PV has been used as an indicator of gut immunity to PV (32). An additional advantage to the use of live attenuated vaccines is the exposure of the vaccinee to forms of the virus present during the course of infection; the action of trypsin in the gut on PV type 3 (PV3) alters antigenicity without reducing the viability of the virus (84). However, use of live attenuated PV vaccines leads to the circulation of vaccine strains and their neurovirulent revertants (73) in the community, and the latter are associated with a risk of vaccine-associated disease in the unimmunized or immunodeficient. At present, a combination of an enhanced-potency inactivated vaccine and attenuated trivalent live vaccines confers the best long-term immunity (31). Although humoral immune defenses have been studied most extensively with regard to the PV vaccines, infection with a live attenuated vaccine also induces cellular immune defenses (8, 112) that are important in reducing the extent of PV infection upon challenge. Although no vaccines exist at present for non-PV enteroviruses, the use of a nonvirulent CVB3 strain to immunize mice against a cardiovirulent CVB3 infection (41) as well as of an inactivated CVB3 presented in an ISCOM format (35) has demonstrated that such vaccines are possible.

PV epitopes have been extensively studied by using antigenic variants and murine monoclonal antibodies (56, 83, 124). This work has defined four primary antigenic sites in the PVs to which neutralizing antibodies bind (82, 88). The determination of the capsid structures of several PV strains (34, 47, 129) has provided a three-dimensional map for the major antigenic sites and has also demonstrated that most residues in neutralizing antigenic sites are located on variable surface loops of the capsid proteins 1B through 1D. The immunogenicity of the sites may be different in humans (82), and at least one site in PV3 is rendered nonneutralizable in strains that can be cleaved by trypsin in the human gut without loss of viability (54). The canyon hypothesis (106) predicts for the majority of picornaviruses a strategy for evading immune surveillance by placing the conserved receptor-binding site within a depressed (protected) region on the capsid surface (see chapter 3). Variability is allowed in the antigenic sites located on the capsid surface and accessible to antibodies (17). While some data exist to define the neutralizing antigenic sites in the CVB viruses (5, 96), the fine localization of neutralizing monoclonal antibody binding sites on the capsids of other enteroviruses awaits crystallographic structural data.

With the exception of neutralizing antigenic site 1 (NAg1), the neutralizing antigen sites of PVs are combinatorial. This limits the ability to mimic the epitope with a single peptide or even with a purified capsid protein (24). One approach to defining antigenic sites has been to create chimeric viruses that display epitopes of different viral serotypes on the capsid (23, 30). One such chimera demonstrated that the location for NAg1 of PVs (the BC loop of VP1) is also an antigenic site for CVBs (96). A portion of the BC loop of CVB4 was inserted in the BC loop of CVB3, rendering the chimeric virus neutralizable by polyclonal CVB4 antiserum. Similar work demonstrated a neutralization epitope for hepatitis A (69) and human rhinovirus type 14 (2). Chimeric PVs and rhinoviruses carrying human immunodeficiency virus type 1 as well as other antigenic sequences have been created (3, 24). While such constructs provide a valuable research tool for definitively characterizing antigenic sites, enterovirus virion structures impose limits on the lengths of foreign epitope sequences that can be expressed (24). However, recent successes in expressing foreign sequences elsewhere in the PV polypeptide (1) suggest that the next generation of chimeric enteroviral vaccine candidates may be able to present foreign epitopes not only on the capsid surface but also as nonstructural peptides.

Other portions of the capsid may also play roles in the humoral antibody response to enteroviruses. By means of the peptide scanning technique (39), oligopeptides have been used to identify epitopes bound by human and murine polyclonal sera. In this manner, Roivanen et al. (100) demonstrated an immunodominant region in PV3 at the amino terminus of capsid protein 1D (amino acids 37 to 53). Interestingly, rabbit antisera raised to this peptide bind cells infected with PVs, CVBs, CVAs, or echoviruses (48). Other peptides from this region (PV1 protein 1D, amino acids 42 to 55 and 71 to 80) can be recognized by human sera containing heterotypic enteroviral IgG; antibodies from these sera, purified by binding to the peptides, bind a variety of enteroviruses (15). The amino terminus of protein 1D, internal in the native PV1 virion, becomes exposed upon attachment to cells (37, 101). Additionally, this region is recognized as antigenic by both murine B and CD4$^+$ T cells (65, 71), inducing anti-PV neutralizing antibodies in mice (71) and rabbits (28). If this region can be shown to be a neutralizing epitope in non-PV enteroviruses, it could represent an important epitope for the production of synthetic vaccines against these enteroviruses.

Enteroviral infections have also been implicated as potentially etiologic in autoimmune diseases (38, 52, 76, 92, 102). An aspect of the autoimmune component of enterovirus-induced diseases such as CVB3-induced murine myocarditis has been attributed to cross-reactivity (mimicry; 25, 123) of antibody to viral and host proteins. A neutralizing monoclonal antibody that binds capsid protein 1D also binds the murine α cardiac myosin heavy chain (10). Various antistreptococcal monoclonal antibodies are able to neutralize CVB3, CVB4, or PV1 and to bind human cardiac myosin as well (25). One of this group of monoclonals bound N-acetyl-β-D-glucosamine, the immunodominant carbohydrate moiety of group A streptococcus, which can be conformationally mimicked by amino acids 102 to 108 in CVB3 capsid protein 1D (111). The pathogenic significance of these specific cross-reactive sites to myosin in myocarditis remains to be convincingly demonstrated (91). Autoimmune disease has been modeled in mice by induction of myocarditis through inoculation with cardiac myosin (90); the CVB3-induced production of heart-specific antibodies (autoantibodies) in specific strains of mice was correlated with the induction of chronic (autoimmune) myocarditis (120). When human myocarditis patients showed elevated titers of antibody to CVB3 and CVB4, patient sera also cross-reacted with heart tissue epitopes (75).

However, the role of humoral autoimmunity to myosin in myocarditis may well be a secondary effect rather than a cause; it may not be surprising that significant lysis of cardiac myocytes releases proteins that then may induce specific autoantibodies. Neu et al. (89) demonstrated that IgG depositions in this disease were not on intact muscle fibers and that autoantibodies did not bind to intact (presumably healthy) cardiac myocytes. Further, reduction of the humoral immune response did not curtail the myosin myocarditis, nor did passive transfer of high-titer myosin autoantibodies induce the disease.

CELL-MEDIATED IMMUNE RESPONSES

Mapping antigenic enteroviral epitopes that are recognized by the cell-mediated immune response and relating them to pathogenesis is still in its infancy. To date, only CVB3 and the PVs have been significantly explored, and in each case, the search for epitope identity has been limited to a specific region of the viral genome and to a few specific murine strains. Owing to the presence of neutralizing-antibody epitopes on capsid proteins, most work has focused on the capsid. As described below, however, antigenic epitopes exist in nonstructural proteins as well; indeed, a search of any of the characterized enteroviral polypeptide sequences that follow the proposed rules (e.g., see references 33, 107, and 113) for predicting epitopes likely to be recognized in class I and II responses will reveal numerous potential epitopes across the viral proteins. However, predicting epitope motifs does not necessarily predict whether they bind MHC molecules or will be active in stimulating immune responses (20).

Leclerc and colleagues (67) mapped and identified a specific oligopeptide sequence in the PV1 capsid protein 1D that was highly antigenic in PV-immunized murine T cells. Amino acids 93 to 116 of capsid protein 1D were antigenic for mice of the $H-2^d$ haplotype (BALB/c and DBA/2) but were not antigenic for $H-2^k$ (C3H/He) or $H-2^b$ (C57BL/6) mice.

When a longer oligopeptide (amino acids 86 to 115) was used to immunize BALB/c mice, not only was the peptide able to raise a response detectable by proliferation of CD4$^+$ T cells in vitro, but it also induced neutralizing antibodies against PV1. Lewis and Feng (71) also demonstrated a colinear T- and B-cell epitope just upstream of that shown by Leclerc et al. (amino acids 70 to 80); interestingly, these 10 amino acids were antigenic in vitro for CD4$^+$ T cells from $H-2^k$ mice (A/J, CBA), and when inoculated, they induced antibodies in $H-2^d$ (BALB/c) and $H-2^b$ (C57BL/6) mice as well. In 1983, Emini and coworkers (28) showed this same region to be antigenic for rabbits. Lewis and Feng demonstrated that T- and B-cell epitopes were located in a common site on the viral protein not normally exposed externally. The fact that Lewis and Feng also demonstrated a relationship between the presence of neutralizing antibody against PV and antibody that binds the amino acid 70 to 80 epitope in human sera shows that the murine results are applicable in an outbred population as well. The data of Leclerc and colleagues (67) also suggested that there was at least one more dominant T-cell epitope in the capsid proteins of PV.

Beck et al. (9) identified a panenteroviral core peptide epitope in the nonstructural protein 2C of CVB3. Their earlier work (6, 7) had demonstrated that one serologically distinct enterovirus could immunize murine T cells, which subsequently would recognize other serologically unrelated enteroviruses in in vitro T-cell proliferation assays. This finding was also demonstrated by Katrak et al. (60) and Leclerc et al. (67) among the three serotypes of PV. Additionally, Beck and colleagues demonstrated that antigens recognized by murine CD4$^+$ T cells reside in both structural and nonstructural CVB3 proteins, a result later confirmed (8) and significantly extended (42, 112) for human peripheral blood T cells. Using highly purified inactivated virions as well as crude virus preparations that contained both structural and nonstructural components, Beck and colleagues (9) described evidence for an epitope that was shared between plant comoviruses and human enteroviruses and was located in the nonstructural proteins. A computer search for peptides of six or more contiguous amino acids detected a possible candidate in protein 2C. Figure 1 displays the identity of the short oligopeptide region in the protein 2C among several different typical picornavirus sequences.

The peptide LEEKGI was antigenic for CD4$^+$ T cells from CVB3-inoculated C3H/HeJ (H-2^k) mice in in vitro T-cell proliferation assays. In addition, T cells from mice inoculated with crude preparations (containing nonstructural proteins) of the plant comovirus bean pod mottle virus proliferated well in response to antigen LEEKGI. The control peptide LERKGT, which differs by two amino acids from that of the enteroviruses and is found in the proteins 2C of cardioviruses (which are not antigenic for enterovirus-primed murine CD4$^+$ T cells in culture; 7), was unable to promote proliferation of CVB3-primed T cells in culture except at very high concentrations (>25 µg/ml). However, the peptide LEEKGI was not antigenic for human peripheral blood lymphocytes taken from volunteers previously shown to have serologic evidence of previous enterovirus infections (9a). Thus, while the exploitation of evolutionary conservation of peptide sequences suggests that using computer analyses of potentially antigenic sites can help in identifying other possible antigenic epitopes, antigenic epitopes identified in nonhuman systems may not be relevant to human disease.

Recent work comparing the sequences derived from the infectious cDNA genomes of a cardiovirulent CVB3 strain and a noncardiovirulent strain (18, 118) demonstrated that 13 amino acids constitute the difference in the polyprotein of these two strains (18). Owing to the well-characterized murine inflammatory response in CVB3-induced murine myocarditis (52, 70, 78, 127), overlapping 9-mer peptides were synthesized across each of the 13 amino acid differences to determine which of these sites may be antigenic for T cells from mice of different haplotypes and susceptibility to CVB3-induced inflammatory heart disease (103). Preliminary results from this study (6a) show that splenocytes derived from C57BL/6 (H-2^b) mice inoculated with the cardiovirulent strain of CVB3 recognize peptides across 4 of the 13 specific loci. Peptides derived from the cardiovirulent strain are antigenic, while peptides from the nonvirulent CVB3 strain, differing by just one amino acid, are not. One locus is located within the same region identified by Mahon et al. (74) in capsid protein 1A of PV, a cross-reactive sequence for PV-immune murine T-cell lines. This region is depicted in Fig. 2.

```
VIRUS              SEQUENCE IN PROTEIN 2C

Comovirus          LISSAPYPLNMAG LEEKGI CFDSQFVFVSTN
CVB3               ..SS......MA. LEEKGI .F.S.FV..STN
PV1                ..S......NMA. LEEKGI .F.S..V..STN
Mengo              ..S......NMA. LE.KG. .F.SQ.V...TN
HRV 14             ..SS......MA. L..KG. .F.S.FV..STN
FMDV               ..S.......MA. LE.KG. .F.S......TN
```

FIGURE 1 Peptide sequence identities in protein 2C of enteroviruses, picornaviruses, and plant comoviruses. Sequences are aligned to the comovirus (cowpea mosaic virus) sequence in protein 2C. Amino acids that vary from those in the cowpea mosaic virus sequence are shown as dots. The box indicates the antigenic LEEKGI sequence in entero- and comoviruses. Mengo, Mengo virus; HRV 14, human rhinovirus type 14; FMDV, foot-and-mouth disease virus. The sequences are based on work by Beck et al. (9).

The capsid 1A proteins of PVs and CVB3 possess a highly antigenic sequence cluster for murine CD4+ T cells within their initial 35 to 40 amino acids. Mahon et al. (74) suggested that this clustering of antigenic sequences for mice of different backgrounds and haplotypes might be useful for promoting a more robust response to a secondary viral infection. It is interesting to speculate whether this might be the dominant, cross-reactive epitope suggested by the data of Leclerc et al. (67); although information from a complete epitope map of the capsid proteins is lacking, this region makes a good candidate. Indeed, secondary enteroviral infections in a murine model suggest that T-cell memory, perhaps employing the CD4+ Th activity stimulated by these peptide sequences, causes a faster T-cell response to secondary enteroviral challenge (6).

Katrak et al. (60) demonstrated that mice inoculated with any PV serotype generated a CD4+ Th cell response against PV as antigen when assayed in in vitro culture. Kutubuddin et al. (65) inoculated mice of three different haplotypes with PV1 and characterized the murine CD4+ T-cell proliferation responses in in vitro culture with purified PV1, the capsid protein 1D, or peptides spanning protein 1D as antigens. Confirming and extending previous observations by others (67) that CD4+ T-cell epitopes can be found close to or overlapping B cell epitopes, Kutubuddin and colleagues showed that CD4+ epitopes clustered by neutralizing antigenic sites 1 and 2 in PV1 capsid protein 1D. Furthermore, recognition of specific epitope sequences was dependent on the murine haplotype. One peptide, comprising amino acids 202 to 221 of protein 1D, was recognized by T cells with either the H-2^d or the H-2^b haplotypes but not with the H-2^k haplotype. However, the adjacent (but nonoverlapping) peptide sequence (amino acids 222 to 241) was recognized by T cells from the H-2^k mouse and not nearly as well or at all by H-2^d or H-2^b mice. Extending their observations to humans, Simons and colleagues (112) demonstrated that at least

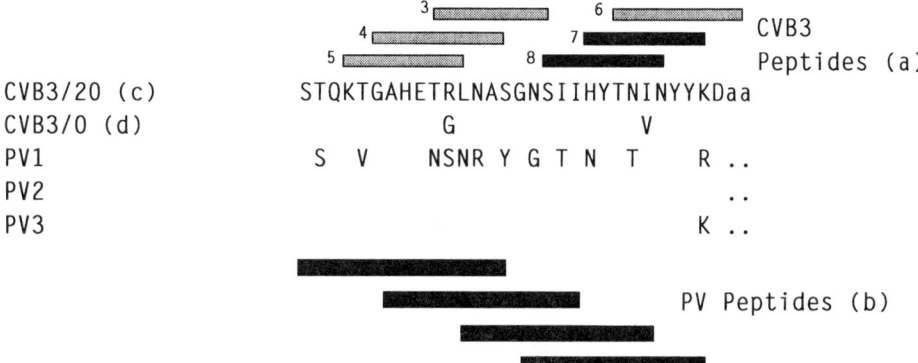

FIGURE 2 Capsid protein 1A sequences in CVB3 and PV1 are antigenic for murine T cells with different haplotypes. Capsid protein 1A sequence is shown from amino acid 6 to 37; lowercase letters represent amino acid residues present in CVB3 but not PV as analyzed by Mahon et al. (74). Dark boxes denote peptides that initiated significant proliferative responses in in vitro cultures. a, CVB3 peptides tested against C57BL/6 (H-2^b) splenocytes (6b); b, PV peptides tested against PV-immune T-cell clones from BALB/c (H-2^d) or CBA (H-2^k) mice (based on Mahon et al. [74]); c, cardiovirulent CVB3 strain (based on Tracy et al. [118]); d, noncardiovirulent CVB3 strain (based on Chapman et al. [18]).

some human CD4+ peripheral blood lymphocyte samples proliferated in response to PV-derived peptides spanning the region between amino acids 161 and 221. Amino acids 244 to 264 in protein 1D were also antigenic for human CD4+ T cells in this study.

The findings that different epitopes are recognized by CD4+ T cells from mice of different haplotypes support the view expressed by Graham et al. (42) and Simons et al. (112) that better vaccine design may result by identifying sequences rich in numerous T-cell epitopes for linkage to B-cell epitopes rather than expecting to find individual CD4+ epitopes recognized by the great majority of an outbred population. Colinear T- and B-cell epitopes have been exploited in attempts to formulate peptide vaccines (36, 68, 81, 94). Multiple antigenic peptides (115) linking T- and B-cell epitopes in linear arrays have been demonstrated to raise both Th and B-cell responses in mice (16), but the authors (16) also noted that specific Th epitopes were recognized better by some strains of mice than others. A cross-reactive, Th-epitope-rich sequence might help circumvent specific epitope recognition problems. Is the protein 1A of enteroviruses such a Th-epitope-rich region? The sequence in PV capsid protein 1A identified by Mahon et al. (74) as having cross-reactive T-cell antigenicity would be an interesting place to start to test this hypothesis.

Auvinen et al. (4) mapped antigenic epitopes in the capsid proteins of CVB3 that were recognized by murine CD4+ T cells. BALB/c mice were inoculated with oligopeptides derived from CVB3 capsid protein sequences, and then T cells were placed in culture with the peptides as antigens. Two primary sites in CVB3 capsid protein 1D that contain CD4+ T-cell epitopes were identified. One site, spanning the CVB3 BC loop (putatively mapped in CVB3 by comparison to solved enteroviral capsid structures; e.g., see references 47 and 105), is in the same relative location as in the PV1 protein (Fig. 3). Interestingly, amino acids 222 to 241 in PV1 protein 1D were also slightly antigenic for C3H/HeJ ($H-2^k$) T cells, suggesting that a significant cluster of CD4+ epitopes also resides within this span of about 40 amino acids in both CVB3 and PV1. This site maps to neutralizing site 2a for polioviruses. These workers also examined regions within CVB3 capsid proteins 1B and 1C. In both proteins, alignment of sequences permits mapping of sites across PV neutralizing sites 2b and 3b, which contain sequences that are antigenic for BALB/c CD4+ T cells. Leclerc et al. (67) and Kutubuddin et al. (65) also defined a primary CD4+ T-cell epitope in this region for both $H-2^d$ and $H-2^k$ mice. These comparative data show that identified CD4+ T-cell epitopes in CVB3 capsid protein 1D are located close to an identified B-cell epitope; a similar B-cell epitope in the same region of CVB4 protein 1D has been demonstrated by Reiman et al. (96). A second site in CVB3 protein 1D, spanning amino acids 189 to 213, was also identified as antigenic for BALB/c mice (51). Kutubuddin and coworkers (65) similarly found this region in PV1 protein 1D (amino acids 202 to 221) to be significantly antigenic for both BALB/c and C57BL/6 CD4+ T cells.

Huber et al. (51) significantly extended their previous work (50) mapping peptide sequences in the CVB3 capsid protein 1D that are antigenic for murine T cells. Using a cardiovirulent strain of CVB3 and a noncardiovirulent derivative of the same strain of virus to infect a BALB/c mouse-derived macrophage cell line, those authors showed a clear difference between the abilities of the two viruses to induce IL-1 and alpha/beta interferon. This finding is also of interest in the context of viral activation of monocytes: Henke et al. (46) have shown that human monocytes exposed in vitro to CVB3 produce a variety of cytokines. In contrast to the noncardiovirulent strain of virus, cardiovirulent CVB3 caused increased levels of both cytokines to be CVB3-inoculated BALB/c mouse mesenteric lymph nodes 7 days postinfection demonstrated that significantly more Th1 than Th2 CD4+ cells were generated. Using overlapping peptides spanning

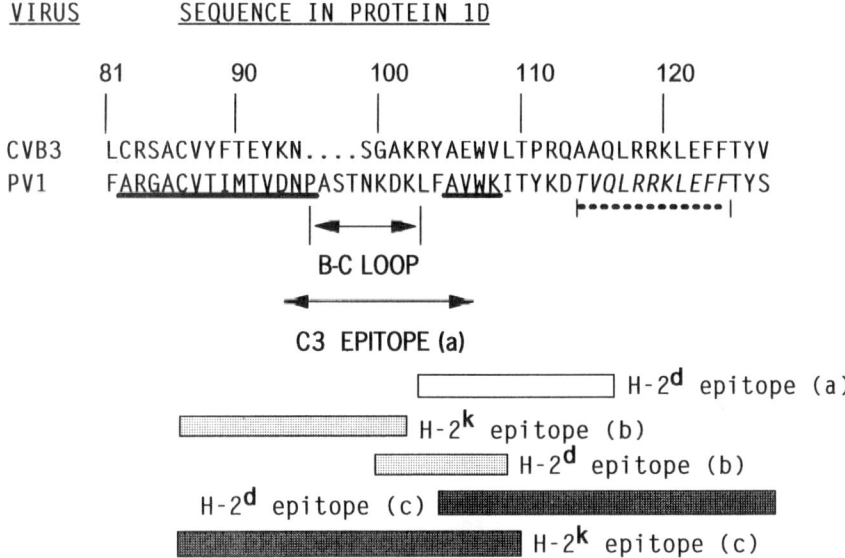

FIGURE 3 Epitopes antigenic for murine T cells cluster near the BC loop in capsid protein 1D of PV1 and CVB3. Amino acid numbering in capsid proteins 1D and PV1 (Mahoney) sequence is based on Kitamura et al. (63); CVB3 sequence is based on Tracy et al. (118). Underline, β-pleated sheet; broken line, α helix; a, based on Leclerc et al. (67); b, based on Kutubuddin et al. (65); c, based on Auvinen et al. (4).

CVB3 capsid protein 1D, they showed that T cells derived from mice inoculated with cardiovirulent CVB3 proliferated in response to multiple peptides, whereas T cells from mice inoculated with the noncardiovirulent CVB3 strain recognized only one of these peptides as antigenic. If, however, the noncardiovirulent-CVB3-infected mice were also given daily injections of IL-2, the T cells derived from these mice proliferated in a pattern essentially identical to that observed for cardiovirulent CVB3-immune T cells. These results clearly demonstrate that virulent and avirulent strains of CVB3 can induce quite different T-cell reactions. These data are consistent with the preliminary results described above (116a) for differential recognition of peptides (differing in a single amino acid) by CVB3-immune CD4$^+$ T cells from C57BL/6 mice. Collectively, the data suggest that differential CD4$^+$ T-cell responses can be generated by strains of an enterovirus that differ by virulence phenotype.

The data obtained by Huber and colleagues suggest that inflammatory disease induction by CVB3, and perhaps other enteroviruses, ultimately hinges on fine control of cytokine production as stimulated by specific viral oligopeptide sequences. It will be of great interest to discover the role(s) each viral epitope plays individually, in concert with other epitopes, and in the context of host genetics in the induction of inflammatory disease. As demonstrated previously (9), specific amino acid alterations in an enterovirus-derived peptide can result in loss of recognition by the responding murine T cell. Although both CD4$^+$ and CD8$^+$ T cells are now recognized as capable of being cytotoxic T lymphocytes (CTL), the responses of CD4$^+$ T cells in in vitro proliferation assays (as described above) have not been extensively examined in terms of whether the primary responding population is Th1 or Th2. In this regard, work by Katrak et al. (60) for PVs and by Huber and colleagues (52) for CVB3 represents a significant step linking in vitro molecular observations with potentially testable pathogenic mechanisms. Research in this area is one of the next significant steps needed for characterizing the responses of murine and human T cells to enteroviral antigens.

While a great deal of effort has been expended on understanding the roles of CTL in the host response to enteroviral (primarily CVB3) infection, these data are in large part descriptive and in many instances are open to different interpretations. The primary model for the study of the role of CTL in enteroviral pathogenesis has been CVB3-induced inflammatory heart disease in mice (52, 70, 121).

Kutubuddin and coworkers (66) demonstrated that exposure of BALB/c mice to PV or capsid protein 1D results in $CD8^+$ CTL. Specific lysis could be shown by using two protein 1D-derived peptides, one spanning amino acids 110 to 120 and the other spanning amino acids 202 to 221. Use of peptides pulsed on target cells demonstrated restriction to the K^d allele. Significantly, a cluster of epitopes recognized by both murine and human $CD4^+$ T cells as well as by neutralizing antibodies maps to the same general sequence in the PV capsid protein 1D (discussed above). Kutubuddin et al. suggest that this may be at least one reason why this specific protein sequence is so antigenic in mice. Will similar clusters of humoral, $CD4^+$ Th, and $CD8^+$ CTL epitopes be found in other enteroviruses?

No $CD8^+$ CTL reactivity to CVB3-infected cardiomyocytes (virus-specific cytotoxicity) has been shown (70, 121), although $CD4^+$ class II MHC-restricted CTL have been demonstrated (29). Huber and colleagues have segregated CTL in experimental murine CVB3 infections into three groups (121). Murine-virus-specific CTL that can lyse syngeneic target cells (not cardiomyocytes) infected with a cardiovirulent CVB3 strain but not cells infected with a noncardiovirulent CVB3 strain have been demonstrated (49). These CTL are $CD4^+$ and class II restricted. So-called metabolic CTL recognize specific antigens produced by cells under stress, such as those induced by a viral infection. It is unclear what role this recognition plays in pathogenesis or how a virulent strain of CVB3 might induce a new antigen whereas a related nonvirulent strain of CVB3 does not (72). Autoimmune CTL are $CD8^+$ class I antigen restricted and have been demonstrated to lyse healthy uninfected cardiomyocytes, causing significant cardiac damage following heart injury as induced by replication of cardiovirulent CVB3 strains (52).

Immunocompromised mice have also been used to study the roles of T cells in CVB3-induced heart disease. Early work demonstrated cardiac damage and persistence of inflammation in the absence of infectious virus, suggesting an immunopathogenic mechanism (125). Hashimoto and Komatsu (44) inoculated athymic nude mice (BALB/c *nu/nu*) deficient in mature T cells with CVB3 and demonstrated that although viral titers were similar among groups, BALB/c *nu/+* or *+/+* mice demonstrated more myocardial disease than *nu/nu* mice. Transfer of splenocytes from BALB/c *nu/+* mice previously inoculated with CVB3 into BALB/c *nu/nu* mice increased the myocarditis (45). Countering these data and suggesting a role for murine T cells in pathogenesis of inflammatory heart disease, Robinson et al. (98) determined that following inoculation with CVB3, BALB/c *nu/nu* and *+/+* mice showed equivalent levels of heart disease and titers of cardiac virus. Schnurr and Schmidt (109) showed that NFR *nu/nu* mice developed disease equivalent in extent to that in their euthymic littermates (*+/nu*). However, virus persisted in *nu/nu* mice with evidence of chronic heart disease. These data suggested that T cells were not involved in pathogenesis but played a role in virus clearance. Recent studies by Chow et al. (21) demonstrated that severe combined immunodeficient (*scid*) mice developed extensive cardiac necrosis with macrophage infiltrates, a fact that supports a protective role for T cells in CVB3 infection. The use of antithymocyte serum to eradicate most T cells or thymectomized mice to study CVB3 infections has given similar contradictory results (43, 61, 128). These apparently conflicting results undoubtedly have some roots in the different strains and ages of mice used as well as in the different strains of CVBs, which differ in cardiovirulence phenotype. It is apparent that T cells can play various roles in both enteroviral clearance and pathogenesis depending on host factors (such as strain, age, sex, preexisting immunities) and viral virulence phenotype. As pointed out by Huber and colleagues (52, 70), CVB3-induced murine inflammatory heart disease is complex and may well result from several mechanisms. Data from studies with T-cell-deficient mice tend to support this judgment.

SUMMARY

The relatively short enteroviral polyprotein and the variety of murine enteroviral pathogenesis models are ideal not only for pursuing the identities of specific antigenic epitopes for T and B lymphocytes but also for asking definitive questions about the roles such epitopes may play in viral disease. Although unexpected, epitopic clusters apparently exist in viral proteins and are recognized by lymphocytes from different strains of mice. What roles do epitope clustering and commonly recognized epitopes play in disease causation? Are epitopes that are recognized by a variety of different haplotypes of potential use for incorporation into viral vaccines, thus making the vaccine antigenically more robust? What are the interactions between the various viral epitopes and T-lymphocyte production of cytokines, and how might these interactions be manipulated to provide more effective vaccines and vaccine vectors? Can mutations engineered in key epitopes significantly diminish or even ablate T-cell recognition of the mutated virus, and will such epitopes remain stable or evolve to a dominant (original?) sequence in the viral population? Will previously unremarked peptide sequences now become antigenic? Such questions can be asked in enterovirus-murine systems and can be used, among other things, to study quasispecies in the realm of virus-host interactions as well as fundamental questions in immunology.

It is a truism that technological developments help drive basic research. It has been barely 10 years since the solution of the first near-atomic crystal structure of a PV and a rhinovirus virion, which permitted three-dimensional depictions of epitopes recognized by antiviral antibodies. Libraries of monoclonal antibodies to virion and nonstructural proteins can be readily constructed in most laboratories. The prices of customized, commercially available oligopeptides have fallen significantly, making possible widespread use of peptides for the mapping and functional analysis of antigenic epitopes recognized by both T and B cells. Infectious cDNA copies of enteroviral genomes and well-defined murine models of enterovirus-induced disease pathogenesis permit genetically controlled studies of virus-immune system interactions. The gate is open to diverse and detailed molecular studies of the interactions between host immune systems and enteroviruses, moving enteroviral immunology from a descriptive, often phenomenologic phase into one of precise experimentation.

ACKNOWLEDGMENTS

This work was supported in part by National Institutes of Health grants HL40303 to S.T. and HL46195 to M.A.B. and by American Heart Association grant 93009360 to S.T.

REFERENCES

1. **Alexander, L., H. H. Lu, and E. Wimmer.** 1994. Polioviruses containing picornavirus type 1 and/or type 2 internal ribosomal entry site elements: genetic hybrids and the expression of a foreign gene. *Proc. Natl. Acad. Sci. USA* **91:**1406–1410.
2. **Altmeyer, R., A. Murdin, J. Harber, and E. Wimmer.** 1991. Construction and characterization of a poliovirus/rhinovirus antigenic hybrid. *Virology* **184:**636–644.
3. **Arnold, G., D. Resnick, Y. Li, A. Zhang, A. Smith, S. Geisler, A. Jacobo-Molina, W. Lee, R. Webster, and E. Arnold.** 1994. Design and construction of rhinovirus chimeras incorporating immunogens from polio, influenza, and human immunodeficiency viruses. *Virology* **198:**403–408.
4. **Auvinen, P., M. Makela, M. Roivainen, M. Kallajoki, R. Vainionpaa, and T. Hyppia.**

1993. Mapping of antigenic sites of coxsackievirus B3 by synthetic peptides. *APMIS* **101**:517–528.
5. **Beatrice, S. T., M. G. Katze, B. A. Zajac, and R. A. Crowell.** 1980. Induction of neutralizing antibodies by the coxsackievirus B3 virion polypeptide, VP2. *Virology* **104**:426–438.
6. **Beck, M., N. Chapman, B. McManus, J. Mullican, and S. Tracy.** 1990. Secondary enterovirus infection in the murine model of myocarditis: pathologic and immunologic aspects. *Am. J. Pathol.* **136**:669–681.
6a. **Beck, M., R. Rubocki, S. Tracy, and N. Chapman.** Unpublished data.
6b. **Beck, M., and S. Tracy.** Unpublished data.
7. **Beck, M., and S. Tracy.** 1989. Murine cell-mediated immune response recognizes an enterovirus group-specific antigen(s). *J. Virol.* **63**:4148–4156.
8. **Beck, M., and S. Tracy.** 1990. Evidence for a group-specific enteroviral antigen(s) recognized by human T cells. *J. Clin. Microbiol.* **28**:1822–1827.
9. **Beck, M., S. Tracy, B. Coller, N. Chapman, G. Hufnagel, J. Johnson, and G. Lomonossoff.** 1992. Comoviruses and enteroviruses share a T cell epitope. *Virology* **186**:238–246.
9a. **Beck, M., S. Tracy, and G. Hufnagel.** Unpublished data.
10. **Beisel, K., J. Srinivasappa, and B. Prabhakar.** 1991. Identification of a putative shared epitope between coxsackievirus B4 and *alpha* cardiac myosin heavy chain. *Clin. Exp. Immunol.* **86**:49–55.
11. **Bendinelli, M., P. G. Conaldi, and D. Matteucci.** 1988. Interactions with the immune system, p. 81–102. *In* M. Bendinelli and H. Friedman (ed.), *Coxsackieviruses, a General Update*. Plenum Press, New York.
12. **Bjorkman, P., M. Saper, B. Samraoui, W. Bennett, J. Strominger, and D. Wiley.** 1987. Structure of the human class I histocompatibility antigen, HLA-A2. *Nature* (London) **329**:506–512.
13. **Brown, J., T. Jardetzky, J. Gorga, L. Stern, R. Urban, J. Strominger, and D. Wiley.** 1993. Three-dimensional structure of the human class II histocompatibility antigen HLA-DR1. *Nature* (London) **364**:33–38.
14. **Burnet, F. M.** 1957. A modification of Jerne's theory of antibody formation. *Aust. J. Sci.* **20**:67–69.
15. **Cello, J., A. Samuelson, P. Stalhandske, B. Svennerholm, S. Jeansson, and M. Forsgren.** 1993. Identification of group-common linear epitopes in structural and non-structural proteins of enteroviruses by using synthetic peptides. *J. Clin. Microbiol.* **31**:911–916.
16. **Chai, S., P. Clavijo, J. Tam, and F. Zavala.** 1992. Immunogenic properties of multiple antigen peptide systems containing defined T and B cell epitopes. *J. Immunol.* **149**:2385–2390.
17. **Chapman, M. S., and M. G. Rossmann.** 1993. Comparison of surface properties of picornaviruses: strategies for hiding the receptor site from immune surveillance. *Virology* **195**:745–756.
17a. **Chapman, N. et al.** Submitted for publication.
18. **Chapman, N., Z. Tu, C. Gauntt, and S. Tracy.** 1994. An infectious cDNA copy of the genome of a non-cardiovirulent coxsackievirus B3 strain: its complete sequence analysis and comparison to the genomes of cardiovirulent coxsackieviruses. *Arch. Virol.*, **135**:115–130.
19. **Cherry, J. D.** 1992. Enteroviruses: polioviruses (poliomyelitis), coxsackieviruses, echoviruses, and enteroviruses, p. 1705–1753. *In* R. Feigin and J. D. Cherry (ed.), *Textbook of Pediatric Infectious Diseases*, 3rd ed. The W. B. Saunders Co., Philadelphia.
20. **Chicz, R., and R. Urban.** 1994. Analysis of MHC-presented peptides: applications in autoimmunity and vaccine development. *Immunol. Today* **15**:155–160.
21. **Chow, L. H., K. Beisel, and B. McManus.** 1992. Enteroviral infection of mice with severe combined immunodeficiency. Evidence for direct viral pathogenesis of myocardial injury. *Lab. Invest.* **66**:24–31.
22. **Christensen, M. L., L. M. Pachman, R. Schneiderman, D. C. Patel, and J. J. M. Friedman.** 1986. Prevalence of coxsackie B virus antibodies in patients with juvenile dermatomyositis. *Arthritis Rheum.* **29**:1365–1370.
23. **Colbere-Garapin, F., C. Christodoulou, R. Crainic, A. C. Garapin, and A. Candrea.** 1988. Addition of a foreign oligopeptide to the major capsid protein of poliovirus. *Proc. Natl. Acad. Sci. USA* **85**:8668–8672.
24. **Crabbe, M., D. Evans, and J. Almond.** 1990. Modeling of poliovirus–HIV-1 antigen chimeras. *FEBS Lett.* **271**:194–198.
25. **Cunningham, M., S. Antone, J. Gulizia, B. M. McManus, V. Fischette, and C. J. Gauntt.** 1992. Cytotoxic and virus neutralizing antibodies cross-react with streptococcal M protein, enterovirus, and human cardiac myosin. *Proc. Natl. Acad. Sci. USA* **89**:1320–1325.
26. **Dausett, J.** 1981. The major histocompatibility complex in man. *Science* **213**:1469–1474.
27. **Davis, M. M., and P. J. Bjorkman.** 1988.

T-cell receptor antigen genes and T-cell recognition. *Nature* (London) **334**:395–402.

28. Emini, E., B. Jameson, and E. Wimmer. 1983. Priming for and induction of anti-poliovirus neutralizing antibodies by synthetic peptides. *Nature* (London) **304**:699–703.
29. Estrin, M., and S. Huber. 1987. Coxsackievirus B3-induced myocarditis autoimmunity is L3T4+ T helper cell and IL-2 independent in BALB/c mice. *Am. J. Pathol.* **127**:335–341.
30. Evans, D., and J. Almond. 1991. Design, construction and characterization of poliovirus antigen chimeras. *Methods Enzymol.* **203**:386–400.
31. Faden, H., L. Duffy, M. Sun, and C. Shuff. 1993. Long-term immunity to poliovirus in children immunized with live attenuated and enhanced-potency inactivated trivalent poliovirus vaccines. *J. Infect. Dis.* **168**:452–454.
32. Faden, H., J. F. Modlin, M. L. Thoms, A. M. McBean, M. B. Ferdon, and P. L. Ogra. 1990. Comparative evaluation of immunization with live attenuated and enhanced-potency inactivated trivalent poliovirus vaccines in childhood: systemic and local immune responses. *J. Infect. Dis.* **162**:1291–1297.
33. Falk, K., O. Rotzschke, S. Stevanovic, J. Gunther, and H. Rammensee. 1991. Allele specific motifs revealed by sequencing of self peptides eluted from MHC molecules. *Nature* (London) **351**:290–296.
34. Filman, D., R. Syed, M. Chow, A. Macadam, P. Minor, and J. Hogle. 1989. Structural factors that control conformational transitions and serotype specificity in type 3 poliovirus. *EMBO J.* **8**:1567–1579.
35. Fohlman, J., N. Ilback, G. Friman, and B. Morein. 1990. Vaccination of BALB/c mice against enteroviral mediated myocarditis. *Vaccine* **8**:381–384.
36. Francis, M. J., G. Z. Hastings, B. E. Clarke, A. L. Brown, C. R. Beddell, D. J. Rowlands, and F. Brown. 1990. Neutralizing antibodies to all seven serotypes of foot-and-mouth disease virus elicited by synthetic peptides. *Immunology* **69**:171–176.
37. Fricks, C. E., and J. M. Hogle. 1990. Cell-induced conformational changes in poliovirus: externalization of the amino terminus of VP1 is responsible for liposome binding. *J. Virol.* **64**:1934–1945.
38. Gautam A., C. Lock, D. Smilek, C. Pearson, L. Steinman, and H. McDevitt. 1994. Minimum structural requirements for peptide presentation by major histocompatibility complex class II molecules: implications in induction of autoimmunity. *Proc. Natl. Acad. Sci. USA* **91**:767–771.
39. Geyson, H., T. Mason, and S. Roda. 1984. Peptides as specific recognition devices, p. 111–119. *In* A. Vaheri, R. Tilton, and A. Balows (ed.), *Rapid Methods and Automation in Microbiology and Immunology*. Springer-Verlag, Berlin.
40. Glimaker, M., A. Samuelson, L. Magnius, A. Ehrnst, P. Olcen, and M. Forsgren. 1992. Early diagnosis of enteroviral meningitis by detection of specific IgM antibodies with a solid-phase reverse immunosorbent test (SPRIST) and mu-capture EIA. *J. Med. Virol.* **36**:193–201.
41. Godeny, E. K., H. Arizpe, and C. Gauntt. 1988. Characterization of the antibody response in vaccinated mice protected against coxsackievirus B3-induced myocarditis. *Viral Immunol.* **4**:305–314.
42. Graham, S., E. Wang, O. Jenkins, and L. K. Borysiewicz. 1993. Analysis of the human T-cell response to picornaviruses: identification of T-cell epitopes close to B-cell epitopes in poliovirus. *J. Virol.* **67**:1627–1637.
43. Grun, J. B., M. Schultz, S. Finkelstein, R. L. Crowell, and B. Landau. 1988. Pathogenesis of acute myocardial necrosis in inbred mice infected with coxsackievirus B3. *Microb. Pathog.* **4**:417–430.
44. Hasimoto, I., and T. Komatsu. 1978. Myocardial changes after infection with coxsackie virus B3 in nude mice. *Br. J. Exp. Pathol.* **59**:13–20.
45. Hashimoto, I., M. Tatsumi, and M. Nakagawa. 1983. The role of T lymphocytes in the pathogenesis of coxsackie virus B3 heart disease. *Br. J. Exp. Pathol.* **64**:497–504.
46. Henke, A., H. Spengler, A. Stelzner, M. Nain, and D. Gemsa. 1992. Lipopolysaccharide suppresses cytokine release from coxsackie virus infected human monocytes. *Res. Immunol.* **143**:65–70.
47. Hogle, J., M. Chow, and D. Filman. 1985. Three-dimensional structure of poliovirus at 2.9 angstrom resolution. *Science* **229**:1358–1365.
48. Hovi, T., and M. Roivanen. 1993. Peptide antisera targeted to a conserved sequence in poliovirus capsid protein VP1 cross-react widely with members of the genus enterovirus. *J. Clin. Microbiol.* **31**:1083–1087.
49. Huber, S., and L. Job. 1983. Differences in cytolytic T-cell response of BALB/c mice infected with myocarditic and non-myocarditic strains of coxsackievirus group B, type 3. *Infect. Immun.* **39**:1419–1425.
50. Huber, S., J. Polgar, A. Moraska, M. Cunningham, P. Schwimmbeck, and P. Schultheiss. 1993. T lymphocyte responses in

CVB3-induced murine mycocarditis. *Scand. J. Infect. Dis. Suppl.* **88:**67–78.
51. **Huber, S. A., J. Polgar, P. Schultheiss, and P. Schwimmbeck.** 1994. Augmentation of pathogenesis of coxsackievirus B3 infections in mice by exogenous administration of interleukin-1 and interleukin-2. *J. Virol.* **68:**195–206.
52. **Huber, S., A. Weller, M. Herzum, P. Lodge, M. Estrin, K. Simpson, and M. Guthrie.** 1988. Immunopathogenic mechanisms in experimental picornavirus-induced autoimmunity. *Pathol. Immunopathol. Res.* **7:**279–291.
53. **Hunt, D., H. Michel, T. Dickinson, J. Shabanowitz, A. Cox, K. Sakaguchi, E. Appella, H. Grey, and A. Sette.** 1992. Peptides presented to the immune system by the murine class II major histocompatibility complex molecule I-Ad. *Science* **256:**1817–1820.
54. **Icenogle, J. P., P. D. Minor, M. Ferguson, and J. M. Hogle.** 1986. Modulation of humoral response to a 12-amino-acid site on the poliovirus virion. *J. Virol.* **60:**297–301.
55. **Iizuka, N., S. Kuge, and A. Nomoto.** 1987. Complete nucleotide sequence of the genome of coxsackievirus B1. *Virology* **156:**64–73.
56. **Jameson, B. A., E. Wimmer, and O. Kew.** 1985. Natural variants of the Sabin type 1 vaccine strain of poliovirus and correlation with a poliovirus neutralization site. *Virology* **143:**337–341.
57. **Jenkins, O., J. D. Booth, P. Minor, and J. W. Almond.** 1987. The complete nucleotide sequence of coxsackievirus B4 and its comparison to other members of the Picornaviridae. *J. Gen. Virol.* **68:**1835–1848.
58. **Jerne, N. K.** 1955. The natural selection theory of antibody formation. *Proc. Natl. Acad. Sci. USA* **41:**849–857.
59. **Kandolf, R., and P. Hofschneider.** 1985. Molecular cloning of the genome of a cardiotropic coxsackie B3 virus: full-length reverse-transcribed recombinant cDNA generates infectious virus in mammalian cells. *Proc. Natl. Acad. Sci. USA* **82:**4818–4822.
60. **Katrak, K., B. Mahon, P. Minor, and K. Mills.** 1989. Cellular and humoral responses to poliovirus in mice: a role for helper T cells in heterotypic immunity to poliovirus. *J. Gen. Virol.* **72:**1093–1098.
61. **Khatib, R., G. Khatib, J. Chason, and A. M. Lerner.** 1983. Alterations in coxsackievirus B4 heart muscle disease in ICR Swiss mice by anti-thymocyte serum. *J. Gen. Virol.* **64:**231–236.
62. **King, M. L., A. Shaikh, D. Bidwell, A. Voller, and J. E. Banatvala.** 1983. Coxsackie B virus-specific IgM responses in children with insulin-dependent (juvenile onset; type I) diabetes mellitus. *Lancet* **i:**1397–1399.
63. **Kitamura, N., B. Semler, P. Rothberg, G. Larsen, C. Adler, A. Dorner, A. Emini, R. Hanecak, J. Lee, S. van der Werf, C. Anderson, and E. Wimmer.** 1981. Primary structure, gene organization, and polypeptide expression of poliovirus RNA. *Nature* (London) **291:**547–553.
64. **Koike, K., C. Taya, T. Kurata, S. Abe, I. Ise, H. Yonekawa, and A. Nomoto.** 1991. Transgenic mice susceptible to poliovirus. *Proc. Natl. Acad. Sci. USA* **88:**951–955.
65. **Kutubuddin, M., J. Simons, and M. Chow.** 1992. Identification of T-helper epitopes in the VP1 capsid protein of poliovirus. *J. Virol.* **66:**3042–3047.
66. **Kutubuddin, M., J. Simons, and M. Chow.** 1992. Poliovirus-specific major histocompatibility complex class II-restricted cytolytic T-cell epitopes in mice localize to neutralizing antigenic regions. *J. Virol.* **66:**5967–5974.
67. **Leclerc, C., E. Deriaud, V. Mimic, and S. van der Werf.** 1991. Identification of a T-cell epitope adjacent to neutralization antigenic site 1 of poliovirus type 1. *J. Virol.* **65:**711–718.
68. **Leclerc, C., G. Przewlocki, M. Schutze, and L. Chedid.** 1987. A synthetic vaccine constructed by copolymerization of B and T cell determinants. *Eur. J. Immunol.* **17:**269–273.
69. **Lemon, S., W. Barclay, M. Ferguson, P. Murphy, L. Jing, K. Burke, D. Wood, K. Katrak, D. Sangar, P. Minor, and J. Almond.** 1992. Immunogenicity and antigenicity of chimeric picornaviruses which express hepatitis A (HAV) sequences: evidence for a neutralizing domain near the amino terminus of VP1 of HAV. *Virology* **188:**285–295.
70. **Leslie, K., R. Blay, C. Haisch, A. Lodge, A. Weller, and S. Huber.** 1989. Clinical and experimental aspects of viral myocarditis. *Clin. Microbiol. Rev.* **2:**191–203.
71. **Lewis, G. K., and C. Feng.** 1992. Intrinsic immunogenicity of an internal VP1 T-B epitope pair of the type 1 poliovirus. *Mol. Immunol.* **29:**1477–1485.
72. **Lutton, C., and C. J. Gauntt.** 1986. Coxsackievirus B3 infection alters plasma membrane of neonatal skin fibroblasts. *J. Virol.* **60:**294–299.
73. **Macadam, A. J., C. Arnold, J. Howlett, A. John, S. Marsden, F. Taffs, P. Reeve, N. Hamada, K. Wareham, J. Almond, N. Cammack, and P. D. Minor.** 1989. Reversion of attenuated and temperature-sensitive phenotypes of the Sabin type 3 strain of polio-

virus in vaccinees. *Virology* **174**:408–414.
74. **Mahon, B., K. Katrak, and K. Mills.** 1992. Antigenic sequences of poliovirus recognized by T cells: serotype-specific epitopes on VP1 and VP3 and cross-reactive epitopes on VP4 defined by using CD4$^+$ T-cell clones. *J. Virol.* **66**:7012–7020.
75. **Maisch, B., E. Bauer, M. Cirsi, and K. Kochsiek.** 1993. Cytolytic cross-reactive antibodies directed against the cardiac membrane and viral proteins in coxsackievirus B3 and B4 myocarditis. *Circulation* **87**(Suppl. 5):IV49–IV65.
76. **Martino, T., P. Liu, and M. Sole.** 1994. Viral infection and the pathogenesis of dilated cardiomyopathy. *Circ. Res.* **74**:182–188.
77. **McKinney, R. E., S. L. Katz, and C. M. Wilfert.** 1987. Chronic enteroviral meningoencephalitis in agammaglobulinemic patients. *Rev. Infect. Dis.* **9**:334–356.
78. **McManus, B., C. Gauntt, and R. Cassling.** 1988. Immunopathological basis of myocardial injury. *Cardiovasc. Clin.* **18**:163–184.
79. **Melnick, J. L.** 1990. Enteroviruses: polioviruses, coxsackieviruses, echoviruses, and newer enteroviruses, p. 549–606. *In* B. Fields and D. Knipe (ed.), *Virology*. Raven Press, New York.
80. **Melnick, J. L., N. Clark, and L. Kraft.** 1950. Immunological reactions of coxsackie viruses. III. Cross-protection tests in infant mice born of vaccinated mothers. Transfer of immunity through the milk. *J. Exp. Med.* **92**:499–505.
81. **Milich, D., J. Hughes, A. McLachlan, G. Thornton, and A. Moriarty.** 1988. Hepatitis B synthetic immunogen comprised of nucleocapsid T-cell sites and an envelope B-cell epitope. *Proc. Natl. Acad. Sci. USA* **85**:1610–1614.
82. **Minor, P. D.** 1990. Antigenic structure of picornaviruses. *Curr. Top. Microbiol. Immunol.* **161**:121–154.
83. **Minor, P. D., M. Ferguson, D. Evans, J. Almond, and J. Icenogle.** 1986. Antigenic structure of polioviruses of serotypes 1, 2 and 3. *J. Gen. Virol.* **67**:1283–1291.
84. **Minor, P. D., M. Ferguson, A. Phillips, D. I. Magrath, A. Huovilainen, and T. Hovi.** 1987. Conservation in vivo of protease cleavage sites in antigenic sites of poliovirus. *J. Gen. Virol.* **70**:1117–1123.
85. **Misbah, S. A., G. Spickett, P. Ryba, J. Hockaday, J. Kroll, C. Sherwood, J. Kurtz, E. Moxon, and H. Chapel.** 1992. Chronic enteroviral meningoencephalitis in agammaglobulinemia: case report and literature review. *J. Clin. Immunol.* **12**:266–270.
86. **Mossman, T. R., and R. L. Coffman.** 1989. TH1 and TH2 cells: different patterns of lymphokine secretion lead to different functional properties. *Annu. Rev. Immunol.* **7**:145–173.
87. **Muir, P., F. Nicholson, A. J. Tilzey, M. Signy, T. A. English, and J. E. Banatvala.** 1989. Chronic relapsing pericarditis and dilated cardiomyopathy: serological evidence of persistent enterovirus infection. *Lancet* **i**:804–807.
88. **Murdin, A. D., and E. Wimmer.** 1989. Construction of a poliovirus type 1/type 2 antigenic hybrid by manipulation of neutralization antigenic site II. *J. Virol.* **63**:5251–5257.
89. **Neu, N., B. Ploier, and C. Ofner.** 1990. Cardiac myosin-induced myocarditis. Heart autoantibodies are not involved in the induction of the disease. *J. Immunol.* **145**:4094–4100.
90. **Neu, N., N. R. Rose, K. Beisel, A. Herskowitz, G. Gurri-Glass, and S. W. Craig.** 1987. Cardiac myosin induces myocarditis in genetically predisposed mice. *J. Immunol.* **139**:3630–3636.
91. **Neuman, D. A.** 1994. Autoimmunity and idiopathic dilated cardiomyopathy. *Mayo Clin. Proc.* **69**:193–195.
92. **Notkins A., T. Onodera, and B. S. Prabhakar.** 1984. Virus-induced autoimmunity, p. 210–215. *In* A. Notkins and M. B. A. Oldstone (ed.), *Concepts in Viral Pathogenesis*. Springer-Verlag, Berlin.
93. **Onorato, I. M., J. F. Modlin, A. M. McBean, M. L. Thoms, G. A. Losonsky, and R. H. Bernier.** 1991. Mucosal immunity induced by enhanced-potency inactivated and oral polio vaccines. *J. Infect. Dis.* **163**:1–6.
94. **Palker, T., T. Mathews, A. Langlois, M. Tanner, M. Martin, R. Scearce, J. Kim, J. Berzofsky, D. Bolognesi, and B. Haynes.** 1989. Polyvalent human immunodeficiency virus synthetic immunogen comprised of envelope gp120 helper cell sites and B cell neutralization epitopes. *J. Immunol.* **142**:3612–3619.
95. **Ramsingh, A., J. Slack, J. Silkworth, and A. Hixson.** 1989. Severity of disease induced by a pancreatropic Coxsackie B4 virus correlates with the H-2Kq locus of the major histocompatibility complex. *Virus Res.* **14**:347–358.
96. **Reimann, B., R. Zell, and R. Kandolf.** 1991. Mapping of a neutralizing antigenic site of coxsackievirus B4 by construction of an antigen chimera. *J. Virol.* **65**:3475–3480.
97. **Ren, R., F. Costantini, E. Gorgacz, J. Lee, and V. Racaniello.** 1990. Transgenic mice expressing a human poliovirus receptor; a new model for poliomyelitis. *Cell* **63**:353–362.
98. **Robinson, J. A., J. B. O'Connell, L. Roeges, E. O. Major, and R. M. Gunnar.** 1981. Coxsackie B3 myocarditis in athymic mice. *Proc. Soc. Exp. Biol. Med.* **166**:80–91.

99. Roivainen, M., M. Agboatwalla, M. Stenvik, T. Rysa, D. S. Akram, and T. Hovi. 1993. Intrathecal immune response and virus-specific immunoglobulin M antibodies in laboratory diagnosis of acute poliomyelitis. *J. Clin. Microbiol.* **31:**2427–2432.

100. Roivainen, M., A. Narvanen, M. Korkolainen, M. Huhtala, and T. Hovi. 1991. Antigenic regions of poliovirus type 3/Sabin capsid proteins recognized by human sera in the peptide scanning technique. *Virology* **180:**99–107.

101. Roivainen, M., L. Piirainen, T. Rysa, A. Narvanen, and T. Hovi. 1993. An immunodominant N-terminal region of VP1 protein of the poliovirion that is buried in crystal structure can be exposed in solution. *Virology* **195:**762–765.

102. Rose, N. R., A. Herskowitz, and D. Neumann. 1993. Autoimmunity in myocarditis: models and mechanisms. *Clin. Immunol. Immunopathol.* **68:**95–99.

103. Rose, N. R., D. A. Neumann, and A. Herskowitz. 1988. Genetics of susceptibility to viral myocarditis in mice. *Pathol. Immunopathol. Res.* **7:**266–278.

104. Rosenthal, A., and E. Shevach. 1973. Function of macrophages in antigen recognition by guinea pig T lymphocytes. Requirement for histocompatible macrophages and lymphocytes. *J. Exp. Med.* **138:**1194–1212.

105. Rossmann, M., E. Arnold, J. Erickson, E. Frankenberger, J. Griffith, H. Hecht, J. Johnson, G. Kamer, M. Luo, A. Mosser, R. Rueckert, B. Sherry, and G. Vriend. 1985. Structure of a human cold virus and functional relationship to other picornaviruses. *Nature* (London) **317:**145–153.

106. Rossmann, M. G., and A. C. Palmenberg. 1988. Conservation of the putative receptor site in picornaviruses. *Virology* **164:**373–382.

107. Rothbard, J., and W. R. Taylor. 1988. A common sequence pattern in T cell epitopes. *EMBO J.* **7:**93–100.

108. Rudensky, A., P. Preston-Hurlburt, S. Hong, A. Barlow, and C. Janeway, Jr. 1991. Sequence analysis of peptides bound to MHC class II molecules. *Nature* (London) **353:**622–627.

109. Schnurr, D. P., and N. J. Schmidt. 1984. Coxsackievirus B3 persistence and myocarditis in NFR nu/nu and +/nu mice. *Med. Microbiol. Immunol.* **173:**1–7.

110. Schwartz, R. S., and S. K. Datta. 1989. Autoimmunity and autoimmune disease, p. 819–866. *In* W. Paul (ed.), *Fundamental Immunology*. Raven Press, New York.

111. Shikhman, A., N. Greenspan, and M. Cunningham. 1993. A subset of mouse monoclonal antibodies cross-reactive with cytoskeletal proteins and group A streptococcal M proteins recognizes N-acetyl-*beta*-D-glucosamine. *J. Immunol.* **151:**3902–3913.

112. Simons, J., M. Kutubuddin, and M. Chow. 1992. Characterization of poliovirus-specific T lymphocytes in the peripheral blood of Sabin-vaccinated humans. *J. Virol.* **67:**1262–1268.

113. Sinigaglia, F., and J. Hammer. 1994. Defining rules for the peptide-MHC class II interaction. *Curr. Opin. Immunol.* **6:**52–56.

114. Strongwater, S. L., K. Dorovini-Zis, R. D. Ball, and T. J. Schnitzer. 1984. A murine model of polymyositis induced by coxsackievirus B1 (Tucson strain). *Arthritis Rheum.* **27:**433–442.

115. Tam, J. P. 1988. Synthetic peptide design: synthesis and properties of a high-density multiple antigenic peptide system. *Proc. Natl. Acad. Sci. USA* **85:**5409–5413.

116. Townsend, A. R. M., F. M. Gotch, and J. Davey. 1985. Cytotoxic T cells recognize fragments of influenza nucleoprotein. *Cell* **42:**457–467.

116a. Tracy, S., M. Beck, R. Rubocki, and N. Chapman. Unpublished data.

117. Tracy, S., N. Chapman, and M. Beck. 1991. Molecular biology and pathogenesis of coxsackie B viruses. *Rev. Med. Virol.* **1:**145–154.

118. Tracy, S., N. Chapman, and Z. Tu. 1992. Coxsackievirus B3 from an infectious cDNA copy of the genome is cardiovirulent in mice. *Arch. Virol.* **122:**399–409.

119. Tracy, S., V. Wiegand, B. McManus, C. Gauntt, M. Pallansch, M. Beck, and N. Chapman. 1990. Molecular approaches to enteroviral diagnosis in idiopathic cardiomyopathy and myocarditis. *J. Am. Coll. Cardiol.* **15:**1688–1694.

120. Traystman, M., and K. Beisel. 1991. Genetic control of coxsackievirus B3-induced heart-specific autoantibodies associated with chronic myocarditis. *Clin. Exp. Immunol.* **86:**291–298.

121. van Houten, N., and S. Huber. 1989. Role of cytotoxic T cells in experimental myocarditis. *Springer Semin. Immunopathol.* **11:**61–68.

122. Vella, C., C. L. Brown, and D. A. McCarthy. 1992. Coxsackievirus B4 infection of the mouse pancreas: acute and persistent infection. *J. Gen. Virol.* **73:**1387–1394.

123. Whitton, J. L., and M. B. A. Oldstone. 1990. Virus-induced immune response inter-

actions: principles of immunity and immunopathology, p. 369–381. *In* B. Fields and D. Knipe (ed.), *Virology*. Raven Press, New York.
124. **Wiegers, K., H. Uhlig, and R. Dernick.** 1989. N-Ag1B of poliovirus type 1: a discontinuous epitope formed by two loops of VP1 comprising residues 96–104 and 141–152. *Virology* **170:**583–586.
125. **Wilson, F. M., Q. R. Miranda, J. Chason, and A. M. Lerner.** 1969. Residual pathologic changes following murine coxsackie A and B myocarditis. *Am. J. Pathol.* **55:**253–265.
126. **Wolfgram, L., K. W. Beisel, A. Herskowitz, and N. R. Rose.** 1986. Variations in the susceptibility of coxsackievirus B3-induced myocarditis among different strains of mice. *J. Immunol.* **136:**1846–1852.
127. **Woodruff, J. F.** 1980. Viral myocarditis. A review. *Am. J. Pathol.* **101:**425–478.
128. **Woodruff, J. F., and J. J. Woodruff.** 1974. Involvement of T lymphocytes in the pathogenesis of coxsackie virus B3 heart disease. *J. Immunol.* **113:**1726–1734.
129. **Yeates, T., D. Jacobson, A. Martin, C. Wychowski, M. Girard, D. Filman, and J. Hogle.** 1991. Three-dimensional structure of a mouse-adapted type 2/type 1 poliovirus chimera. *EMBO J.* **10:**2231–2241.
130. **Zaman, S., B. Carlsson, A. Morikawa, S. Jeansson, I. Narayanan, K. Thiringer, F. Jalil, and L. Hanson.** 1993. Poliovirus antibody titres, relative affinity, and neutralising capacity in maternal milk. *Arch. Dis. Child.* **68:**198–201.
131. **Zinkernagel, R. M., and P. C. Doherty.** 1974. Restriction of in vitro T cell-mediated cytotoxicity in lymphocytic choriomeningitis within a syngeneic or semiallogeneic system. *Nature* (London) **248:**701–702.

CLINICAL MANIFESTATIONS

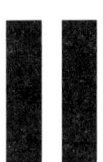

POLIOMYELITIS AND POLIOVIRUS IMMUNIZATION

John F. Modlin

9

Poliomyelitis is an acute, febrile illness characterized by aseptic meningitis and weakness or paralysis of one or more extremities. It is a disease of immense historical importance and contemporary interest. Prior to the advent of polio immunization, infection with one or more of the three poliovirus serotypes was universal, although recognized poliomyelitis occurred in only a small fraction of infected persons. After the first appearance of epidemic poliomyelitis approximately 100 years ago, subsequent annual summertime epidemics in northern Europe and the United States galvanized public attention and concern unlike any other acute infectious disease had done. The development and implementation of safe and effective polio vaccines in the 1950s are widely cited as crowning achievements of modern medicine. Today, poliomyelitis due to wild-type poliovirus infection no longer occurs in the Western Hemisphere, and the challenge before the international health community is the eradication of poliomyelitis from the rest of the world.

This chapter reviews the historical background, pathophysiology, and clinical manifestations of poliomyelitis as well as current issues regarding both inactivated and live, attenuated poliovirus vaccines. Detailed discussions of the epidemiology, virology, and molecular biology of poliovirus infection can be found elsewhere in this book.

HISTORY OF POLIOMYELITIS AND DEVELOPMENT OF POLIOVIRUS VACCINES

Although evidence exists that poliomyelitis has afflicted humans since antiquity, recorded references prior to the 18th century are difficult to find. The first unambiguous description in English is a biographical narrative of the acute paralysis and resulting lameness suffered by Sir Walter Scott in the second year of his life, ca. 1772 (116). The first medical description is recorded in the second edition of *A Treatise on Diseases of Children*, published in 1789 by Michael Underwood, a London pediatrician and obstetrician (206). Referring to the disease only as the "debility of the lower extremities," Underwood carefully described the predilection for children between 1 and 5 years of age and the relationship of lower-limb weakness to acute illness. However, Underwood made no reference to outbreaks of disease.

John F. Modlin, Departments of Pediatrics and Medicine, Dartmouth Medical School, Dartmouth-Hitchcock Medical Center, Lebanon, New Hampshire 03756.

Poliomyelitis in the 19th Century

Further independent descriptions were added by Giovanni Monteggia in 1813 and by John Shaw, a London surgeon, in 1823. However, the pathologic nature of the limb "debility" was not understood at the time. The Scottish neurologist Abercrombie was the first to speculate (in 1828) that the lesion was located in the anterior segment of the gray matter of the spinal cord (1). This postulate was advanced in 1840 by Jacob von Heine, a German practitioner of orthopedics and physical medicine (72). Heine's monograph, which may be the first series of poliomyelitis case reports, carefully describes the clinical features of the acute disease in young children and promotes management of long-term paresis with exercise and metal braces.

During the second half of the 19th century, the convergence of new developments in clinical microscopy, pathology, and bacteriology engendered profound changes in concepts of the origins of human disease that had been entrenched for centuries. The development of histologic techniques allowed Cornil, working in 1872 in the laboratory of Jean-Marie Charcot, to demonstrate that residual paralysis was accompanied by atrophy of the anterolateral columns of the spinal cord, thus confirming the postulates of Abercrombie and Heine (32). Charcot himself later showed that paralysis was accompanied by a loss of motor nerve cells within the anterior horns of the cord (26), and this finding gave rise to the pathologic term "poliomyelitis" (from the Greek *polios* for "gray" and *myelos* for "spinal cord").

Meanwhile, several clusters of poliomyelitis cases were reported from Norway, Sweden, and France. The first of these, an account of 12 cases in 1868, was initially mistaken for spinal meningitis (114). Bergenholtz is credited with a report of 13 cases of poliomyelitis that occurred in northern Sweden in the summer of 1881, although the paper was delivered verbally and never published. A slightly larger outbreak occurred near Lyons, France, in 1885 (31).

The obscurity of poliomyelitis came to an end in 1890 with a report to the Tenth International Medical Congress in Berlin by Karl Oskar Medin, the prominent Swedish pediatrician. Medin, who was professor of pediatrics at the Karolinska Institute, had studied the clinical features of poliomyelitis intensely during an epidemic of 44 cases in Stockholm in the summer of 1887. Medin recognized that the illness began with a systemic phase that often failed to progress to neurologic paresis, and he developed the classification of disease that became widely used for decades afterwards. The eponym "Heine-Medin disease," which was introduced by his pupil Ivar Wickman in 1907 to honor Medin's contributions, was widely applied throughout Europe and North America during the early 20th century.

In the United States, Putnam and Taylor noted a brief reference to 26 cases of poliomyelitis in suburban Boston during the summer of 1893 (163). The next year, Charles Caverly described 132 cases with 18 deaths in the Otter Creek Valley near Rutland, Vermont, the largest outbreak known to have occurred up to that time (207). Caverly's report is notable for careful observations regarding the age distribution of the population affected, the predominance of males among those affected, the concurrent feature of aseptic meningitis, and the acute and long-term effects of poliomyelitis.

These early outbreaks heralded the increasingly larger epidemics of the 20th century, including a country-wide epidemic of more than 1,000 cases in Sweden in 1905 (219) and 1,200 cases in New York City in 1907 (154), and the spread of disease throughout Europe and the United States. It became apparent during these larger epidemics that poliomyelitis (i) was clearly a contagious disease; (ii) affected children, adolescents, and young adults as well as young infants; (iii) occurred mainly in economically advantaged and often remotely distributed populations; and (iv) frequently caused a minor illness without central nervous system (CNS) symptoms. This last fact proved crucial to understanding the contagious nature of poliomyelitis and the observation that disease occurred in the absence of exposure to paralytic cases.

Scientific Advances in the 20th Century

DISCOVERY OF THE POLIOVIRUSES

In a series of experiments conducted in 1908 and 1909, Karl Landsteiner and E. Popper convincingly demonstrated that the etiologic agent of poliomyelitis was a "filterable virus." In these experiments, they induced flaccid paralysis and the characteristic spinal cord lesions in a *Cynocephalus* monkey by intraperitoneal injection of neural tissue from a human patient with a fatal case (110). This discovery evoked immediate interest worldwide. Within months, Simon Flexner and his colleagues at the Rockefeller Institute replicated the transmission of virus and disease from humans to monkeys and went on to demonstrate serial passage of virus in monkeys (52), fulfilling one of Koch's postulates.

EPIDEMIOLOGIC STUDIES AND POPULATION IMMUNITY

The investigations of the 1894 Vermont outbreak by Charles Caverly and of the 1905 Swedish epidemic by Ivar Wickman represent the earliest descriptions of epidemic poliomyelitis that use basic epidemiologic methods. The concept of acquired population immunity was first proposed by the Swedish pediatrician Wernstedt in 1912, when he observed that epidemic disease did not revisit the same geographic area soon after a prior epidemic (215). Early virologic studies at the Swedish State Bacteriological Institute found that polioviruses could be isolated from children with abortive disease and from asymptomatic contacts during epidemics and that the number of these healthy carriers exceeded the number of typical poliomyelitis cases, underscoring the importance of individuals without neurologic disease in the spread of disease (102). Also, it was discovered that serum antibodies ("germicidal substances"), which inactivated polioviruses, were produced in the course of infection (53, 137).

It was the work of Wade Hampton Frost that firmly established that widespread immunity in the population was acquired as a result of previously unrecognized infection. In a series of formal epidemiologic studies conducted from 1910 to 1912 during epidemics in the midwestern and northeastern United States, Frost found that exposure to poliomyelitis was widespread but that the incidence of clinical disease was limited to those susceptible to infection, i.e., infants and young children (55). These concepts were strongly supported by the simultaneous demonstration by Anderson and Frost (5) and investigators at the Rockefeller Institute (159) that the majority of healthy adults had serum antibodies to poliovirus.

The epidemic that swept the northeastern United States in 1916 caused more than 9,000 cases in New York City alone. Observations made by the Public Health Service during this epidemic verified Frost's views of general population immunity and the role of asymptomatic persons in the spread of infection. This epidemic also demonstrated that imposition of strict quarantine procedures and severe travel restrictions had little or no effect on the spread of disease (154).

The subsequent observation that polioviruses could be isolated from the gastrointestinal tract focused attention on the role of fecal excretion in the community spread of poliovirus infection. In time, the concept emerged that asymptomatic infections far outnumbered cases of disease during epidemics and that asymptomatic persons, who were most often infants and young children, served as the reservoir for epidemic spread of polioviruses (123). Surveillance of municipal sewage for polioviruses in the 1940s proved a useful means of tracking the seasonal and geographic patterns of poliovirus infection (126, 158).

Serologic surveys in the 1930s and 1940s helped define the basis for the observed differences in the behavior of epidemics in different geographic locations and social conditions. Evidence of immunity was found in 80 to 100% of adults tested, with generally lower levels in children (157). These investigations progressed dramatically with the adaptation of the Lansing poliovirus strain to mice, which allowed easier and more accurate assessment of antibody titers to type 2 virus (67). Using the mouse protection assay, Thomas Turner and colleagues at Johns Hopkins demonstrated the rapid acquisition of antibody at an early age among children in an underprivileged section of Baltimore (205). In time, it would be shown that the risk of infection was universal, but children living with poor sanitary conditions acquired infection at a much earlier age than children from higher socioeconomic levels. This realization explained the enigmatic shift of poliomyelitis from an endemic disease involving only young infants to an epidemic disease affecting children and young adults as well. Serologic surveys conducted by Paul and Riordan in a remote Eskimo population 15 to 20 years following an outbreak of poliomyelitis showed that immunity persisted for at least two decades and perhaps for life (155). The cultivation of polioviruses in cell culture allowed the development of neutralization assays for all three poliovirus types, thus greatly enhancing the information gained from serologic surveys.

EXPERIMENTAL INFECTION AND THE PATHOGENESIS OF POLIOMYELITIS

The concept of poliomyelitis as a systemic disease dates to the 1888 observation of Rissler, a Norwegian pathologist, that extraneural lesions, principally enlargement of lymphoreticular tissue, were present throughout the bodies of patients dying of acute poliomyelitis (169). Within a few years of first isolating the virus, Landsteiner, working with colleagues at the Pasteur Institute, demonstrated that virus could be recovered from both the upper respiratory tract and the mesenteric lymph nodes of patients with fatal disease (109). Other European scientists isolated polioviruses from the oropharynx (200) and intestinal washings (102) and also demonstrated evidence of experimental infection via the gastrointestinal tract (101). However, these early discoveries were overlooked; instead, it was widely held that polioviruses were transmitted directly from the nasopharynx to the CNS via the olfactory nerve (42, 51). This misconception was fostered by the view that polioviruses were predominately neurotropic and by the unfortunate fact that rhesus monkeys, which were universally used as experimental animals, are relatively insusceptible to mucosal infection. Adherence to this dogma is said to have delayed progress in understanding the mode of transmission and the pathophysiology of poliomyelitis for more than a generation (81, 154).

A 1935 report of spontaneous poliomyelitis in two chimpanzees in a German zoo suggested to Howard Howe and David Bodian at Johns Hopkins that these primates would be more susceptible than those more distantly related to humans. Howe and Bodian convincingly showed that chimpanzees could be infected via the oral route and would subsequently develop paralytic disease (86).

Renewed interest in the role of oropharyngeal and gastrointestinal replication in the pathogenesis of poliomyelitis was also sparked by the isolation of viruses from the oropharynx and the gastrointestinal system in patients and contacts during epidemics (107, 203) and the demonstration that virus was shed in the feces for many weeks after acute infection.

Initial attempts to isolate polioviruses from the blood of patients with paralytic disease were generally unsuccessful (209). However, studies with primates demonstrated that virus appeared in blood within 5 days of feeding and prior to the onset of neurologic symptoms (12, 80). Subsequently, viremia was demonstrated in humans during the incubation period or prodromal symptoms of the minor stage of illness (83).

CULTIVATION AND CHARACTERIZATION OF POLIOVIRUSES

The adaptation of polioviruses to rodents proved to be a substantial advance, freeing many laboratories of their dependence on expensive and cumbersome primates. The initial and apparently successful 1935 report of Brodie and colleagues (21) in passaging polioviruses in irradiated mice was not widely accepted. However, within a few years, Armstrong demonstrated that the Lansing strain could be adapted to cause encephalitis in cotton rats after a number of passages (6). Later, the rat-adapted strain was passaged to mice (7). The attempts of contemporary investigators were not always as successful (98). It ultimately became apparent that rodent adaptation was dependent on the poliovirus type, with type 2 strains being more readily passaged in rodent CNS tissue.

In 1936, Sabin and Olitsky produced the first unequivocal evidence that polioviruses could be grown in vitro when they propagated the MV poliovirus strain in human embryonic CNS tissue (181). A decade later, Enders, Weller, and Robbins, working at the Children's Hospital in Boston, succeeded in growing Lansing strain poliovirus in human embryonic tissues and demonstrating the direct cytopathic effect of the virus in monolayers of these cells (45). This achievement is widely acknowledged as the landmark event that opened the door to further characterization of the virus, better understanding of the pathophysiology of poliomyelitis, and development of successful vaccines within the subsequent decade.

The existence of more than one type of poliovirus was first deduced by Burnet and Macnamara in 1931, when they demonstrated that monkeys who had recovered from infection with a strain recovered in Melbourne subsequently developed disease when given the virulent MV strain and also showed that the two strains differed qualitatively in in vitro neutralization tests (23). These results were confirmed by Paul and Trask at Yale (156), and the two virus groups were respectively designated Lansing-like and Brunhilde-like, the latter in reference to the name of a laboratory chimpanzee (154). A third type was predicted from the studies of Bodian et al. at Johns Hopkins in 1949 (18). Subsequently, the existence of three types and no more was verified by the testing of poliovirus strains collected worldwide by a collaborative group organized by the National Foundation for Infantile Paralysis (201).

TREATMENT OF ACUTE POLIOMYELITIS

The modern era of poliomyelitis therapy began with William Osler's dictum that paralyzed patients should receive only bed rest and passive management of affected limbs; thus were the noxious medical practices of earlier times rejected (145). A treatise by the Boston physician Robert Lovett reflects the more enlightened management precepts of the period, i.e., bed rest, warm baths, and gentle massage of the affected limbs (118).

Intrathecal and intravenous injection of human immune serum was widely practiced following a 1915 report from France claiming improved outcome in a group of 30 cases (136). The use of human convalescent-phase serum had been encouraged by the demonstration that convalescent-phase serum protected monkeys from experimental disease (53). Trials of serum therapy were carried out in New York and Boston during the epidemic of 1916. Because the natural history of poliomyelitis was not well understood at that time and the principles of the controlled clinical trial did not exist, enthusiasm for serum therapy persisted until the early 1930s, when well-controlled trials proved this form of treatment to be of little benefit (106). In 1948, it was shown that serum antibodies were already present when CNS symptoms occurred (68), further demonstrating the futility of serum therapy.

One of the first true advances in the management of acute respiratory paralysis was the invention of the Drinker negative-pressure ventilator, or iron lung, at the Harvard School of Public Health (44) and its development at several Boston hospitals (43). The earliest devices were powered by vacuum cleaners and fitted with portholes originally made for boats to allow access to the body of the patient within.

Progress in the management of the persistently paralyzed patient was also made during this period. The tenet of rigid immobilization of even mildly involved extremities for long periods gave way to the influential practices of Sister Elizabeth Kenny, who used warm, moist packs and prolonged physical therapy (161).

EARLY ATTEMPTS TO PREVENT POLIOMYELITIS

Several well-intentioned but flawed attempts to prevent transmission of poliomyelitis bear mentioning. In the mid-1930s, interest developed in the use of astringent nasal sprays that were purported to block transmission of virus from the nasal mucosa to the CNS (see above). A controlled trial of zinc sulfate nasal spray in Toronto demonstrated the futility of this practice (202). After polioviruses were isolated from houseflies trapped during periods of epidemic disease (182, 210), insect control programs that used dichlorodiphenyltrichoroethane trichloroethane (DDT) in urban areas were tried, with little success (125, 147).

The first clearly successful effort in preventing poliomyelitis was the demonstration that serum immunoglobulin protected against paralytic disease for up to 5 weeks during epidemic periods (65).

Development of Poliovirus Vaccines

It may be a surprise to most physicians practicing today that both inactivated and live, attenuated poliovirus vaccines were tested in human subjects in the mid-1930s. A vaccine consisting of a 10% suspension of poliovirus-infected monkey spinal cord that had been inactivated with formalin was reported by Maurice Brodie at New York University to successfully protect rhesus monkeys against challenge with virulent virus (20). This vaccine was rapidly given to more than 3,000 California children in 1935. Although no harmful effects were reported (22), the safety and effectiveness of this vaccine remain rather obscure, and additional human studies were never performed. In the same year, a live vaccine consisting of a 4% suspension of monkey cord "inactivated" by treatment with sodium ricinoleate was given to several thousand children after brief testing in monkeys (103). The acute paralysis that occurred in about 1/1,000 vaccinees shortly after administration during a nonepidemic period represents the first known cases of vaccine-associated poliomyelitis, some of which were fatal. This well-intended but premature and disastrous experiment generated vitriolic criticism (113) and set back the cause of poliomyelitis immunization by a decade.

INACTIVATED (SALK-TYPE) VACCINE

By the end of World War II, there existed sufficient knowledge of the pathophysiology of poliovirus infections and sufficient will and resources at the National Foundation for Infantile Paralysis to mount a concerted vaccine effort. Jonas Salk built on his experience with formalin-inactivated influenza vaccines in the Army to produce the first successful poliovirus vaccine, which was first administered to paralyzed patients in a home for crippled children in Pennsylvania in 1952 (185). In 1954, the inactivated vaccine was tested in a monumental, placebo-controlled trial involving more than 1.8 million U.S. schoolchildren. This trial was conducted under the leadership of Thomas Francis at the University of Michigan. On April 12, 1955, it was announced to the public that the Salk vaccine had achieved a protective efficacy of more than 50%, with no adverse events attributed to vaccination. With the rapid distribution of the Salk-type vaccine that ensued, the incidence of paralytic poliomyelitis fell from 13.9 cases per 100,000 in 1954 to 0.5 cases per 100,000 in 1961.

LIVE, ATTENUATED POLIOVIRUS VACCINES

The passage of polioviruses in mice may be viewed as the first step toward the development of live, attenuated poliovirus vaccines. In 1946, Max Theiler reported that Lansing strain virus passaged more than 50 times in rats and mice was avirulent for rhesus monkeys. By the early 1950s, Koprowski et al. demonstrated that type 2 virus attenuated in cotton rats was immunogenic in a small number of volunteers (105). Enders, Weller, and Robbins showed that cell culture passage reduced the virulence of type 1 poliovirus (46). By the time the Salk vaccine was under investigation in the Francis field trial, several independent investigators were testing live, attenuated polioviruses with the goal of maintaining sufficient gastrointestinal replication to induce immunity with viruses that remained avirulent for monkeys (179). Several of these strains were extensively tested in humans in a number of international locations. Ultimately, between August 1961 and March 1962, three monovalent strains developed by Albert Sabin were licensed for use in the United States. Within the next 2 years, more than 100 million oral poliovirus vaccine (OPV) doses were given in the United States via community programs (Sabin Sundays) organized by local health departments and medical societies. Trivalent OPV, which was introduced in 1964, has been the principal poliovirus vaccine used in the United States and many other locations.

ADVERSE VACCINE EVENTS

Within weeks of the successful termination of the Francis field trial in 1955, hundreds of thousands of doses of Salk vaccine were produced by five different commercial manufacturers. Unfortunately, 7 of 17 lots distributed by Cutter Laboratories were incompletely inactivated, resulting in 79 cases of type 1 poliomyelitis among recipients and another 105 cases among their contacts.

The administration of millions of OPV doses in the mass campaigns from 1962 to 1964 produced the first cases of OPV-associated paralytic disease. These cases, which were mostly due to the type 3 strain, were recognized because they occurred in low-risk adults during nonepidemic periods (73).

PATHOPHYSIOLOGY AND IMMUNITY IN POLIOVIRUS INFECTIONS

Transmission

Humans are the only source of poliovirus infection. Infectious virus can be recovered from the feces of 92 to 97% of persons with primary infection. The virus is shed in the oropharynx for 1 to 3 weeks and in the feces for an average of 5 to 8 weeks. During reinfection, oropharyngeal virus shedding is rare, and the period of gastrointestinal shedding is reduced to less than 3 weeks, with lower titers than are shed during primary infection. Humans are infected as a result of ingestion of material contaminated with feces or oropharyngeal secretions of close contacts, usually family or household members. Only small amounts of infectious virus are necessary to cause infection. Experimental studies with OPV virus suggest that fewer than 100 50% tissue culture infectious doses ($TCID_{50}$) will induce infection in most nonimmune infants (131); approximately 1 $TCID_{50}$ is all that is required when virus is introduced directly into the gastrointestinal tract (104).

Pathogenesis

Ingested polioviruses implant in the oropharynx and small bowel; the small bowel appears to be a more efficient site of replication (15). Humans ingesting >10^6 $TCID_{50}$ of OPV virus regularly shed virus in both oropharyngeal secretions and feces, while doses of <10^5 $TCID_{50}$ result in only fecal shedding (176). Although the site of initial virus replication (i.e., mucosal cells or lamina propria) has never been satisfactorily determined, maximal replication in these locations is found in submucosal lymphoid tissue, where up to 10^8 $TCID_{50}$ of polioviruses per g may be detected in Peyer's patches. Spread of naturally occurring poliovirus infection to regional lymph nodes gives rise to a minor viremia, which is transient and clinically silent and during which virus spreads to systemic reticuloendothelial tissue including lymph nodes, bone marrow, liver, and spleen (16). Viral replication is contained at this stage during the majority of infections, resulting in subclinical infection. In a minority of cases (fewer than 10%), further replication of virus in reticuloendothelial tissue leads to a major viremia, which coincides with the onset of the clinical symptoms associated with the minor illness 3 to 7 days after transmission (82). Among Sabin strain polioviruses, only type 2 causes viremia (84).

The path by which polioviruses reach the CNS has long been in contention, and the issue remains unsettled. When it was demonstrated that viremia precedes paralysis in humans and chimpanzees, the long-held concept of direct invasion of the CNS via the nasal mucosa and olfactory nerve gave way to the view that dissemination is hematogenous (14). While the requirement for viremia is probably correct, the precise mechanism by which the virus breaches the blood-brain barrier remains unresolved. A recent study using transgenic mice bearing the gene for the human poliovirus receptor found that spinal cord involvement can be blocked by sciatic nerve section after virus is injected intramuscularly (165) (see chapter 3). This suggests that virus replication in skeletal muscle precedes transport of virus to the cord via the peripheral nerve (17, 97), a concept consistent with the myotropic nature of other enteroviruses and the clinical observation of intense myalgias preceding the onset of paralysis in affected patients. Poliovirus disease in extraneural sites such as the myocardium is almost certainly the result of viremic spread.

Polioviruses are recoverable from the spinal cord during the first several days of paralysis but diminish to undetectable levels within the first week. In contrast, the histopathologic lesions may persist for months. These consist of inflammatory infiltrates and neuronal necrosis, characteristically distributed within the gray matter of the anterior horn of the spinal cord and the motor nuclei of the pons and medulla (11). The severity of clinical paralysis depends more on the intensity of the lesions than on their distribution.

Immunity to Poliovirus Infection

Immunity to poliovirus infection is type specific; cross-protection between the three serotypes is low if it exists at all. Reinfection with the same serotype occurs upon exposure to live poliovirus, regardless of whether prior immunity is based on infection with naturally occurring polioviruses, infection with live attenuated viruses, or administration of inactivated poliovirus vaccine (IPV). Following household exposure to wild-type virus, 20 to 50% of naturally immune (57), 30 to 50% of OPV-immune, and 90 to 100% of IPV-immune persons are reinfected, as defined by virus excretion from the gastrointestinal tract or a rise in antibody titer. Reinfections are universally asymptomatic and are rarely associated with oropharyngeal virus excretion.

HUMORAL IMMUNITY

Type-specific serum neutralizing antibodies are made in response to natural infection and to immunization with either OPV or IPV. Antibodies made in response to natural infection appear to persist for life (153). Neutralizing antibodies alone protect against disease but not against infection (66). Preexisting humoral antibody prevents or reduces oropharyngeal shedding of poliovirus upon reinfection but has only a minor effect on fecal shedding (14, 57, 75, 115, 119, 144, 212). Prior IPV vaccination has some effect on the duration and titer of virus shed in the feces, but the difference is small enough to be epidemiologically and biologically insignificant (58, 119, 144, 212). In most IPV vaccinees, small challenge doses readily induce reinfection (75, 144).

SECRETORY ANTIBODY RESPONSE AND MUCOSAL IMMUNITY

Poliovirus-specific immunoglobulin A (IgA) appears in nasopharyngeal and intestinal secretions 1 to 3 weeks after natural infection or administration of OPV (141). Secretory IgA antibody persists for at least 5 to 6 years at low levels and, unlike humoral antibody, is not boosted significantly upon rechallenge with OPV (143). The degree of protection conferred by local IgA antibody is relative. Upon rechallenge, high secretory IgA titers inhibit virus replication, while lower titers permit replication; virus shedding is dependent on the challenge dose (75, 144). Challenge studies suggest that the intestinal immunities induced by OPV and natural infection are equivalent (61).

CLINICAL FEATURES OF POLIOMYELITIS

Acute Illness

The manifestations of infection by polioviruses range from inapparent illness to flaccid paralysis and death. More than 90% of naturally occurring poliovirus infections are inapparent. Acute clinical poliomyelitis is traditionally separated into two distinct phases: the minor illness, with an incubation period of 3 to 7 days, and the major illness, with onset of symptoms generally 9 to 12 days after exposure (85). The minor illness, coinciding with viremia, consists of nonspecific symptoms such as fever, headache, sore throat, anorexia, and listlessness. Overall, 4 to 8% of infected persons experience symptoms of the minor illness, and the majority resolve their illness within 1 to 2 days without further symptoms.

MAJOR ILLNESS

The major illness is associated with symptoms of CNS involvement, which has been variously estimated to occur in 0.1 to 1% of all patients with poliovirus infections (128, 135). About one-third of young children who develop the major illness experience a biphasic illness (the so-called dromedary pattern), with symptoms of the minor illness preceding onset of CNS disease; adults usually develop CNS disease without the preceding minor illness (78, 214). The major illness is heralded by the abrupt onset of fever, headache, vomiting, and meningismus. Cerebrospinal fluid pleocytosis is present at this early stage. Approximately one-third of cases of CNS disease are limited to aseptic meningitis, which resolves within 5 to 10 days (i.e., nonparalytic poliomyelitis).

The motor weakness is generally preceded by intense myalgias of the involved limb(s) and muscles of the axial skeleton. The muscle pain is relieved by exercise; patients may pace nervously in an attempt to work off the pain. The hallmark of poliomyelitis is asymmetric motor weakness, which develops 1 to 2 days into the major illness. The severity of disease ranges from weakness of a single extremity to complete quadriplegia. Proximal limb muscles are more involved than distal, and legs are more commonly involved than arms. Any combination of limbs may be affected, but the most common patterns are one leg, one arm, or both legs. The deep tendon reflexes, which were initially brisk, become absent. The pace of development of the paresis ranges from several hours to several days, most commonly requiring over 2 to 3 days.

Cranial nerve involvement (i.e., bulbar poliomyelitis) occurs in 5 to 35% of paralytic cases. Any of the motor cranial nerves can be involved, the 9th and 10th nerves being the most common. Bulbar paralysis results in dysphagia, nasal speech, dyspnea, difficulty with secretions, anxiety, and respiratory compromise. Involvement of respiratory and vasomotor nuclei is less common but may portend a fatal outcome due to hypoventilation, blood pressure lability, and cardiac arrhythmias.

COMPLICATIONS

Respiratory failure from paralysis of the diaphragm and intercostal muscles represents the most serious complication of paralytic poliomyelitis. Aspiration pneumonia, pulmonary edema, myocarditis, paralytic ileus, gastric dilatation, and ileus of the bladder may also complicate acute paralytic disease.

Differential Diagnosis

PARALYTIC DISEASE DUE TO NONPOLIO ENTEROVIRUSES

Sporadic cases of paralytic disease that are clinically indistinguishable from poliomyelitis but are caused by a number of nonpolio enterovirus serotypes have been widely reported. Only two serotypes have been known to cause epidemic disease: coxsackievirus A7 virus, which has caused small outbreaks of paralytic disease in the former USSR (208), South Africa, and Scotland (63), and enterovirus 71, which caused large outbreaks in eastern Europe in the late 1970s (188).

GUILLAIN-BARRE SYNDROME
The disease most often confused with acute poliomyelitis is Guillain-Barre syndrome, which, unlike poliomyelitis, causes paralysis that is classically ascending in nature, symmetrical, and accompanied by sensory abnormalities in approximately 80% of cases and that characteristically persists for 2 weeks or longer. Sensory loss in poliomyelitis is very rare. In addition, the cerebrospinal fluid pleocytosis noted during the major illness of poliomyelitis is uncharacteristic of the Guillain-Barre syndrome, which is associated with a normal cerebrospinal fluid leukocyte count and an elevated protein concentration.

OTHER DISEASES
A number of other conditions, including transverse myelitis, botulism, tick paralysis, epidural abscess, cord tumors, and hysteria, produce acute paralysis. However, each of these clinical entities has features that readily separate it from acute poliomyelitis.

Risk Factors

AGE
Although it is widely believed that adults are more susceptible to paralytic complications, there is probably little correlation of age with severity of disease after the decline of maternal antibody (128, 135).

PREGNANCY
Studies during outbreaks in the United States indicate that infected pregnant women have an increased risk of developing paralytic disease (4, 148, 213). However, there is no evidence that either naturally occurring polioviruses (189) or attenuated polioviruses (71) cause congenital defects.

IMMUNODEFICIENCY
Persons with B-cell immunodeficiency, primarily young children with X-linked immunodeficiency syndromes, have an increased risk of CNS disease when they are infected with either naturally occurring or attenuated polioviruses. These patients may develop acute paralysis or may have an atypical course with an incubation period of several months, prolonged febrile illness, chronic meningitis, and progressive neurologic dysfunction that includes both upper and lower motor neurons (36, 222).

EXERCISE
Strenuous exercise substantially increases the risk and severity of poliomyelitis. This effect has been well documented clinically (79), and experimental infections with other enteroviruses provide supportive evidence (56). Exercise during the minor illness has no effect (173), but exercise during the early stages of the major illness is detrimental (174).

INJECTIONS OR TRAUMA
Paralytic poliomyelitis tends to localize in a limb that has been the site of a recent intramuscular injection or injury (62, 76, 197). Observations in cases of experimental poliomyelitis confirm this association but do not fully explain the mechanism of the provoking effect (13, 165, 204).

TONSILLECTOMY
Surgical removal of the tonsils during the incubation period of poliomyelitis markedly increases the risk of bulbar disease (146). The mechanism may be similar to the provoking effect of injections on spinal poliomyelitis.

Prognosis

Paralysis most often progresses for 1 to 3 days after onset, rarely more than a week, halting about the time the patient becomes afebrile

(175). Most patients with limb paresis experience some recovery of function in the weeks to months after acute disease. Some estimate of the eventual outcome can be made by a month after onset, when most reversible weakness will have resolved. Very little additional recovery of strength can be expected after 9 months. Residual motor deficits, ranging from minor debility to permanent, flaccid paralysis, remain in about two-thirds of initially paralyzed patients.

Overall mortality for spinal poliomyelitis is about 4 to 6%. During the poliomyelitis epidemics 40 to 50 years ago, bulbar polio caused a mortality of 20 to 60% when respiratory assistance was required. With modern intensive care, deaths from temporary respiratory paralysis should be less common.

Postpoliomyelitis Syndrome
Some patients who recover from paralytic poliomyelitis experience new onset of muscle weakness, pain, atrophy, and fatigue many years after the acute illness (35) (see chapter 16). Typically, the involved muscles are the same as those affected during the original illness, but weakness may also occur in previously unaffected limb muscles. Progression of new symptoms is gradual, and as a result, affected individuals are seldom disabled (34). Population-based studies suggest that postpoliomyelitis syndrome affects 20 to 30% of previously paralyzed patients (164). The risk of progressive weakness peaks between 25 and 35 years after acute poliomyelitis. While the cause is unknown, some authorities believe that late progression of muscle weakness is a result of physiologic attrition of motor units innervating muscles already less innervated as a result of earlier acute infection (96).

POLIOVIRUS VACCINES

Live, Attenuated Poliovirus Vaccine (OPV)
Separate, monovalent OPV vaccines were licensed for routine use in this country in 1961 and 1962. Trivalent OPV, which was introduced in 1964, is now the only formulation available in the United States. Although the minimum potency standards of the Food and Drug Administration are $10^{5.5}$, $10^{4.5}$, and $10^{5.2}$ $TCID_{50}$ for poliovirus types 1, 2, and 3, respectively, the formulation distributed by the sole domestic manufacturer (Lederle Laboratories, Wayne, N.J.) exceeds the Food and Drug Administration standard, containing $10^{6.5}$, $10^{5.4}$, and $10^{6.3}$ $TCID_{50}$, respectively (152). The unequal contribution of each type to the trivalent preparation represents a balanced formulation designed to account for the more efficient replication of type 2 OPV virus in the gastrointestinal tract, which, if type 2 virus is given in equal concentrations with types 1 and 3, will interfere with the replication of types 1 and 3 (170).

HUMORAL ANTIBODY RESPONSE
An optimal immune response requires three doses separated by at least 2 months. In the United States, trivalent OPV was routinely administered to infants at 2, 4, and 12 to 18 months of age until a recent advisory committee encouraged reducing the age at the third dose to 6 months. A fourth dose is routinely administered at 4 to 6 years of age. Assessment of the immune response to the initial dose at 2 months of age is obscured somewhat by the presence of maternal antibody. However, by 6 months of age, which is 2 months after the second dose, 86 to 100% of infants possess serum antibody to all three poliovirus serotypes (70, 122). The prevalence of antibody to all three types is more than 96% at 2 months after the third dose (122). Type 2 OPV produces higher seroconversion rates and higher antibody titers than types 1 and 3. Detectable serum antibody to all three types persists in 84 to 98% of vaccinees 5 years after primary immunization (108). The degree to which reexposure to vaccine virus helps to maintain detectable antibody in the population is unknown, but studies in the United States and Japan suggest that boosts in antibody titer occur as a result of community spread of OPV viruses (8, 138).

SECRETORY ANTIBODY RESPONSE

Secretory IgA poliovirus antibody appears in oropharyngeal and duodenal secretions 1 to 3 weeks after OPV immunization (141) and persists for at least 5 to 6 years (142). IgA antibody is also secreted in human colostrum, where it interferes with the serum antibody response in breast-fed neonates receiving OPV (64) but not in infants older than 1 month (38).

OPV EFFICACY

Three decades of OPV use in the United States provide overwhelming evidence of the effectiveness of OPV in preventing poliomyelitis. Interestingly, however, the efficacy of OPV has never been tested under conditions of exposure to natural polioviruses in the United States. OPV efficacy was evaluated during a type 1 poliovirus outbreak in Taiwan in the early 1980s. During this outbreak, vaccine efficacies were estimated to be 82, 96, and 98% for one, two, and three or more doses, respectively (100).

TRANSMISSION OF OPV VIRUSES

Vaccinees shed OPV virus in the feces for 1 to 6 weeks or longer after feeding and from the oropharynx for 1 to 3 weeks. As with the naturally occurring polioviruses, the abilities of OPV viruses to spread among household contacts appear to be inversely related to the age of the index infected person (usually a vaccinee) (19, 60) and to be enhanced by crowding and poor hygiene within households (60). Spread of vaccine virus to community contacts occurs less readily (9). Type 3 OPV virus may spread more easily than other serotypes (60).

The spread of vaccine virus to unimmunized children is considered to be advantageous, especially in areas in which vaccine acceptance levels are low. The importance of this "back door" method of protecting the community is uncertain. Investigation of an outbreak in Taiwan suggested that unimmunized children had little or no protection against paralytic disease, despite OPV immunization levels of 83 to 98% among young children (100). Outbreaks have also been recorded in Oman and South Africa in locations with high prior OPV coverage (187, 196). On the other hand, a recent seroprevalence study in Houston and Detroit found that 11 to 42% of 11- to 35-month-old children had antibody, despite having received no OPV (27).

However, there are also potential disadvantages associated with transmission of OPV viruses. It is now recognized that a high proportion of OPV viruses shed in the feces of recent vaccinees contain mutations that have reverted to the neurovirulence genotype at one important locus in the 5' noncoding region of the genome (see below) (129). The risk, if any, that these revertant viruses pose relative to the risk involved with direct administration of OPV is unknown.

OPV-ASSOCIATED POLIOMYELITIS

Although naturally occurring poliovirus infection has been eradicated in the United States, an average of eight cases of neurologic disease that are caused by OPV viruses occur annually (139, 162, 195). Approximately 45% of OPV-associated poliomyelitis cases occur among recent OPV vaccinees (195). Most patients among OPV recipients are infants, and 80 to 90% of cases occur following the first feeding of OPV. A similar number of OPV-associated poliomyelitis cases (approximately 48%) is reported to occur among direct contacts of recent OPV recipients (195). These cases occur most often among parents, other family members, baby-sitters, or other associates of the family who have close contact with a recent OPV vaccinee. Similar to the OPV recipient patients, most are contacts of infants who have received their first OPV dose, for which it is well established that the titer of virus shed in the feces and the duration of fecal virus shedding are greater than those following subsequent OPV doses (60). In addition, a few cases (i.e., 5%) of community contact paralytic poliomyelitis are known to occur (195). OPV-like viruses have been isolated from individuals who report no identifiable exposure to OPV or to a recent OPV recipient. OPV types 2 and 3 have been recovered from vaccine-associated cases more frequently than has type 1.

About 10 to 15% of reported paralytic poliomyelitis cases occur among OPV recipients or contacts of OPV recipients who are immunodeficient (195). Most patients have either isolated B-cell immunodeficiency or severe combined immunodeficiency syndrome (124). The majority of infections in immunocompromised children and adults have been associated with type 2 OPV virus (195), although it is presumed that all live vaccine and naturally occurring polioviruses represent an increased risk.

The risk of paralytic disease depends on the method used to calculate risk; the overall risk is estimated to be 1 case per 2.5 million doses distributed. For immunologically competent infants, the annual rate of vaccine-associated disease is 7.6/10 million, and for adults, it is 0.45/10 million household contacts of children <6 years old (195). The risk of OPV-related paralytic disease in patients with hereditary immunodeficiencies is estimated to be 10,000 times the risk in healthy children (222). However, the risk is relative; although most children with X-linked agammaglobulinemia receive OPV, only about 2.5% develop poliomyelitis (223). Children with severe combined immunodeficiency syndrome have also inadvertently received OPV without ill effects (117).

The mechanism by which the OPV viruses cause rare cases of paralytic disease is not fully understood. It is well known that OPV virus readily undergoes mutation during its brief period of intestinal replication and that isolates that are neurovirulent for primates can be recovered (see above) (177). Most OPV recipients shed polioviruses that have reverted to the naturally occurring genotype at a specific locus in the 5' noncoding region of the genome, which is strongly associated with attenuation for each of the three OPV serotypes (129) (see chapter 2). However, because the attenuated Sabin strains differ from their virulent parent strains at multiple genetic loci and because the genetic basis for loss of neurotropism among the Sabin strains remains to be fully delineated, it is not entirely certain which mutational events are most important in producing reversion to neurovirulence. The reader is referred to chapter 2 in this volume as well as another excellent review (2) and several primary manuscripts (3, 47, 130, 193) for a more thorough understanding of the molecular bases of poliovirus neurovirulence and attenuation.

IPV

IPV is prepared by inactivation of well-characterized wild-type poliovirus seed strains by the method originally developed by Jonas Salk, i.e., 1:1,000 formalin treatment for 12 to 14 days at 37°C. The potency of the first IPV preparations, which was directly related to viral antigen content, varied widely until minimum standards were set in 1968. Within the past decade, the adoption of continuous cell lines and microcarrier systems for virus cultivation has made possible the production of IPVs of higher potency, which have largely supplanted the older, less potent vaccines. These enhanced-potency vaccines were first introduced in The Netherlands, France, and Canada in the early 1980s. The first enhanced-potency IPV licensed in the United States (in 1987) was produced in human diploid cells. The vaccine now available, which is distributed by Connaught-Merieux, is produced in Vero cells. Like most other new IPVs, this vaccine contains 40, 8, and 32 D-antigen units for poliovirus serotypes 1, 2, and 3, respectively.

The recommended primary series for enhanced-potency IPV is the same as for OPV, i.e., three doses administered at 2, 4, and 6 to 18 months of age. Currently, IPV is recommended as the preferred poliomyelitis vaccine for persons who are immunodeficient and for previously unvaccinated adults (25).

HUMORAL ANTIBODY RESPONSE

The serologic response to IPV is directly related to vaccine potency. The enhanced-potency vaccines are far more immunogenic than the earlier IPV formulations. When given according to the same schedule, the former produce seroconversion rates that are equal to and mean antibody titers that are superior to those of OPV. Neutralizing antibodies to all three types are detectable in 99% of recipients after two doses and in 100% after the third dose (122, 190). A large boost in antibody titer follows the third dose (122). At 20 months of age, titers to types 1 and 3 are higher than in OPV-immunized children, while titers to type 2 are equivalent. Detectable antibody persists at protective levels for at least 5 years, although geometric mean titers decline considerably (199).

IPV EFFICACY
Like that of OPV, the efficacy of IPV for preventing poliomyelitis is high but not 100%. In 1959, prior to distribution of OPV, 5,267 cases of paralytic polio occurred in the United States. Although 65% of these patients had received no vaccine, 18% had received one or two doses, 14% had received three doses, and 3% had received four doses of IPV. The overall vaccine efficacies for (lower-potency) IPV were estimated to be 91 and 95%, respectively, for three and four doses. Data regarding vaccine efficacy of enhanced-potency IPV are few. A case control study in Senegal indicated lower-than-expected protection rates of 36 and 89% for recipients of one and two doses, respectively (171).

MUCOSAL IMMUNITY AND TRANSMISSION OF LIVE POLIOVIRUSES TO CONTACTS
IPV-immunized children develop little or no measurable secretory antibody (141). When challenged with live polioviruses, IPV-immunized children shed the challenge virus in their feces at a higher rate and a higher titer and for a longer period than do OPV-immunized children (144), indicating a greater potential for asymptomatic infection and transmission of circulating polioviruses to unimmunized contacts.

Although this is widely cited as a disadvantage of IPV, there is evidence that widespread use of IPV results in protection that extends to unvaccinated persons in the community. From 1958 to 1961, when only IPV was used in the United States, a herd effect (54) was observed in which the number of observed cases of poliomyelitis was consistently lower than the number expected if only vaccinated persons derived protection (194). In The Netherlands, where IPV has been used exclusively since 1957 and where approximately 95% of the population are fully immunized, there is little evidence of endemic persistence of wild-type strains despite the frequent importation of wild-type polioviruses (10, 186).

IPV recipients exhibit a different shedding pattern than nonimmune persons during epidemic or endemic poliovirus transmission. Studies during polio epidemics in Iowa and Missouri (28, 29) and in Rhode Island (119) and during natural circulation of wild-type virus in Louisiana (59) showed that IPV had the effect of reducing community transmission of polioviruses, while there was little effect on transmission within the household once poliovirus was introduced. This effect may be due to the marked reduction of pharyngeal shedding of poliovirus in reinfected IPV recipients, which is probably the important mode of community spread (211), whereas IPV has little effect in preventing spread within families, where fecal-oral spread may be a more important mode of transmission (60, 212).

Poliovirus Vaccination Strategy and Public Policy in the United States
Both the American Academy of Pediatrics Committee on Infectious Diseases and the U.S. Public Health Service Advisory Committee on Immunization Practices recommend relying primarily on OPV for routine use among infants while reserving IPV for special situations, including vaccination of immunocompromised persons and previously unimmunized adults (24, 25, 30). The continued annual occurrence of paralytic disease among recipients of OPV and the resulting liability issues for both vaccine manufacturers and pediatric practitioners

have perpetuated controversy over the current U.S. policy of exclusive use of OPV for routine immunization. Strong positions have been taken by those who favor continuing the policy of exclusive use of OPV (180) and those who favor a change to exclusive use of IPV (183, 184).

The advocates of OPV cite the following advantages of live vaccines relative to inactivated vaccines: (i) they are easy to produce and relatively inexpensive; (ii) they are easy to administer; (iii) they enhance overall immunization coverage in the community by transmission of vaccine viruses to susceptible contacts; and (iv) they induce intestinal immunity, which may limit the community spread of naturally occurring polioviruses. Proponents of IPV tout the safety of these products and the solid immunity they induce. However, the exclusive use of IPV would certainly enhance the likelihood of the introduction and circulation of naturally occurring polioviruses and would increase the risk of disease among unimmunized persons (77).

SEQUENTIAL IPV-OPV IMMUNIZATION

An alternative strategy is to administer IPV and OPV sequentially, i.e., one or two doses of IPV followed by two or more doses of OPV. The benefits of this approach would be the prevention of OPV-associated neurologic disease among recipients and the reduction of risk to contacts of OPV recipients and children with immunodeficiencies (121). A secondary benefit might be a reduction in the cost of OPV as a result of diminished liability exposure. Recent studies have confirmed that the sequential use of enhanced-potency IPV and OPV produces serum neutralizing antibody titers that are equal or superior to those produced by either OPV alone or IPV alone given according to the same schedule (50, 132).

In 1988, an expert panel convened by the Institute of Medicine reviewed the current epidemiology of poliomyelitis and the current data regarding both OPV and enhanced-potency IPV. This committee reaffirmed continued routine use of OPV alone for the present but indicated a preference for introduction of a sequential schedule involving one or two doses of IPV prior to administration of OPV whenever IPV could effectively be combined with a diphtheria-tetanus-pertussis (DTP) vaccine containing an acellular pertussis component (89). Quadrivalent formulations combining IPV with DTP are available in some countries and are currently undergoing trials in the United States.

POLIOMYELITIS IN THE DEVELOPING WORLD

The existence of poliomyelitis was ignored for many years in developing countries because polio was considered an epidemic disease of wealthier nations. In the 1960s and 1970s, lameness surveys of schoolchildren in more than 20 nations revealed lower-limb paralysis prevalence rates of 2 to 11/1,000, figures that reflect poliomyelitis incidence rates that equal or exceed those of the peak epidemic years in the United States (74, 140). Most cases of paralytic poliomyelitis in developing countries occur in children between the ages of 6 months and 2 years. The majority of cases are caused by type 1 poliovirus. Despite the high incidence of poliomyelitis, the level of public concern is often low because of the nonepidemic disease pattern, the high prevalence of other physical disabilities in poor communities, and the fact that paralysis occurs in early childhood, when it may not be immediately recognized. Many children in developing countries remain unprotected because current poliomyelitis immunization programs fail to reach them or because the administered polio vaccines fail to produce adequate immunity to all three poliovirus serotypes.

Worldwide Initiatives toward Control of Poliomyelitis

In 1974, the World Health Organization founded the Expanded Program on Immunization (EPI) to provide monetary and technical support for basic immunization against several childhood diseases worldwide. The EPI has produced substantial progress by applying several strategies to the control of poliomyelitis, including routine immunization programs, national immunization days, and intensified surveillance and response to outbreaks (87, 221). By 1983, an international conference in Bellagio, Italy, articulated the vision of worldwide poliomyelitis eradication (172), and in 1985, the Pan American Health Organization resolved to eradicate poliomyelitis from the Western Hemisphere, a goal that was achieved by 1991 with the aid of substantial support from Rotary International, the United Nation's Children's Fund, the United States Agency for International Development, the World Bank, and the Rockefeller Foundation. By the early 1990s, approximately 80% of children in most countries had received a basic course of three OPV doses, and the reported incidence of poliomyelitis had steadily declined to approximately 15,000 cases per year (compared with an estimated 600,000 cases per year in the prevaccine era) (87).

Despite this progress, wild-type polioviruses continue to circulate and cause disease in approximately 38% of the 211 nations of the world (87). Sub-Saharan Africa and South Asia remain regions with high rates of endemic disease. The EPI recommendations are intended to be universal, but polio vaccines fail to reach many children because of interrupted vaccine supplies, problems in delivery from central stores to the final locations for immunization, and disruptions in the cold chain necessary to maintain the potency of OPV. Low population acceptance remains the dominant cause of low immunization rates. In addition, continued civil strife, poor political support, and inadequate funding continue to hamper efforts to control poliomyelitis and represent the major obstacles to the World Health Assembly goal of worldwide eradication of poliomyelitis by the year 2000 (87, 220).

Use of Poliomyelitis Vaccines in the Developing World

OPV is used almost exclusively in underdeveloped nations because of its lower cost and ease of administration. The superior secretory immunity in the gastrointestinal tract induced by OPV is considered an advantage because of high rates of exposure to wild-type polioviruses. Transmission of OPV virus from immunized to nonimmune contacts, an event that is thought to be aided by poor sanitation and crowded living conditions, is also considered an advantage of OPV. However, the contribution of fecal transmission of OPV virus to the protection of unimmunized contacts in developing countries has been difficult to document (218). Furthermore, this concept has been challenged by observations during a large poliomyelitis outbreak in one developing country, Taiwan, in which unimmunized children did not appear to be protected despite prevailing OPV immunization levels of 83 to 98% in young children (99).

The EPI recommendation of three OPV doses in the first year of life (at 6, 10, and 14 weeks of age) supplanted the previously nonuniform immunization schedules used in most developing countries. In 1985, the EPI schedule was amended to include a dose of trivalent OPV given shortly after birth; this practice provides an opportunity to administer at least one dose of vaccine to a child who may not present for routine health maintenance care later (48). Even though the passively acquired maternal antibody to polioviruses present in the infant's circulation and in maternal colostrum reduces vaccine virus replication in the gastrointestinal tract and therefore blunts the immune response in some infants, infants who receive OPV at birth are more likely to have antibody to all three poliovirus types at 4 months of age (41).

EFFICACY OF OPV IN DEVELOPING COUNTRIES

Unfortunately, in many tropical countries, the full recommended series of OPV may fail to produce active immunity to all three poliovirus serotypes in a significant proportion of infants. In Vellore, India, for example, John and Jayabal found seroconversion rates of 35, 76, and 48% to serotypes 1, 2, and 3, respectively, after two OPV doses among seronegative children 3 months to 6 years of age (95). Data from Singapore (40), Nigeria (92), The Gambia (69), Brazil (37), and Gaza (111) confirm that three or fewer doses of OPV do not provide optimal protection to young children in developing counties. Overall seroconversion rates after three OPV doses in these locations average 73, 90, and 70% for types 1, 2, and 3, respectively (152). In Israel and Brazil, the poor response has been cited as a contributing factor to outbreaks of poliomyelitis despite relatively high immunization rates prior to the appearance of epidemic disease (111, 127, 151). Studies conducted during type 1 poliomyelitis outbreaks in Oman and The Gambia found vaccine efficacy to be in the range of 80 to 90% (39, 196). During a type 3 poliomyelitis outbreak in Brazil, vaccine efficacy was estimated to be 55% (150).

Low OPV seroconversion rates and efficacy are not uniformly observed in developing regions. During the type 1 poliovirus outbreak in Taiwan, vaccine efficacies for OPV were estimated to be 82, 96, and 98 for one, two, and three or more doses, respectively (100). Similarly, surveillance from 1982 through 1987 in Bombay, where type 1 poliomyelitis is endemic, confirmed that the efficacy of three doses of OPV is greater than 90% (49).

REASONS FOR LOWER RESPONSE TO OPV

The reasons for the lower potency of OPV in tropical areas remain incompletely understood. Many explanations have been considered, including (i) OPV stability, potency, volume, and formulation; (ii) inadequate replication of vaccine virus due to interference from passively acquired maternal serum antibodies, breast milk antibodies, competition from other enteroviruses, or intercurrent diarrheal disease; and (iii) poor antibody response of the host because of malnutrition (152). Both vaccine formulation and the effect of concurrent diarrheal illnesses have emerged as important factors.

The OPV vaccines distributed to most developing countries only marginally meet the 1988 EPI minimum potency standards of 10^6, 10^5, and $10^{5.5}$ $TCID_{50}$ for types 1, 2, and 3, respectively. Vaccines meeting but not exceeding these levels are 3-, 2.5-, and 7-fold less potent for serotypes 1, 2, and 3, respectively, than OPV distributed in the United States (152). These small differences appear to be important. Patriarca et al. demonstrated that a twofold increase in the type 3 component increased the seroconversion rate from 16 to 42% among type 3 seronegative Brazilian children given one dose of trivalent OPV (151). Although reformulation of OPV has recently been shown to enhance responses to types 1 and 3 polioviruses (217), the overall responses to type 1 and type 3 remain suboptimal, in part because of interference from more efficient replication of the type 2 vaccine virus (151).

Diarrheal disease at the time of immunization reduces rates of seroconversion with OPV. One study conducted in Brazil and The Gambia (216) and another conducted in Bangladesh (134) have each convincingly shown reduced seroconversion rates to types 2 and 3 OPV, while the response to type 1 was not affected. The impact of diarrhea on seroconversion persists despite the administration of three or four OPV doses.

Conversely, intercurrent enterovirus infections do not appear to be responsible for diminished OPV seroconversion rates (88, 93). It is still uncertain whether investigational live, attenuated rotavirus vaccines will interfere when they are administered simultaneously with OPV (152, 166). Breast feeding may interfere with the response to OPV in the newborn infant, but there is little evidence that it does so in infants 2 months of age and older (38, 64, 94, 160). Similarly, malnourished infants and children develop adequate antibody responses to OPV compared with the responses in healthy subjects (88, 95). OPV is heat labile, losing approximately $10^{0.5}$ $TCID_{50}$/day at 37°C (120, 192). Although loss of potency has occasionally been implicated as a cause of vaccine failure (149), improvements in training and advances in technology that ensure proper storage temperatures have meant fewer documented breaches in the cold chain (152).

STRATEGIES TO IMPROVE POLIOVIRUS IMMUNITY

The adoption of aggressive programs such as pulse immunization in epidemic areas and supplemental National Vaccination Days on which all children receive live oral vaccine regardless of vaccination history has been an effective approach in some locations (91, 178). Seroconversion rates during mass campaigns are higher than those with routine immunization (167), possibly because the OPV virus spreads or because the campaigns are conducted during the dry season, when diarrheal disease is less prevalent. In Cuba and Brazil, twice-yearly mass campaigns have been credited with rapid abatement of circulation of naturally occurring polioviruses and disappearance of disease (33, 168).

Reformulation of OPV distributed under EPI to achieve a content closer to the U.S. standard is expected to enhance seroconversion rates but will take several years to accomplish. Seroconversion rates also improve when five doses of OPV are used in the first year of life (90). Unfortunately, the delivery of multiple doses of OPV in the first year of life to children in many underdeveloped areas is impractical.

Although enhanced-potency IPV is highly immunogenic among children in developing areas (191, 198), the costs associated with production and delivery and the requirement for injection have made sole use of IPV an undesirable alternative in developing countries. However, enhanced-potency IPV has been used as a supplement to OPV immunization in Israel, where type 1 poliovirus continued to cause epidemic disease in Gaza despite relatively good rates of OPV coverage (111, 112), and in Cote d'Ivoire, where IPV administered at 9 months of age markedly enhanced seroconversion rates among infants given OPV at 2, 3, and 4 months of age (133).

SUMMARY

Epidemic paralytic poliomyelitis is a disease that has both appeared and disappeared during the past 120 years. The clinical, epidemiologic, and scientific foundations for the control of poliomyelitis were laid in the first half of the 20th century, and eradication has since been achieved through routine immunization programs that use two very effective vaccines, each of which possesses unique advantages and disadvantages. The relative merits of these vaccines and other immunization strategies continue to be debated in the developed world, where infections with virulent, wild-type polioviruses no longer occur. There is now reason to hope that the Herculean effort to rid the remaining nations of the earth of poliomyelitis by the year 2000 will succeed.

REFERENCES

1. **Abercrombie, J.** 1828. *Pathological and Practical Researches on Diseases of the Brain and Spinal Cord*. Waugh and Innes, Edinburgh.
2. **Almond, J. W.** 1987. The attenuation of poliovirus neurovirulence. *Annu. Rev. Microbiol.* **41:**154–180.
3. **Almond, J. W., G. D. Westrop, D. M. Evans, et al.** 1987. Studies on the attenuation of the Sabin type 3 oral polio vaccine. *J. Virol. Methods* **17:**183–189.
4. **Anderson, G. W., G. Anderson, and A. Skaar.** 1952. Poliomyelitis in pregnancy. *Am. J. Hyg.* **55:**127.
5. **Anderson, J. F., and W. H. Frost.** 1911. Abortive cases of poliomyelitis: an experimental demonstration of specific immune bodies in their blood-serum. *JAMA* **56:**633–639.
6. **Armstrong, C.** 1939. The experimental transmission of poliomyelitis to the eastern cotton rat, *Sigmodon hispidus hispidus*. *Public Health Rep.* **54:**1719–1721.
7. **Armstrong, C.** 1939. Successful transfer of the Lansing strain of poliomyelitis virus from the cotton rat to the white mouse. *Public Health Rep.* **54:**2302–2305.

8. **Bass, J. W., S. B. Halsted, and G. W. Fischer.** 1978. Oral polio vaccine: effect of booster vaccination one to 14 years after primary series. *JAMA* **239:**2252–2255.
9. **Benyesh-Melnick, M.** 1967. Studies of the immunogenicity, communicability and genetic stability of oral poliovaccine administered during the winter. *Am. J. Epidemiol.* **86:**112–136.
10. **Bijkerk, H.** 1979. Poliomyelitis epidemic in the Netherlands. *Dev. Biol. Stand.* **43:**195–206.
11. **Bodian, D.** 1949. Histopathologic basis of the clinical findings in poliomyelitis. *Am. J. Med.* **6:**563.
12. **Bodian, D.** 1952. Pathogenesis of poliovirus in normal and passively immunized primates after virus feeding. *Fed. Proc.* **11:**462.
13. **Bodian, D.** 1954. Viremia in experimental poliomyelitis. II. Viremia and the mechanism of the "provoking" effect of injections or trauma. *Am. J. Hyg.* **60:**358.
14. **Bodian, D.** 1954. Viremia in experimental poliomyelitis. I. General aspects of infection after intravascular inoculation with strains of high and low invasiveness. *Am. J. Hyg.* **60:**339.
15. **Bodian, D.** 1955. Emerging concepts of poliomyelitis infection. *Science* **122:**105.
16. **Bodian, D.** 1956. Poliovirus in chimpanzee tissues after virus feeding. *Am. J. Hyg.* **64:**187.
17. **Bodian, D., and H. A. Howe.** 1940. An experimental study of the role of neurones in the dissemination of poliomyelitis virus in the nervous system. *Brain* **63:**135.
18. **Bodian, D., I. M. Morgan, and H. A. Howe.** 1949. Differentiation of three types of poliomyelitis virus. III. The grouping of fourteen strains into three immunological types. *Am. J. Hyg.* **49:**234.
19. **Bottiger, M., S. Gard, and B. Zetterberg.** 1966. Vaccination with attenuated type 1 poliovirus, the Chat strain. II. Transmission of virus in relation to age. *Acta Paediatr. Scand.* **55:**416–421.
20. **Brodie, M.** 1934. Active immunization in monkeys against poliomyelitis with germicidally inactivated virus. *Science* **79:**594–595.
21. **Brodie, M., S. A. Goldberg, and P. Stanley.** 1935. Transmission of the virus of poliomyelitis to mice. *Science* **81:**319.
22. **Brodie, M., and W. H. Park.** 1935. Active immunization against poliomyelitis. *JAMA* **105:**9.
23. **Burnet, F. M., and J. Macnamara.** 1931. Immunological differences between strains of poliomyelitic virus. *Br. J. Exp. Pathol.* **12:**57–61.
24. **Centers for Disease Control.** 1982. Recommendations of the Immunization Practices Advisory Committee: poliomyelitis prevention. *Morbid. Mortal. Weekly Rep.* **31:**22–26, 31–34.
25. **Centers for Disease Control.** 1987. Poliomyelitis prevention: enhanced-potency inactivated poliomyelitis vaccine—supplementary statement. *Morbid. Mortal. Weekly Rep.* **36:**795–798.
26. **Charcot, J.-M.** 1872. Groupe des myopathies de cause spinale; paralysie infantile. *Rev. Phot. Hop.* (Paris) **4:**1–36.
27. **Chen, R., M. Hanfling, and S. Hausinger.** 1992. Extent of secondary spread of oral polio vaccine virus spread in inner-city pre-school children, abst. 1403. *Program Abstr. 32nd Intersci. Conf. Antimicrob. Agents Chemother.*
28. **Chin, T. D. Y., and W. M. Marine.** 1961. The changing pattern of poliomyelitis observed in two urban epidemics. *Public Health Rep.* **76:**553–563.
29. **Chin, T. D. Y., W. M. Marine, and E. C. Hall.** 1961. Poliomyelitis in Des Moines, Iowa, 1959. The influence of Salk vaccination on the epidemic pattern and spread of the virus in the community. *Am. J. Hyg.* **74:**67–94.
30. **Committee on Infectious Diseases, American Academy of Pediatrics.** 1994. *Report of the Committee on Infectious Diseases, 23rd ed.* American Academy of Pediatrics, Elk Grove Village, Ill.
31. **Cordier, S.** 1988. Relation d'une épidémie de paralysie atrophique de l'enfance. *Lyon Med.* **48:**5–12.
32. **Cornil, V.** 1863. Paralysie infantile; cancer les seins; autopsie; altérations de la moelle épinière, des nerfs et des muscles; généralisation du cancer. *C. R. Soc. Biol.* (Paris) **5:**187.
33. **Cruz, R. R.** 1984. Cuba: mass polio vaccination program, 1962–1982. *Rev. Infect. Dis.* **6(2):**408–412.
34. **Dalakas, M. C., G. Elder, and M. Hallet.** 1986. A long-term follow-up study of patients with post-poliomyelitis neuromuscular symptoms. *N. Engl. J. Med.* **314:**959–963.
35. **Dalakas, M. C., J. L. Sever, and D. L. Madden.** 1984. Late postpoliomyelitis muscular atrophy: clinical, virologic, and immunologic studies. *Rev. Infect. Dis.* **6(2):**S562–S567.
36. **Davis, L. E., D. Bodian, and D. Price.** 1977. Chronic progressive poliomyelitis secondary to vaccination of an immunodeficient child. *N. Engl. J. Med.* **297:**241.
37. **de Brito Bastos, N. C., E. S. de Carvalho, H. Schatzmayr, A. Homma, and J. Chaves.** 1974. Antipoliomyelitis program in Brazil: a serologic study of immunity. *Bull. PAHO* **8:**54–65.
38. **DeForest, A.** 1973. The effect of breast-feeding on the antibody response of infants to trivalent oral poliovirus vaccine. *J. Pediatr.* **83:**93–95.

39. **Deming, M. S., K. O. Jaiteh, and M. W. Otten.** 1992. Epidemic poliomyelitis in The Gambia following the control of poliomyelitis as an endemic disease. II. Clinical efficacy of trivalent oral polio vaccine. *Am. J. Epidemiol.* **135:**393–408.
40. **Domok, I., M. S. Balayan, and O. A. Fayinka.** 1974. Factors affecting the efficacy of live poliovirus vaccine in warm climates. *Bull. W.H.O.* **51:**333–347.
41. **Dong, D.-X., X.-M. Hu, W.-J. Liu, et al.** 1986. Immunization of neonates with trivalent oral poliomyelitis vaccine (Sabin). *Bull. W.H.O.* **64:**853–860.
42. **Draper, G.** 1935. *Infantile Paralysis*, 2nd ed. Appleton-Century, New York.
43. **Drinker, P., and C. F. McKhann.** 1929. The use of a new apparatus for the prolonged administration of artificial respiration; a fatal case of poliomyelitis. *JAMA* **92:**1658.
44. **Drinker, P., and L. A. Shaw.** 1929. Apparatus for prolonged administration of artificial respiration; design for adults and children. *J. Clin. Invest.* **7:**229.
45. **Enders, J. F., T. H. Weller, and F. C. Robbins.** 1949. Cultivation of the Lansing strain of poliomyelitis virus in cultures of various human embryonic tissue. *Science* **109:**85–87.
46. **Enders, J. F., T. H. Weller, and F. C. Robbins.** 1952. Alterations in pathogenicity for monkeys of Brunhilde strain of poliovirus following cultivation in human tissues. *Fed. Proc.* **11:**467.
47. **Evans, D. M., G. Dunn, P. D. Minor, et al.** 1985. Increased neurovirulence associated with a single nucleotide change in a noncoding region of the Sabin type 3 poliovaccine genome. *Nature* (London) **314:**548–550.
48. **Expanded Programme on Immunization.** 1985. Global Advisory Group. *Weekly Epidemiol. Rec. W.H.O.* **60:**13–16.
49. **Expanded Programme on Immunization.** 1988. Poliomyelitis surveillance and vaccine efficacy. *Weekly Epidemiol. Rec. W.H.O.* **63:**249–251.
50. **Faden, H., J. F. Modlin, M. L. Thoms, A. M. McBean, M. B. Ferndon, and P. L. Ogra.** 1990. Comparative evaluation of immunization with live attenuated and enhanced potency inactivated trivalent poliovirus vaccines in childhood: systemic and local immune responses. *J. Infect. Dis.* **162:**1291–1297.
51. **Flexner, S., and P. F. Clark.** 1912–1913. A note on the mode of infection in epidemic poliomyelitis. *Proc. Soc. Exp. Biol. Med.* **10:**1.
52. **Flexner, S., and P. A. Lewis.** 1909. The transmission of poliomyelitis to monkeys. *JAMA* **53:**1639.
53. **Flexner, S., and P. A. Lewis.** 1910. Experimental poliomyelitis in monkeys; active immunization and passive serum protection. *JAMA* **54:**1780.
54. **Fox, J. P., L. Elveback, and W. Scott.** 1971. Herd immunity: basic concept and relevance to public health immunization practices. *Am. J. Epidemiol.* **94:**179–189.
55. **Frost, W. H.** Epidemiologic studies of acute anterior poliomyelitis. *Hyg. Lab. Bull.* **90:**1913.
56. **Gatmaitan, B. G., J. L. Chason, and A. M. Lerner.** 1970. Augmentation of the virulence of murine coxsackievirus B-3 myocardiopathy by exercise. *J. Exp. Med.* **131:**1121–1136.
57. **Gelfand, H. M., D. R. LeBlanc, and J. P. Fox.** 1957. Studies on the development of natural immunity to poliomyelitis in Louisiana. II. Description and analysis of episodes of infection observed in study group households. *Am. J. Hyg.* **65:**367–385.
58. **Gelfand, H. M., D. R. LeBlanc, and J. P. Fox.** 1959. Studies on the development of natural immunity to poliomyelitis in Louisiana. III. The serologic response to commercially produced "Salk vaccine" of children totally or partially susceptible to poliovirus infection. *Am. J. Hyg.* **70:**303–311.
59. **Gelfand, H. M., D. R. LeBlanc, and L. Potash.** 1959. Studies on the development of natural immunity to poliomyelitis in Louisiana. IV. Natural infections with polioviruses following immunization with a formalin-inactivated vaccine. *Am. J. Hyg.* **70:**312–327.
60. **Gelfand, H. M., L. Potash, and D. R. LeBlanc.** 1959. Intrafamilial and interfamilial spread of living vaccine strains of polioviruses. *JAMA* **170:**2039–2048.
61. **Ghendon, Y. U. Z., and I. I. Sanakoyeva.** 1961. Comparison of the resistance of the intestinal tract to poliomyelitis virus (Sabin's strains) in person after naturally and experimentally acquired immunity. *Acta Virol.* (Prague) **5:**265–273.
62. **Greenberg, M., H. Abramson, and H. M. Cooper.** 1952. The relation between recent injections and paralytic poliomyelitis in children. *Am. J. Public Health* **42:**142.
63. **Grist, N. R., and E. J. Bell.** 1970. Enteroviral etiology of the paralytic poliomyelitis syndrome. *Arch. Environ. Health* **21:**382.
64. **Halsey, N., and A. Galazka.** 1985. The efficacy of DPT and oral poliomyelitis immunization schedules initiated from birth to 12 weeks of age. *Bull. W.H.O.* **63:**1151–1169.
65. **Hammon, W. M., L. I. Coriell, and J. Stokes, Jr.** 1952. Evaluation of Red Cross

gamma globulin as a prophylactic agent for poliomyelitis. *JAMA* **150:**139.
66. **Hammon, W. M., L. L. Coriell, P. F. Wehrle, and J. J. Stokes.** 1953. Evaluation of Red Cross gamma globulin as a prophylactic agent for poliomyelitis. IV. Final report of results based on clinical diagnoses. *JAMA* **151:**1272–1285.
67. **Hammon, W. M., and E. M. Izumi.** 1942. Poliomyelitis mouse neutralization test, applied to acute and convalescent sera. *Proc. Soc. Exp. Biol. Med.* **49:**242.
68. **Hammon, W. M., and E. C. Roberts.** 1948. Serum neutralizing antibodies to the infecting strain of virus in poliomyelitis patients. *Proc. Soc. Exp. Biol. Med.* **69:**256–258.
69. **Hanlon, P., L. Hanlon, V. Marsh, et al.** 1987. Serological comparisons of approaches to polio vaccination in The Gambia. *Lancet* **i:**800–801.
70. **Hardy, G. E., C. C. Hopkins, and C. C. Linneman.** 1970. Trivalent oral poliovirus vaccine: a comparison of two infant immunization schedules. *Pediatrics* **45:**444–448.
71. **Harjulehto, T., T. Aro, T. Hovi, and L. Saxen.** 1989. Congenital malformations and oral poliovirus vaccination during pregnancy. *Lancet* **i:**771–772.
72. **Heine, J.** 1940. *Beobachtungen über Lähmungszustände der unteren Extremitäten und deren Behandlung.* Köhler, Stuttgart, Germany.
73. **Henderson, D. A., J. J. Witte, L. Morris, and A. D. Langmuir.** 1964. Paralytic disease associated with oral poliovaccines. *JAMA* **190:**153–160.
74. **Henderson, R. H.** 1984. The Expanded Programme on Immunization of the World Health Organization. *Rev. Infect. Dis.* **6(2):**475–479.
75. **Henry, J. L., E. S. Jaikaran, and J. R. Davies.** 1966. A study of polio vaccination in infancy: excretion following challenge with live virus by children given killed or living poliovaccine. *J. Hyg.* **64:**105–120.
76. **Hill, A. B., and J. Knowelden.** 1950. Inoculation and poliomyelitis: a statistical investigation in England and Wales in 1949. *Br. Med. J.* **2:**1.
77. **Hinman, A. R., J. P. Koplan, W. A. Orenstein, E. W. Brink, and B. M. Nkowane.** 1988. Live or inactivated poliovirus vaccine: an analysis of the benefits and risks. *Am. J. Public Health* **78:**291–295.
78. **Horstmann, D. M.** 1949. Clinical aspects of acute poliomyelitis. *Am. J. Med.* **6:**592.
79. **Horstmann, D. M.** 1950. Acute poliomyelitis. Relation of physical activity at the time of onset to the course of the disease. *JAMA* **142:**236.
80. **Horstmann, D. M.** 1952. Poliomyelitis in the blood of orally infected monkeys and chimpanzees. *Proc. Soc. Exp. Biol. Med.* **79:**417.
81. **Horstmann, D. M.** 1985. The poliomyelitis story: a scientific hegira. *Yale J. Biol. Med.* **58:**79–90.
82. **Horstmann, D. M., and R. W. McCollum.** 1953. Poliomyelitis virus in human blood during the "minor" illness and asymptomatic infection. *Proc. Soc. Exp. Biol. Med.* **82:**434.
83. **Horstmann, D. M., R. W. McCollum, and A. D. Mascola.** 1954. Viremia in human poliomyelitis. *J. Exp. Med.* **99:**355–369.
84. **Horstmann, D. M., E. M. Opton, and R. Klemperer.** 1964. Viremia in infants vaccinated with oral poliovirus vaccine (Sabin). *Am. J. Hyg.* **79:**47.
85. **Horstmann, D. M., and J. R. Paul.** 1947. The incubation period in human poliomyelitis and its implications. *JAMA* **135:**11.
86. **Howe, H. A., and D. Bodian.** 1941. Poliomyelitis in the chimpanzee; a clinical pathological study. *Bull. Johns Hopkins Hosp.* **69:**149–181.
87. **Hull, H. F., N. A. Ward, B. P. Hull, J. B. Milstien, and C. de Quadros.** 1994. Paralytic poliomyelitis: seasoned strategies, disappearing disease. *Lancet* **343:**1331–1337.
88. **Idris, M. Z., A. Mathur, P. Sharma, U. C. Chaturvedi, and N. L. Sharma.** 1980. Oral polio vaccination and factors affecting its efficacy. *Indian J. Med. Res.* **71:**671–678.
89. **Institute of Medicine, National Academy of Sciences.** 1988. *An Evaluation of Poliomyelitis Vaccine Policy Options.* National Academy of Sciences, Washington, D.C.
90. **John, T. J.** 1976. Antibody response of infants in tropics to five doses of oral polio vaccine. *Lancet* **i:**812.
91. **John, T. J.** 1984. Poliomyelitis in India: prospects and problems of control. *Rev. Infect. Dis.* **6(2):**438–441.
92. **John, T. J., and S. Christopher.** 1975. Oral polio vaccination of children in the tropics. II. Antibody response in relation to vaccine virus infection. *Am. J. Epidemiol.* **102:**414–421.
93. **John, T. J., and S. Christopher.** 1975. Oral polio vaccination of children in the tropics. III. Intercurrent enterovirus infections, vaccine virus take and antibody response. *Am. J. Epidemiol.* **102:**422–428.
94. **John, T. J., L. V. Devarajan, L. Luther, and P. Vijayarathnam.** 1976. Effect of breast-feeding on seroresponse of infants to oral poliovirus vaccination. *Pediatrics* **57:**47–53.

95. John, T. J., and P. Jayabal. 1972. Oral polio vaccination of children in the tropics: I. The poor seroconversion rates and the absence of viral interference. *Am. J. Epidemiol.* **96:**263–269.
96. Johnson, R. T. 1984. Late progression of poliomyelitis paralysis: discussion of pathogenesis. *Rev. Infect. Dis.* **6**(2):S568–S569.
97. Jubelt, B., G. Gallez-Hawkins, and O. Narayan. 1980. Pathogenesis of human poliovirus infection in mice. II. Age dependency of paralysis. *J. Neuropathol. Exp. Neurol.* **39:**149.
98. Kessel, J. F., and F. D. Stimpert. 1940. Attempts to transmit poliomyelitis virus to rodents. *Proc. Soc. Exp. Biol. Med.* **45:**665–667.
99. Kim-Farley, R. J., K. J. Bart, L. B. Schonberger, et al. 1984. Poliomyelitis in the USA: virtual elimination of disease caused by wild virus. *Lancet* **ii:**1315–1317.
100. Kim-Farley, R. J., G. Rutherford, P. Lichfield, et al. 1984. Outbreak of paralytic poliomyelitis, Taiwan. *Lancet* **ii:**1322–1324.
101. Kling, C., G. Levaditi, and P. Lépine. 1929. La pénétration du virus poliomyélitique à travers la muqueuse du tube digestif chez le singe et sa conservation dans l'eau. *Bull. Acad. Med.* (Paris) **102:**158.
102. Kling, C., A. Petterson, and W. Wernstedt. 1912. Experimental and pathological investigation. The presence of the microbe of infantile paralysis in human beings. *Commun. Inst. Med. Etat Stockholm* **3:**5.
103. Kolmer, J. A. 1935. Susceptibility and immunity in relation to vaccination in acute anterior poliomyelitis. *JAMA* **105:**1956–1962.
104. Koprowski, H. 1956. Immunization against poliomyelitis with living attenuated virus. *Am. J. Trop. Med. Hyg.* **5:**440–452.
105. Koprowski, H., G. A. Jervis, and T. W. Norton. 1952. Immune responses in human volunteers upon oral administration of a rodent-adapted strain of poliomyelitis virus. *Am. J. Hyg.* **55:**108–126.
106. Kramer, S. D., W. L. Aycock, C. I. Soloman, and C. L. Thenebe. 1932. Convalescent serum therapy in preparalytic poliomyelitis. *N. Engl. J. Med.* **206:**432.
107. Kramer, S. D., B. Hoskwith, and L. H. Grossman. 1939. Detection of the virus of poliomyelitis in the nose and throat and gastrointestinal tract of human beings and monkeys. *J. Exp. Med.* **69:**49–67.
108. Krugman, R. D., G. E. Hardy, and C. Sellers. 1977. Antibody persistence after primary immunization with trivalent oral poliovirus vaccine. *Pediatrics* **60:**80–82.
109. Landsteiner, K., C. Levaditi, and C. Pastia. 1911. Etude expérimentale de la poliomyélite aiguë (maladie de Heine-Medin). *Ann. Inst. Pasteur* **25:**805.
110. Landsteiner, K., and E. Popper. 1908. Mikroscopische Präparate von einem Menschlichen und zwei Affenrückemarken. *Wein Klin. Wochenschr.* **21:**1830.
111. Lasch, E. E., Y. Abed, K. Abdulla, et al. 1984. Succesful results of a program combining live and inactivated poliovirus vaccines to control poliomyelitis in Gaza. *Rev. Infect. Dis.* **6:**467–470.
112. Lasch, E. E., Y. Abed, O. Marcus, C. B. Gerichter, and J. L. Melnick. 1986. Combined live and inactivated poliovirus vaccine to control poliomyelitis in a developing country—five years after. *Dev. Biol. Stand.* **65:**137–143.
113. Leake, J. P. 1935. Poliomyelitis following vaccination against the disease. *JAMA* **105:**2152.
114. Leegaard, C. 1914. Die akute Poliomyelitis in Norwegen. *Dtsch. Z. Nervenheilkd.* **53:**145–262.
115. Lipson, M. J., F. C. Robbins, and W. A. Woods. 1956. The influence of vaccination upon intestinal infection of family contacts of poliomyelitis patients. *J. Clin. Invest.* **35:**722.
116. Lockhart, J. G. 1837. *Memoirs of the Life of Sir Walter Scott, Bart.* Carey Lean and Blanchard, Philadelphia.
117. Lopez, C., W. D. Biggar, and B. H. Park. 1974. Nonparalytic poliovirus infections in patients with severe combined immunodeficiency disease. *J. Pediatr.* **84:**497–502.
118. Lovett, R. W. 1916. *The Treatment of Infantile Paralysis.* P. Blakeston's Sons, Philadelphia.
119. Marine, W. M., T. D. Y. Chin, and C. R. Gravelle. 1962. Limitation of fecal and pharyngeal poliovirus excretion in Salk-vaccinated children. *Am. J. Hyg.* **76:**173–195.
120. Mauler, R., and H. Gruschkau. 1978. On stability of oral poliovirus vaccines. *Dev. Biol. Stand.* **41:**267–270.
121. McBean, A. M., and J. F. Modlin. 1987. Rationale for the sequential use of inactivated poliovirus vaccine and live attenuated poliovirus vaccine for routine use in the United States. *Pediat. Infect. Dis. J.* **6:**881–887.
122. McBean, A. M., M. L. Thoms, and P. Albrecht. 1988. The serologic response to oral polio vaccine and enhanced potency inactivated polio vaccines. *Am. J. Epidemiol.* **128:**615–628.
123. McClure, G. Y., and A. D. Langmuir. 1942. Search for carriers in an outbreak of acute anterior poliomyelitis in a rural community. *Am. J. Hyg.* **35:**285.
124. McKinney, R. E., S. L. Katz, C. M. Wilfert, R. E. McKinney, Jr., S. L. Katz, and C. M. Wilfert. 1987. Chronic enterovi-

ral meningoencephalitis in agammaglobulinemic patients. *Rev. Infect. Dis.* **9:**334–356.
125. Melnick, J. L. 1947. Fly-abatement studies in urban poliomyelitis epidemics during 1945. *Public Health Rep.* **62:**910–922.
126. Melnick, J. L. 1947. Poliomyelitis virus in urban sewage in epidemic and nonepidemic times. *Am. J. Hyg.* **45:**240–253.
127. Melnick, J. L. 1981. Combined use of live and killed vaccines to control poliomyelitis in tropical areas. *Dev. Biol. Stand.* **47:**265–273.
128. Melnick, J. L., and N. Ledinko. 1951. Social serology: antibody levels in a normal young population during an epidemic of poliomyelitis. *Am. J. Hyg.* **54:**354.
129. Minor, P., G. Dunn, N. Begg, A. Murdin, J. Thipphawong, and L. Barreto. 1993. Poliovirus vaccination schedules and reversion to virulence, abstr. 1426. *Program Abstr. 33rd Intersci. Conf. Antimicrob. Agents Chemother.*
130. Minor, P. D., A. John, M. Ferguson, and J. P. Icenogle. 1986. Antigenic and molecular evolution of the vaccine strain of type 3 poliovirus during the period of excretion by a primary vaccinee. *J. Gen. Virol.* **67:**693–706.
131. Minor, T. E., C. I. Allen, A. A. Tsiatis, D. B. Nelson, and D. J. D'Alessio. 1981. Human infective dose determinations for oral poliovirus type 1 vaccine in infants. *J. Clin. Microbiol.* **13:**388–389.
132. Modlin, J. F., I. M. Onorato, A. M. McBean, et al. 1990. The humoral immune response to type 1 oral poliovirus vaccine in children previously immunized with enhanced potency inactivated poliovirus vaccine or live oral poliovirus vaccine. *Am. J. Dis. Child.* **144:**480–484.
133. Morinere, B. J., F. P. L. van Loon, P. H. Rhodes, et al. 1993. Immunogenicity of a supplemental dose of oral versus inactivated poliovirus vaccine. *Lancet* **341:**1545–1550.
134. Myaux, J. A., L. Unicomb, A. Uzma, et al. Diarrhoea contributes to a poor serological response to oral polio vaccination. Submitted for publication.
135. Nathanson, N., and J. R. Martin. 1979. The epidemiology of poliomyelitis: enigmas surrounding its appearance and disappearance. *Am. J. Epidemiol.* **110:**672.
136. Netter, A. 1915. La sérothérapie de la poliomyélite; nos résultats chez 30 malades; indications, techniques; incidents possibles. *Gaz. Med. Paris* **86:**88.
137. Netter, A., and C. Levaditi. 1910. Action microbicide exercée sur la virus de la poliomyélite aiguë par le sérum des sujets antérieurement atteints de paralysie infantile; sa constatation dans le sérum d'un sujet qui a présenté une forme abortive. *C. R. Soc. Biol.* (Paris) **68:**855.
138. Nishio, O., Y. Ishihara. and K. Sakae. 1984. The trend of acquired immunity with live poliovirus vaccine and the effect of revaccination: follow-up of vaccinees for ten years. *J. Biol. Stand.* **12:**1–10.
139. Nkowane, B. M., S. C. F. Wassilak, and W. A. Orenstein. 1987. Vaccine-associated paralytic poliomyelitis: United States: 1973 through 1984. *JAMA* **257:**1335–1340.
140. Ofusu-Amaah, S. 1984. The challenge of poliomyelitis in tropical Africa. *Rev. Infect. Dis.* **6(2):**318–320.
141. Ogra, P. L. 1968. Immunoglobulin response in serum and secretions after immunization with live and inactivated poliovaccine and natural infection. *N. Engl. J. Med.* **279:**893–900.
142. Ogra, P. L. 1984. Mucosal immune response to poliovirus vaccines in childhood. *Rev. Infect. Dis.* **6(2):**S361–S368.
143. Ogra, P. L., and D. T. Karzon. 1971. Formation and function of poliovirus antibody in different tissues. *Prog. Med. Virol.* **13:**157.
144. Onorato, I. M., J. F. Modlin, A. M. McBean, M. L. Thoms, G. A. Losonsky, and R. Bernier. 1991. Mucosal immunity induced by enhanced potency IPV and OPV. *J. Infect. Dis.* **163:**1–6.
145. Osler, W. 1892. *Principles and Practice of Medicine.* Young and Pentland, Edinburgh.
146. Paffenbarger, R. S. 1957. The effect of prior tonsillectomy on incidence and clinical type of acute poliomyelitis. *Am. J. Hyg.* **66:**131.
147. Paffenbarger, R. S., and J. Watt. 1953. Poliomyelitis in Hidalgo County, Texas, 1948. Epidemiologic observations. *Am. J. Hyg.* **58:**269–287.
148. Paffenbarger, R. S., and V. D. Wilson. 1955. Previously tonsillectomy and current pregnancy as they affect risk of poliomyelitis. *Ann. N.Y. Acad. Sci.* **61:**856–868.
149. Pan American Health Organization. 1985. Polio outbreak in Honduras. *Expanded Programme Immunization Newsl.* **7:**1–4.
150. Pan American Health Organization. 1986. Polio in Brazil's northeast. *Expanded Programme Immunization Newsl.* **8:**3–4.
151. Patriarca, P. A., F. Laender, G. Palmeira, et al. 1988. Randomised trial of alternative formulations of oral poliovaccine in Brazil. *Lancet* **1:**429–433.
152. Patriarca, P. A., P. F. Wright, and T. J. John. 1991. Factors affecting the immunogenicity of oral poliovirus vaccine in developing countries. *Rev. Infect. Dis.* **13:**926–939.

153. **Paul, J. P.** 1951. Antibodies to three different antigenic types of poliomyelitis virus in sera from North Alaskan Eskimos. *Am. J. Hyg.* **54:**275–285.
154. **Paul, J. R.** 1971. *History of Poliomyelitis.* Yale University Press, New Haven, Conn.
155. **Paul, J. R., and J. T. Riordan.** 1950. Observations on serological epidemiology. *Am. J. Hyg.* **52:**202–212.
156. **Paul, J. R., and J. D. Trask.** 1933. A comparative study of recently isolated human strains and a passage strain of poliomyelitis virus. *J. Exp. Med.* **58:**513–529.
157. **Paul, J. R., and J. D. Trask.** 1935. The neutralization test in poliomyelitis; comparative results with four strains of the virus. *J. Exp. Med.* **61:**447–464.
158. **Paul, J. R., J. D. Trask, and C. S. Culotta.** 1939. Poliomyelitic virus in sewage. *Science* **90:**258–259.
159. **Peabody, F. W., G. Draper, and A. R. Dochez.** 1912. *A Clinical Study of Acute Poliomyelitis.* Monograph no. 4. Rockefeller Institute of Medical Research, New York.
160. **Plotkin, S. A., M. Katz, R. E. Brown, and J. S. Pagano.** 1966. Oral poliovirus vaccination in newborn African infants. The inhibitory effect of breast-feeding. *Am. J. Dis. Child.* **111:**27–30.
161. **Pohl, J. F., and E. Kenny.** 1943. *The Kenny Concept of Infantile Paralysis and Its Treatment.* Bruce, Minneapolis.
162. **Prevots, D. R., R. W. Sutter, P. M. Strebel, R. E. Weibel, and S. L. Cochi.** 1994. Completeness of reporting for paralytic poliomyelitis, United States, 1980 through 1991. *Arch. Pediatr. Adolesc. Med.* **148:**479–485.
163. **Putnam, J. J., and E. W. Taylor.** 1893. Is acute poliomyelitis unusually prevalent this season. *Boston Med. Surg. J.* **129:**509–519.
164. **Ramlow, J., M. Alexander, and R. LaPorte.** 1992. Epidemiology of the postpolio syndrome. *Am. J. Epidemiol.* **136:**769–786.
165. **Ren, R., and V. R. Rancaniello.** 1992. Poliovirus spreads from muscle to the central nervous system by neural pathways. *J. Infect. Dis.* **166:**747–752.
166. **Rennels, M.** 1994. Concurrent administration of oral rhesus rotavirus reassortant vaccines (at 4×10^5 pfu) and OPV did not result in significant immune interference, abstr. H62. *Abstr. 34th Intersci. Conf. Antimicrob. Agents Chemother.*
167. **Richardson, G., R. Linkins, and M. Eames.** 1993. Immunogenicity of oral poliovirus vaccine (OPV) given in mass campaigns versus routine immunization programs, abstr. 1237. *Program Abstr. 33rd Intersci. Conf. Antimicrob. Agents Chemother.*
168. **Risi, J. B.** 1984. The control of poliomyelitis in Brazil. *Rev. Infect. Dis.* **6(2):**400–403.
169. **Rissler, J.** 1888. Zur Kenntniss der Veranderungen des Nervensystems bei Poliomyelitis anterior acuta. *Nord. Med. Ark.* **20:**1.
170. **Robertson, H. E.** 1962. Community-wide use of a "balanced" trivalent oral poliovirus vaccine (Sabin). *Can. J. Public Health* **53:**179–191.
171. **Robertson, S. E., H. P. Traverso, J. A. Drucker, et al.** 1988. Clinical efficacy of a new, enhanced-potency, inactivated poliovirus vaccine. *Lancet* **i:**897–899.
172. **Rockefeller Foundation.** 1984. *Protecting the World's Children: Vaccines and Immunization.* Rockefeller Foundation, Bellagio, Italy.
173. **Russell, W. R.** 1947. Poliomyelitis: the preparalytic stage, and the effect of physical activity on the severity of paralysis. *Br. Med. J.* **2:**1023.
174. **Russell, W. R.** 1949. Paralytic poliomyelitis: the early symptoms, and the effect of physical activity on the course of disease. *Br. Med. J.* **1:**465.
175. **Russell, W. R., and M. Fischer-Williams.** 1954. Recovery of muscular strength after poliomyelitis. *Lancet* **i:**330.
176. **Sabin, A. B.** 1955. Behavior of chimpanzee-avirulent poliomyelitis viruses in experimentally infected human volunteers. *Am. J. Med. Sci.* **230:**1.
177. **Sabin, A. B.** 1957. Properties and behavior of orally administered attenuated poliovirus vaccine. *JAMA* **164:**1216–1223.
178. **Sabin, A. B.** 1984. Strategies for elimination of poliomyelitis in different parts of the world with use of oral poliovirus vaccine. *Rev. Infect. Dis.* **6(2):**391–396.
179. **Sabin, A. B.** 1985. Oral polio vaccine: history of its development and use and current challenge to eliminate poliomyelitis from the world. *J. Infect. Dis.* **151:**420–436.
180. **Sabin, A. B.** 1987. Commentary: is there a need for a change in poliomyelitis immunization policy? *Pediatr. Infect. Dis. J.* **6:**887–889.
181. **Sabin, A. B., and P. K. Olitsky.** 1936. Cultivation of poliovirus *in vitro* in human embryonic nervous tissue. *Proc. Soc. Exp. Biol. Med.* **34:**357–359.
182. **Sabin, A. B., and R. Ward.** 1941. Flies as carriers in human poliomyelitis virus. *Science* **94:**590.
183. **Salk, D.** 1980. Eradication of poliomyelitis in the United States. II. Experience with killed poliovirus vaccine. *Rev. Infect. Dis.* **2:**243–257.

184. **Salk, J.** 1987. Commentary: poliomyelitis vaccination—choosing a wise policy? *Pediatr. Infect. Dis. J.* **6:**889–893.
185. **Salk, J. E.** 1953. Studies in human subjects on active immunization against poliomyelitis. I. A preliminary report of experiments in progress. *JAMA* **151:**1081–1098.
186. **Schaap, G. J. P., H. Bijkerk, and R. A. Coutinho.** 1984. The spread of wild poliovirus in the well-vaccinated Netherlands in connection with the 1978 epidemic. *Prog. Med. Virol.* **29:**124–140.
187. **Schoub, B. D.** 1992. Poliomyelitis outbreak in Natal/KwaZulu, South Africa, 1987–1988. II. Immunity aspects. *Trans. R. Soc. Trop. Med. Hyg.* **86:**83–85.
188. **Shindarov, L. M., M. P. Chumakov, and M. K. Voroshilova.** 1979. Epidemiological, clinical, and pathomorphological characteristics of epidemic poliomyelitis-like disease caused by enterovirus 71. *J. Hyg. Epidemiol. Microbiol. Immunol.* **23:**284.
189. **Siegel, M., and M. Greenberg.** 1956. Poliomyelitis in pregnancy: effect on fetus and newborn infant. *J. Pediatr.* **49:**280–288.
190. **Simoes, E. A., and T. J. John.** 1986. The antibody response of seronegative infants to inactivated poliovirus vaccine of enhanced potency. *J. Biol. Stand.* **14:**127–131.
191. **Simoes, E. A. F., B. Padmini, M. C. Steinhoff, M. Jadhav, and T. J. John.** 1995. Antibody response of infants to two doses of inactivated poliovirus vaccine of enhanced potency. *Am. J. Dis. Child.* **139:**977–980.
192. **Sokhey, J., C. K. Gupta, B. Sharma, and H. Singh.** 1988. Stability of oral polio vaccine at different temperatures. *Vaccine* **6:**12–13.
193. **Stanway, G., P. J. Hughes, R. C. Mountford, et al.** 1984. Comparison of the complete nucleotide sequences of the genomes of the neurovirulent poliovirus P3/Leon/37 and its attenuated Sabin vaccine derivative P3/Leon 12a1b. *Proc. Natl. Acad. Sci. USA* **81:**1539–1543.
194. **Stickle, G.** 1964. Observed and expected poliomyelitis in the United States, 1958–1961. *Am. J. Public Health* **1964:**1222–1229.
195. **Strebel, P. M., R. W. Sutter, and S. L. Cochi.** 1992. Epidemiology of poliomyelitis in the United States one decade after the last reported case of indigenous wild virus-associated disease. *Clin. Infect. Dis.* **14:**568–579.
196. **Sutter, R. W.** 1991. An outbreak of paralytic poliomyelitis in Oman: evidence for widespread transmission among fully vaccinated children. *Lancet* **338:**715–720.
197. **Sutter, R. W.** 1992. Attributable risk of DTP (diphtheria and tetanus toxins and pertussis vaccine) injection in provoking paralytic poliomyelitis during a large outbreak in Oman. *J. Infect. Dis.* **165:**444–449.
198. **Swartz, T. A., E. Ben-Porath, Z. Ben-Yshai, et al.** 1981. A controlled trial with inactivated poliovaccine. *Dev. Biol. Stand.* **47:**199–206.
199. **Swartz, T. A., M. Roumiantzeff, L. Peyron, et al.** 1986. Use of a combined DTP-polio vaccine in a reduced schedule. *Dev. Biol. Stand.* **65:**159–166.
200. **Taylor, E., and H. L. Amoss.** 1917. Carriage of the virus of poliomyelitis, with subsequent development of the infection. *J. Exp. Med.* **26:**745–754.
201. **The Committee on Typing of the National Foundation for Infantile Paralysis.** 1951. A cooperative program for the typing of one hundred strains. *Am. J. Hyg.* **54:**191–274.
202. **Tisdall, F. F., A. Brown, R. D. deFries, M. A. Ross, and A. H. Sellers.** 1937. Zinc sulphate nasal spray in the prophylaxis of poliomyelitis; observations of a group of 4,713 children age 3–10 years, during an epidemic in Toronto. *Can. J. Public Health* **28:**523.
203. **Trask, J. D., A. J. Vignec, and J. R. Paul.** 1937. Isolation of poliomyelitis virus from human stools. *Proc. Soc. Exp. Biol. Med.* **38:**147–149.
204. **Trueta, J., and R. Hodes.** 1954. Provoking and localizing factors in poliomyelitis. *Lancet* **1:**998.
205. **Turner, T. B., L. E. Young, and E. S. Maxwell.** 1945. Mouse-adapted Lansing strain of poliomyelitis virus: neutralizing antibodies in serum of healthy children. *Am. J. Hyg.* **42:**119–127.
206. **Underwood, M.** 1789. *A Treatise on Diseases of Children with General Directions for the Management of Infants from the Birth*, 2nd ed. Mathews, London.
207. **Vermont State Department of Public Health.** 1924. *Infantile Paralysis in Vermont*. Vermont Printing Co., Brattleboro.
208. **Voroshilova, M. K., and M. P. Chumakov.** 1959. Poliomyelitis-like properties of AB-IV-coxsackie A7 group of viruses. *Prog. Med. Virol.* **2:**106.
209. **Ward, R., D. M. Horstmann, and J. L. Melnick.** 1946. The isolation of poliovirus from human extra-neural sources; search for virus in the blood of patients. *J. Clin. Invest.* **25:**284–286.
210. **Ward, R., J. L. Melnick, and D. M. Horstmann.** 1945. Poliomyelitis virus in fly-contaminated food collected at an epidemic.

211. **Wehrle, P. F., O. Carbonaro, and P. A. Day.** 1961. Transmission of polioviruses. III. Prevalence of polioviruses in pharyngeal secretions of infected household contacts of patients with clinical disease. *Pediatrics* **27**:762–764.
212. **Wehrle, P. F., R. Reichert, and O. Carbonaro.** 1958. Influence of prior active immunization on the presence of poliomyelitis virus in the pharynx and stools of family contacts of patients with paralytic poliomyelitis. *Pediatrics* **21**:353–361.
213. **Weinstein, L., W. L. Aycock, and R. F. Feemster.** 1951. Relation of sex, pregnancy, and menstruation to susceptibility in poliomyelitis. *N. Engl. J. Med.* **245**:54.
214. **Weinstein, L., A. Shelokov, and R. Seltser.** 1952. A comparison of the clinical features of poliomyelitis in adults and children. *N. Engl. J. Med.* **246**:296.
215. **Wernstedt, W.** 1912. Some epidemiologic experiences from the great epidemic of infantile paralysis which occurred in Sweden in 1911. *Commun. Inst. Med. Etat Stockholm* **3**:235–267.
216. **WHO Collaborative Study Group on Oral Poliovirus Vaccine.** 1992. Effect of diarrhea on seroconversion to oral poliovirus vaccine, abstr. 1401. *Program Abstr. 32nd Intersci. Conf. Antimicrob. Agents Chemother.*
217. **WHO Collaborative Study Group on Oral Poliovirus Vaccine.** 1992. A randomized trial of alternative formulations of oral poliovirus vaccine (OPV) in Brazil and The Gambia, abstr. 916. *Program Abstr. 32nd Intersci. Conf. Antimicrob. Agents Chemother.*
218. **WHO Collaborative Study Group on Oral Poliovirus Vaccine.** 1993. Effect of secondary spread of oral polio vaccine (OPV) virus on seroconversion rates to poliovirus in Brazil and The Gambia, abstr. 1428. *Program Abstr. 33rd Intersci. Conf. Antimicrob. Agents Chemother.*
219. **Wickman, I.** 1907. Beiträge zur Kenntnis der Heine-Medinschen Krankheit (Poliomyelitis acuta und verwandter Erkrankungen). Karger, Berlin.
220. **World Health Organization.** 1988. Global eradication of poliomyelitis by the year 2000. *Weekly Epidemiol. Rec. W.H.O.* **63**:161–162.
221. **Wright, P. F., R. J. Kim-Farley, C. A. de Quadros, et al.** 1991. Strategies for the global eradication of poliomyelitis by the year 2000. *N. Engl. J. Med.* **325**:1774–1779.
222. **Wyatt, H. V.** 1973. Poliomyelitis in hypogammaglobulinemics. *J. Infect. Dis.* **128**:802.
223. **Wyatt, H. V.** 1975. Risk of live poliovirus in immunodeficient children. *J. Pediatr.* **87**:152.

PERINATAL ENTEROVIRUS INFECTIONS

Mark J. Abzug

10

Neonates represent a population at great risk for severe enteroviral disease. In addition, the potential adverse effects of enteroviral infections during pregnancy—for the pregnant woman, the placenta, and the fetus—are beginning to be understood. Polioviruses were the first enteroviruses to be recognized as a concern during pregnancy and the first month of life; subsequently, the pathogenicity of the nonpoliovirus enteroviruses during this high-risk period has also been appreciated. This chapter summarizes information about the effects of enteroviral infections during gestation and the neonatal period.

EPIDEMIOLOGY

In the prevaccine era, paralytic poliomyelitis occurred during pregnancy in apparent excess of age-adjusted expected rates, suggesting a predisposition among pregnant women (10, 13, 18, 44, 61, 123). This increased rate was not associated with a specific trimester. Mortality from poliomyelitis among pregnant women was higher than that among nonpregnant females in some series but not others and was greatest in the last trimester of gestation

and in the puerperium in some series (18, 61). Sequelae, including residual paralysis, among survivors were similar to those among nonpregnant women (18). Although poliovirus infection of the fetus has been documented, examples of fetal poliovirus infection or abnormal fetal development due to poliovirus infection were infrequent. More common was an indirect effect of maternal poliomyelitis on the health of the fetus, occasionally leading to fetal wastage, particularly in the first two trimesters (13, 18, 23, 32, 44, 61, 128). An increased incidence of premature delivery was also correlated with maternal poliomyelitis (113).

A high rate of neonatal poliomyelitis occurred following exposure to mothers who had poliomyelitis during the period from 1 week prior to delivery to 4 weeks after delivery; the incidence of clinical poliomyelitis in neonates born to mothers with poliomyelitis at delivery was nearly 40% (128). The incubation period was often shorter (<11 days) than in typical acquired poliomyelitis (128). A minority of affected newborns had symptoms at birth or at less than 5 days of age, suggesting intrauterine infection (14, 18, 32). The remainder presumably acquired infection via contact with maternal blood or secretions at or following delivery. Nonmaternal sources of

---

Mark J. Abzug, Department of Pediatrics, Section of Infectious Diseases, University of Colorado School of Medicine, and The Children's Hospital, Denver, Colorado 80218.

neonatal infection were also occasionally implicated (114). Although relatively high transmission rates were observed in neonates born to mothers with symptoms of poliomyelitis near the time of delivery (18, 114), neonatal poliomyelitis in the absence of concurrent maternal disease or following maternal disease with onset more than 7 days prior to delivery was relatively uncommon (<0.01% incidence) (128) and was generally associated with a longer incubation period (11 to 28 days). Neonatal poliomyelitis overall was relatively uncommon compared to the incidence of poliomyelitis in later childhood; this relative rarity was perhaps related to protection by maternal antibody. Neonatal poliomyelitis is currently extremely uncommon in countries with widespread vaccination but continues to occur in regions with underimmunized populations (128).

Infections of pregnant women by the nonpoliovirus enteroviruses occur frequently. In a seroepidemiologic study, Brown and Karunas found a 42% rate of infection during pregnancy in a population evaluated prospectively over a 10-year period, and many of the infections were asymptomatic (28). Sever et al. serologically identified a 9% incidence of coxsackie B virus infection during pregnancy (111). Cherry et al. isolated enteroviruses from throat or rectal specimens of 4% of pregnant women near the time of delivery during summer and fall (the peak incidence period in Northern Hemisphere temperate climates) and documented maternal serologic evidence of enteroviral infection in 25% of pregnant women during the 3-month period before and after delivery. Neonatal infections were identified by culture in 5% of infants and by serology in 7% of infants; both symptomatic and asymptomatic maternal and neonatal infections were observed (34). Although maternal vaginal cultures were negative in this study, growth of enteroviruses from cervical specimens of ill pregnant women and of mothers of infected sick newborns has been documented (71, 104, 105). Amstey et al. reported a 10-year retrospective review of virology laboratory data that showed that 7.7% of documented enteroviral infections occurred in individuals ≥17 years of age, with 90% of these occurring in the childbearing years between 17 and 39. Fourteen of the 40 infections identified in adult females, including 3 with growth of enteroviruses from cervical specimens, were in pregnant women. None of the neonates born to these 14 women had demonstrable sequelae of the maternal infections (9). Other studies documented a 3 to 4% prevalence of echovirus excretion among adults of childbearing age or in pregnant women during community outbreaks; this excretion was frequently associated with minimal or no symptoms (85). In addition to maternal shedding in the cervix, rectum, and throat, potential sources of exposure of neonates to enteroviruses include other family members and nursery contacts. Abzug et al. reported high rates of viral illness in the peripartum period among family contacts of a group of enterovirus-infected neonates, including mothers (65%), siblings (58%), and fathers (14%) (5).

Numerous episodes of sporadic nosocomial transmission in hospital nurseries and nursery outbreaks of enterovirus infections (echoviruses and coxsackieviruses) that resulted in symptomatic (commonly, respiratory, gastrointestinal, or neurologic symptoms) and asymptomatic infections in full-term and premature infants have been described (21, 27, 60, 71, 75, 84, 91, 93, 100, 125). Coxsackievirus B5 and echovirus 11 have been implicated in several of these outbreaks (27, 71, 72, 75, 84, 93, 100). Rare outbreaks have involved a coinfecting virus, such as respiratory syncytial virus (125). Vertically infected neonates were the sources of several outbreaks, and there was evidence that hospital staff contributed to nosocomial spread; in other outbreaks, infected adults were thought to have introduced virus into the nursery (84, 85). Risk factors for infection in the hospital setting include intensive care, low birth weight or prematurity, and instrumentation of the oropharynx or nasopharynx (27, 75, 100). Nosocomial cases are characterized by later onset of illness, milder courses, and a lower mortality rate than for the index, vertically infected cases (84).

Neonatal nonpoliovirus enteroviral infections are common. Jenista et al. demonstrated viral acquisition in 13% of infants <1 month of age in one community during the summer and fall seasons, with 21% of infected newborns developing illness. Infection was associated with lower socioeconomic status and lack of breastfeeding (68, 69). Enteroviruses were responsible for the majority (65%) of <3-month-old infant admissions to the hospital for suspected sepsis in the summer and fall in the same community (36). Enteroviruses were the most frequently identified pathogen causing meningitis between days 8 and 29 of life in another large series, accounting for at least one-third of all cases of neonatal meningitis (112). Estimated attack rates indicate that the incidence of enteroviral disease in newborns and young infants is comparable to or exceeds symptomatic neonatal infections caused by herpes simplex virus, cytomegalovirus, and *Streptococcus agalactiae* (68, 72, 84). Centers for Disease Control and Prevention surveillance data demonstrated a male/female ratio for symptomatic infants <2 months of age of 1.4:1 (see also chapter 1), with viral isolates being echoviruses in 51% of children, coxsackie B viruses in 45%, and coxsackie A viruses in 4% (90).

PATHOGENESIS

The pathogenesis of perinatal enteroviral infections is incompletely understood. Evidence for in utero infection includes pathologic demonstration of enteroviruses and/or their effects in fetal tissues (17, 29, 46, 63), abnormal fetal development associated with serologic indication of enterovirus infection (28, 49), and documentation of neonatal infection and illness within the first hours of life (24, 29, 71, 72, 74, 84, 98). Pathologic changes and/or identification of virus in placentas suggests that fetal infections may occur via transplacental infection. Placental changes seen with echovirus, coxsackie A virus, and coxsackie B virus infections include placentitis, villitis, villous necrosis, villous sclerosis, intervillositis, decreased vascularity, thrombosis, hemorrhage, leukostasis, and fibrosis (16, 25, 47, 115). Garcia et al. described findings of hematogenous placentitis in 17 of 19 placentas that were culture positive for enteroviruses. Macroscopic changes included opalescence and/or meconium staining of the membranes and umbilical cord and thrombus formation on the maternal surface of the placenta. Microscopic findings involving placentas and umbilical vessels included villous inflammation, villous necrosis, diffuse vasculitis, and thrombosis, similar to findings associated with placentitis from other viruses. In some cases, placental detachment with hemorrhage had occurred (46, 47). Isolation of enterovirus from the placenta without pathologic changes has also been reported (27).

Transplacental transmission of polioviruses has been studied in a number of animal models. Administration of murine-adapted polioviruses to pregnant mice induced high rates of abortion with frequent infection of abortuses but without apparent infection of delivered liveborns (30, 77). Increased susceptibility of pregnant animals to polioviruses was observed in several of these models. Knox (77) found an increase in maternal susceptibility as pregnancy advanced, and Byrd (30) observed a shorter incubation period in pregnant mice than in nonpregnant controls. In contrast, Weaver did not find evidence of transplacental infection or of increased susceptibility among pregnant mice infected with Lansing strain poliovirus (122).

Other investigators have obtained various results when investigating gestational infection with nonpoliovirus enteroviruses in animal models. Dalldorf and Gifford found that both maternal and perinatal mortality due to coxsackie B1 virus infection increased the later in murine gestation that inoculation occurred. Although there was significant mortality among litters born to dams inoculated with coxsackie B1 virus, virus was rarely recoverable from fetuses procured prior to delivery. Maternal infection with coxsackie A8 virus had no effect on perinatal outcome (39). Soike demonstrated multiorgan infection of the fetus with coxsackie B3 virus, with appreciable fetal viral titers, in the latter third of pregnancy, although viral infection was no longer detectable by 6 days after maternal infection. Viral infection was associated with increased stillbirth and neonatal mortality rates (116). Selzer was unable to document fetal infection following maternal infection with coxsackie A9 and A18 viruses in middle gestation and found low-titer transient infection of fetuses after maternal inoculation with coxsackie B3 and B4 viruses. The last two agents were associated with an increased abortion rate (110). Modlin et al. found a high rate of abortion and evidence of placental or fetal infection after maternal infection with coxsackie B1 virus in early pregnancy. After maternal infection in late gestation, transplacental infection occurred inconsistently, and fetal viral titers were relatively low (less than placental titers) and transient. A high rate of perinatal mortality was nevertheless observed, often with viral culture positivity, suggesting infection during or shortly after birth. An increase in susceptibility of dams to viral infection during the third trimester of pregnancy was also observed (87, 88). Gicheva demonstrated modest-titer transient placental and fetal infection with coxsackie A13 virus, with greater fetal titers following maternal inoculation in the last half of gestation (51). Porcine enteroviruses infect the embryo and fetus and induce abortions in swine (40, 62).

In some models in which fetal infection was documented, histologic or anatomic effects of viral infection in the fetus were also observed. For example, coxsackie B virus-induced fetal myocarditis has been reported (108), and Gauntt et al. reported the development of porencephaly in 4% of surviving neonatal mice transplacentally infected during the second trimester with a temperature-sensitive strain of coxsackie B3 virus (50).

Abzug et al. developed a model of gestational enteroviral infection that involved a murine enterovirus, Theiler's murine encephalomyelitis virus, in its natural host. High-titer infections developed in placentas and fetuses after maternal inoculation in early gestation, while late-gestation inoculations generally infected placentas but not fetuses (7, 8). Following early-gestation inoculation, virus was first localized in multifunctional trophoblastic giant cells and was subsequently heavily concentrated in the maternally derived decidua layer, the fetally derived spongiotrophoblast layer, and, especially, the labyrinth, the region of the placenta in which maternal-fetal vascular exchange occurs (1, 8). The normal vasculature of the labyrinth was often replaced by hyaline and hemorrhagic tissue after early-gestation Theiler's murine encephalomyelitis virus infection, with associated infiltration of monocytes or macrophages (2). Fetuses infected in early gestation contained virus in the heart and great vessels, brain, lung, and liver. In late gestation, virus was present in the decidua and spongiotrophoblast layers but was generally restricted from the labyrinth, which maintained normal histology, and from fetuses (7, 8). The development of this placental barrier during gestation appears to be best explained by anatomic factors within the placenta (2).

Although the route of infection of the human fetus has been assumed to be transplacental (129), there is no direct evidence for this (9). Amstey et al. were unable to demonstrate transplacental passage of coxsackie B3 virus or echovirus 11 in an in vitro perfusion system with human placental lobules, despite use of high viral titers in the maternal infusate (9). Alternatively, enteroviruses may ascend from an infected vagina or cervix, penetrate the fetal membranes, and infect amnion cells and/or amniotic fluid. This possibility is supported by the infectability of both amnion cells (9) and amniotic fluid by enteroviruses. Several case reports describe cultivation of enteroviruses from amniotic fluid, often in association with maternal symptoms suggestive of chorioamnionitis and with fetal demise (72, 94, 115).

In a small number of cases of neonatal disease, evidence for intrauterine infection is well documented. Enteroviruses have been cultivated from umbilical cord blood (24, 71), and coxsackievirus antigen was identified in myocardia of neonates dying within hours after birth (29). Philip and Larson reported a newborn who developed overwhelming infection and died within 3.5 h of birth; echovirus 19 was cultured from multiple organs in this newborn (98). Detection of serum neutralizing immunoglobulin M (IgM) antibody on the first day of life was also used to document intrauterine infection (21). On the basis of development of symptoms and/or detection of viremia in the first 1 to 2 days of life, it was estimated that approximately 22% of newborns with fatal coxsackie B virus infections and 11% with echovirus infections had intrauterine infections (12, 72, 74, 83, 84). Likewise, poliovirus is suspected to be transplacentally transmitted in late gestation, but during infection with nonpoliovirus enteroviruses, the placental barrier may protect against transplacental viremia in most cases (18, 32, 84). The majority of enterovirus (poliovirus and nonpoliovirus)-infected newborns are thus presumed to be infected intrapartum or postnatally via exposure to maternal blood, vaginal secretions, or oropharyngeal secretions or feces of mothers or other infectious contacts (61, 81, 84, 85).

An important risk factor for development of symptomatic enteroviral infection among exposed neonates is a low serum titer of maternally acquired neutralizing antibody. Although passive antibody is protective against development of illness, it does not necessarily protect from infection (86, 89, 91, 93, 100). Cord blood neutralizing antibody titers are frequently lower than corresponding titers in maternal serum, and neutralization titers in symptomatic neonates are often lower than contemporaneous maternal titers (4, 58). Studies of mice show that neonates born to coxsackie B3 virus-infected dams had a lower mortality rate if maternally derived antibody was present (87) and, in other experiments, that passively administered antibody protects sucklings from fatal infection by coxsackie B3 virus (101). Passive humoral immunity may also protect against human neonatal poliomyelitis, perhaps explaining its overall low frequency (18) but increased occurrence in association with maternal poliomyelitis at term, when the neonate may be exposed to high titers of virus without benefit of maternal antibody (which either has not yet formed or is delayed in crossing to the fetus) (114). The route of delivery has not been shown to affect the incidence or course of neonatal enteroviral infection (poliovirus or nonpoliovirus); cases following cesarean section are well described (18, 84, 86, 93).

The pathology of neonatal enteroviral infections has been studied in numerous animal models. In several of these, newborn mice were more susceptible to effects of enteroviruses than were older mice (127); neonatal mice inoculated with coxsackie B viruses frequently developed widespread disease with high mortality, while older animals developed localized disease with less morbidity (74). This increased susceptibility appeared to be related to deficiencies in both humoral and cellular immunity in the neonate (101). Coxsackie A viruses inoculated into neonatal mice infected skeletal and cardiac muscle, with inflammatory changes only in the former, and caused flaccid paralysis; in contrast, coxsackie B viruses infected a broader range of tissues, including pancreas, liver, cardiac and skeletal muscle, brain, spinal cord, and brown fat, with inflammation or necrosis produced in most infected tissues, and they induced spastic paralysis (64). Peripheral inoculation of coxsackie B viruses into suckling mice caused myocarditis and destruction of spinal cord anterior horn cells, the latter indistinguishable from the lesions of poliomyelitis (73, 74). Gauntt et al. inoculated neonatal and suckling mice intracranially with coxsackie B3 virus and related temperature-sensitive mutants, inducing hydranencephaly or porencephaly in a high percentage of survivors. Neonates were more susceptible to the effects of virus than were sucklings (50).

Pathology of the human fetus infected in utero with enteroviruses has been described in several reports. Extensive pathologic findings in cases of echovirus-induced intrauterine death included acute adrenal hemorrhage, congestion, cytolysis, and necrosis; hepatic congestion, hemorrhage, thrombosis, fibroplasia, cytolysis, and necrosis; cerebral edema, perivascular lymphocytic inflammation, and subarachnoid hemorrhage; pulmonary congestion and inflammation; and intramuscular hemorrhage. Disseminated intravascular coagulation was felt to play a role in pathogenesis (46, 115). Enteroviruses, primarily echoviruses and coxsackie B viruses, have been isolated from or identified by immunofluorescence, immunohistochemistry, and electron microscopy in placentas and fetal brain, heart, liver, kidneys, adrenal glands, and spleen (15, 46). Detection of coxsackie B virus antigen in fetal myocardium was described in association with myocardial interstitial inflammation and fibrosis, muscle fiber necrosis, and, in one report, endocardial and epicardial inflammation and fibrosis (17, 29). Coxsackie A virus infection was associated with evidence of mild, focal inflammation in fetal brain (subarachnoid space) and heart (16).

Pathologic findings in cases of human neonatal poliomyelitis have included polioencephalomyelitis with inflammation involving the spinal cord and, variably, the brainstem, cerebellum, midbrain, and/or cerebral cortex. Spinal cord abnormalities have included characteristic inflammatory infiltrates and neuronal degeneration in the anterior horn. Significant myocarditis has also been described in neonates infected with poliovirus (14).

Multiorgan involvement has been characteristic of the pathology observed in neonates who died from severe nonpoliovirus enteroviral disease. Common features included pneumonitis; hepatic necrosis; encephalitis; myocarditis; and adrenal inflammation, hemorrhage, infarct, and/or necrosis (24, 31, 33, 72, 81, 126). Virus has been isolated at autopsy from blood, peritoneal fluid, liver, lung, heart, brain, spinal cord, kidney, and spleen (31, 72–74, 81, 86). Hearts from neonates with coxsackie B virus infections showed pancarditis, with cardiomegaly, myocardial fiber disruption, necrosis, and interstitial infiltration by neutrophils and mononuclear cells; virus has frequently been isolated from cardiac tissue (72, 126). Pulmonary findings included interstitial and alveolar inflammation, hyaline membranes, hemorrhage, or thrombosis. Livers from patients infected with echoviruses or coxsackie B viruses have shown central hemorrhagic necrosis with variable amounts of inflammation; hepatic involvement may reflect viral infection and/or heart failure (72, 86). In severe cases, the majority of the liver may be necrotic (63, 98). Giant cell transformation has also been reported (35). Pathology of the central nervous system has included leptomeningeal inflammation; hemorrhage; microglial and astrocytic proliferative infiltrates; perivascular cuffing; and necrosis in the cerebrum (white matter or gray matter), basal ganglia, brainstem, cerebellum, and spinal cord (72, 126). Pancreatic islet cell inflammation and focal necrosis have been observed after coxsackie B virus infection (72, 119, 126), and renal medullary hemorrhage and gastrointestinal hemorrhage have been seen with echovirus-induced hepatitis and coagulopathy (86, 93). Erythrophagocytosis has been reported in association with echovirus disease (93), and splenic necrosis was reported with coxsackie B virus and echovirus infections (24, 74).

The reasons that enteroviruses often cause more serious disease in the newborn (in humans and animal species) than in older children and adults are incompletely understood. In part, this difference may be related to enhanced susceptibility of neonatal tissues to enteroviral infection, as observed in animals. A reduced neonatal immune response may also be a contributing factor (74, 86) (see chapter 8).

CLINICAL PRESENTATIONS

Spontaneous Abortion and Stillbirth

Maternal poliovirus infection during gestation is associated with an increased risk of fetal loss, stillbirth, intrauterine growth retardation, and prematurity, particularly when maternal infection occurs early in pregnancy (18, 61, 114). Fetal loss was greatest with maternal infection in the first trimester, occurring in almost half of clinically affected pregnancies in one series (114), and with severe maternal disease, although fetal loss with mild, nonparalytic maternal illness was also observed (61). Survival of the fetus or neonate could be threatened by compromise of maternal respiration or circulation, particularly in the bulbar form of poliomyelitis (114). Pathologic evidence of a direct effect of poliovirus on the fetus or the stillborn was generally lacking, although poliovirus was infrequently recovered from the placenta and the fetus (18, 114).

Evidence that nonpoliovirus enteroviruses are causes of abortion or stillbirth is derived primarily from case reports; broad population-based studies indicating such a risk are lacking (9). Basso et al. (15) and Garcia et al. (46) reported several cases of abortion between the third and fifth months of pregnancy and stillbirths during the ninth month associated with enteroviral infection; echovirus 27, echovirus 33, coxsackievirus B2, and coxsackievirus B6 were implicated by placental and/or fetal cultures (brain, liver, heart, kidney, adrenal glands, and/or spleen). Nielsen et al. (94) and Skeels et al. (115) described in utero deaths at 28 weeks and 39 weeks during maternal illnesses suggestive of chorioamnionitis; amniotic fluid cultures grew echoviruses 27 and 11, respectively (94, 115). Freedman described a stillborn delivered to a woman with echovirus 11 infection; virus was not cultivated from fetal tissues and histologic evidence of fetal viral infection was not found (45). Brady and Purdon isolated a coxsackie A virus from blood, cerebrospinal fluid, heart, liver, and spleen of a stillborn infant delivered shortly after a maternal influenzalike illness (26), and Batcup et al. isolated coxsackie A9 from the mother's placenta but not from the organs of a stillborn infant following maternal meningitis (16). Coxsackie A3 virus was implicated in the in utero infection of twins, causing stillbirth of one infant and neonatal death in the other (12), and coxsackie A16 virus infection was associated with a spontaneous abortion in the first trimester (95). In several population-based studies, echovirus 9 epidemics were not associated with an increase in spontaneous abortions or stillbirths (19, 82, 103).

Fetal death from coxsackievirus-associated myocarditis has been reported. Bates described a stillborn infant delivered in the eighth month who had calcific pancarditis and hydrops and whose myocardial cells were positive for coxsackievirus B3 antigen by immunofluorescence (17). Burch et al. similarly detected coxsackie B virus antigens in myocardia by immunofluorescence in association with histologic myocarditis in three stillborns delivered at 5, 6, and 8 months of pregnancy and in two newborns who died on the first day of life after 5- and 9-month gestations (29).

Congenital Anomalies

No increase in congenital defects following maternal poliovirus infection has been observed (114).

In the large seroepidemiologic study by Brown and Karunas (28), the overall rate of nonpoliovirus enteroviral infection in pregnancies that produced babies with congenital anomalies was the same as for pregnancies resulting in normal infants. However, serologic evidence of maternal infection with certain enteroviruses was associated with specific types of abnormalities. Fetal cardiovascular anomalies were associated with first-trimester maternal coxsackie B3 and B4 viral infections (frequently asymptomatic), urogenital abnormalities were associated with coxsackie B2 and B4 viral infections, and gastrointestinal lesions were associated with coxsackie A9 viral infections. Despite these associations, no seasonality pattern was identifiable for the birth defects (28). Koskimies et al. identified increases in titer of serum antibody to coxsackie B5 virus more frequently during pregnancy in mothers of children with congenital anomalies than in control mothers, although increases in antibody titer were not associated with abnormalities of a particular organ system (78). Numerous investigators were unable to find an association between maternal gestational echovirus 9 infections during large community epidemics and congenital anomalies in the offspring (19, 76, 82, 97, 103). Likewise, coxsackie B virus epidemics have not been associated with increases in congenital heart disease (96).

Several other associations of intrauterine enteroviral infections and abnormal offspring have been suggested on the basis of more circumstantial data. Gauntt et al. (49) assayed ventricular cerebrospinal fluids from 28 neonates with severe congenital central nervous system defects for antibodies to coxsackie B viruses. The cerebrospinal fluids of four infants (two with hydranencephaly, one with meningocele and hydrocephalus, and one with hydrocephalus with aqueductal stenosis) contained neutralizing antibody; one contained IgM antibody to coxsackie B6 virus. No fluids were viral culture positive (49). A cluster of infants born in a 2-year period in a circumscribed area in Ohio with a syndrome including hypoplastic right cardiac ventricle and associated intracardiac and extracardiac defects was linked to enteroviral infection by the spring or summer conception of the majority of infants, high titers of serum antibody titers against coxsackie B viruses and echoviruses in the local population, and visualization by electron microscopy of possible enteroviral particles in cardiac tissue from one infant (11). Congenital infection with polioviruses and nonpoliovirus enteroviruses has been epidemiologically implicated as a possible cause of schizophrenia, but direct evidence of such an association is lacking (41, 118). Most recently, the PCR has been used to test amniotic fluids for enteroviruses, and evidence for infection was found in several fluids from babies born with central nervous system and/or cardiac anomalies (97a). Only a small number of control patients were tested.

Neonatal Poliomyelitis

Poliomyelitis in the newborn may be difficult to diagnose. The age range at clinical presentation extends from birth to 28 days; the majority present between 5 and 21 days of life. Among reported cases, paralytic disease is frequent, but fever is variable. Other symptoms may include anorexia, lethargy, and, in a few patients, diarrhea. Cerebrospinal fluid frequently reveals mild pleocytosis (≤ 500 cells per mm^3). One-half of reported newborns died, and another quarter had residual paralysis; however, these findings likely include some degree of reporting bias (18, 117).

Nonpoliovirus Enteroviral Neonatal Illnesses

Clinical presentations of nonpoliovirus enteroviral infections in the neonate range from asymptomatic to benign undifferentiated febrile illness to severe disease, with manifestations including sepsis, meningoencephalitis, hepatitis, and myocarditis (5, 84). Most newborns infected with enteroviruses are asymptomatic (68). The majority of symptomatic infants are full term, have had uncomplicated births and neonatal courses prior to onset of enterovirus disease, and become ill in the summer or fall (in Northern Hemisphere temperate climates) (5, 72, 81). Maternal history often (59 to 68%) reveals symptoms consistent with a viral illness, e.g., fever or respiratory symptoms, during the week prior to delivery or shortly thereafter; some mothers have peripartum fever and abdominal pain mimicking chorioamnionitis-endometritis, abruptio placentae, or appendicitis (5, 72, 80, 81, 84, 86). These symptoms may be severe enough to prompt cesarean section or laparotomy (86, 93). There is also a high incidence of viral symptoms in other family members prior to the neonate's illness (5). Onset of symptoms in the infant may occur throughout the newborn period, with some cases manifesting as early as day 1 of life. Presenting symptoms and signs include fever in the majority (often $\geq 39°C$; hypothermia may also occur), irritability, anorexia, lethargy, diminished perfusion, rash, jaundice, respiratory findings (tachypnea, cough, grunting, retracting, wheezing, rhinorrhea), apnea, abdominal distension, and emesis. Rash, usually macular or maculopapular, is a frequent sign (38 to 41%) and has been observed as early as the time of birth (Fig. 1) (5, 81, 83). Diarrhea, while frequent in some series and occasionally bloody or severe, is most often not a prominent feature (5, 72, 81). Central nervous system involvement, documented by cerebrospinal fluid examination or autopsy, is most often accompanied only by nonspecific findings such as lethargy or irritability but may occasionally cause focal neurologic findings such as focal seizures (72) or other specific findings, e.g., bulging fontanelle, complex seizures, nuchal rigidity, or reduced consciousness (74, 106).

Laboratory features may include either a normal leukocyte count or leukocytosis, elevated band count, abnormal cerebrospinal fluid (pleocytosis, with usually <500 but sometimes up to several thousand leukocytes per mm^3 and not uncommonly with a predominance of polymorphonuclear cells; elevated protein or depressed glucose in a minority), chest radiograph infiltrates, abnormal urinalyses, elevated transaminases and/or increased bilirubin, thrombocytopenia, and evidence of disseminated intravascular coagulation (5, 72, 81). Electrocardiograms reveal tachycardia and diffusely decreased voltage in patients with myocarditis (72).

Most patients have benign courses with spontaneous resolution of fever in 3 days on average and of other symptoms within approximately 7 days without significant residual problems (5, 72, 81). Some patients exhibit a biphasic course of illness (72, 74). A minority of infants have more severe and prolonged courses, with complications dominated by single-system disease or multisystem involvement. Findings may include meningoencephalitis, myocarditis, hepatitis, thrombocytopenia, bleeding, and/or pneumonitis (Fig. 1). Encephalitis may be severe, with necrosis and resultant neurologic compromise (57). Myocarditis may occur as an isolated finding or may accompany central nervous system or hepatic disease (80). Manifestations consist of arrhythmias, including supraventricular tachycardia; cardiomegaly; congestive heart failure; and/or associated pericarditis (54, 117, 125). Hepatic involvement may present as acute hepatic necrosis and failure (86). Severe coagulopathy may develop in association with hepatic failure or as a result of disseminated intravascular coagulation (72) (Fig. 1). Pneumonia may be a primary manifestation and can be rapidly progressive (12, 24, 33). Other reported complications include myositis (117), necrotizing enterocolitis (81, 125), and hyponatremia with inappropriate antidiuretic hormone secretion in the presence of meningitis and parotitis (72, 81).

Substantial mortality rates have been reported, e.g., 7% (72), 11% (81), and 63% (84), with 83% mortality in patients with severe hepatitis and coagulopathy (84), although these estimates were generally derived from retrospective data or summaries of literature reports. No fatalities were reported in one prospectively studied population (5). Most reported deaths due to enterovirus infection have occurred in infants ≤4 weeks of age (12). In patients who die, disease may be rapidly progressive, biphasic, or gradually progressive (72). Mortality appears to be most associated with the presence of myocarditis or hepatic disease (72, 84). Cases of sudden infant death syndrome have also been linked to enteroviral infections (90).

Factors associated with severe neonatal disease vary among different studies but include early age of illness onset (particularly during the first day[s] of life), maternal illness shortly before or at delivery, prematurity, multisystem disease, severe hepatitis-hepatic necrosis, positive serum viral culture, specific infecting serotype (e.g., echovirus 11), and absence of antibody to the infecting serotype (4, 5, 72, 80, 81, 84, 86, 89). In some series, coxsackie B viruses have been associated with increased mortality (81). The associations of early age of illness onset and maternal peripartum illness with more severe disease suggest that severe in-

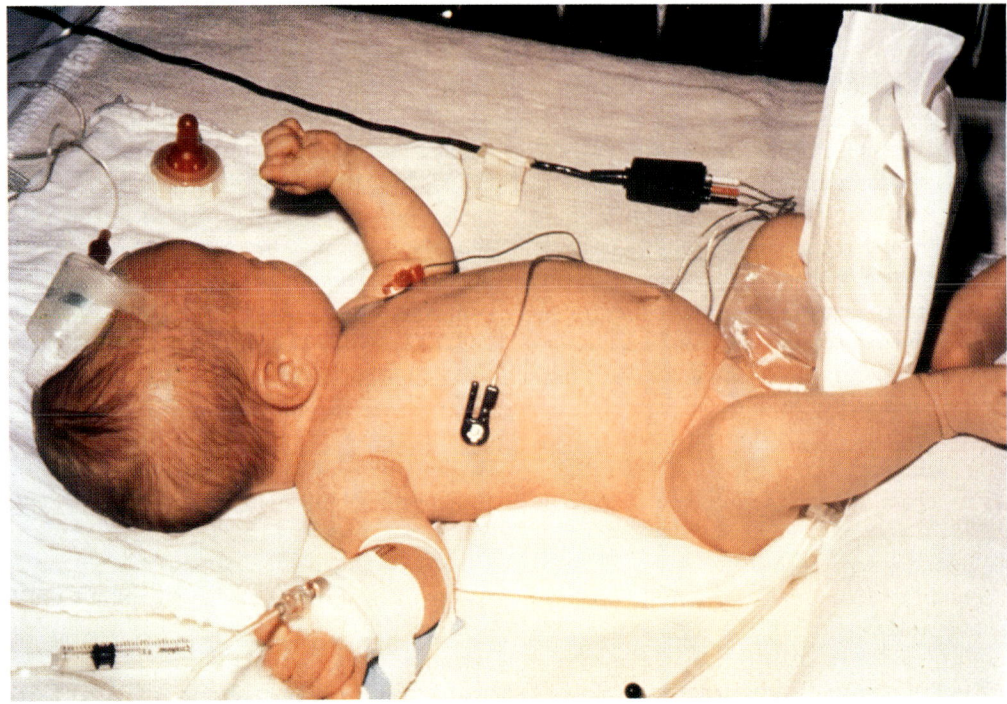

FIGURE 1 One-week-old infant with overwhelming sepsis due to echovirus 11. A typical maculopapular rash is seen on the trunk and extremities. This child recovered from virus-induced disseminated intravascular coagulation, meningoencephalitis, pneumonia, and renal impairment but died at age 3 months of hepatic failure. Infection was likely acquired in utero. This baby is profiled in the preface to this book.

fections are more likely to be acquired prenatally (5, 72, 86). It is unclear to what degree prematurity predisposes to more severe clinical course or enteroviral infections predispose to premature delivery (84). Prolonged multisystem illness beginning at 3 weeks of life has been observed in a young infant with severe combined immunodeficiency disease (79).

Sequelae of neonatal enteroviral infections may include residual hepatic, cardiac, or neurologic dysfunction. Although hepatic disease may persist well into infancy, the long-term natural history of a surviving infant seems to be one of gradual improvement in liver function and normal growth and development (3). Neonatal enteroviral myocarditis may rarely evolve into chronic, calcific myocarditis with chronic heart failure and dysrhythmias (54); however, most survivors of neonatal enteroviral myocarditis do not appear to have long-term cardiac dysfunction (117). Data on the long-term outcomes for young infants with central nervous system infection are conflicting, and most studies have not focused specifically on disease in the newborn period. Some follow-up studies of neonates and infants with meningitis have reported long-term morbidity, including delayed speech and language development; spasticity, hypotonicity, and/or motor weakness; intellectual deficits; seizure disorders; microcephaly; and ocular abnormalities (42, 53, 72, 109, 124), while other studies revealed no sequelae compared to controls (20, 60, 102) (see chapter 13). Infants with features of encephalitis, such as seizures, twitching, decerebrate posturing, or focal neurologic abnormalities, may be at increased risk of sequelae, e.g., decreased intelligence, motor abnormalities, and hydrocephalus (42, 57, 59, 109). One large study of infants and children <2 years of age found no association between acute neurologic complications and long-term sequelae and showed similar overall neurodevelopmental outcome for patients and controls (106, 107). At the other extreme, another study detected delays in development and in receptive and expressive language skills among infants previously infected with enteroviruses, whether symptomatically or asymptomatically, in the neonatal period (67).

Enteroviruses shown to cause neonatal infections are primarily coxsackie B viruses and echoviruses; some data suggest that the echoviruses cause the majority of neonatal disease (85). Coxsackie A viruses are implicated less often than echoviruses and coxsackie B viruses as causes of neonatal disease (81), a fact that may in part reflect the difficulty in laboratory diagnosis of the coxsackie A viruses (see chapter 17). Although many serotypes of enteroviruses cause disease in the newborn, certain ones are frequently implicated, such as coxsackieviruses B2 through B5 and echoviruses 6, 11, and 19 (72, 80, 81, 84, 86). Other serotypes reported less commonly include coxsackieviruses A3, A9, A14, and B1 and echoviruses 2 through 5, 7, 9, 14, 16 through 19, 21, 22, and 31 (4, 12, 60, 72, 79, 81, 84, 126). Disease patterns tend to correlate with the group of infecting enterovirus, but there is a great deal of overlap. Severe echovirus infections are characterized by hepatic necrosis and coagulopathy, while severe coxsackie B virus disease is associated with myocarditis (72, 84, 86). However, myocarditis may occur with echovirus infection, hepatic disease may result from coxsackie B virus infection, and meningoencephalitis or pneumonia may accompany infection by either group (72, 84, 126). It is not known what factors account for the increased virulence of certain strains in the newborn, e.g., echovirus 11 (84).

A number of conditions, such as herpes simplex infection, other viral infections (e.g., adenovirus or cytomegalovirus infection), bacterial infection (e.g., sepsis, meningitis, urinary tract infection, omphalitis), metabolic disorders, and congenital structural heart disease, may mimic neonatal enteroviral infections (5). In patients with evidence of meningitis, diagnostic considerations include bacterial infection, syphilis, toxoplasmosis, rubella, cytomegalovirus, and herpes simplex virus (81). Coinfection by enteroviruses and bacteria may also occur (5, 81).

DIAGNOSIS

Viral culture is the standard technique for diagnosis of neonatal enteroviral infections (see chapter 17 for review of diagnosis). The highest-yield specimens in the newborn are rectum or stool (positive in 91 to 93% of patients) and cerebrospinal fluid (positive in 62 to 83% of patients). Other sites with significant positivity include nasopharynx or throat (52 to 67%), serum (25 to 47%), and urine (24 to 47%) (5, 37, 81). Cultures of mucosal sites may identify either colonized or infected symptomatic newborns; cultures of body fluids such as serum or cerebrospinal fluid are more likely to distinguish infected infants from colonized ones (37, 68). Viral titers of 10^1 to 10^4 50% tissue culture infective doses $(TCID_{50})$/ml in serum and 10^1 to 10^2 $TCID_{50}$/ml in urine have been documented in newborns (4, 66). Echoviruses are more likely than coxsackieviruses to be cultivated from the blood of neonates and young infants (4, 37). Positive serum cultures are also more likely from newborns with early age of illness onset (≤5 days of life) and/or low serum neutralizing antibody titer (4). Cerebrospinal fluid may have a normal cytologic and chemical profile despite being culture positive or may have a profile that mimics that of bacterial meningitis (5, 81). Viral cultures of maternal rectal or cervical specimens frequently yield the same virus as that obtained from neonatal specimens, and maternal serum may contain a significant titer of neutralizing antibody to the neonatal viral isolate (4, 74, 81).

Abzug et al. demonstrated that the PCR (amplification of viral RNA) performed on serum and urine from neonates has a high yield, approaching 90%, which is significantly greater than the yield of serum and urine viral culture (5, 6, 81). This test maintained high sensitivity (and specificity) for several days of illness and produced results within hours rather than in the several or more days required for tissue culture (6) (see chapter 17).

Other diagnostic techniques that have been used with neonates include enzyme immunoassay and counterimmunoelectrophoresis to detect IgM antibodies to coxsackie viruses (43, 55, 56) and neutralization assay to detect IgM antibody to a variety of enteroviruses; the last assay has limited sensitivity and specificity in young infants (48, 99).

TREATMENT

Symptomatic newborns most often require hospitalization both for diagnostic evaluation and for empiric treatment of possible bacterial and/or herpes simplex virus infection, because the symptoms of enteroviral infection are nonspecific. In addition, supportive care may be required for manifestations of severe enteroviral infection (5, 81). This care may include respiratory support, cardiovascular pharmacotherapy, and blood product administration; exchange transfusions and plasmapheresis have also been tried in severe cases (35, 93). Prolonged hospitalization may be necessary for infants with serious disease (5).

Currently, specific antiviral therapy is not available for enteroviral infections, although candidate therapies are in development (see chapter 18). Immunoglobulin has for several reasons been considered a potential therapeutic agent for neonates with enteroviral disease. Absence of type-specific antibody is a risk factor for symptomatic neonatal enteroviral infection, commercial immunoglobulin contains neutralizing antibodies to commonly circulating serotypes, and immunoglobulin has been successfully used therapeutically for hypogammaglobulinemic patients with severe or chronic enteroviral infections (4, 31, 38, 58, 89, 91). In several reported cases, intramuscular or intravenous immunoglobulin was administered as empiric therapy for neonates with severe disease (22, 70, 120, 126). No definitive conclusions can be drawn from these uncontrolled experiences. A small randomized trial of intravenous immunoglobulin (750 mg/kg of body weight) given to symptomatic enterovirus-infected infants in the first 2 weeks of life showed modest boosts of titers of serum neutralizing antibody to patient viral isolates among infants receiving immunoglobulin. Immunoglobulin therapy was associated with subtle clinical benefits without affecting major clinical endpoints. Treatment with immunoglobulin did not reduce subsequent frequency of viremia and viruria in the treated patients as a whole, although receipt of immunoglobulin containing a high titer ($\geq$1:800) of neutralizing antibody to patients' own isolates was associated with faster cessation of viremia and viruria (4). These findings suggest that future studies should evaluate repeated higher doses of immunoglobulin or lots containing high neutralizing antibody titers to selected serotypes. Infusion of maternal plasma, likely to contain a high antibody titer to a neonate's viral isolate if maternal infection preceded neonatal infection, remains an untested therapeutic possibility.

Fulminant hepatic failure due to neonatal enteroviral infection has been treated in several novel ways. Selective decontamination of the intestine with nonabsorbable oral antibiotics was used to reduce endotoxemia (exacerbated by ineffective hepatic clearance), with consequent control of disseminated intravascular coagulation and thrombocytopenia (121). Peritoneovenous shunting was used to control intractable ascites in another patient until hepatic failure resolved (52). Orthotopic liver transplantation has been performed with success; hepatitis did not recur in the transplanted liver despite continued viremia and immune suppression posttransplantation (35).

PREVENTION

Because transplacental maternal neutralizing antibody protects against symptomatic neonatal enteroviral illness, a number of attempts to provide prophylaxis by administering exogenous antibody have been undertaken. This strategy was first utilized during poliomyelitis epidemics, when intramuscular immunoglobulin was administered to prevent secondary cases in hospital nurseries (18). Another approach involved intramuscular administration of convalescent-phase serum containing neutralizing antibody to echovirus 11 to newborns exposed to this virus in the nursery; no conclusions about efficacy could be drawn, owing to a low infection rate among the exposed infants (91). Intramuscular immunoglobulin has also been administered to abort nursery outbreaks of echovirus infection. Concomitant infection control measures, such as restricting new admissions or closing units to new admissions and visitors during the outbreak period, cohorting and isolating affected infants, and using gown-and-glove precautions, make conclusions about the efficacy of prophylactic immunoglobulin in this setting difficult (31, 75, 92, 93, 125). Some nosocomial outbreaks have had no observable benefit from immunoglobulin prophylaxis (75). A number of nursery outbreaks have responded to infection control maneuvers alone, while other outbreaks, including ones caused by echovirus 11, have resolved without use of immunoglobulin or any specific infection control maneuvers except for handwashing and surveillance cultures (65). The latter may be necessary because of the significant rate of asymptomatic infection in nursery outbreaks (125).

Unlike pregnant women presenting with other obstetrical complications, those presenting with symptoms and signs indicative of enteroviral infection do not require emergent delivery unless monitoring indicates fetal compromise or unless obstetrical emergencies cannot be excluded. Rather, because of the importance of transplacentally acquired neutralizing antibody, it may be advantageous for pregnancy to continue, allowing the fetus to acquire protective maternal antibody prior to delivery (89). A strategy of passive immunoprophylaxis of newborns born to mothers with enteroviral infections diagnosed within the few days prior to delivery, similar to what is done for varicella-zoster virus exposure, is a logical but untested approach to reducing the morbidity and mortality of neonatal enteroviral infections (117).

REFERENCES

1. **Abzug, M. J.** 1993. Identification of trophoblastic giant cells as the initial principal target of early gestational murine enterovirus infection. *Placenta* **14:**137–148.
2. **Abzug, M. J.** Characterization of the placental barrier to murine enterovirus infection. *Placenta*, in press.
3. **Abzug, M. J.** Unpublished data.
4. **Abzug, M. J., H. L. Keyserling, M. L. Lee, M. J. Levin, and H. A. Rotbart.** *Clin. Infect. Dis.*, in press.
5. **Abzug, M. J., M. J. Levin, and H. A. Rotbart.** 1993. Profile of enterovirus disease in the first two weeks of life. *Pediatr. Infect. Dis. J.* **12:**820–824.
6. **Abzug, M. J., M. Loeffelholz, and H. A. Rotbart.** Diagnosis of neonatal enterovirus infection by polymerase chain reaction. *J. Pediatr.*, in press.
7. **Abzug, M. J., H. A. Rotbart, and M. J. Levin.** 1989. Demonstration of a barrier to transplacental passage of murine enteroviruses in late gestation. *J. Infect. Dis.* **159:**761–765.
8. **Abzug, M. J., H. A. Rotbart, S. A. Magliato, and M. J. Levin.** 1991. Evolution of the placental barrier to fetal infection by murine enteroviruses. *J. Infect. Dis.* **163:**1336–1341.
9. **Amstey, M. S., R. K. Miller, M. A. Menegus, and P. A. di Sant'Agnese.** 1988. Enterovirus in pregnant women and the perfused placenta. *Am. J. Obstet. Gynecol.* **158:**775–782.
10. **Aycock, W. L.** 1941. The frequency of poliomyelitis in pregnancy. *N. Engl. J. Med.* **225:**405–408.
11. **Baetz-Greenwalt, B., N. B. Ratliff, and D. S. Moodie.** 1983. Hypoplastic right-sided heart complex: a cluster of cases with associated congenital birth defects. A new syndrome? *J. Pediatr.* **103:**399–401.
12. **Baker, D. A., and C. A. Phillips.** 1980. Maternal and neonatal infection with coxsackievirus. *Obstet. Gynecol.* **55:**12S–15S.
13. **Baker, M. E., and I. G. Baker.** 1947. Acute poliomyelitis in pregnancy. Report of thirty cases. *Minn. Med.* **30:**729–758.
14. **Baskin, J. L., E. H. Soule, and S. D. Mills.** 1950. Poliomyelitis of the newborn. *Am. J. Dis. Child.* **80:**10–21.

15. Basso, N. G. S., M. E. F. Fonseca, A. G. P. Garcia, J. A. T. Zuardi, M. R. Silva, and H. Outani. 1990. Enterovirus isolation from foetal and placental tissues. *Acta Virol.* **34:**49–57.
16. Batcup, G., P. Holt, M. H. Hambling, L. M. Gerlis, and M. R. Glass. 1985. Placental and fetal pathology in coxsackie virus A9 infection: a case report. *Histopathology* **9:**1227–1235.
17. Bates, H. R. 1970. Coxsackie virus B3 calcific pancarditis and hydrops fetalis. *Am. J. Obstet. Gynecol.* **106:**629–630.
18. Bates, T. 1955. Poliomyelitis in pregnancy, fetus, and newborn. *Am. J. Dis. Child.* **90:**189–195.
19. Bell, E. J., C. A. C. Ross, and N. R. Grist. 1975. ECHO 9 infection in pregnant women with suspected rubella. *J. Clin. Pathol.* **28:**267–269.
20. Bergman, I., M. J. Painter, E. R. Wald, D. Chiponis, A. L. Holland, and H. G. Taylor. 1987. Outcome in children with enteroviral meningitis during the first year of life. *J. Pediatr.* **110:**705–709.
21. Berkovich, S., and E. M. Smithwick. 1968. Transplacental infection due to ECHO virus type 22. *J. Pediatr.* **72:**94–96.
22. Black, S. 1983. *Program Abstr. 23rd Intersci. Conf. Antimicrob. Agents Chemother.*, abstr. 314, p. 140.
23. Bowers, V. M., and D. N. Danforth. 1953. The significance of poliomyelitis during pregnancy. *Am. J. Obstet. Gynecol.* **65:**34–39.
24. Boyd, M. T., S. W. Jordan, and L. E. Davis. 1987. Fatal pneumonitis from congenital echovirus type 6 infection. *Pediatr. Infect. Dis. J.* **6:**1138–1139.
25. Boyd, P. A. 1987. Placenta and umbilical cord, p. 67–73. *In* J. W. Keeling (ed.), *Fetal and Neonatal Pathology.* Springer-Verlag, New York.
26. Brady, W. K., and A. Purdon. 1986. Intrauterine fetal demise associated with enterovirus infection. *South. Med. J.* **79:**770–772.
27. Brightman, V. J., T. F. McNair Scott, M. Westphal, and T. R. Boggs. 1966. An outbreak of coxsackie B-5 virus infection in a newborn nursery. *J. Pediatr.* **69:**179–192.
28. Brown, G. C., and R. S. Karunas. 1971. Relationship of congenital anomalies and maternal infection with selected enteroviruses. *Am. J. Epidemiol.* **95:**207–217.
29. Burch, G. E., S. C. Sun, K. C. Chu, R. S. Sohal, and H. L. Colcolough. 1968. Interstitial and coxsackievirus B myocarditis in infants and children. *JAMA* **203:**1–8.
30. Byrd, C. L. 1950. The influence of infection with Lansing strain poliomyelitis virus on pregnant mice. *J. Neuropathol. Exp. Neurol.* **9:**202–203.
31. Carolane, D. J., A. M. Long, P. A. McKeever, S. J. Hobbs, and A. P. Roome. 1985. Prevention of spread of echovirus 6 in a special care baby unit. *Arch. Dis. Child.* **60:**674–676.
32. Carter, H. M. 1956. Congenital poliomyelitis. Report of a case. *Obstet. Gynecol.* **8:**373–374.
33. Cheeseman, S. H., M. S. Hirsch, E. W. Keller, and D. E. Keim. 1977. Fatal neonatal pneumonia caused by echovirus type 9. *Am. J. Dis. Child.* **131:**1169.
34. Cherry, J. D., F. Soriano, and C. L. Jahn. 1968. Search for perinatal viral infection. A prospective, clinical, virologic, and serologic study. *Am. J. Dis. Child.* **116:**245–250.
35. Chuang, E., E. S. Maller, M. A. Hoffman, R. L. Hodinka, and S. M. Altschuler. 1993. Successful treatment of fulminant echovirus 11 infection in a neonate by orthotopic liver transplantation. *J. Pediatr. Gastroenterol. Nutr.* **17:**211–214.
36. Dagan, R., C. B. Hall, K. R. Powell, and M. A. Menegus. 1989. Epidemiology and laboratory diagnosis of infection with viral and bacterial pathogens in infants hospitalized for suspected sepsis. *J. Pediatr.* **115:**351–356.
37. Dagan, R., J. A. Jenista, S. L. Prather, K. R. Powell, and M. A. Menegus. 1985. Viremia in hospitalized children with enterovirus infections. *J. Pediatr.* **106:**397–401.
38. Dagan, R., S. Prather, K. Powell, and M. A. Menegus. 1983. Neutralizing antibodies to non-polio enteroviruses in human immune serum globulin. *Pediatr. Infect. Dis. J.* **2:**454–456.
39. Dalldorf, G., and R. Gifford. 1954. Susceptibility of gravid mice to coxsackie virus infection. *J. Exp. Med.* **99:**21–27.
40. Dilovski, M., and D. Ognianov. 1975. Isolation and identification of a virus causing abortions and stillbirths in swine (preliminary report). *Vet. Med. Nauki* **12:**52–53.
41. Eagles, J. M. 1992. Are polioviruses a cause of schizophrenia? *Br. J. Psychiatry* **160:**598–600.
42. Farmer, K., B. A. MacArthur, and M. M. Clay. 1975. A follow-up study of 15 cases of neonatal meningoencephalitis due to coxsackie virus B5. *J. Pediatr.* **87:**568–571.
43. Feldman, R. G., J. Bryant, K. N. Ives, and N. C. W. Hill. 1987. A novel presentation of coxsackie B2 virus infection during pregnancy. *J. Infect.* **15:**73–76.
44. Fox, M. J., and F. H. Belfus. 1950. Poliomyelitis in pregnancy. *Am. J. Obstet. Gynecol.* **59:**1134–1139.
45. Freedman, P. S. 1979. Echovirus 11 infec-

46. Garcia, A. G. P., N. G. D. S. Basso, M. E. F. Fonseca, and H. N. Outani. 1990. Congenital echo virus infection-morphological and virological study of fetal and placental tissue. *J. Pathol.* **160:**123–127.
47. Garcia, A. G. P., N. G. D. S. Basso, M. E. F. Fonseca, J. A. T. Zuardi, and H. N. Outanni. 1991. Enterovirus associated placental morphology: a light, virological, electron microscopic and immunohistologic study. *Placenta* **12:**533–547.
48. Gaudin, O. G., B. Pozzetto, M. Aouni, and A. Ros. 1989. Detection of neutralizing IgM antibodies in the diagnosis of enterovirus infections. *J. Med. Virol.* **28:**200–205.
49. Gauntt, C. J., R. J. Gudvangen, Y. W. Brans, and A. E. Marlin. 1985. Coxsackievirus group B antibodies in the ventricular fluid of infants with severe anatomic defects in the central nervous system. *Pediatrics* **76:**64–68.
50. Gauntt, C. J., D. C. Jones, H. W. Huntington, H. M. Arizpe, R. J. Gudvangen, and R. M. DeShambo. 1984. Murine forebrain anomalies induced by coxsackievirus B3 variants. *J. Med. Virol.* **14:**341–355.
51. Gicheva, T. A. 1988. Modelling coxsackie-virus infection in pregnant mice in long-term experiment. *J. Hyg. Epidemiol. Microbiol. Immunol.* **32:**439–445.
52. Gillam, G. L., K. B. Stokes, J. McLellan, and A. L. Smith. 1986. Fulminant hepatic failure with intractable ascites due to an echovirus 11 infection successfully managed with a peritoneo-venous (LeVeen) shunt. *J. Pediatr. Gastrenterol. Nutr.* **5:**476–480.
53. Gonzalez-del-Rey, J. A., R. C. Baker, A. W. Kummer, and J. R. Schultz. 1991. Neurodevelopmental outcome of infants with enteroviral meningitis in the first three months of life, abstr. 1018, p. 172A. *Abstr. Soc. Pediatr. Res. 1991.*
54. Goren, A., M. Kaplan, J. Glaser, and M. Isacsohn. 1989. Chronic neonatal coxsackie myocarditis. *Arch. Dis. Child.* **64:**404–406.
55. Haddad, J., J. P. Gut, M. J. Wendling, D. Astruc, M. Jernite, G. Obert, and J. Messer. 1993. Enterovirus infections in neonates. A retrospective study of 21 cases. *Eur. J. Med.* **2:**209–214.
56. Haddad, J., F. Keller, U. Simeoni, J. P. Gut, J. Messer, and D. Willard. 1988. Meningomyocardite à virus coxsackie B4 en périnatologie. *Arch. Fr. Pediatr.* **45:**259–261.
57. Haddad, J., J. Messer, J. P. Gut, D. Chaigne, D. Christmann, and D. Willard. 1990. Neonatal echovirus encephalitis with white matter necrosis. *Neuropediatrics* **21:**215–217.
58. Hammond, G. W., H. Lukes, B. Wells, L. Thompson, D. E. Low, and M. Cheang. 1985. Maternal and neonatal neutralizing antibody titers to selected enteroviruses. *Pediatr. Infect. Dis. J.* **4:**32–35.
59. Haynes, R. E., H. G. Cramblett, M. D. Hilty, P. H. Azimi, and J. Crews. 1972. ECHO virus type 3 infections in children: clinical and laboratory studies. *J. Pediatr.* **80:**589–595.
60. Helin, I., A. Widell, S. Borulf, M. Walder, and U. Ulmsten. 1987. Outbreak of coxsackievirus A-14 meningitis among newborns in a maternity hospital ward. *Acta Paediatr. Scand.* **76:**234–238.
61. Horn, P. 1955. Poliomyelitis in pregnancy. A twenty-year report from Los Angeles County, California. *J. Am. Acad. Obstet. Gynecol.* **6:**121–137.
62. Huang, J., R. F. Gentry, and A. Zarkower. 1980. Experimental infection of pregnant sows with porcine enterovirus. *Am. J. Vet. Res.* **41:**469–473.
63. Hughes, J. R., C. M. Wilfert, M. Moore, K. Benirschke, and E. de Hoyos-Guevara. 1972. Echovirus 14 infection associated with fatal neonatal hepatic necrosis. *Am. J. Dis. Child.* **123:**61–67.
64. Hyypiä, T., M. Kallajoki, M. Maaronen, G. Stanway, R. Kandolf, P. Auvinen, and H. Kalimo. 1993. Pathogenetic differences between coxsackie A and B virus infections in newborn mice. *Virus Res.* **27:**71–78.
65. Isaacs, D., A. R. Wilkinson, R. Eglin, S. R. M. Dobson, P. L. Hope, and E. R. Moxon. 1989. Conservative management of an echovirus 11 outbreak in a neonatal unit. *Lancet* **i:**543–545.
66. Jahn, C. L., and J. D. Cherry. 1966. Mild neonatal illness associated with heavy enterovirus infection. *N. Engl. J. Med.* **274:**394–395.
67. Jenista, J. A., L. E. Dalzell, P. W. Davidson, and M. A. Menegus. 1984. Outcome studies of neonatal enterovirus infection, abstr. 808, p. 230A. *Abstr. Soc. Pediatr. Res. 1984.*
68. Jenista, J. A., K. R. Powell, and M. A. Menegus. 1984. Epidemiology of neonatal enterovirus infection. *J. Pediatr.* **104:**685–690.
69. Jenista, J. A., S. A. Prather, and M. A. Menegus. 1983. Determinants of severity of neonatal enterovirus infection. *Am. J. Dis. Child.* **137:**532.
70. Johnston, J. M., and J. C. Overall. 1989. Intravenous immunoglobulin in disseminated neonatal echovirus 11 infection. *Pediatr. Infect. Dis. J.* **8:**254–256.

71. Jones, M. J., M. Kolb, H. J. Votava, R. L. Johnson, and T. F. Smith. 1980. Intrauterine echovirus type 11 infection. *Mayo Clin. Proc.* **55:**509–512.
72. Kaplan, M. H., S. W. Klein, J. McPhee, and R. G. Harper. 1983. Group B coxsackievirus infections in infants younger than three months of age: a serious childhood illness. *Rev. Infect. Dis.* **5:**1019–1032.
73. Kibrick, S., and K. Benirschke. 1956. Acute aseptic myocarditis and meningoencephalitis in the newborn child infected with coxsackie virus group B, type 3. *N. Engl. J. Med.* **255:**883–889.
74. Kibrick, S., and K. Benirschke. 1958. Severe generalized disease (encephalohepatomyocarditis) occurring in the newborn period and due to infection with coxsackie virus, group B. Evidence of intrauterine infection with this agent. *Pediatrics* **22:**857–874.
75. Kinney, J. S., E. McCray, J. E. Kaplan, D. E. Low, G. W. Hammond, G. Harding, P. F. Pinsky, M. J. Davi, S. F. Kovnats, P. Riben, W. J. Martone, L. B. Schonberger, and L. J. Anderson. 1986. Risk factors associated with echovirus 11' infection in a hospital nursery. *Pediatr. Infect. Dis. J.* **5:**192–197.
76. Kleinman, H., J. T. Prince, W. E. Mathey, A. B. Rosenfield, J. E. Bearman, and J. T. Syverton. 1962. ECHO 9 virus infection and congenital abnormalities: a negative report. *Pediatrics* **29:**261–269.
77. Knox, A. W. 1950. Infection and immunity in offspring of mice inoculated during gestation with murine poliomyelitis virus. *Proc. Soc. Exp. Biol. Med.* **74:**792–796.
78. Koskimies, O., K. Lapinleimu, and L. Saxén. 1978. Infections and other maternal factors as risk indicators for congenital malformations: a case-control study with paired serum samples. *Pediatrics* **61:**832–837.
79. Krous, H. F., D. Dietzman, and C. G. Ray. 1973. Fatal infections with echovirus types 6 and 11 in early infancy. *Am. J. Dis. Child.* **126:**842–846.
80. Kulhanjian, J. 1992. Fever, hepatitis and coagulopathy in a newborn infant. *Pediatr. Infect. Dis. J.* **11:**1069.
81. Lake, A. M., B. A. Lauer, J. C. Clark, R. L. Wesenberg, and K. McIntosh. 1976. Enterovirus infections in neonates. *J. Pediatr.* **89:**787–791.
82. Landsman, J. B., N. R. Grist, and C. A. C. Ross. 1964. Echo 9 virus infection and congenital malformations. *Br. J. Prev. Soc. Med.* **18:**152–156.
83. McLean, D. M., W. L. Donohue, C. E. Snelling, and J. C. Wyllie. 1961. Coxsackie B5 virus as a cause of neonatal encephalitis and myocarditis. *Can. Med. Assoc. J.* **85:**1046–1048.
84. Modlin, J. F. 1986. Perinatal echovirus infection: insights from a literature review of 61 cases of serious infection and 16 outbreaks in nurseries. *Rev. Infect. Dis.* **8:**918–926.
85. Modlin, J. F. 1988. Echovirus infections of newborn infants. *Pediatr. Infect. Dis. J.* **7:**311–312.
86. Modlin, J. F. 1988. Fatal echovirus 11 disease in premature neonates. *Pediatrics* **66:**775–780.
87. Modlin, J. F., and M. Bowman. 1987. Perinatal transmission of coxsackievirus B3 in mice. *J. Infect. Dis.* **156:**21–25.
88. Modlin, J. F., and C. S. Crumpacker. 1982. Coxsackievirus B infection in pregnant mice and transplacental infection of the fetus. *Infect. Immun.* **37:**222–226.
89. Modlin, J. F., B. F. Polk, P. Horton, P. Etkind, and E. Crane. 1981. Perinatal echovirus infection: risk of transmission during a community outbreak. *N. Engl. J. Med.* **305:**368–371.
90. Morens, D. M. 1978. Enteroviral disease in early infancy. *J. Pediatr.* **92:**374–377.
91. Nagington, J. 1982. Echovirus 11 infection and prophylactic antiserum. *Lancet* **ii:**446.
92. Nagington, J., J. Walker, G. Gandy, and J. J. Gray. 1983. Use of normal imunoglobulin in an echovirus 11 outbreak in a special-care baby unit. *Lancet* **ii:**443–446.
93. Nagington, J., T. G. Wreghitt, G. Gandy, N. R. C. Roberton, and P. J. Berry. 1978. Fatal echovirus 11 infections in outbreak in special-care baby unit. *Lancet* **ii:**725–728.
94. Nielsen, J. L., G. K. Berryman, and G. D. V. Hankins. 1988. Intrauterine fetal death and the isolation of echovirus 27 from amniotic fluid. *J. Infect. Dis.* **158:**501–502.
95. Ogilvie, M. M., and C. F. Tearne. 1980. Spontaneous abortion after hand-foot-and-mouth disease caused by coxsackie virus A16. *Br. Med. J.* **ii:**1527–1528.
96. Overall, J. C. 1972. Intrauterine virus infections and congenital heart disease. *Am. Heart J.* **84:**823–833.
97. Peterson, J. C., and L. Glicklich. 1960. The effect of ECHO 9 infection on the fetus. *Am. J. Dis. Child.* **100:**779–780.
97a. Petitjean, J., F. Tron-Laporte, M. Dommerques, F. Freymuth, F. Daffos, J. C. Pons, Y. Dumez, G. Bercau, J. F. Oury, and P. Lebon. 1994. Involvement of enteroviruses in fetal infections, p. 200. *Program Abstr. Prog. Clin. Virol.*
98. Philip, A. G. S., and E. J. Larson. 1973.

Overwhelming neonatal infection with ECHO 19 virus. *J. Pediatr.* **82**:391–397.
99. **Pozzetto, B., O. G. Gaudin, M. Aouni, and A. Ros.** 1989. Comparative evaluation of immunoglobulin M neutralizing antibody response in acute-phase sera and virus isolation for the routine diagnosis of enterovirus infection. *J. Clin. Microbiol.* **27**:705–708.
100. **Rabkin, C. S., E. E. Telzak, M. S. Ho, J. Goldstein, Y. Bolton, M. Pallansch, L. Anderson, E. Kilchevsky, S. Solomon, and W. J. Martone.** 1988. Outbreak of echovirus 11 infection in hospitalized neonates. *Pediatr. Infect. Dis. J.* **7**:186–190.
101. **Rager-Zisman, B., and A. C. Allison.** 1973. The role of antibody and host cells in the resistance of mice against infection by coxsackie B-3 virus. *J. Gen. Virol.* **19**:329–338.
102. **Rantakallio, P., A. L. Saukkonen, and U. Krause.** 1970. Follow-up study of 17 cases of neonatal coxsackie B5 meningitis and one with suspected myocarditis. *Scand. J. Infect. Dis.* **2**:25.
103. **Rantasalo, I., K. Penthinen, L. Saxen, and A. Ojala.** 1960. Echo 9 virus antibody status after an epidemic period and the possible teratogenic effect of the infection. *Ann. Paediatr. Fenn.* **6**:175–184.
104. **Reyes, M. P., E. M. Ostrea, J. Roskamp, and A. M. Lerner.** 1983. Disseminated neonatal echovirus 11 disease following antenatal maternal infection with a virus-positive cervix and virus-negative gastrointestinal tract. *J. Med. Virol.* **12**:155–159.
105. **Reyes, M. P., D. Zalenski, F. Smith, F. M. Wilson, and A. M. Lerner.** 1986. Coxsackievirus-positive cervices in women with febrile illnesses during the third trimester in pregnancy. *Am. J. Obstet. Gynecol.* **155**:159–161.
106. **Rorabaugh, M. L., L. E. Berlin, F. Heldrich, K. Roberts, L. A. Rosenberg, T. Doran, and J. F. Modlin.** 1993. Aseptic meningitis in infants younger than 2 years of age: acute illness and neurologic complications. *Pediatrics* **92**:206–211.
107. **Rorabaugh, M. L., L. E. Berlin, L. Rosenberg, M. Rossman, M. Allen, and J. F. Modlin.** 1992. Absence of neurodevelopmental sequelae from aseptic meningitis, abstr. 1047, p. 177A. *Abstr. Soc. Pediatr. Res. 1992.*
108. **Rosenberg, H. S.** 1987. Cardiovascular effects of congenital infections. *Am. J. Cardiovasc. Pathol.* **1**:147–156.
109. **Sells, C. J., R. L. Carpenter, and C. G. Ray.** 1975. Sequelae of central-nervous-system enterovirus infections. *N. Engl. J. Med.* **293**:1–4.
110. **Selzer, G.** 1969. Transplacental infection of the mouse fetus by coxsackie viruses. *Isr. J. Med. Sci.* **5**:125–127.
111. **Sever, J. L., R. J. Huebner, and G. A. Costellano.** 1963. Serologic diagnosis "en masse" with multiple antigens. *Am. Rev. Respir. Dis.* **88**:342.
112. **Shattuck, K. E., and T. Chonmaitree.** 1992. The changing spectrum of neonatal meningitis over a fifteen-year period. *Clin. Pediatr.* **31**:130–136.
113. **Siegel, M., and M. Greenberg.** 1955. Incidence of poliomyelitis in pregnancy. Its relations to maternal age, parity and gestational period. *N. Engl. J. Med.* **253**:841–847.
114. **Siegel, M., and M. Greenberg.** 1956. Poliomyelitis in pregnancy: effect on fetus and newborn infant. *J. Pediatr.* **49**:280–288.
115. **Skeels, M. R., J. J. Williams, and F. M. Ricker.** 1981. Perinatal echovirus infection. *N. Engl. J. Med.* **305**:1529.
116. **Soike, K.** 1967. Coxsackie B-3 virus infection in the pregnant mouse. *J. Infect. Dis.* **117**:203–208.
117. **Spector, S. A., and R. C. Straube.** 1983. Protean manifestations of perinatal enterovirus infections. *West. J. Med.* **138**:847–851.
118. **Squires, R. F.** 1992. Are polioviruses a cause of schizophrenia? *Br. J. Psychiatry* **161**:427.
119. **Ujevich, M. M., and R. Jaffe.** 1980. Pancreatic islet cell damage. Its occurrence in neonatal coxsackievirus encephalomyocarditis. *Arch. Pathol. Lab. Med.* **104**:438–441.
120. **Valduss, D., D. L. Murray, P. Karna, K. Lapour, and J. Dyke.** 1993. Use of intravenous immunoglobulin in twin neonates with disseminated coxsackie B1 infection. *Clin. Pediatr.* **32**:561–563.
121. **van Saene, H. K. F., C. P. Stoutenbeek, R. Faber-Nijholt, and J. J. M. van Saene.** 1992. Selective decontamination of the digestive tract contributes to the control of disseminated intravascular coagulation in severe liver impairment. *J. Pediatr. Gastroenterol. Nutr.* **14**:436–442.
122. **Weaver, H. M., and G. Steiner.** 1944. Acute anterior poliomyelitis during pregnancy. *Am. J. Obstet. Gynecol.* **47**:495–505.
123. **Weinstein, L., W. L. Aycock, and R. F. Feemster.** 1951. The relation of sex, pregnancy and menstruation to susceptibility in poliomyelitis. *N. Engl. J. Med.* **245**:54–58.
124. **Wilfert, C. M., R. J. Thompson, T. R. Sunder, A. O'Quinn, J. Zeller, and J. Blacharsh.** 1981. Longitudinal assessment of children with enteroviral meningitis during the first three months of life. *Pediatrics* **67**:811–815.

125. **Wilson, C. W., D. K. Stevenson, and A. M. Arvin.** 1989. A concurrent epidemic of respiratory syncytial virus and echovirus 7 infections in an intensive care nursery. *Pediatr. Infect. Dis. J.* **8:**24–29.
126. **Wong, S. N., A. Y. C. Tam, T. H. K. Ng, W. F. Ng, C. Y. Tong, and T. S. Tang.** 1989. Fatal coxsackie B1 virus infection in neonates. *Pediatr. Infect. Dis. J.* **8:**638–641.
127. **Woodruff, J. F.** 1980. Viral myocarditis. *Am. J. Pathol.* **101:**427–479.
128. **Wyatt, H. V.** 1979. Poliomyelitis in the fetus and the newborn. A comment on the new understanding of the pathogenesis. *Clin. Pediatr.* **18:**33–38.
129. **Zeichner, S. L., and S. A. Plotkin.** 1988. Mechanisms and pathways of congenital infections. *Clin. Perinatol.* **15:**163–188.

NONPOLIO ENTEROVIRUSES AND THE FEBRILE INFANT

Ron Dagan and Marilyn A. Menegus

11

HISTORICAL BACKGROUND

Our understanding of the clinical picture of nonpolio enteroviruses is based on fewer than 50 years of research. The era of enteroviruses began when Dalldorf et al. (19) isolated a new virus from the feces of two children with paralysis during an epidemic of poliomyelitis in 1948, in Coxsackie, N.Y. These viruses were subsequently classified as group A coxsackieviruses. Shortly thereafter, the group B coxsackieviruses (10, 38) were discovered; they, too, were recovered from patients who appeared to have poliomyelitis. Additional enteroviruses were soon isolated from patients with aseptic meningitis (35, 37) and from healthy children (24, 26, 37, 42). These novel agents were called enteric cytopathogenic human orphan (ECHO) viruses (9) because their association with disease was unclear and they were primarily isolated from stool. The association of nonpolio enteroviruses with acute febrile illness was still far from being established.

The contribution of nonpolio enteroviruses to acute illness and to hospitalization of children, particularly young infants, has been studied with increasing frequency over the last 30 years. Enteroviruses are now recognized as a leading cause of acute febrile illness among young children and infants and the most common cause of aseptic meningitis in countries that currently immunize against mumps. Despite the importance of nonpolio enteroviruses in the etiology of acute febrile illness in the first months of life, the clinical spectrum of acute febrile enteroviral disease is frequently not well defined and not sufficiently emphasized in clinical practice. Therefore, this chapter focuses on the epidemiology, clinical features, and laboratory aspects of nonpolio enteroviral infection in infants, primarily those less than 3 months of age.

EPIDEMIOLOGY

The epidemiology of enteroviruses in general is covered elsewhere in this book (chapter 1). Infants and young children make up a substantial portion of the enterovirus-susceptible population, because they still lack the repertoire of antibodies acquired by repeated exposures to enterovirus during early childhood. Further, the large number of susceptible children, as well as the nonhygienic behavior common to this age group, favors efficient

---

Ron Dagan, Pediatric Infectious Disease Unit, Soroka University Medical Center, and Faculty of Health Sciences, Ben-Gurion University of the Negev, Beer-Sheva, Israel.   *Marilyn A. Menegus,* Department of Microbiology, University of Rochester Medical Center, Rochester, New York 14642.

Human Enterovirus Infections, Edited by Harley A. Rotbart,
© 1995 American Society for Microbiology, Washington, DC 20005

transmission among young children. However, similar to poliovirus infections, most nonpoliovirus infections are asymptomatic (36). Thus, a multiplicity of factors has to be taken into account when the frequency and type of symptomatic enteroviral infections in childhood are being considered. These factors are divided into three main categories: (i) factors associated with the virus, i.e., serotype, strain, virulence, and inoculum size; (ii) extrinsic factors such as portal of entry and inoculum size; and (iii) intrinsic host factors such as genetic background, age, sex, immune competence, and previous experience with specific serotypes (expressed as immune status). In temperate climates, enteroviral infections occur primarily in summer and fall, as noted in chapter 1. As might be expected, febrile disease in young children and infants follows a similar seasonal pattern, with increased rates of infection among those living under poor hygenic and overcrowded conditions.

Most of the epidemiologic data on disease and infection come from studies of well-defined clinical entities such as acute flaccid paralysis, aseptic meningitis, hand-foot-and-mouth syndrome, or acute hemorrhagic conjunctivitis. However, probably the most common presentation of symptomatic enteroviral infection in young children and infants is simply febrile illness. Because of the nonspecific nature of acute febrile illness, its epidemiology is very difficult to characterize. Furthermore, since more than one serotype may be circulating during one season and since all serotypes can cause a nonspecific febrile illness, more than one enteroviral febrile episode per patient per season may occur, further complicating epidemiologic assessments. This problem was exemplified in a description of three successive outbreaks of acute febrile illness caused by different serotypes (coxsackievirus B4 and echoviruses 9 and 16) during the same season (39, 49). During this outbreak, more than one febrile episode was observed in some patients, with the episodes separated by short intervals and with each one caused by a different serotype.

Only a few studies attempt to define in detail the epidemiology of acute febrile illness in children and infants. In one study, a cohort of newborns in Rochester, N.Y., was enrolled and monitored for 1 month during a single enterovirus season. The risk of acquiring an enterovirus was not associated with prematurity, neonatal or maternal complications, gender, illness exposure, size of the household, or recent use of polio vaccine in a household member (27, 28). The only factors predicting infection were low socioeconomic status (defined by such characteristics as single mother, maternal age of <20 years, and household income) and bottle feeding (defined as lack of breast-feeding). Socioeconomic status was correlated with the lack of breast-feeding, that is, poorer mothers tended to bottle feed, but breast-feeding was associated with lower infection rates within every socioeconomic level. Breast-feeding, however, did not decrease the risk of hospitalization for symptomatic enteroviral infection (27). Among 75 infected infants observed in this study, the only factors found to determine the severity of infection, that is, asymptomatic versus symptomatic, were the virus serotype isolated and the presence of cord blood antibody. The distribution of serotypes was clearly different when asymptomatic patients were compared with symptomatic patients (Table 1). The risk of symptomatic disease varied for each serotype, e.g., 54% for echovirus 5 and 0% for echovirus 22. Interestingly, other epidemiologic (45) and virologic (46) evidence also suggests that echovirus 22 may be biologically distinct from other enteroviruses. It is also interesting to note that three-quarters of the antibody-negative infants with group B coxsackievirus infections and one antibody-negative infant with echovirus 11 infection were asymptomatic. These viruses are the ones most often reported to be associated with fatal neonatal disease (see chapter 10). Apparently, such infections are not invariably severe.

The presence of passively transferred maternal antibody to the infecting serotype clearly influenced the clinical expression of

TABLE 1 Frequency of symptomatic enteroviral infections in cord blood antibody-positive and -negative young infants infected with enteroviruses

Enteroviral serotype	No. symptomatic/no. infected		
	Antibody[a]		All infants
	Positive	Negative	
Echovirus 3	0/3	0/2	0/5
Echovirus 4		2/2	2/2
Echovirus 5	0/4	7/9	7/13
Echovirus 9		1/4	1/4
Echovirus 11		0/1	0/1
Echovirus 13	0/1		0/1
Echovirus 22	0/17		0/17
Echovirus 30	0/1	2/7	2/8
Coxsackievirus A9	0/2	0/5	0/7
Coxsackievirus B1		0/2	0/2
Coxsackievirus B4	0/2	1/2	1/4
Unidentified	—[b]	—[b]	3/11
All	0/30 (0%)	13/34 (38%)	16/75 (21%)

[a] Antibody titers were ≥1:10 (positive) or <1:10 (negative) by plaque reduction neutralization versus the infecting serotype.
[b] Antibody status not determined.

infection in the infants. None of the 13 symptomatic infants had detectable antibodies, whereas 30 of the 51 asymptomatically infected neonates had a neutralizing antibody titer of at least 1:10 for the infecting serotype (28). The risk of symptomatic infection was zero (zero of 30 infected) when antibodies were present and 38% (13 of 34 infected) when antibodies were not detected ($P < 0.001$). The presence of transplacentally acquired maternal antibody thus appears to be one factor but not the only factor involved in averting symptomatic infection.

Enteroviruses play an important role in morbidity requiring hospitalization or emergency room visits during the first months of life. When a cohort of 586 newborns was studied during the 1981 enterovirus season in Rochester, N.Y., the risk of enterovirus infection was 12.8% (75 of 586). For those infected, the risk of admission to the hospital was 21% (16 of 75). Four percent (24 of 586) of the entire cohort was readmitted to the hospital during the first month of life; 66% (16 of 24) were enterovirus positive. Of infants admitted for suspected sepsis, 14 of 17 (82%) were enterovirus positive (27). In 1982, when an active surveillance system was used to determine enterovirus-associated hospitalization rates, 1% of infants born live between June 1 and October 1 in the counties surrounding Rochester and Syracuse, N.Y., were readmitted in the first month of life. Suspected sepsis accounted for 60% of these admissions; a nonpolio enterovirus was isolated in 60% of the suspected sepsis episodes (26a).

Sanders and Cramblett (44) in 1968, and Linnemann et al. (34) in 1974 were the first to suggest that enteroviruses may play an important role in febrile young infants hospitalized for suspected sepsis. This observation was further extended in later studies to demonstrate that enteroviruses are the major cause of hospitalization of young infants (younger than 2 to 3 months) for suspected sepsis during the summer and fall (1, 4, 6, 11, 12, 31, 33).

In a 2-year prospective study set up to determine the organisms associated with hospitalization for suspected sepsis, 233 previously healthy infants younger than 3 months of age with suspected sepsis were studied in Rochester, N.Y., during the years 1982 through 1984 (11). Bacterial infection was found in 19 infants (8%), viral infection was found in 138

(59%), and concomitant bacterial-viral infection was found in 14 (2%) (Table 2). Enteroviruses accounted for 33% of all hospitalizations. Hospitalization occurred in two peaks, the first from July to October (summer and fall peak) and the second from December to April (winter and early spring peak). Enteroviruses accounted for 65% of the 103 infants hospitalized during the summer-fall peak (Fig. 1). No significant year-to-year variations were observed. Although extrapolation to other geographic areas is not automatic, a similar predominance of enteroviruses was observed over a 2-year period among 248 infants younger than 2 months of age with suspected sepsis in southern Israel (10a).

No population-based infection rates have been established for older infants and children with acute nonspecific febrile illness or for children with febrile nonspecific rashes.

PATHOGENESIS

The primary portal of entry of enteroviruses is the mouth (36), and in some cases, the respiratory tract may play a secondary role (7) (see chapter 1). In addition, specific viruses (like enterovirus 70) appear to be spread by fomites as well as by direct inoculation of conjunctiva from contaminated fingers. We know most about the pathogenesis of the polioviruses, and it seems that the pathogenesis of the nonpolio enteroviruses is similar, at least in the initial stages of infection. During later stages, the target organs vary, resulting in the heterogeneous clinical picture associated with nonpolio enteroviral infections (7). The classic description of the pathogenesis of enteroviral infections was provided by Cherry (7) and Melnick and Ågren (36). After exposure, the time to onset of symptoms ranges from less than 2 days to several weeks. It is not clear if and how this incubation period varies among the various enteroviral serotypes. During the first few days, a chain of events occurs (Fig. 2) that begins with penetration to and replication in lymphoid tissue of the pharynx and gut (such as tonsils, lymph nodes, and Peyer's patches). Thereafter, viruses reach the bloodstream, causing viremia. It is unclear whether viremia is in the form of free virions or infected mononuclear cells or both (see below). During stages of the viremia, the patient may be asymptomatic. Viruses thus reach the various target organs (central nervous system, liver, respiratory tract, myocardium, skin, mucous membranes, and others), where further replication occurs. Despite many common clinical features, enteroviruses vary considerably in their organ tropism.

Symptoms usually appear on or about day 3, and their peak coincides with the peak of the viremia. However, organ-specific symp-

TABLE 2 Bacteria and viruses detected in previously healthy infants less than 3 months of age with suspected sepsis[a]

Organism(s) detected	Positive infants		Comment
	No.	%	
Bacterial	23[b]	10	
Viruses	143[c]	61	
Enteroviruses	78	33	Virus isolated from blood or CSF of 48 infants
Echovirus	49		
Coxsackievirus B	21		
Other	8		
Respiratory syncytial	35	15	
Influenza	14	6	
Other	16	7	

[a] The 233 infants were tested in Rochester, N.Y.
[b] Two infants with concomitant enteroviral infections and two infants with concomitant infection with other viruses.
[c] Four infants with concomitant bacterial infections and five infants with dual viral infections.

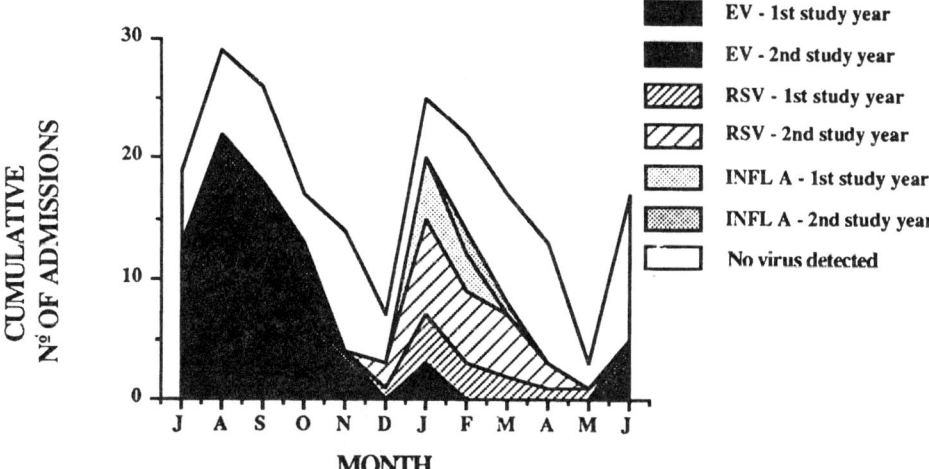

FIGURE 1 Cumulative number of admissions per month during 2 years of study. EV, enteroviral infection; INFL A, influenza virus A; RSV, respiratory syncytial virus. Reproduced with permission from reference 11.

toms, primarily central nervous system symptoms, often occur later during the course of infection, suggesting either that seeding occurs during the peak of the viremia or that for some organs, infection is delayed. This biphasic-fever phenomenon is illustrated in the case of a 5-week-old infant infected with coxsackievirus B5 (Fig. 3). The cessation of viremia correlates with the development of neutralizing antibody, and within a few days, full recovery usually occurs.

Evidence for the association of the peak of the viremia with the peak of symptoms can be drawn from several studies. In a preliminary study conducted at the clinical microbiology laboratory at the University of Rochester Medical Center, enteroviruses were isolated from 14 (45%) of 31 serum specimens obtained from neonates with enteroviral infection on admission to hospital (41). In an extension of this earlier study that was conducted during the summer and fall of 1982 (14), blood culture for enteroviruses was positive in 21 (44%) of 48 of children aged 2 days to 14 years who were hospitalized with enteroviral infection.

There is evidence to suggest that during viremia, enteroviruses are found in free virions and in infected mononuclear cells, which may enhance the ability of the viruses to spread to various organs. In a study conducted to determine the fraction of blood in which enteroviruses are found during symptomatic viremia, enteroviruses were isolated from 11 (39%) of 28 symptomatic pediatric patients (40). In 11 patients with positive blood cultures, an enterovirus was isolated from serum in 7 (64%), from mononuclear cell fraction in 9 (82%), and from granulocyte or plasma-mixed leukocyte fractions in only 30%. This suggests that during viremia, enteroviruses are transported both intracellularly by mononuclear cells (lymphocytes or monocytes) and extracellularly in serum. This notion is also supported by the in vitro finding that nonpolio enteroviruses replicate in mononuclear cells (16, 20, 22). Further, more replication occurs in monocyte-enriched populations than in mixed leukocyte populations (16).

The presence of viremia was inversely related to the presence of enterovirus in cerebrospinal fluid (CSF). As noted above, all enteroviruses are not equal. Group B coxsackieviruses and echoviruses differ markedly in their abilities to infect various animal species, in their pathogenicities, and in their abilities to replicate in different types of cell cul-

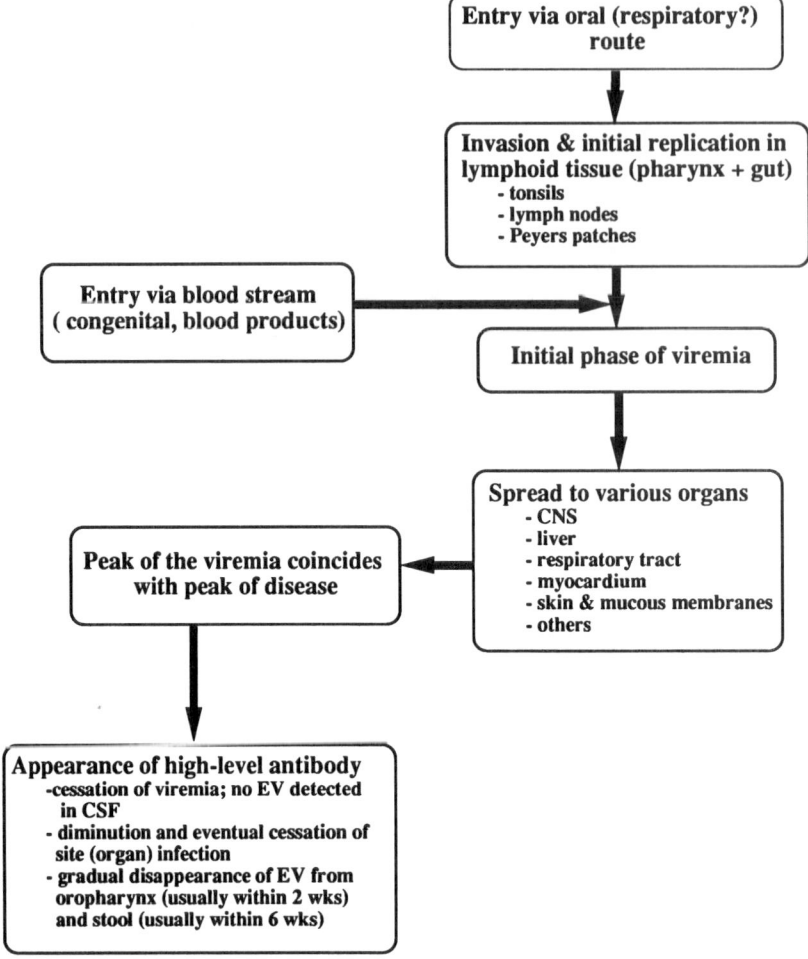

FIGURE 2 Chain of events in enteroviral (EV) infections. CNS, central nervous system.

tures. Therefore, it is somewhat surprising that the clinical picture encountered with these viruses in very young infants is so uniform. When laboratory findings were compared, however, we noted significant differences between group B coxsackievirus- and echovirus-infected infants. The site-specific virus isolation rate, particularly recovery from blood and CSF, was the first striking difference noted (Table 3) (12). Infants with echovirus infection were viremic upon presentation twice as often as those with group B coxsackievirus infection. In contrast, the CSF was virus positive three times more often in infants presenting with group B coxsackievirus infection than in those with echovirus infection. In other words, infants <3 months of age who were hospitalized with echovirus infection were usually viremic with negative CSF upon presentation, whereas those with group B coxsackievirus infection usually had negative blood culture but positive CSF. These results suggest differences in tissue tropism between the two groups. However, exceptions seem to occur. In our series, echovirus 30 appeared equivalent in its central nervous system tropism to that of the group B coxsackieviruses (7, 13) (see also chapter 13).

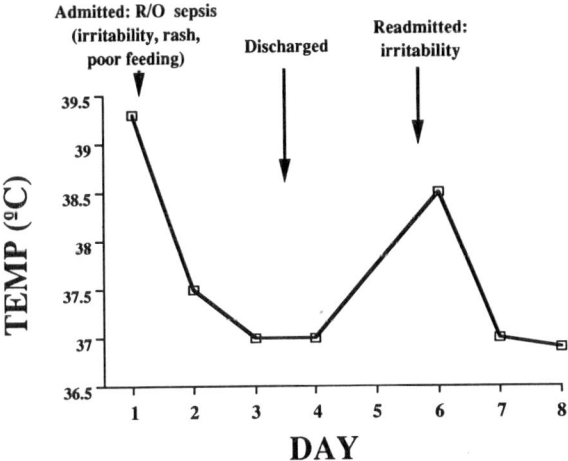

FIGURE 3 Coxsackievirus B5 infections in a 5-week-old infant. WBC, leukocytes; R/O, rule out.

We also noted differences in the blood and CSF mononuclear cell counts between group B coxsackievirus- and echovirus-infected infants (Table 4). Echovirus infections were associated with a low blood lymphocyte and monocyte count and with a normal to very slightly elevated CSF leukocyte count, whereas group B coxsackievirus infections were associated with a normal to moderately elevated blood mononuclear cell count but a distinct elevation of the CSF leukocyte count. The elevation in the lymphocyte and monocyte counts in CSF was more pronounced than that of polymorphonuclear cell counts. Even greater differences were noted when only viremic infants were compared.

The finding that enteroviral infection is associated with depressed blood mononuclear cell counts, particularly during the viremic phase of the infection, is similar to the experimental findings of Gomez et al. (23), who demonstrated a marked decrease in the absolute mononuclear cell counts of mice infected with coxsackievirus B3.

In vivo observations of differences in the ways various enteroviruses interact with mononuclear cells were substantiated by in vitro assays on replication of selected

TABLE 3 Frequency of positive blood and CSF cultures in echovirus- and group B coxsackievirus-infected infants

Type of enteroviral infection	No. positive/no. tested (% positive)		P^a
	CSF[b]	Blood	
Echoviruses	8/36 (22)	43/61 (70)	<0.001
Group B coxsackieviruses	13/19 (68)	10/25 (40)	0.03
P_a	0.01	0.003	

[a]Calculated by chi-square test.
[b]Grossly bloody (≥1,000 erythrocytes per mm^3) specimens and specimens from viremic infants with ≥100 erythrocytes per mm^3 were excluded.

TABLE 4 Blood and CSF leukocytes in infants <3 months of age hospitalized with symptomatic enteroviral infections: comparison of echovirus- and group B enteroviruses-infected infants

Leukocyte population	No. of cells/mm³ ± SD (range) in infected infants					
	Blood			CSF[a]		
	Group B coxsackievirus (n = 22)	Echovirus (n = 53)	P[b]	Group B coxsackievirus (n = 18)	Echovirus (n = 43)	P[b]
Total	13,900 ± 7,600 (5,800–41,000)	8,900 ± 3,000 (4,000–14,200)	<0.005	320 ± 318 (3–1,240)	29 ± 87 (6–439)	<0.001
Polymorphonuclear and band-form cells	4,030 ± 2,242 (1,624–12,710)	4,436 ± 1,828 (1,173–9,504)	NS	85 ± 118 (0–438)	14 ± 52 (0–272)	<0.025
Lymphocytes	7,069 ± 3,720 (1,215–15,244)	3,110 ± 1,658 (476–6,110)	<0.001	69 ± 66 (0–203)	4 ± 9 (0–83)	<0.001
Monocytes	1,614 ± 1,288 (448–6,150)	520 ± 383 (0–1,875)	<0.001	173 ± 172 (0–570)	7 ± 20 (0–162)	<0.001

[a] Only CSF samples that were not bloody (≤1,000 erythrocytes per mm³) were selected.
[b] Calculated by the Student t test.

nonpolio enteroviruses in human blood mononuclear cells (3, 16, 20, 22, 47). Although the methods were not strictly comparable, the data suggest that echoviruses replicate in human blood mononuclear cells, whereas coxsackieviruses are inactivated in these cells. In fact, as shown in Fig. 4 (16), three distinct patterns are observed. In one pattern, titers increase substantially within 5 days. This is exemplified by echoviruses 11 and 5. In the second pattern, titers remain constant throughout the incubation period, as can be seen with echovirus nine and coxsackievirus A9. In the final pattern, titers rapidly decrease to undetectable levels, as with coxsackieviruses B3 and B4.

Thus, we have speculated that the various enteroviruses produce disease in young infants by different pathogenic mechanisms and that, in some way, their interactions with mononuclear leukocytes are key differentiating features.

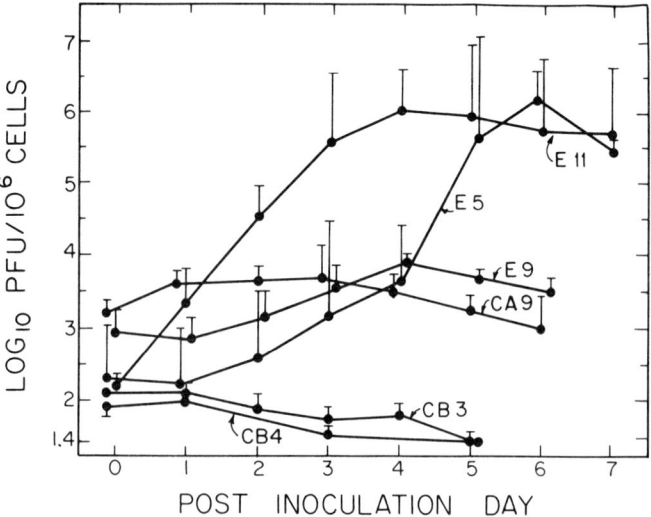

FIGURE 4 Replication of coxsackie virus A9, B3, and B4 and echovirus 5, 9, and 11 in mixed blood mononuclear cells from healthy adult donors. Values are means ± deviations. Reprinted from reference 16.

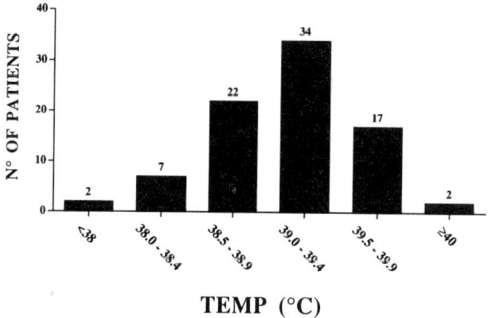

FIGURE 5 Peak temperature on day of admission in previously healthy infants less than 3 months of age hospitalized with enteroviral infection. Data are from reference 12.

CLINICAL PRESENTATIONS

Clinical descriptions of enteroviral disease are frequently developed through retrospective surveys of laboratory data and include children of all ages. Studies of this kind tend to overemphasize severe disease or well-defined clinical entities and rarely address asymptomatic or mildly symptomatic infection. In addition, such studies are often prompted by outbreaks and focus on disease caused by a single enteroviral serotype. For these reasons, our knowledge of the course and consequences of enteroviral infection in very young infants is limited.

Nonspecific febrile illness is the most common manifestation of enteroviral infections. All enteroviral types can cause this clinical presentation, but the frequency may vary considerably among individual viruses. In young children, onset of illness is usually abrupt, without prodrome, and the most common symptoms are fever and irritability (7, 12–14, 17, 32, 34, 44). In older children, common complaints include headache, sore throat (or "scratchy" throat), nausea and abdominal discomfort, a few loose stools, and myalgia. The fever tends

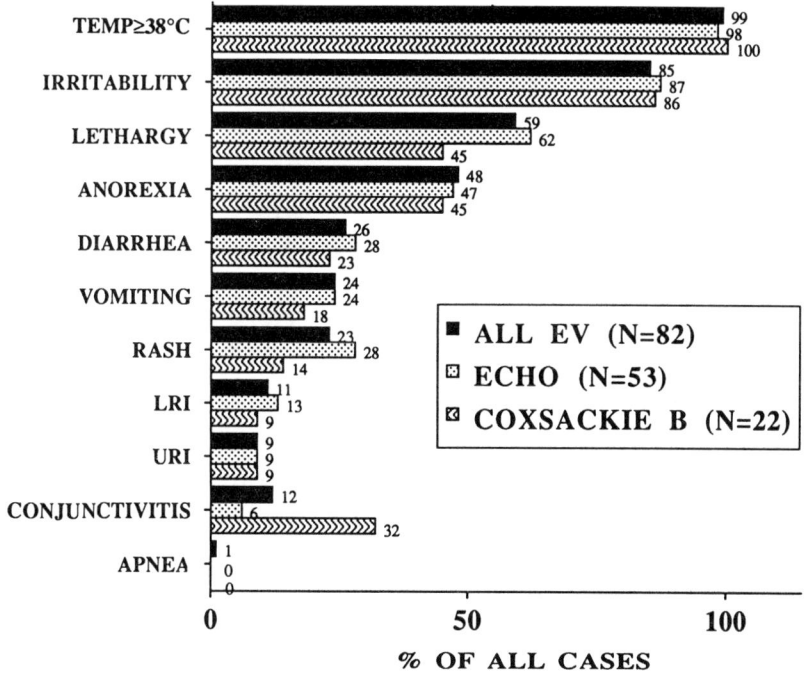

FIGURE 6 Clinical features of 82 hospitalized infants less than 3 months old with enteroviral (EV) infection. Data are from reference 12. LRI, lower respiratory tract infection; URI, upper respiratory tract infection.

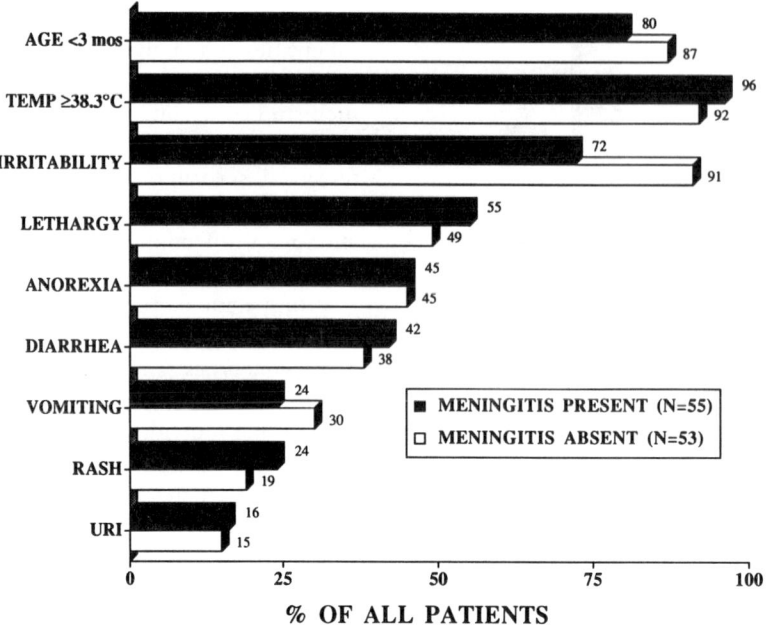

FIGURE 7 Clinical presentation of 108 hospitalized infants with enteroviral infection. URI, upper respiratory tract infection. Data are from reference 13.

to be high. In a series of studies done in Rochester, N.Y., during enterovirus seasons in 1982 through 1983, 62% of infants younger than 3 months of age who were hospitalized with enteroviral infections had temperatures of ≥39°C (Fig. 5). This pattern was also observed by others (7, 32). The fever may be biphasic, with an intervening afebrile period of 1 to 3 days (Fig. 3).

Figure 6 illustrates the clinical features of the febrile infant with enteroviral infection. Irritability, often alternating with lethargy, is the second most common manifestation. Irritability usually correlates with the height of the fever and disappears or decreases markedly within 3 to 4 days. When biphasic fever is noted, irritability usually recurs. High temperature and irritability were also associated with the presence of viremia. In a series of 48 hospitalized children with enteroviral infections, fever of ≥38°C occurred in 95% of 21 viremic children versus 67% of 26 nonviremic children ($P = 0.02$), and irritability occurred in 71 and 41%, respectively (14).

About one-half of the children have histories of poor feeding. These infants typically resume normal feeding patterns within 48 h. Either diarrhea or vomiting is noted in a quarter of the infants; both are generally mild and are not usually the reason for hospitalization. An erythematous macular or maculopapular rash is seen in about one-quarter of the infants. Mild conjunctivitis may also be observed. Signs of upper respiratory tract infection and signs and symptoms consistent with lower respiratory tract infection with or without radiologic evidence of pneumonia occur infrequently.

The clinical manifestations of enteroviral infection are strikingly similar (Fig. 6), despite the serotype-dependent differences in pathogenesis described in the previous section. On the basis of these clinical features, one cannot predict the presence or absence of enteroviral meningitis (Fig. 7). Furthermore, there is considerable overlap in the signs and symptoms caused by the various viruses that are associated with febrile illness in young infants. The distinctive as well as overlapping features of

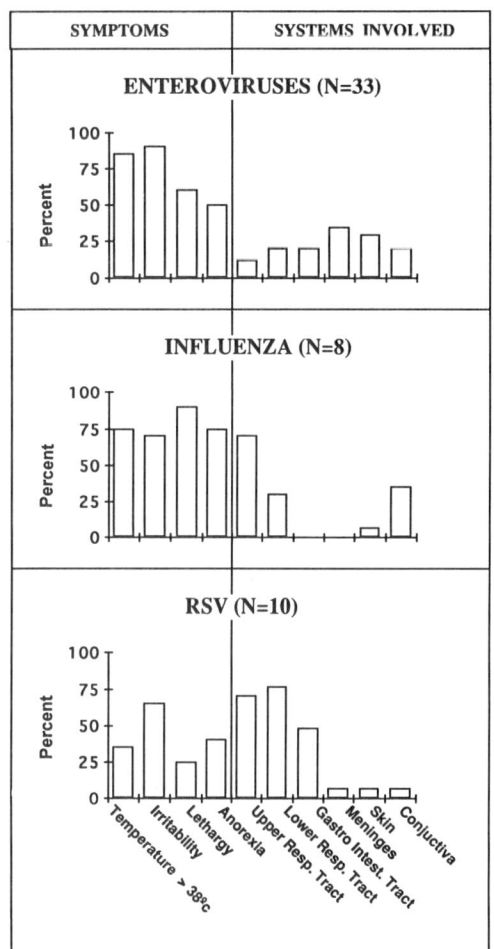

FIGURE 8 Main clinical features and organ involvement in hospitalized febrile infants less than 3 months of age. Comparison is between infants infected with enteroviruses, influenza virus, and respiratory syncytial virus (RSV).

disease caused by enteroviruses, respiratory syncytial virus, and influenza viruses in the young infant are illustrated in Fig. 8.

The nonspecific nature of the illness in young infants together with the high fever and the remarkable irritability prompts the hospitalization of many enterovirus-infected infants, usually for "suspected bacterial sepsis" or "to rule out bacterial sepsis." In most American academic institutions, such infants have a "septic workup," including blood, CSF, and urine cultures for bacteria. Pending these culture results, most are treated with parenteral antibiotics for at least 2 to 3 days. In fact, the majority of infants under 3 months of age who are hospitalized with suspected sepsis during the summer and fall have enteroviral infections, as noted above in the section on epidemiology. It is impossible to distinguish on clinical grounds alone between infants with enteroviral infections and those with bacterial infections. However, an attempt was made to predict the absence of bacterial infections among infants younger than 3 months of age who were hospitalized for suspected sepsis by using the following criteria to categorize infants as low risk: (i) normal blood count and urinalysis and (ii) absence of soft tissue, skeletal, or ear infections (17). Nonpolio enteroviruses were isolated from 42% of 144 infants categorized as being at low risk for bacterial infection but from only 18% of 89 infants at high risk for bacterial infection ($P < 0.01$) (17). Clearly, there is also overlap in the clinical features associated with viral and bacterial infections in young children.

Duration of signs and symptoms in young children varies from less than 24 h to more than a week, but the usual duration is 3 to 4 days. A severe or even fatal course may occur, but this is rare and generally is seen only in neonates infected in the first week of life (see chapter 10).

DIAGNOSIS

Despite the increasing emphasis on rapid diagnostic techniques for direct detection of viral antigens and nucleic acid, virus isolation in cell culture remains the only reliable way of demonstrating most enteroviruses in clinical specimens. Attempts to develop nonculture detection methods are based in part on the belief that isolation is slow and cannot be achieved within a clinically useful time frame (see chapter 17). However, enteroviruses can often be isolated within several days and usually in less than a week (7, 15, 25). Traditionally, two tissue culture systems are used: human diploid

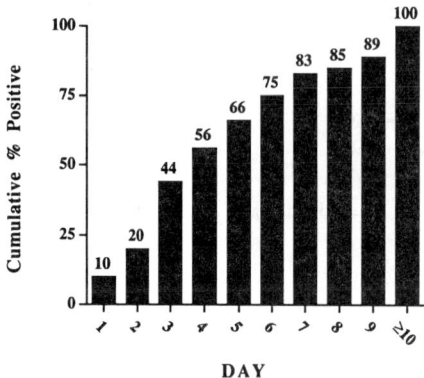

FIGURE 9 Recovery of echoviruses from clinical specimens in combination of CMK, HEL, RD, and GM cells. Data are from reference 15.

fibroblasts and primary monkey kidney cells. During June through October of 1982 and 1983, we studied the impact of adding two new cell lines, buffalo green monkey kidney (BGM) cells and human rhabdomyosarcoma (RD) cells, to the more traditional cell combination (15). Of the 2,558 specimens submitted to our laboratory, an enterovirus was isolated from 417 (16%). Of the 417 positive specimens, 77 (18%) were positive only in the additional cell lines (BGM or RD), and 146 specimens (35%) were positive in BGM and RD cells at least 1 day before they were positive in the traditional cell combination. BGM cells contributed by increasing both the speed and the number of isolations of group B coxsackieviruses, whereas RD cells increased the speed and number of isolations for some but not all of the echoviral serotypes.

The speed of isolation for echoviruses is presented in Fig. 9. Twenty percent of the positive specimens were reported by day 2, and 56% were reported by day 4. The speed was greater for group B coxsackieviruses (74% by day 2 and 95% by day 3) than for echoviruses. Overall, 42% of enterovirus-positive specimens were reported by day 2, and 61% were reported by day 4 when these four cell lines were used (15).

These numbers show that many enteroviruses are rapidly isolated. The sensitivity (defined as the percentage of infants with true enteroviral infection who will be culture positive) of viral cultures for the diagnosis of enteroviral diseases is not known. Some suggestion that culture is a sensitive test in young symptomatic infants can be derived from our studies of infants less than 3 months of age who were hospitalized with suspected sepsis during the months of July through October of 1981 through 1983 (Table 5). The sensitivity was at least 65% in young infants from whom specimens were obtained from at least two sites. In fact, the sensitivity is likely to be higher, since 13% of the culture-negative infants had other diagnoses explaining their illness. Because of the obvious difficulties of establishing the sensitivity of a test that itself is used as a "gold standard," the question of sensitivity is likely to remain poorly defined. Possible reasons for the inability to isolate enteroviruses by virus culture may be low concentrations of viruses in specimens (the nonstool specimens in particular) (5, 48) and the inability of some enteroviruses (especially some coxsackievirus A strains) to grow in the cell types commonly used for culture (36). The PCR in conjunction with culture may be a

TABLE 5 Frequency of enterovirus isolation

Study date[a]	Infants' ages (days)	No. of consecutive infants[b]		Reference
		Studied	Positive (%)	
1981	≤29	17	14 (82)	26a
1982	≤90	46	30 (65)	18
1983	≤90	58	40 (69)	10a

[a]July through October in each year.
[b]Infants hospitalized for suspected sepsis from whom culture specimens were obtained from at least two sites (feces, throat, CSF, or blood).

TABLE 6 Enterovirus isolation from infants <3 months of age who had symptomatic enteroviral infection

Virus isolated	No. of infants	No. (%) of infants positive			
		Throat	Feces	CSF	Blood
Echovirus	53	24 (47)	43 (81)	16 (30)	28[a] (64)
Group B coxsackievirus	22	19 (86)	22 (100)	15 (68)	7 (32)
Other or unidentified enterovirus	7	3 (43)	7 (100)	3 (43)	4 (57)
All	82	47 (57)	72 (88)	34 (41)	39[a] (53)
		74 (90)[a]		56 (68)[b]	

[a]Throat and feces.
[b]CSF and blood. Blood was not tested for nine infants.

more sensitive means of enterovirus detection (43) (see chapter 17).

Other methods of increasing sensitivity include treating cells with iododeoxyuridine (2), inoculating animals (5, 36), and performing serology tests for the enteroviral serotypes prevalent in the community during the same calendar year (5). The specificity of viral culture in diagnosing enteroviral disease (defined as the percentage of infants for whom the isolated enterovirus represents the true etiology of the illness) depends on the site from which the virus was isolated (see chapter 17). The most specific site should be the one that is most associated with acute symptoms. Blood, CSF, and fluid from blisters are generally accepted as specific sites, because virus is isolated from these sites only during acute infection (8, 14, 36). A fecal specimen, on the other hand, is the least specific, especially during outbreaks, because many young children shed virus from stool (21, 30). The specificity of throat culture is not established, but it probably lies somewhere between that of body fluids and that of fecal specimens.

Our isolation rates from different sites are presented in Table 6. As expected, fecal specimens were the most frequently positive. Enteroviruses were isolated from blood, CSF, or both in 68% of patients, providing a specific diagnosis of enteroviral disease in the majority of infants.

As discussed earlier in this chapter, the isolation of enterovirus from different components of blood was studied (40). We found that while plasma with mixed leukocytes or a polymorphonuclear cell suspension provides poor yields, good results are obtained by culturing serum or a mononuclear cell suspension (obtained by Ficoll-Hypaque separation from anticoagulated blood). We compared 51 pairs of serum and mononuclear cells from young infants with symptomatic enteroviral infections. Sixteen sera (31%) and 21 mononuclear cell suspensions (41%) were positive. In four instances (8%), only serum was positive, and in nine instances (18%), only the mononuclear cells were positive. Thus, if the best yield is desired, both specimens should be obtained and cultured.

Using routine virus culture alone, we showed that physicians will act on a definitive diagnosis of neonatal enteroviral disease promptly enough to shorten hospital stay (28). Throat and rectal swabs, CSF, and blood for virus culture were collected on admission from all neonates <29 days of age who were hospitalized for suspected sepsis in the summer of 1982 in Monroe County. Infants for whom a positive blood or CSF virus isolation report was available by day 2 of hospitalization were discharged an average of 2 days before those infants for whom no culture report was known before day 3 (2.7 versus 4.7 days). There were also concomitant decreases in the use of parenteral fluids, antibiotics, and isolation rooms.

In summary, virus culture of specimens from multiple sites, perhaps with the addition of PCR techniques, can provide a sensitive, rapid, often specific diagnosis of enteroviral disease in symptomatic young infants.

TREATMENT

Antiviral treatment for enteroviruses is discussed in chapter 18. To date, no specific antiviral agent is licensed for this entity, which is self-limited and usually benign. When the course of illness seems severe and rapidly deteriorating, immunoglobulin administration (intravenous is preferable when possible) may be reasonable, since neutralizing antibodies to many enteroviruses are present in various serum immunoglobulin preparations (18, 29). Although no evidence exists to show a beneficial effect from such treatment, the administration of serum immunoglobulins may prevent continuation of enteroviral seeding via viremia. When bacterial infection cannot be ruled out, appropriate antibiotics should be administered until bacterial cultures are shown to be negative or enteroviral etiology is demonstrated. Maintaining adequate feeding and fluids and preventing excessive temperature fluctuations are important.

REFERENCES

1. **Allison, J. E., G. L. Kasel, and W. P. Glezen.** 1978. Etiology of suspected sepsis in infants, abstr. 180. *Program Abstr. 18th Intersci. Conf. Antimicrob. Agents Chemother.*
2. **Benton, W. H., and R. L. Ward.** 1982. Induction of cytopathogenicity in mammalian cell lines challenged with culturable enteric viruses and its enhancement by 5-iododeoxyuridine. *Appl. Environ. Microbiol.* **13:**861–868.
3. **Berg, R. B.** 1961. Multiplication of echo 6 virus in suspensions of human leukocytes. *Proc. Soc. Exp. Biol. Med.* **108:**742–744.
4. **Berkowitz, C. D., N. Uchiyama, S. B. Tully, R. D. Marble, M. Spencer, M. T. Stein, and D. P. Orr.** 1985. Fever in infants less than two months of age: spectrum of diagnoses and predictor of outcome. *Pediatr. Emerg. Care* **1:**128–135.
5. **Berlin, L. E., M. L. Rorabaugh, F. Heldrich, K. Roberts, T. Doran, and J. F. Modlin.** 1993. Aseptic meningitis in infants <2 years of age: diagnosis and etiology. *J. Infect. Dis.* **168:**888–892.
6. **Black, S. B., M. Grossman, R. Levin, and R. Manalo.** 1984. Fever in the first two months of life. *Clin. Res.* **32:**107A.
7. **Cherry, J. D.** 1992. Enteroviruses: polioviruses (poliomyelitis), coxsackieviruses, echoviruses and enteroviruses, p. 1705–1753. *In* R. D. Feigin and J. D. Cherry, (ed.), *Textbook of Pediatric Infectious Diseases*, 3rd ed., The W. B. Saunders Co., Philadelphia.
8. **Chonmaitree, T., M. A. Menegus, and K. R. Powell.** 1982. The clinical relevance of "CSF viral culture." A two year experience with aseptic meningitis in Rochester, N.Y. *JAMA* **247:**1843–1847.
9. **Committee on the Enteroviruses, National Foundation for Infantile Paralysis.** 1957. The enteroviruses. *Am. J. Public Health* **47:**1556–1566.
10. **Curnen, E. C., E. W. Shaw, and J. L. Melnick.** 1949. Disease resembling nonparalytic poliomyelitis associated with a virus pathogenic for infant mice. *JAMA* **141:**894–901.
10a. **Dagan, R.** Unpublished data.
11. **Dagan, R., C. B. Hall, K. R. Powell, and M. A. Menegus.** 1989. Epidemiology and laboratory diagnosis of infection with viral and bacterial pathogens in infants hospitalized for suspected sepsis. *J. Pediatr.* **115:**351–356.
12. **Dagan, R., J. A. Jenista, and M. A. Menegus.** 1985. Clinical epidemiological and laboratory aspects of enterovirus infections in young infants, p. 123–151. *In* L. de la Maza and E. M. Peterson (ed.), *Medical Virology IV*, Lawrence Erlbaum Associates Inc., Hillsdale, N.J.
13. **Dagan, R., J. A. Jenista, and M. A. Menegus.** 1988. Association of clinical presentation, laboratory findings and virus serotypes with the presence of meningitis in hospitalized infants with enterovirus infections. *J. Pediatr.* **113:**975–978.
14. **Dagan, R., J. A. Jenista, S. L. Prather, K. R. Powell, and M. A. Menegus.** 1985. Viremia in hospitalized children with enterovirus infection. *J. Pediatr.* **106:**397–401.
15. **Dagan, R., and M. A. Menegus.** 1986. A combination of four cell types for rapid detection of enteroviruses in clinical specimens. *J. Med. Virol.* **19:**219–228.
16. **Dagan, R., and M. A. Menegus.** 1992. Replication of enteroviruses in human mononuclear cells. *Isr. J. Med. Sci.* **28:**369–372.
17. **Dagan, R., K. R. Powell, C. B. Hall, and M. A. Menegus.** 1985. Identification of infants unlikely to have serious bacterial infection although hospitalized for suspected sepsis. *J. Pediatr.* **107:**855–860.
18. **Dagan, R., S. L. Prather, K. R. Powell, and M. A. Menegus.** 1983. Neutralizing antibodies to nonpolio enteroviruses in human immune serum globulin. *Pediatr. Infect. Dis.*

19. **Dalldorf, G., G. M. Sickles, H. Plager, and R. Gifford.** 1949. A virus recovered from the feces of "poliomyelitis" patients pathogenic for suckling mice. *J. Exp. Med.* **89:**567–582.
20. **Denman, A. M., B. Zisman-Rager, and D. A. J. Tyrrell.** 1974. Replication and inactivation of different viruses by human lymphocyte preparations. *Infect. Immun.* **9:**373–376.
21. **Gelfand, H. M., A. H. Holguin, G. E. Marchetti, and P. M. Feorino.** 1963. A continuing surveillance of enterovirus infections in healthy children in six United States cities. I. Viruses isolated during 1960 and 1961. *Am. J. Hyg.* **78:**358–375.
22. **Ghann, J. W., E. C. Hayes, J. Z. Smith, and C. M. Wilfert.** 1979. Echovirus 33 replication in human peripheral white blood cells. *J. Med. Virol.* **3:**291–299.
23. **Gomez, M. P., M. P. Reyes, F. Smith, L. K. Ho, and A. M. Lerner.** 1980. Coxsackievirus B3 positive mononuclear leukocytes in peripheral blood of Swiss and athymic mice during infections. *Proc. Soc. Exp. Biol. Med.* **165:**107–113.
24. **Hammon, W. M., E. H. Ludwig, G. Sather, and D. S. Yohn.** 1957. Comparative studies on patterns of family infections with polioviruses and ECHO virus type 1 on an American military base in the Philippines. *Am. J. Public Health* **47:**802–811.
25. **Herrmann, E. C., Jr.** 1967. Experience in providing a viral diagnostic laboratory compatible with medical practice. *Mayo Clin. Proc.* **42:**112.
26. **Honig, E. I., J. L. Melnick, P. Isacson, R. Parr, I. L. Myers, and M. Walton.** 1956. An epidemiological study of enteric virus infections: poliomyelitis, coxsackie, and orphan (ECHO) viruses isolated from normal children in two socioeconomic groups. *J. Exp. Med.* **103:**247–262.
26a. **Jenista, J. A.** Unpublished data.
27. **Jenista, J. A., K. R. Powell, and M. A. Menegus.** 1984. Epidemiology of neonatal enterovirus infection. *J. Pediatr.* **104:**685–690.
28. **Jenista, J. A., S. P. Prather, K. R. Powell, and M. A. Menegus.** 1983. Virus cultures in the reduction of neonatal morbidity. *Pediatr. Res.* **17:**224A.
29. **Johnston, J. M., and J. C. Overall, Jr.** 1989. Intravenous immunoglobulin in disseminated neonatal echovirus-11 infection. *Pediatr. Infect. Dis. J.* **8:**254–256.
30. **Kogon, A., I. Spigland, T. G. Frothingham, L. Elveback, C. Williams, C. E. Hall, and J. P. Fox.** 1974. The virus watch program: a continuing surveillance of viral infections in metropolitan New York families. VII. Observations on viral excretion, sero-immunity, intrafamilial spread and illness association in coxsackie and echovirus infections. *Am. J. Epidemiol.* **89:**51–61.
31. **Krober, M. S., J. W. Bass, J. M. Powell, F. R. Smith, and D. S. Y. Seto.** 1985. Bacterial and viral pathogens causing fever in infants less than 3 months old. *Am. J. Dis. Child.* **139:**889–892.
32. **Lake, A. M., B. A. Lauer, J. G. Clark, R. L. Wasenberg, and K. McIntosh.** 1976. Enterovirus infections in neonates. *J. Pediatr.* **89:**787–791.
33. **Leggiadro, R. J., and B. T. Darras.** 1983. Viral and bacterial pathogens of suspected sepsis in young infants. *Pediatr. Infect. Dis.* **2:**287–289.
34. **Linnemann, C. C., J. Steichen, W. G. Sherman, and G. M. Schiff.** 1974. Febrile illness in early infants associated with ECHO virus infection. *J. Pediatr.* **84:**49–54.
35. **Melnick, J. L.** 1954. Application of tissue culture methods to epidemiological studies of poliomyelitis. *Am. J. Public Health* **44:**571–580.
36. **Melnick, J. L.** 1989. Enteroviruses, p. 191–203. *In* A. S. Evans (ed.), *Viral Infections of Humans—Epidemiology and Control*, 3rd ed. Plenum Medical Book Co., N.Y.
37. **Melnick, J. L., and K. Ågren.** 1952. Poliomyelitis and coxsackieviruses isolated from normal infants in Egypt. *Proc. Soc. Exp. Biol. Med.* **81:**621–624.
38. **Melnick, J. L., E. W. Shaw, and E. C. Curnen.** 1949. A virus from patients diagnosed as non-paralytic poliomyelitis or aseptic meningitis. *Proc. Soc. Exp. Biol. Med.* **71:**344–349.
39. **Nishmi, M., and Y. Yodfat.** 1973. Successive overlapping outbreaks of a febrile illness associated with coxsackie virus type B4 and echo virus type 9 in a kibbutz. *Isr. J. Med. Sci.* **9:**895–899.
40. **Prather, S. L., R. Dagan, J. A. Jenista, and M. A. Menegus.** 1984. The isolation of enteroviruses from blood: a comparison of four processing methods. *J. Med. Virol.* **14:**221–227.
41. **Prather, S. L., J. A. Jenista, and M. A. Menegus.** 1984. The isolation of nonpolio enteroviruses from serum. *Diagn. Microbiol. Infect. Dis.* **2(4):**353–357.
42. **Ramos-Alvarez, M., and A. B. Sabin.** 1954. Characteristics of poliomyelitis and other enteric viruses recovered in tissue culture from healthy American children. *Proc. Soc. Exp. Biol. Med.* **87:**655–661.
43. **Rotbart, H.** 1991. Nucleic acid detection sys-

tems for enteroviruses. *Clin. Microbiol. Rev.* **4:**156–168.
44. **Sanders, D. Y., and H. G. Cramblett.** 1968. Viral infections in hospitalized neonates. *Am. J. Dis. Child.* **116:**251–256.
45. **Sato, N., H. Sato, and R. Kawana.** 1972. Ecological behavior of 6 coxsackie B and 29 ECHO serotypes as revealed by serologic survey of general populations in Aomori, Japan. *Jpn. J. Med. Sci. Biol.* **25:**355–368.
46. **Seal, L. A., and R. M. Jamison.** 1984. Evidence for secondary structure within the virion of RNA of echovirus-22. *J. Virol.* **50:**641–644.
47. **Wallace, R. E.** 1969. Susceptibility of human lymphoblasts to viral infection *in vitro*. *Proc. Soc. Exp. Biol. Med.* **130:**702–710.
48. **Wilfert, C. M., S. Nusinoff-Lehrman, and S. L. Katz.** 1983. Enteroviruses and meningitis. *Pediatr. Infect. Dis.* **2:**359–363.
49. **Yodfat, Y., and M. Nishmi.** 1973. Epidemiologic and clinical observations in six outbreaks of viral disease in a kibbutz 1968–1971. *Am. J. Epidemiol.* **97:**415–423.

RESPIRATORY INFECTIONS

Tasnee Chonmaitree and Linda Mann

12

Respiratory infections are the most frequent and universal illnesses suffered by children and adults. On average, a child experiences two to seven episodes and an adult experiences one to three episodes of respiratory illness per year, most of them caused by viruses (50, 93). A variety of viruses contribute to the etiology of respiratory tract infection in a given population, and patients with acute respiratory syndromes of diverse etiologies frequently present with clinically similar symptoms. The more commonly known viruses associated with respiratory disease include respiratory syncytial virus, parainfluenza viruses, influenza viruses, adenoviruses, rhinoviruses, and enteroviruses. (In this chapter, the term enteroviruses refers to nonpolio enteroviruses excluding hepatitis A virus, i.e., to coxsackie A and B viruses, echoviruses, and enterovirus types 68 through 71.)

Evidence that enteroviruses cause respiratory disease has been obtained from three main sources: (i) surveys of patients during outbreaks of respiratory disease, with or without parallel study of healthy subjects; (ii) longitudinal studies of populations during both health and illness; and (iii) experimental inoculation of susceptible hosts with the viruses.

Enteroviral infections are exceedingly common, and the spectrum of disease is protean. The contribution to respiratory disease of enteroviruses relative to that of other respiratory viruses cannot be assessed with accuracy, since enteroviruses are frequently carried asymptomatically in the gastrointestinal tract for a long time. Hence, viruses identified in patient specimens are not always responsible for a concomitant illness. The importance of enteroviruses to respiratory disease can, however, be estimated from the numerous reports on the viral etiology of respiratory disease. Worldwide, enteroviruses appear to account for 2 to 15% of all viruses that cause upper and lower respiratory tract diseases (13, 39, 44, 65, 88, 94, 112). The higher percentage represents their contribution to upper respiratory tract infection; they are less frequently associated with lower respiratory tract disease. At The University of Texas Medical Branch (UTMB) Clinical Virology Laboratory, enteroviruses were isolated from 1.7% of 3,119 respiratory specimens submitted for viral culture over a 10-year period (1984 through 1993). This number accounts for 6.4% (54 of 838) of all viruses isolated from respiratory specimens submitted during the same period (89a).

Tasnee Chonmaitree, Pediatric Infectious Diseases Division, University of Texas Medical Branch, The Children's Hospital, Galveston, Texas 77555-0371. *Linda Mann,* Department of Pathology, Clinical Microbiology Division, University of Texas Medical Branch, Galveston, Texas 77555-0743.

Human Enterovirus Infections, Edited by Harley A. Rotbart,
© 1995 American Society for Microbiology, Washington, DC 20005

Of all clinical syndromes reported to be associated with enteroviral infections, respiratory disease accounts for 14 to 21%. In a study by the World Health Organization of data collected from 1967 through 1974 (56), respiratory disease (excluding pleurodynia) accounted for 15% of cases (6,234 of 41,540). Of respiratory diseases 12.4% were caused by coxsackie type A viruses, 20.3% were caused by coxsackie type B viruses, and 12.6% were caused by echoviruses. In the United States, surveillance of enteroviral disease (1970 through 1979) by the Centers for Disease Control (12) has shown that respiratory disease is the second most common clinical syndrome and accounts for 21% of overall disease. In this report, respiratory disease includes upper respiratory tract syndromes (tonsillitis, croup, epiglottitis, etc.) and lower respiratory tract syndromes (pneumonia, pleurodynia, etc). Data collected at UTMB hospitals for 10 years agree with national and worldwide data. Between 1984 and 1993, 647 infants and children were diagnosed as having enteroviral infection; 93 (14.4%) of these patients presented with respiratory symptoms. Table 1 shows the clinical diagnoses of these 93 patients and the serotypes of the associated enteroviruses.

EPIDEMIOLOGY

Respiratory disease associated with enteroviruses is distributed worldwide (56). Corresponding to the seasonal variation of enteroviral disease in general, peak incidence occurs during summer and fall in temperate climates and year-round in the tropics (15, 90) (see chapter 1). During the peak enterovirus season, numerous outbreaks of specific types of enteroviruses associated with respiratory disease have been reported in the general population and in crowded communities such as military bases, children's homes, and orphanage nurseries (63, 95, 101, 102). Many studies have reported enteroviruses as the most important cause of acute respiratory disease, especially upper respiratory tract infections during the summer and fall months (8a, 40, 65, 79). Ten years of experience at the UTMB Clinical Virology Laboratory (Table 2) reveals a similar pattern in which enteroviruses are responsible for a higher proportion of respiratory disease during the summer and fall months.

Enteroviruses spread from person to person. Although the fecal-oral route is the common mode of spread for this virus group in general, studies of respiratory infection induced by certain types of enteroviruses in adult volunteers have shown that intranasal or aerosol administration more effectively induces respiratory infection (10, 70, 105). Results have suggested the importance of fomite transmission: infected volunteers who have cold symptoms shed virus either in large drops upon

TABLE 1 Respiratory diagnosis in 93 patients and associated types of nonpolio enteroviruses at UTMB clinical laboratory, 1984 through 1993[a]

Clinical diagnosis[b]	No. of cases	Coxsackievirus A	Coxsackievirus B	Echovirus and enterovirus type(s)
Upper respiratory tract infection (common cold, congestion, cough)	43	9	1, 2, 3, 4	1, 3, 5, 6, 7, 8, 9, 11, 14, 16, 18, 20, 21, 25, 30
Otitis media	11		2, 3, 4, 5	9, 11
Pharyngotonsillitis	2		1	11
Respiratory distress, apnea	12	9	3, 4	1, 7, 9, 5, 14, 20
Croup	5	9	5	1, 9, 11, 18
Pneumonia	12	9	5	6, 11, 16, 18, 22, 30
Bronchiolitis, wheezing, asthma	8		5	6, 11, 14, 22, 29, 71

[a]During this period, 647 infants and children were diagnosed with nonpolio enteroviral infections as determined by isolation of the virus from throat swab, nasal wash, middle ear fluid, cerebrospinal fluid rectal swab, and/or stool specimens. Respiratory disease accounted for 14.4% (93 of 647 patients) of all enteroviral disease.
[b]From UTMB Clinical Virology Laboratory requisition forms. One case of bronchitis was associated with an untyped enterovirus.

TABLE 2 Respiratory specimens submitted and positive for viruses, UTMB Clinical Laboratory, 1984 through 1993[a]

Parameter	Jan	Feb	Mar	Apr	May	June	July	Aug	Sep	Oct	Nov	Dec	Total
No. of specimens submitted[b]	603	433	362	237	139	100	92	102	110	146	244	551	3,119
% positive for any virus	30	27	24	30	22	22	24	19	14	16	24	34	27
% of virus-positive isolates identified as enteroviruses[c]	2	1	2	6	16	23	23	16	27	25	12	5	6.4

[a] Data are from reference 89a.
[b] Nasal wash, nasal wash combined with throat swab, or nasopharyngeal aspirate.
[c] Only nonpolio enteroviruses are included.

sneezing or into handkerchiefs upon blowing their noses. Airborne transmission is not significant (10). Infected volunteers with respiratory symptoms shed more virus in nasal secretions than in throat secretions, saliva, or feces. In natural infections, pharyngeal shedding may exceed nasal shedding (8a, 119a). In a surveillance study, virus was shed in respiratory secretions alone in one-fourth of individuals infected with coxsackieviruses and in one-third of those infected with echoviruses (82). In the same study, however, respiratory shedding (often with concomitant fecal excretion) was more common in coxsackievirus infections (48%) than in echovirus infections (32%). When fecal excretion occurred, it was of a relatively long duration (e.g., up to 70 days) and lasted longer during coxsackieviral infection than during echoviral infection (82).

In respiratory disease associated with enteroviruses, contagiousness depends on type of contact and viral serotype involved. Studies have shown that coxsackievirus A21 can be transmitted from one volunteer to another by regular personal contact (10, 64); however, the rate of transmission is relatively low. Contagiousness within households is generally high. Continuous surveillance of viral infections within families has documented an infection rate of up to 80% (34, 58, 82) (see chapter 1). Rates of intrahousehold spread of coxsackieviruses A and B are higher than that of echoviruses (82). Family size also plays a role. Infected families were slightly larger, with more children between 5 and 9 years of age; young children are thought to introduce the virus into the family. In other crowded environments, such as children's homes and orphanage nurseries (63, 101, 102), similarly high rates of infectivity (52 to 74%) were reported among resident children during coxsackievirus outbreaks. Within a community, horizontal spread between households is more difficult to document than spread within households (32). Some viral serotypes, such as coxsackievirus A21, are less contagious among infants (70), though serologic studies demonstrate infection later in life.

PATHOGENESIS AND PATHOLOGY

Respiratory diseases associated with enteroviruses are usually mild and self-limited. Therefore, opportunities to study the pathogenesis and pathology of these diseases have been limited. Furthermore, very few animal models have been available for the study of enteroviral respiratory disease. Thus, knowledge of disease mechanisms comes mainly from studies of adult volunteers infected with representative strains of enteroviruses that are associated with respiratory disease, such as coxsackievirus A21 and echovirus type 11 (10, 64, 70, 89, 103, 105).

Like any respiratory virus, enterovirus usually infects the respiratory tract via the respiratory route. A higher rate of infection occurs after direct inoculation (drops or swab) into the nasal septum or conjunctiva than after inoculation into the oropharynx (10, 105). In an adult volunteer study, administration of coxsackievirus A21 (10^5 50% tissue culture infective doses) by enteric coated capsules to nine volunteers produced no evidence of illness or serologic response, although virus was recovered from six volunteers (70). After the virus enters the body via the respiratory route, replication appears to occur primarily in the nasopharynx. Evidence for this hypothesis comes from a study of adult volunteers who received the virus by inoculation into the nostril (10). The mean titer of virus shed in nasal secretions 1 to 6 days following challenge was more than 100-fold higher than that of virus shed in throat secretions or saliva. In natural infection, however, a small study done more than three decades ago and a large recent study indicate that virus may be more recoverable from throat than nasal secretions (8a, 119a). This may indicate that natural infection originates via pharyngeal "inoculation" of infected secretions. Although virus was also shed in the feces, this was less frequent, and the virus occurred in lower concentrations.

The incubation period is generally short, between 1 to 3 days (70, 101, 105). The period of viremia is assumed to be brief, since it could not be demonstrated in adult volunteers for whom blood and urine samples were obtained daily for 4 days after virus challenge. Early symptoms include nasal obstruction, postnasal discharge, headache, and occasional fever. Rhinorrhea occurs at 48 h after onset of symptoms. Lower respiratory tract symptoms occur more frequently in volunteers given a higher inoculum dose (70), and when these symptoms occur, they usually follow the onset of rhinorrhea. By day 5 after onset, remission of all symptoms begins, and symptoms progressively decline to near normal after 1 week.

The rate of infection is generally related to age and presence of preexisting antibody. Younger children and nonimmune persons are more likely to be infected (63). Subclinical infection is very common. Approximately one-half to two-thirds of adult volunteers and of children infected during natural disease outbreaks do not manifest any symptoms (32, 82, 105). A community surveillance program has shown a higher percentage of echoviral diseases than coxsackieviral diseases to be subclinical (82).

Pathogenesis of intraoral disease, such as herpangina, differs from that of respiratory tract disease. Experimental infection in rhesus monkeys with coxsackievirus A4 has shown that after oral inoculation, the virus multiplies in the lower part of the alimentary tract, enters the bloodstream, and then multiplies in the oropharynx (110). Lesions characteristic of herpangina develop and persist for 2 to 7 days in the oropharynx. Following intravenous inoculation, viremia is the source of extensive secondary viral multiplication in the upper and lower parts of the alimentary tract. In monkeys infected with smaller doses of virus, only traces of virus were detected in the throat, blood, and feces.

Immunity

Serum antibody to various types of enteroviruses develops with age, presumably as a result of previous infections (see chapter 8). Preexisting neutralizing antibody plays a significant role in protection against disease, and antibody titers correlate inversely with rate of infection and degree of clinical illness (70). The antibody levels required for disease protection depend on inoculum dose, route of inoculation, and viral serotype. During an outbreak of respiratory disease associated with coxsackieviruses B3 and B4, preexisting neutralizing antibody levels of 1:20 or more were found to be protective (63). On the other hand, in experimental coxsackievirus A21 infection, volunteers with preexisting titers of 1:124 to 1:1,600 manifested a slight illness typical of secondary response (64). Nasal antibody titers of >1:100 protect against reinfection (70).

In children or volunteers without preexisting neutralizing antibody, primary infection induces seroconversion in 66 to 100% of cases (10, 70, 84). Primary antibody response mainly consists of a delayed rise in levels of immunoglobulin M (IgM), which can be detected within 15 to 40 days; IgG and IgA have also been found in primary response (89). In secondary (repeated) infection, IgG represents the major type of immune response, and seroconversion occurs in approximately one-third of cases (101). While nasal neutralizing antibody is infrequently found, the presence of this antibody correlates with a reduction in the frequency of nasal viral shedding (105). Presence of serum antibody correlates with a reduction in viral shedding and a shortening of the duration of clinical illness. The significance of hemagglutination-inhibiting antibody is unclear. In the absence of neutralizing antibody, this antibody response seems to be transient (64).

Pathology

Most respiratory diseases associated with enteroviruses are mild, and their pathologies have therefore not been well described. Pathologic data are available only for fetal pneumonitis (9, 37, 117). In this illness, the infected lungs are grossly firm, granular, and hyperaerated, with occasional presence of pleural fluid. Focal or diffuse interstitial pneumonitis or diffuse bronchopneumonia can be observed microscopically, with atelectasis, interstitial lymphoid hyperplasia, diffuse intra-alveolar infiltrates with mostly mononuclear cells, intra-alveolar hemorrhage, and occasional intravascular thrombi (see chapter 10).

CLINICAL PRESENTATIONS

Common Cold

The common cold is an acute, mild, undifferentiated upper respiratory tract disease which generally lasts 3 to 6 days and is characterized by nasal congestion, rhinorrhea, and sneezing, with no or minimal fever or sore throat. The syndrome is sometimes accompanied by general malaise and cough. Although the viral etiology of summer cold is certainly diverse, numerous reports have linked summer cold outbreaks to a variety of coxsackieviruses and echoviruses (36, 57, 60, 63, 72, 79, 82, 101, 102). Moreover, undifferentiated upper respiratory tract disease is probably the most common respiratory manifestation of enteroviruses (56, 57, 113).

Among enteroviruses, coxsackievirus A21 (Coe virus) is an important cause of mild respiratory tract disease in military personnel worldwide (8, 52, 73, 85, 99). This enteroviral serotype has also been used as a representative strain to induce upper respiratory tract disease in adult volunteers (10, 64, 70, 89). Other coxsackieviruses of the A group that have been associated with cold symptoms include coxsackieviruses A9, 10, and 24 (56, 70, 82). Coxsackieviruses B1 through B5 have frequently been implicated as causes of upper respiratory infections, especially in outbreaks in children's homes and orphanage nurseries (11, 56, 57). Of coxsackievirus group B infections associated with clinical disease, more than two-thirds appear to be mild respiratory disease (57, 82, 113). Several types of echoviruses, including types 1 through 3, 5 through 9, 11, 14, 16, 18, 20, 21, 22, 25, and 30, and enterovirus types 68 and 71 have been reported to be associated with upper respiratory tract disease (29, 33, 36, 53, 56, 70, 78, 79, 105, 107, 113). Echovirus type 11 has been used as a representative echovirus to induce upper respiratory tract disease in adult volunteers (70, 105). The serotypes of enteroviruses noted in association with the common cold and other respiratory diseases are shown in Table 3.

Otitis Media

Acute inflammation of the middle ear is generally a complication of upper respiratory tract infection. In the usual course, a child who is suffering an upper respiratory tract infection for a few days suddenly develops fever, irritability, otalgia, and hearing loss. Examination with the pneumatic otoscope reveals a hyperemic, opaque tympanic membrane of poor mobility. Purulent otorrhea may be present.

Although acute otitis media is generally considered a bacterial disease, studies from the past decade have shown a strong association between acute otitis media and viral infection of the respiratory tract (26, 61, 81, 106). Approximately 28 to 46% of children with acute otitis media have documented viral respiratory tract infection, and viruses can be detected in 8 to 25% of middle ear fluids from these patients (23, 30). Although infections with respiratory viruses such as respi-

TABLE 3 Coxsackievirus and echovirus types associated with respiratory disease

Clinical syndrome	Coxsackievirus type A	Coxsackievirus type B	Echovirus and enterovirus types
Common cold	9, 10, 21, 24	1–5	1–3, 5–9, 11, 14, 16, 18, 20, 21, 22, 25, 30, 68, 71
Pharyngitis	Probably all	1–5	Probably all; mainly 2, 4, 6, 9, 10, 11, 16, 19, 25, 30, 71
Herpangina	1–10, 16, 22	1–5	6, 9, 11, 16, 17, 22, 25
Croup	9	4, 5	1, 4, 9, 11, 18, 21, 71
Bronchitis		1, 3, 4	8, 12–14, 19
Bronchiolitis		1–5	6, 14, 68, 71
Infectious asthma	Many	3, 4, 5	11, 15, 18, 22, 29, 71
Pneumonia	9, 16, 21	1–5	6, 7, 9, 11, 12, 16–20, 22, 30, 68, 71
Pleurodynia	1, 2, 4, 6, 9, 10, 16	1–6	1–3, 6–9, 11, 12, 14, 16–19, 23–25, 30

ratory syncytial virus, adenoviruses, and influenza viruses impart a greater risk for otitis media than does infection with enteroviruses (62), 16% of children with respiratory infection caused by enteroviruses developed otitis media. In an earlier report of respiratory illness (coryza) associated with an echovirus (36), mild, diffuse erythema of the tympanic membrane occurred later in the illness in five of six infants. One of these infants developed purulent otitis media as a complication. Virologic studies at UTMB of patients with acute otitis media have shown that enteroviruses account for approximately 15% of all viruses isolated from nasopharyngeal secretions of these patients (Fig. 1). Serotypes of enteroviruses isolated from nasopharyngeal secretions and middle ear fluids of children with acute otitis media are shown in Table 4.

Pharyngitis, Pharyngotonsillitis, and Tonsillitis

Pharyngitis is an acute inflammatory illness of the mucous membranes and underlying structures of the throat. This inflammation also frequently involves the nasopharynx, tonsils, uvula, and soft palate. The onset of pharyngitis is usually sudden, with fever and the complaint of sore throat accompanied by anorexia. On examination, fever is almost always present, and the pharynx is erythematous with or without follicular, ulcerative, or petechial lesions and/or generalized or circumscribed exudates. Cervical lymphadenitis is commonly present. Pharyngitis associated with enteroviral infection is self-limited, lasting 3 to 6 days (15, 16). A clinical syndrome, acute lymphonodular pharyngitis, associated with coxsackievirus A10 has been described as occurring during an outbreak (111). The distinctive, raised, micronodular lesions of this syndrome occur primarily in the pharynx. The lesions are not vesicular, but whitish or yellowish. All lesions regress at approximately the same time without ulceration. The associated symptoms include fever, malaise, anorexia, and mild headache. No rhinorrhea, cough, or gingivitis is present. The course ranges from 4 to 14 days.

Pharyngitis is a very common manifestation of enteroviral infection, and probably all enteroviruses on occasion cause mild pharyngitis (15). Enteroviral pharyngitis is often associated with exanthem or more severe manifestations such as aseptic meningitis. Nevertheless, numerous outbreaks of enteroviral infections, and of coxsackievirus type B infections in particular, with fever and pharyngitis as the predominant clinical syndrome have been reported (63, 95, 101, 111). The most common enteroviruses associated with pharyngitis are coxsackieviruses A9 and B1 through B5; echovirus types 2, 4, 6, 9, 10, 11, 16, 19, 25, and 30; and enterovirus 71 (15, 19–21, 36, 48, 75, 76, 77, 80, 95, 109, 111, 115).

Herpangina

Herpangina is a fairly common acute febrile illness characterized by papular, vesicular, and

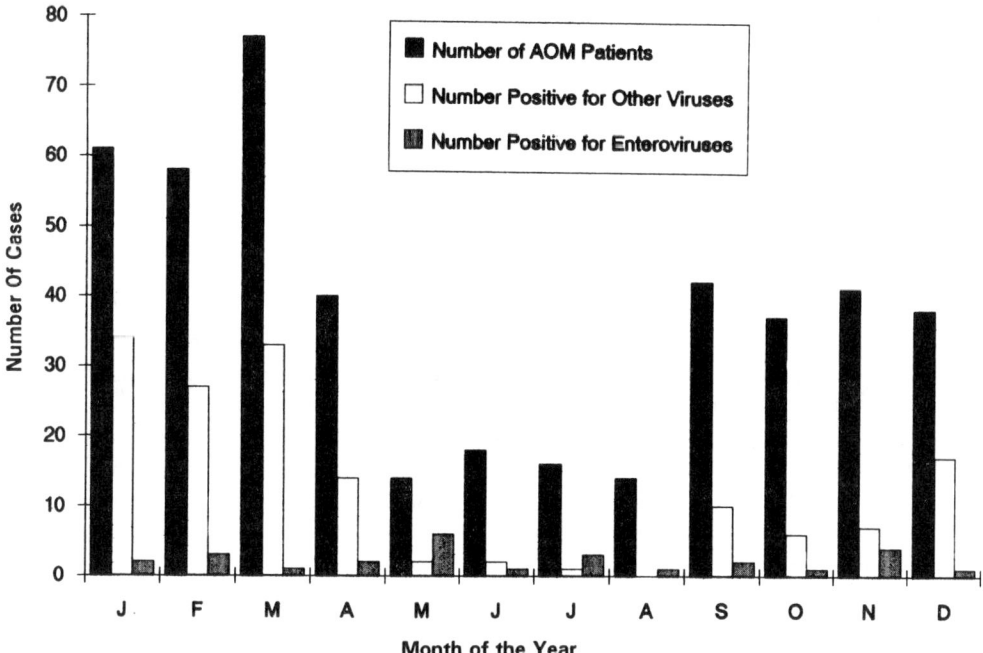

FIGURE 1 Viral infections in acute otitis media (AOM) patients by month of the year. Between 1990 and 1992, of the 432 patients with AOM who were studied at UTMB, Galveston, 168 (39%) had documented viral infections of the respiratory tract. Of the 168 virus strains, 25 were nonpolio enteroviruses.

ulcerative lesions on the anterior tonsillar pillars, soft palate, uvula, tonsils, and posterior pharyngeal mucous membrane (17, 22, 98). Although the illness was well described by Zahorsky (121, 122) in 1920 and 1924, the viral etiology was not established until 1951, when Huebner et al. (67) first described association of the disease with coxsackie A viral infection. Since then, epidemic and sporadic cases of herpangina have been reported in association with numerous types of coxsackie A and B viruses and echoviruses (Table 3).

The onset of herpangina is relatively sudden, without evidence of prodromal manifestations. Fever is generally the initial symptom observed. The temperature rises rapidly and varies from low grade to 41°C (106°F). The temperature tends to be higher in younger patients, who may also become irritable, listless, or anorexic; sore throat and drooling occur in approximately 25 to >50% of the patients. Headache and generalized muscle pains are less frequently noted. Diarrhea and coryza have been reported infrequently.

TABLE 4 Serotypes of nonpolio enteroviruses isolated from patients with acute otitis media

Isolates from:		Reference(s)
Middle ear fluid	Nasopharyngeal secretion or throat swab	
Coxsackievirus A9	Coxsackievirus A9	30, 59
Coxsackieviruses B4 and B5	Coxsackieviruses B1–B5	3, 26, 30, 31, 63, 101, 116
Echovirus types 11 and 25	Echovirus types 1, 6, 7, 9, 11, 22, 25, 30	4, 30
	Enterovirus 71	30, 53

Within 24 to 48 h after the initial nonspecific symptoms appear, characteristic throat lesions appear. These consist of small (1 to 2 mm in diameter), grayish white papulovesicular lesions with surrounding areolas of erythema. The lesions (2 to 15 in number, with an average of 5 per patient) are usually discrete. Over a 2- to 3-day period, vesicles become larger (3 to 4 mm wide), rupture, and assume an ulcerative appearance with grayish yellow coloration (17, 98). Each vesicular and ulcerative lesion is surrounded by an erythematous ring that varies in size up to 10 mm in diameter. The lesions are most commonly found on the anterior tonsillar pillars. They also appear on the soft palate, uvula, tonsils, posterior pharyngeal wall, and, occasionally, posterior buccal surfaces or tip of the tongue. Lesions are not generally observed on the gingiva or anterior buccal mucosa.

Although herpangina occasionally occurs in association with other manifestations of enteroviral diseases such as exanthem or aseptic meningitis (83, 96), in most cases, fever and oropharyngeal lesions are the main manifestations. The disease runs a benign self-limited course, with fever lasting from 1 to 4 days.

Routine laboratory study is of little value in herpangina. The total leukocyte count may be normal or slightly elevated. The differential count is most often normal (17, 98). Certain types of causative enteroviruses can be isolated from throat swabs or swabs of lesions. Isolation of the virus from rectal swabs may give an indirect clue to the etiologic agent.

The classic appearance of the oropharyngeal lesions helps differentiate this illness from herpes stomatitis. Ulcerative lesions in the oropharynx caused by herpes simplex virus typically involve the more anterior buccal mucosa, inner lips, tongue, gingiva, and sublingual mucosa (98).

Croup

Croup is an acute respiratory illness characterized by various degrees of inspiratory stridor, cough, and hoarseness resulting from obstruction in the larynx. The clinical syndrome of croup includes acute laryngitis, laryngotracheitis, laryngotracheobronchitis, laryngotracheobronchopneumonitis, and spasmodic croup (18). The onset of the disease is usually gradual, with initial symptoms of coryza, cough, and sore throat. Fever usually occurs within the first 24 h after onset and is followed within 12 to 48 h by upper-airway obstructive signs and symptoms. The cough becomes "croupy" or "barking," and evidence of inspiratory stridor gradually increases. The child's voice then becomes hoarse. The speed of progression and the final degree of upper-airway obstruction may vary from mild, with a gradual return to normal within 3 to 7 days, to severe, with respiratory distress, hypoxia, and cyanosis lasting as long as 7 to 14 days. In general, the illnesses associated with enteroviral infection are milder than those associated with parainfluenza and influenza viruses (15). The most important infection in the differential diagnosis is acute epiglottitis, which is generally bacterial in origin. In acute epiglottitis, there is no croupy cough, but a swollen, cherry red epiglottis is present. Lateral neck radiograph helps differentiate these two conditions.

An association between enteroviral infection and symptoms of croup has been noted sporadically (15, 18, 53, 72, 78, 100). An outbreak of croup due to echovirus type 11 in a day nursery has been reported (100). Coxsackieviruses A9, B4, and B5; echovirus types 1, 4, 9, 11, 18, and 21; and enterovirus 71 have also been found in association with croup (15, 18, 53, 72, 78, 100).

Bronchitis

Acute bronchitis is an acute febrile illness characterized by cough and rhonchi. The prodromal period, which lasts 1 to 2 days, is characterized by fever and upper respiratory tract symptoms. Onset of cough can be insidious or abrupt. Initially, the cough is dry and harsh. It becomes looser as the disease progresses, and purulent sputum can be expectorated. Rhonchi are audible on examination of the chest. Chest pain may be experienced. The acute tracheobronchial symptoms generally last 4 to 6 days and are followed by an afebrile recovery period characterized by cough and expectoration that lasts 1 to 2 weeks.

Bronchitis can be a sporadic manifestation of enteroviral infection. It has been reported in infections associated with coxsackieviruses B1, B3, and B4 and with echovirus types 8, 12, 13, 14, and 19 (13, 15, 36, 38, 46, 102).

Bronchiolitis
Acute bronchiolitis is an infantile illness characterized by symptoms of upper respiratory tract infection and signs of obstructive airway disease. Initial symptoms include fever, copious nasal discharge, cough, irritability, anorexia, and restlessness. Symptoms usually progress in severity over a 3- to 7-day period, when onset of wheezing becomes recognizable. Examination reveals fever, labored breathing, and audible wheezing. Although the disease is commonly associated with respiratory syncytial virus, parainfluenza viruses, or adenovirus (118), sporadic cases of bronchiolitis associated with enteroviruses have been described (13, 46, 53, 77). In rare reports that link this syndrome to specific types of enteroviruses, coxsackieviruses type B and enteroviruses 68 and 71 are mentioned (53, 77, 107).

Infectious Asthma
An asthmatic attack is an acute episode of illness characterized by reversible bronchospasm (wheezing). It is often precipitated by viral infection associated with many common respiratory viruses. Onset of asthma precipitated by viral respiratory infection is insidious, with gradual increases in frequency and severity of cough and wheezing over a few days. The signs and symptoms of asthma include cough, which sounds light and is nonproductive early in the course of an attack; wheezing, tachypnea, and dyspnea, with prolonged expiration and use of accessory muscles of respiration; cyanosis; hyperinflation of the chest; tachycardia; and abdominal pain. Enteroviruses have been sporadically found in association with virus-induced asthma (27, 42, 47, 55, 66, 92, 97).

Among the specified serotypes associated with this syndrome are coxsackieviruses B3, B4, and B5 and echovirus types 11, 15, 18, and 22 (27, 47, 66, 92, 97, 102). Coxsackievirus B5 and echovirus type 18 have been isolated from stool specimens from patients who developed poliomyelitislike illness a few days following an acute attack of asthma (7).

Pneumonia
The clinical symptoms of pneumonia that are caused by enteroviruses are indistinguishable from those that are caused by other viruses. Unlike the onset of bacterial pneumonia, the onset of viral pneumonia is generally gradual, following 1 to 2 days of coryza, decreased appetite, and low-grade fever. In older children and adults, myalgia is often prominent. Respiratory prodomes are followed by increasing fretfulness, respiratory congestion, cough, fever, and respiratory distress (tachypnea, tachycardia, nasal flaring, and retraction). In young infants, apneic spells and cyanosis may occur.

Physical findings include diminished local percussion or breath sounds and fine rales (diffuse or localized). If pneumonia associated with bronchiolitis or bronchospasm occurs, then hyperresonance or wheezing can be detected. Cough is usually nonproductive. The patient can also be dehydrated from fever, hyperventilation, and low fluid intake.

Radiographic findings are usually more generalized than those that typify bacterial pneumonia; bilateral perihilar-parabronchial infiltrates are common. Air trapping, patchy areas of consolidation, and subsegmental atelectasis are also common. Pleural effusion is uncommon.

In earlier studies of respiratory infections in children, enteroviruses were associated with pneumonia in 1 to 7% of cases (13, 15, 45, 51, 54). In a small, more recent study of viral pneumonia in the first month of life, enteroviruses were associated with pneumonia in 6 (15%) of 40 cases (2). Pneumonia associated with enteroviral infection has been reported both in outbreaks (6, 46, 87) and as sporadic cases (9, 15, 37, 49, 71, 117, 120). Specific virus types include coxsackieviruses A9, A16, and B1 through B5; echovirus types 6, 7, 9, 11, 12, 16 through 20, 22, and 30; and enteroviruses 68 and 71 (9, 15, 37, 49, 53, 57, 71, 78, 107, 117, 120). Fatal pneumonia has been associated with infection caused by coxsackieviruses A9, A16, B1, and B5 and echovirus types 6, 9, 11, and 17 (9, 14, 37, 45, 49, 71, 86, 117, 120).

Pleurodynia

Pleurodynia (Bornholm disease) is an acute febrile illness with severe pain of the chest and upper abdomen that is muscular in origin. Other names that refer to this syndrome include epidemic myalgia, devil's grippe, epidemic diaphragmatic spasm, and epidemic benign pleurisy (15). The disease often occurs as an epidemic, but sporadic cases also occur. The incubation period is approximately 4 days. Onset of fever and pain is usually sudden. Typical pain involves chest or upper abdomen and occasionally other areas of the body. The pain is frequently severe and is associated with profuse sweating. The patient may be pale, as if in shock. The pain is spasmodic and usually lasts from 15 to 30 min, but it may last for hours. During spasms, respiration is compromised, and breathing is rapid and shallow. The pain may be aggravated by sudden movement with coughing or deep inspiration. Other constitutional symptoms such as anorexia, nausea, vomiting, headache, and sore throat may be observed.

On physical examination, some degree of tenderness is present in areas of pain, but frank myositis with muscle swelling is not observed. Pleural friction rubs may be noted on auscultation, and they may come and go with the pain episodes. Breath sounds are otherwise clear. Upper respiratory tract signs suggesting viral infection may be present. Chest radiograph is normal, and this finding usually differentiates pleurodynia from pneumonia. When pain is localized in the abdomen, the disease has to be differentiated from acute surgical conditions such as appendicitis or peritonitis. Acute symptoms usually wane after 1 to 3 days. Recurrent pain episodes may appear several days later.

Coxsackieviruses B1 through B6 have long been established as causes of this illness because of their characteristic myotropism. The major types are coxsackieviruses B3 and B5 (15, 35, 41, 43, 56). Coxsackievirus B1 and echovirus type 20 have been reported to cause pleurodynia outbreaks among athletic teams (69, 114). Other enterovirus types associated with sporadic occurrences of pleurodynia include coxsackieviruses A1, A2, A4, A6, A9, A10, and A16 and echovirus types 1 through 3, 6 through 9, 11, 12, 14, 16 through 19, 23 through 25, and 30 (5, 15, 35, 41, 43, 56, 69, 74, 114).

LABORATORY DIAGNOSIS

Conventional viral culture remains the mainstay for laboratory diagnosis of enteroviral infections of the respiratory tract (see chapter 17). For most patients with respiratory illness, enteroviral infection is only part of the differential diagnosis, which includes other viral respiratory infections, and conventional viral culture is a cost-effective method of detecting most enteroviruses as well as other viral agents in respiratory specimens. Cell culture can detect most enteroviruses except some strains of coxsackieviruses A that require inoculation of newborn mice for isolation. The cell types used most widely to grow enteroviruses include primary monkey (rhesus, cynomolgus, or African green) kidney and human diploid fibroblastic lines such as MRC-5 (24) (see chapter 17). Other cell types include continuous human heteroploid cells (HeLa and HEp-2), primary or diploid human embryonic kidney, human fetal kidney, human amnion, human rhabdomyosarcoma, chicken embryo, and the buffalo green monkey line of African green monkey cells (24, 91, 108). Use of multiple appropriate cell lines increases yield and enhances the speed of enteroviral isolation. The majority of the isolates are detected within 3 to 7 days (25) by observation of cell cultures for characteristic cytopathic effects. A specific identification of the serotype can be accomplished by virus neutralization with intersecting virus antiserum pools (87). If only vaccine polioviruses need to be separated from nonpolio enteroviruses, a simple neutralization test can be performed with pooled antisera to the three types of poliovirus (91). Another highly sensitive and specific method of separating nonpolio enteroviruses from polioviruses is the PCR technique with a single set of primers selected from a region of the poliovirus genome (1) (see chapter 17).

For most respiratory viruses, the specimen of choice is a nasal wash or nasopharyngeal aspirate. As noted above, the data as to whether enteroviruses are more readily recovered from nasal or from throat specimens are conflicting. Depending on study design, higher virus titers have been found in nasal specimens (volunteer studies) or throat specimens (natural infections). Direct comparisons in natural infections have been between nasal swabs and throat swabs only: comparisons between nasal wash and throat swabs for enteroviral diagnosis have not been performed (8a, 10, 105, 119a), nor have gargle (throat wash) specimens been studied. We recommend both nasal wash and throat swab (or gargle) cultures to evaluate respiratory illness during enterovirus season. The throat swab may be added to the nasal wash specimen (by immersing the swab and then squeezing out the tip against the sides of the vial and discarding the swab) to reduce the cost to that of a single culture. Isolation of enteroviruses is more likely when specimens are collected early in the course of the illness. As in the case of central nervous system disease, isolation of enteroviruses from rectal swabs or stool can provide rapid but only indirect evidence of enteroviral infection in respiratory disease (28, 119).

Until recently, good specific monoclonal antibodies for enteroviruses were not widely available, and identification of presumptive enteroviruses to serotype depended on neutralization reactions, often performed in a state or reference laboratory. While direct antigen detection and centrifugation-enhanced rapid culture techniques such as shell vial assays have become important for other viral respiratory pathogens such as respiratory syncytial virus and influenza A virus for which specific antiviral therapies are available, similar assays are not widely used for enteroviruses from respiratory sources (68). The reasons for this lack of development of direct or rapid tests for enteroviral respiratory infections include (i) the lack of specific antiviral agents for therapy, (ii) the large number of enteroviral serotypes, and (iii) the relative rapidity of conventional virus culture techniques. While PCR assay of cerebrospinal fluid is promising for the diagnosis of aseptic meningitis due to enteroviruses (104), the technique has not yet been widely used for detection of enteroviruses in respiratory specimens.

TREATMENT

Because of the mild and self-limited nature of respiratory disease caused by enteroviruses, specific treatment is not generally indicated. Supportive and symptomatic treatment depends on the spectrum and severity of clinical manifestations involved. Prolonged and severe disease in an immunocompromised host may be an indication for a specific investigational antiviral therapy or exogenously administered immunoglobulin. Specific drugs under investigation for treatment of enteroviral infection are discussed in chapter 18 of this volume.

REFERENCES

1. **Abraham, R., T. Chonmaitree, J. McCombs, B. Prabhakar, P. T. Lo Verde, and P. L. Ogra.** 1993. Rapid detection of poliovirus by reverse transcription and polymerase chain amplification: application for differentiation between poliovirus and nonpoliovirus enteroviruses. *J. Clin. Microbiol.* **31:**395–399.
2. **Abzug, M. J., A. C. Beam, E. A. Gyorkos, and M. J. Levin.** 1990. Viral pneumonia in the first month of life. *Pediatr. Infect. Dis. J.* **9:**881–885.
3. **Adlington, P., and J. R. Davies.** 1969. Virus studies in secretory otitis media. *J. Laryngol. Otol.* **83:**161–173.
4. **Arola, M., T. Ziegler, and O. Ruuskanen.** 1990. Respiratory virus infection as a cause of prolonged symptoms in acute otitis media. *J. Pediatr.* **116:**697–701.

5. **Bell, E. J., and N. R. Grist.** 1970. Echoviruses, carditis, and acute pleurodynia. *Lancet* **i:**326–328.
6. **Berkovich, S., and J. Pangan.** 1968. Recoveries of virus from premature infants during outbreaks of respiratory disease: the relation of ECHO virus type 22 to disease of the upper and lower respiratory tract in the premature infant. *Bull. N.Y. Acad. Med.* **44:**377–387.
7. **Blomquist, H. K., and B. Bjorksten.** 1980. Poliomyelitis-like illness associated with asthma. *Arch. Dis. Child.* **55:**61–63.
8. **Bloom, H. H., K. M. Johnson, M. A. Mufson, and R. M. Chanock.** 1962. Acute respiratory disease associated with coxsackie A21 virus infection. II. Incidence in military personnel: observations in a nonrecruit population. *JAMA* **179:**120–125.
8a. **Blum, D.,** et al. Unpublished observations.
9. **Boyd, M. T., S. W. Jordan, and L. E. Davis.** 1987. Fatal pneumonitis from congenital echovirus type 6 infection. *Pediatr. Infect. Dis. J.* **6:**1138–1139.
10. **Buckland, F. E., M. L. Bynoe, and D. A. J. Tyrell.** 1965. Experiments on the spread of colds. II. Studies in volunteers with coxsackievirus A21. *J. Hyg.* **63:**327–343.
11. **Carmichael, J., R. McGuckin, and P. S. Gardner.** 1968. Outbreak of coxsackie type B2 virus in a children's home in Newcastle-upon-Tyne. *Br. Med. J.* **ii:**532–533.
12. **Centers for Disease Control.** 1981. Enterovirus surveillance report, 1970–1979, p. 14. Centers for Disease Control, Atlanta.
13. **Chanock, R. M., and R. H. Parrott.** 1965. Acute respiratory disease in infancy and childhood: present understanding and prospects for prevention. *Pediatrics* **36:**21–39.
14. **Cheeseman, S. H., M. S. Hirsch, E. W. Keller, and D. E. Keim.** 1977. Fatal neonatal pneumonia caused by echovirus type 9. *Am. J. Dis. Child.* **131:**1169.
15. **Cherry, J. D.** 1992. Enteroviruses: polioviruses (poliomyelitis), coxsackieviruses, echoviruses, and enteroviruses, p. 1705–1753. *In* R. D. Feigin and J. D. Cherry (ed.), *Textbook of Pediatric Infectious Diseases*, 3rd ed. The W. B. Saunders Co., Philadelphia.
16. **Cherry, J. D.** 1992. Pharyngitis (pharyngitis, tonsillitis, tonsillopharyngitis, and nasopharyngitis), p. 159–166. *In* R. D. Feigin and J. D. Cherry (ed.), *Textbook of Pediatric Infectious Diseases*, 3rd ed. The W. B. Saunders Co., Philadelphia.
17. **Cherry, J. D.** 1992. Herpangina, p. 230–232. *In* R. D. Feigin and J. D. Cherry (ed.), *Textbook of Pediatric Infectious Diseases*, 3rd ed. The W. B. Saunders Co., Philadelphia.
18. **Cherry, J. D.** 1992. Croup (laryngitis, laryngotracheitis, spasmodic croup, and laryngotracheobronchitis), p. 209–220. *In* R. D. Feigin and J. D. Cherry (ed.), *Textbook of Pediatric Infectious Diseases*, 3rd ed. The W. B. Saunders Co., Philadelphia.
19. **Cherry, J. D., A. M. Lerner, J. O. Klein, and M. Finland.** 1963. Coxsackievirus A9 infections with exanthems: with particular reference to urticaria. *Pediatrics* **31:**819–823.
20. **Cherry, J. D., A. M. Lerner, J. O. Klein, and M. Finland.** 1963. ECHO 11 virus infections associated with exanthems. *Pediatrics* **32:**509–516.
21. **Cherry, J. D., A. M. Lerner, J. O. Klein, and M. Finland.** 1963. Coxsackie B5 infections with exanthems. *Pediatrics* **31:**455–462.
22. **Cherry, J. D., and C. L. Jahn.** 1965. Herpangina: The etiologic spectrum. *Pediatrics* **36:**632–634.
23. **Chonmaitree, T.** 1990. Viral otitis media. *Pediatr. Ann.* **19:**522–532.
24. **Chonmaitree, T., C. D. Baldwin, and H. L. Lucia.** 1989. Role of the virology laboratory in diagnosis and management of patients with central nervous system disease. *Clin. Microbiol. Rev.* **2:**1–14.
25. **Chonmaitree, T., C. Ford, C. Sanders, and H. L. Lucia.** 1988. Comparison of cell cultures for rapid isolation of enteroviruses. *J. Clin. Microbiol.* **26:**2576–2580.
26. **Chonmaitree, T., V. M. Howie, and A. L. Truant.** 1986. Presence of respiratory viruses in middle ear fluids and nasal wash specimens from children with acute otitis media. *Pediatrics* **77:**698–702.
27. **Chonmaitree, T., and M. A. Lett-Brown.** 1992. Variations in histamine, IgE and interferon concentrations in nasal secretions and sera of children with asthma associated with viral or mycoplasma infection. *Pediatr. Allergy Immunol.* **3:**16–2.
28. **Chonmaitree, T., M. A. Menegus, and K. R. Powell.** 1982. The clinical relevance of "CSF viral culture." A two-year experience with aseptic meningitis in Rochester, NY. *JAMA* **247:**1843–1847.
29. **Chonmaitree, T., M. A. Menegus, E. M. Schervish-Swierkosz, and E. Schwalenstocker.** 1981. Enterovirus 71 infection: report of an outbreak with two cases of paralysis and a review of the literature. *Pediatrics* **67:**489–493.
30. **Chonmaitree, T., M. J. Owen, J. A. Patel, D. Hedgpeth, D. Horlick, and V. M. Howie.** 1992. Effect of viral respiratory tract infection on outcome of acute otitis media. *J. Pediatr.*

120:856–862.
31. Chonmaitree, T., J. A. Patel, R. Garofalo, T. Uchida, T. Sim, M. J. Owen, and V. M. Howie. Role of leukotriene B4 and interleukin-8 in acute bacterial and viral otitis media. Submitted for publication.
32. Clemmer, D. I., F. Li, D. R. LeBlanc, and J. P. Fox. 1966. An outbreak of subclinical infection with coxsackievirus B3 in southern Louisiana. *Am. J. Epidemiol.* **83:**123–129.
33. Connolly, J. H., J. D. Russell, F. L. Robinson, and D. A. Canavan. 1985. Echovirus type 7 outbreak in Northern Ireland during 1984. *Ulster Med. J.* **54:**191–95.
34. Cooney, M. K., C. E. Hall, and J. P. Fox. 1972. The Seattle virus watch. III. Evaluation of isolation methods and summary of infections detected by virus isolations. *Am. J. Epidemiol.* **96:**286–305.
35. Cramblett, H. G., H. L. Moffet, J. P. Black, H. Shulenberger, A. Smith, and C. T. Colonna. 1964. Coxsackie virus infections: clinical and laboratory studies. *J. Pediatr.* **64:**406–414.
36. Cramblett, H. G., L. Rosen, R. H. Parrott, J. A. Bell., R. J. Huebner, and N. B. McCullough. 1958. Respiratory illness in six infants infected with a new recognized echo virus. *Pediatrics* **21:**168–177.
37. Craver, R. D., and R. Gohd. 1990. Fatal pneumonitis caused by echovirus 17. *Pediatr. Infect. Dis. J.* **9:**453–454.
38. Crovari, P., F. M. Chiossi, and A. Vannucci. 1969. An outbreak of acute respiratory disease due to echovirus 19. *G. Ig. Med. Prev.* **10:**163–175.
39. de Arruda, E., F. G. Hayden, J. F. McAuliffe, M. A. de Sousa, S. B. Mota, M. I. McAuliffe, F. C. Geist, E. P. Carvalho, M. C. Fernandes, R. L. Guerrant, and J. M. Gwaltney, Jr. 1991. Acute respiratory viral infections in ambulatory children of urban northeast Brazil. *J. Infect. Dis.* **164:**252–258.
40. Denny, F. W., A. M. Collier, and F. W. Henderson. 1986. Acute respiratory infections in day care. *Rev. Infect. Dis.* **8:**527–532.
41. Dery, P., M. I. Marks, and R. Shapera. 1974. Clinical manifestations of coxsackievirus infections in children. *Am. J. Dis. Child.* **128:**464–468.
42. Disney, M. E., R. Matthews, and J. D. Williams. 1971. The role of infection in the morbidity of asthmatic children admitted to hospital. *Clin. Allergy* **1:**399–406.
43. Domok, I., and E. Molnar. 1960. An outbreak of meningoencephalomyocarditis among newborn infants during the epidemic of Bornholm disease of 1958 in Hungary. *Ann. Paediatr.* **194:**102–114.
44. Doraisingham, S., and A. E. Ling. 1986. Patterns of viral respiratory tract infections in Singapore. *Ann. Acad. Med. Singapore* **15:**9–14.
45. Downham, M. A., P. S. Gardner, J. McQuillin, and J. A. Ferris. 1975. Role of respiratory viruses in childhood mortality. *Br. Med. J.* **1:**235 239.
46. Eckert, H. L., B. Portnoy, M. A. Salvatore, and R. Ressler. 1967. Coxsackie virus infection in infants with acute lower respiratory disease. *Pediatrics* **39:**526–531.
47. Ehrnst, A., and M. Eriksson. 1993. Epidemiological features of type 22 echovirus infection. *Scand. J. Infect. Dis.* **25:**275–281.
48. Evans, A. S., and E. C. Dick. 1964. Acute pharyngitis and tonsillitis in University of Wisconsin students. *JAMA* **190:**699.
49. Flewett, T. H. 1965. Histological study of two cases of coxsackie B virus pneumonia in children. *J. Clin. Pathol.* **18:**743–746.
50. Fox, J. P., C. E. Hall, M. K. Cooney, R. E. Luce, and R. A. Kronmal. 1972. The Seattle virus watch. II. Objectives, study population and its observation, data processing and summary of illnesses. *Am. J. Epidemiol.* **96:**270–285.
51. Foy, H. M., M. K. Cooney, A. J. Maletzky, and J. T. Grayston. 1973. Incidence and etiology of pneumonia, croup and bronchiolitis in preschool children belonging to a prepaid medical care group over a four-year period. *Am. J. Epidemiol.* **97:**80–92.
52. Fukumi, H., F. Nishikawa, T. Sonoguchi, and T. Shimizu. 1961. Isolation of Coe virus and some sero-epidemiological surveys of Coe virus infections. *Jpn. J. Med. Sci. Biol.* **14:**21–25.
53. Gilbert, G. L., K. E. Dickson, M. J. Waters, M. L. Kennett, S. A. Land, and M. Sneddon. 1988. Outbreak of enterovirus 71 infection in Victoria, Australia, with a high incidence of neurologic involvement. *Pediatr. Infect. Dis. J.* **7:**484–488.
54. Glezen, W. P., F. A. Loda, W. A. Clyde, Jr., R. J. Senior, C. I. Sheaffer, W. G. Conley, and F. W. Denny. 1971. Epidemiologic patterns of acute lower respiratory disease of children in a pediatric group practice. *J. Pediatr.* **78:**397–406.
55. Gregg, I., M. Horn, E. Brain, J. M. Inglis, and S. J. Yealland. 1975. Proceedings: the role of viral infection in asthma and bronchitis. *Tubercle* **56:**171.
56. Grist, N. R., E. J. Bell, and F. Assaad. 1978. Enteroviruses in human disease. *Prog. Med. Virol.* **4:**114–157.
57. Hable, K. A., E. J. O'Connell, and E. C. Herrmann, Jr. 1970. Group B coxsackieviruses

as respiratory viruses. *Mayo Clin. Proc.* **45:**170–176.
58. Hall, C. E., M. K. Cooney, and J. P. Fox. 1970. The Seattle virus watch program. I. Infection and illness experience of virus watch families during a communitywide epidemic of echovirus type 30 aseptic meningitis. *Am. J. Public Health Nations Health* **60:**1456–1465.
59. Halsted, C., M. L. Lepow, N. Balassanian, J. Emmerich, and E. Wolinsky. 1968. Otitis media. Clinical observations, microbiology, and evaluation of therapy. *Am. J. Dis. Child.* **115:**542–551.
60. Hamre, D., A. P. Connelly, Jr., and J. J. Procknow. 1966. Virologic studies of acute respiratory disease in young adults. IV. Virus isolations during four years of surveillance. *Am. J. Epidemiol.* **83:**238–249.
61. Henderson, F. W., A. M. Collier, M. A. Sanyal, J. M. Watkins, D. L. Fairclough, W. A. Clyde, Jr., and F. W. Denny. 1982. A longitudinal study of respiratory viruses and bacteria in the etiology of acute otitis media with effusion. *N. Engl. J. Med.* **306:**1377–1383.
62. Henderson, F. W., and G. S. Giebink. 1986. Otitis media among children in day care: epidemiology and pathogenesis. *Rev. Infect. Dis.* **8:**533–538.
63. Hierholzer, J. C., S. R. Mostow, and W. R. Dowdle. 1972. Prospective study of a mixed coxsackie virus B3 and B4 outbreak of upper respiratory illness in a children's home. *Pediatrics* **49:**744–752.
64. Holmes, M. J., T. R. Allen, A. F. Bradburne, and E. J. Stott. 1971. Studies of respiratory viruses in personnel at an Antarctic base. *J. Hyg.* **69:**187–199.
65. Horn, M. E., E. Brain, I. Gregg, S. J. Yealland, and J. M. Inglis. 1975. Respiratory viral infection in childhood. A survey in general practice, Roehampton 1967–1972. *J. Hyg.* **74:**157–168.
66. Horn, M. E., and I. Gregg. 1973. Role of viral infection and host factors in acute episodes of asthma and chronic bronchitis. *Chest* **63** (Suppl.):44S–48S.
67. Huebner, R. J., R. M. Cole, E. A. Beeman, J. A. Bell, and J. H. Peers. 1951. Herpangina: etiological studies of a specific infectious disease. *JAMA* **145:**628–633.
68. Hughes, J. H. 1993. Physical and chemical methods for enhancing rapid detection of viruses and other agents. *Clin. Microbiol. Rev.* **6:**150–175.
69. Ikeda, R. M., S. F. Kondracki, P. D. Drabkin, G. S. Birkhead, and D. L. Morse. 1993. Pleurodynia among football players at a high school. An outbreak associated with coxsackievirus B1. *JAMA* **270:**2205–2206.
70. Jackson, G. G., and R. L. Muldoon. 1973. Viruses causing common respiratory infections in man. II. Enteroviruses and paramyxoviruses. *J. Infect. Dis.* **128:**387–469.
71. Jahn, C. L., O. L. Felton, and J. D. Cherry. 1964. Coxsackie B1 pneumonia in an adult. *JAMA* **189:**236–237.
72. Johnson, K. M., H. H. Bloom, B. Forsythe, M. A. Mufson, P. A. Webb, and R. M. Chanock. 1963. The role of enteroviruses in respiratory disease. *Am. Rev. Respir. Dis.* **88:**240–245.
73. Johnson, K. M., H. H. Bloom, M. A. Mufson, and R. M. Chanock. 1962. Acute respiratory disease associated with coxsackie A21 virus infection. I. Military personnel: observation in a recruit population. *JAMA* **179:**112–119.
74. Kantor, F. S., and G. D. Hsiung. 1962. Pleurodynia associated with echo virus type 8. *N. Engl. J. Med.* **266:**661–663.
75. Karzon, D. T., and A. L. Barron. 1962. An epidemic of aseptic meningitis syndrome due to Echo virus type 6. I. Correlation of enterovirus isolation with illness. *Pediatrics* **29:**409–417.
76. Karzon, D. T., and A. L. Barron. 1962. An epidemic of aseptic meningitis syndrome due to Echo virus type 6. II. Clinical study. *Pediatrics* **29:**418–431.
77. Kendall, E. J. C., G. T. Cook, and D. M. Stone. 1960. Acute respiratory infections in children. Isolation of coxsackie B virus and adenovirus during a survey in a general practice. *Br. Med. J.* **2:**1180–1184.
78. Kennett, M. L., C. J. Birch, F. A. Lewis, A. P. Yung, S. A. Locarnini, and I. D. Gust. 1974. Enterovirus type 71 infection in Melbourne. *Bull. W.H.O.* **51:**609–615.
79. Kepfer, P. D., K. A. Hable, and T. F. Smith. 1974. Virus isolation rates during summer from children with acute upper respiratory tract disease and healthy children. *Am. J. Clin. Pathol.* **61:**1–5.
80. Kibrick, S. 1964. Current status of coxsackie and ECHO viruses in human disease. *Prog. Med. Virol.* **6:**27–70.
81. Klein, B. S., F. R. Dollete, and R. H. Yolken. 1982. The role of respiratory syncytial virus and other viral pathogens in acute otitis media. *J. Pediatr.* **101:**16–20.
82. Kogon, A., I. Spigland, T. E. Frothingham, L. Elveback, C. Williams, C. E. Hall, and J. P. Fox. 1969. The virus watch program: a continuing surveillance of viral infections in metropolitan New York families. VII. Observations on viral excretion, seroimmunity,

intrafamilial spread and illness association in coxsackie and echovirus infections. *Am. J. Epidemiol.* **89:**51–61.
83. **Kravis, L. P., K. Hummeler, M. Sigel, and H. I. Lecks.** 1953. Herpangina: clinical and laboratory aspects of an outbreak caused by group A coxsackie viruses. *Pediatrics* **11:**113–119.
84. **Lang, D. J., T. R. Cate, R. B. Couch, V. Knight, and K. M. Jackson.** 1965. Response of volunteers to inoculation with hemagglutinin-positive and hemagglutinin-negative variants of coxsackie A-21 virus. *J. Clin. Invest.* **44:**1125–1131.
85. **Lennette, E. H., V. L. Fox, N. J. Schmidt, and J. O. Culver.** 1958. The Coe virus: an apparently new virus recovered from patients with mild respiratory disease. *Am. J. Hyg.* **68:**272–287.
86. **Lerner, A. M., J. O. Klein, H. S. Levin, and M. Finland.** 1960. Infections due to coxsackie virus group A, type 9, in Boston, 1959, with special reference to exanthems and pneumonia. *N. Engl. J. Med.* **263:**1265–1272.
87. **Lim, K. A., and M. Benyesh-Melnick.** 1960. Typing of viruses of combinations of antiserum pools. Application to typing of enterovirus (coxsackie and ECHO). *J. Immunol.* **84:**309–317.
88. **Loda, F. A., W. P. Glezen, and W. A. Clyde, Jr.** 1972. Respiratory disease in group day care. *Pediatrics* **49:**428–437.
89. **Magee, W. E., and O. V. Miller.** 1970. Individual variability in antibody response of human volunteers to infection of the upper respiratory tract by coxsackie A-21 virus. *J. Infect. Dis.* **122:**127–138.
89a. **Mann, L., and T. Chonmaitree.** Unpublished data.
90. **Melnick, J. L.** 1990. Enteroviruses: polioviruses, coxsackieviruses, echoviruses, and newer enteroviruses, p. 549–605. *In* B. N. Fields and D. M. Knipe (ed.), *Virology*, 2nd ed. Raven Press, New York.
91. **Menegus, M. A.** 1991. Enteroviruses, p. 943–947. *In* A. Balows, W. J. Hausler, Jr., K. L. Herrmann, H. D. Isenberg, and H. J. Shadomy (ed.), *Manual of Clinical Microbiology*, 5th ed. American Society for Microbiology, Washington, D.C.
92. **Mitchell, I., H. Inglis, and H. Simpson.** 1976. Viral infection in wheezy bronchitis and asthma in children. *Arch. Dis. Child.* **51:**707–711.
93. **Monto, A. S., and B. M. Ullman.** 1974. Acute respiratory illness in an American community: the Tecumseh study. *JAMA* **227**(2):164–169.
94. **Mufson, M. A., H. E. Krause, H. E.** mycoplasma pneumoniae and bacteria associated with lower respiratory tract disease among infants. *Am J. Epidemiol.* **91:**192–202.
95. **Murphy, A. M., and R. Simmul.** 1964. Coxsackievirus B4 virus infections in New South Wales during 1962. *Med. J. Aust.* **ii:**443–445.
96. **Nakayama, T., T. Urano, M. Osano, Y. Hayashi, S. Sekine, T. Ando, and S. Makino.** 1989. Outbreak of herpangina associated with coxsackievirus B3 infection. *Pediatr. Infect. Dis. J.* **8:**495–498.
97. **Oehling, A., I. Antepara, and C. E. Baena Cagnani.** 1981. The viral factor in the etiology of acute asthma attacks in children. *Allergol. Immunopathol.* **9:**29–36.
98. **Parrott, R. H., S. Ross, F. G. Burke, and E. C. Rice.** 1951. Herpangina: clinical studies of a specific infectious disease. *N. Engl. J. Med.* **245:**275–280.
99. **Pereira, M. S., and H. G. Pereira.** 1959. Coe virus: properties and prevalence in Great Britain. *Lancet* **ii:**539–541.
100. **Philipson, L., and T. Wesslen.** 1958. Recovery of cytopathogenic agent from patients with non-diphtheritic croup and from day-nursery children. I. Properties of the agent. *Arch. Gesamte Virusforsch.* **8:**77–94.
101. **Ray, C. G., K. L. Plexico, H. A. Wenner, and T. D. Chin.** 1967. Acute respiratory illness associated with coxsackie B4 virus in children. *Pediatrics* **39:**220–226.
102. **Roberts, A. N., R. C. Rendtorff, and B. D. Hale.** 1965. Association of coxsackievirus B3 with epidemic respiratory illness in an orphanage nursery. *Am. J. Epidemiol.* **82:**123–134.
103. **Rossen, R. D., W. T. Butler, T. R. Cate, C. F. Szwed, and R. B. Couch.** 1965. Protein composition of nasal secretion during respiratory virus infection. *Proc. Soc. Exp. Biol. Med.* **119:**1169–1176.
104. **Rotbart, H. A.** 1991. Nucleic acid detection systems for enteroviruses. *Clin. Microbiol. Rev.* **4:**156–168.
105. **Saliba, G. S., S. L. Franklin, and G. G. Jackson.** 1968. Echo-11 as a respiratory virus: quantitation of infection in man. *J. Clin. Invest.* **47:**1303–1313.
106. **Sarkkinen, H., O. Ruuskanen, O. Meurman, H. Puhakka, E. Virolainen, and J. Eskola.** 1985. Identification of respiratory virus antigens in middle ear fluids of children with acute otitis media. *J. Infect. Dis.* **151:**444–448.
107. **Schieble, J. H., V. L. Fox, and E. H. Lennette.** 1967. A probable new human picor-

navirus associated with respiratory diseases. *Am. J. Epidemiol.* **85**:297–310.
108. **Schnurr, D.** 1992. Enteroviruses, p. 351–364. *In* E. H. Lennette (ed.), *Laboratory Diagnosis of Viral Infections,* 2nd ed. Marcel Dekker, Inc., New York.
109. **Siegel, W., F. J. Spencer, D. J. Smith, J. M. Toman, W. F. Skinner, and M. B. Marx.** 1963. Two new variants of infection with coxsackie virus group B, type 5, in young children. A syndrome of lymphadenopathy, pharyngitis and hepatomegaly or splenomegaly, or both, and one of pneumonia. *N. Engl. J. Med.* **268**:1210–1216.
110. **Šimková, A., and A. Petrovicová.** 1972. Experimental infection of rhesus monkeys with coxsackie A 4 virus. *Acta Virol.* **16**:250–257.
111. **Steigman, A. J., M. M. Lipton, and H. Braspennickx.** 1962. Acute lymphonodular pharyngitis: a newly described condition due to coxsackie A virus. *J. Pediatr.* **61**:331–336.
112. **Steinhoff, M. C., B. Padmini, T. J. John, J. Kingsley, and S. M. Pereira.** 1985. Viral etiology of acute respiratory infections in South Indian children. *Indian J. Med. Res.* **81**:349–353.
113. **Stott, E. J.** 1975. The importance of picornavirus infections in respiratory disease of man and other mammals. *Dev. Biol. Stand.* **28**:65–85.
114. **Sudman, J. H., and R. A. Gunn.** 1988. *Pleurodynia Outbreak among Athletic Teams, Ohio.* Field Epidemiology Report No. 88-09, p. 1–10. Centers for Disease Control, Atlanta.
115. **Suzuki, N., K. Ishikawa, T. Horiuchi, M. Schibazaki, and K. Soda.** 1980. Age-related symptomatology of ECHO 11 virus infection in children. *Pediatrics* **65**:284–286.
116. **Tilles, J. G., J. O. Klein, R. L. Jao, J. E. Haslam, Jr., M. Feingold, S. S. Gellis, and M. Finland.** 1967. Acute otitis media in children: serologic studies and attempts to isolate viruses and mycoplasmas from aspirated middle-ear fluids. *N. Engl. J. Med.* **277**:613–618.
117. **Toce, S. S., and W. J. Keenan.** 1988. Congenital echovirus 11 pneumonia in association with pulmonary hypertension. *Pediatr. Infect. Dis. J.* **7**:360–362.
118. **Welliver, R. C., and J. D. Cherry.** 1992. Bronchiolitis and infectious asthma, p. 245–254. *In* R. D. Feigin and J. D. Cherry (ed.), *Textbook of Pediatric Infectious Diseases,* 3rd ed. The W. B. Saunders Co., Philadelphia.
119. **Wildin, S., and T. Chonmaitree.** 1987. The importance of the virology laboratory in the diagnosis and management of viral meningitis. *Am. J. Dis. Child.* **141**:454–457.
119a.**Wigand, R., and A. B. Sabin.** 1962. Properties of epidemic strains of ECHO type 9 virus and observations on the nature of human infection. *Arch. Gesamte Virusforsch.* **11**:683–701.
120. **Wright, H. T., Jr., B. H. Landing, E. H. Lennette, and R. M. McAllister.** 1963. Fatal infection in an infant associated with coxsackie virus group A, type 16. *N. Engl. J. Med.* **268**:1041–1044.
121. **Zahorsky, J.** 1920. Herpetic sore throat. *South. Med. J.* **13**:871–872.
122. **Zahorsky, J.** 1924. Herpangina (a specific infectious disease). *Arch. Pediatr.* **41**:181–184.

MENINGITIS AND ENCEPHALITIS

Harley A. Rotbart

13

Central nervous system (CNS) infection by the enteroviruses (EVs) has been recognized since antiquity because of the dramatic physical effects of the prototypic EVs, the polioviruses. Today, though eradicated from the Americas and much of the developed world, poliomyelitis continues to be a World Health Organization target priority in developing countries (see chapter 9). The most vexing clinical syndromes caused by the nonpolio EVs also result from infection of the CNS. This chapter will review the two most common CNS EV infections, meningitis and encephalitis. Other neurologic syndromes have also been associated with nonpolio EV infections, including paralytic myelitis (indistinguishable from that due to polioviruses) due to coxsackievirus A7, EV70, and EV71, among others (4, 42, 46, 48, 117). Cerebellar ataxia has occasionally been associated with EV infections, as have Guillain-Barre syndrome and transverse myelitis. These latter three associations are weakened by the difficulty in distinguishing pathogenicity of a throat or stool isolate from coincidental viral shedding, which may occur for weeks to months after EV infections (see chapter 17).

The term "aseptic meningitis" refers to a clinical syndrome of meningeal inflammation in which common bacterial agents cannot be identified in the cerebrospinal fluid (CSF) (118, 119). Implicit in the definition of aseptic meningitis is the benignity of the clinical course and the absence of signs of parenchymal brain involvement. When the brain itself is prominently involved in an inflammatory process, "encephalitis" is the appropriate term; it reflects a potentially much more severe natural history. Many patients exhibit less discrete signs and symptoms and are described as having "meningoencephalitis." The EVs are the most common cause of aseptic meningitis in the United States as well as an important cause of encephalitis.

EPIDEMIOLOGY

The overall epidemiology of the EVs is reviewed in chapters 1 and 9. More than 7,000 cases of aseptic meningitis are reported in the United States annually (18, 20); the actual incidence, including unreported cases, may be as much as 10-fold higher (see below). The vast majority of cases are due to viral infections; however, infections caused by nonviral pathogens, including certain bacteria (which are not readily seen by stains and/or do not grow in standard culture systems), mycoplasmas, and

Harley A. Rotbart, University of Colorado School of Medicine and The Children's Hospital of Denver, Denver, Colorado 80262.

fungi, may present identically to viral aseptic meningitis (102). Autoimmune diseases, malignancies, and reactions to certain drugs are occasionally manifested as aseptic meningitis as well. The first viruses recognized to cause meningitis, mumps virus, lymphocytic choriomeningitis virus, and poliovirus, are uncommon causes in developed countries today (Table 1). Initial series of aseptic meningitis included identification of a specific etiologic agent in only 25% of cases (3, 98).

With the discovery in 1948 of the group B coxsackieviruses (30), and the advent in 1949 of tissue culture (37), which permits convenient and efficient identification of the polioviruses and echoviruses, EVs quickly emerged as the leading recognizable cause of aseptic meningitis (Table 1). More recent series include identification of a specific viral pathogen in as many as 55 to 70% of cases when consistent diagnostic methodology is applied (8, 11, 68, 69, 78). Application of PCR to the diagnosis of aseptic meningitis has resulted in increased identification of the EVs (see below and chapter 17). At least two-thirds of all culture-negative CSF specimens from patients with aseptic meningitis are positive for EV by PCR (101, 108). All of these data suggest that as many as 75,000 cases of EV meningitis occur in the United States each year, more than 10 times the number actually reported to the Centers for Disease Control and Prevention, and that nonpolio EVs account for 85 to 95% of all cases of aseptic meningitis for which an etiologic agent is identified (Table 1). The overall epidemiology of aseptic meningitis mirrors that of the EVs (Fig. 1) because of the striking numeric dominance of the latter among the etiologic agents.

Conversely, aseptic meningitis is the syndrome most commonly identified in association with EV infections (75, 82), a fact due to the age distribution of EV meningitis, which affects very young children disproportionately (126), and to the difficulty of clinically distinguishing aseptic from bacterial meningitis in this age group. Hence, viral cultures, particularly of the CSF, are commonly ob-

TABLE 1 Viral causes of aseptic meningitis in selected large series

Investigator(s) (reference)	Yr	No. of cases	EVs P	EVs NPE	Arboviruses	Mumps	Herpes	LCM	Other	None	Consistent methodology[b]
Rasmussen (98)	1941–1946	374				15.3		11.2	No	73.5	Yes
Adair et al. (3)	1947–1952	480				13.3	5.3	9.7	No	74.8	Yes
Meyer et al. (78)	1953–1958	430	8.8	29.8	0.7	15.8	1.4	8.8	No	29	Yes
Lepow et al. (69)	1955–1958	407	7	41		8			No	46	Yes
Lennette et al. (68)	1958	368	2	57		9	1		Yes[c]	31	Yes
Buescher et al. (11)	1958–1963	374	4.8	38.5	0.8	7.5	0.5	1.9	Yes[d]	43.5	Yes
Deibel et al. (31–34, 43)	1972–1979	2,382	0.5	24	1.4	1.2	2.7	0.5	Yes[e]	68.3	No
Berlin et al.[g]	1986–1990	274	0.007	61.3					Yes[f]	38.4	Yes

[a] Abbreviations: P, polioviruses; NPE, nonpolio EVs; LCM, lymphocytic choriomeningitis virus.
[b] Consistent methodology: virologic and/or serologic studies performed by a single laboratory, with most or all specimens subjected to all tests.
[c] 1% adenovirus.
[d] <1% each of measles virus, Epstein-Barr virus, influenza A virus.
[e] 1.4% influenza A virus; 1% adenovirus; <1% each of measles virus, cytomegalovirus, varicella-zoster virus, rubella virus, influenza B virus, parainfluenza virus, and respiratory syncytial virus.
[f] <1% adenovirus (one case).

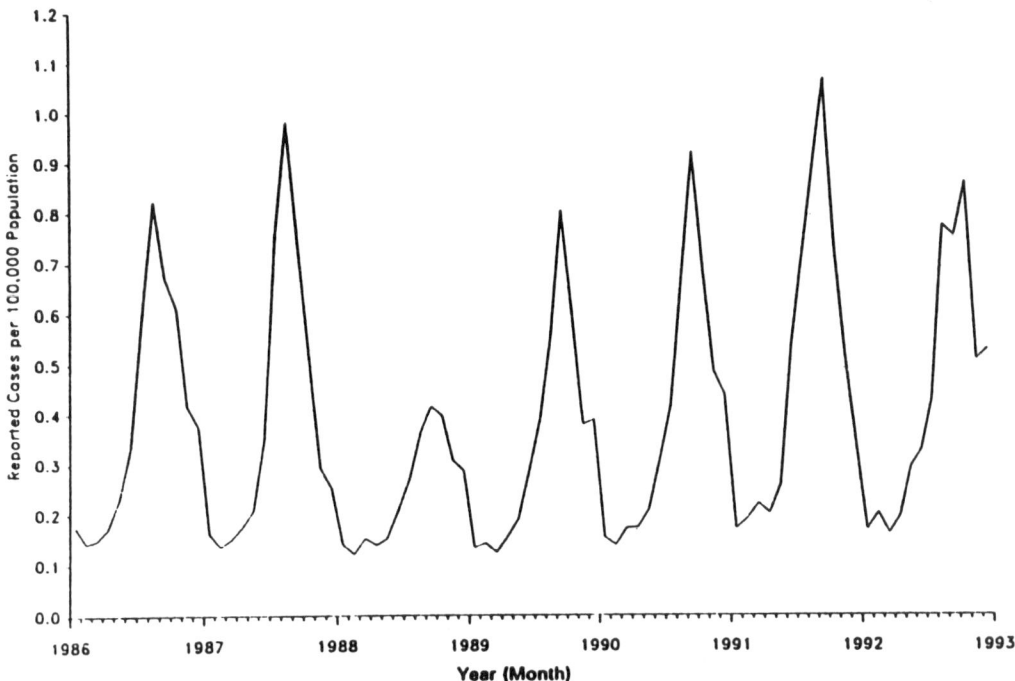

FIGURE 1 Seasonal occurrence of aseptic meningitis in the United States from 1986 through 1992, as reported to the Centers for Disease Control and Prevention (20). The striking predominance of cases during the summer months reflects the predominance of EVs as etiologic agents in aseptic meningitis.

tained from children with meningitis, and EVs are frequently identified (125, 126). Viral cultures are less likely to be performed with non-CNS infections, even in young infants, despite a high incidence of EV-associated systemic disease without concomitant CNS involvement (see chapter 11).

The true incidence of EV encephalitis is difficult to determine because the isolation of any virus from the CSF of patients with encephalitis is rare and because of a reluctance to do brain biopsies (122). For the estimated 20,000 cases of viral encephalitis in the United States each year, herpes simplex virus is the most commonly identified pathogen, but it accounts for only 10% of cases (122). Arboviruses and EVs are probably the next most common causes; for most cases of viral encephalitis, a specific etiologic agent is never identified. PCR is already proving to be a significant improvement over culture in herpes simplex virus and EV encephalitis (see below and chapter 17) and should help to more precisely define the relative significance of these pathogens in patients with encephalitis.

Children are the primary victims of CNS EV infections (126). In a large Finnish cohort (96), the annual incidence of viral meningitis was 219/100,000 children less than 1 year of age but only 19/100,000 children between the ages of 1 and 4 years. The incidence dropped even further with increased age. The vast majority of identified viral pathogens were EVs. Other surveys of meningitis and encephalitis have revealed a similar skew toward young infants (8, 114); an incidence peak among young school age children, aged 5 to 10 years, has also been reported in several studies (29, 99, 130); occasional outbreaks of CNS EV infections occur predominantly among adults (64, 85). A possible explanation for these seemingly conflicting age incidence findings may lie in the recent history of particular serotypes in the geographic area studied. Serotypes with patterns of endemicity, occurring with significant incidence every year, are most likely to affect only the youngest children. This group is the most susceptible to these serotypes for the same reason that it is most susceptible to many common infections: the absence of previous exposure and immunity. Older children are more likely to predominate as patients in an outbreak of a serotype that has not been present in a community for several years, as a reservoir of susceptible children, born since the last appearance of that serotype, has been created. Although EVs are the most common cause of aseptic meningitis among adults as well, the usual incidence and severity of this disease and the vigor with which a specific viral etiology is sought are all diminished in older age groups. When a serotype is introduced into a community that has many susceptible adults, perhaps because it has been many years since that serotype last appeared or because an antigenic variant of a common serotype has emerged, the large number of affected adults will spark renewed interest and increased efforts toward specific diagnosis.

Among the many EV serotypes that cycle from year to year, certain serotypes are more commonly associated with aseptic meningitis than others. Among the most common U.S. EV isolates during the years 1970 through 1983 are found the most common EV causes of meningitis, since isolates from patients with meningitis dominate the specimens submitted for typing each year (113). The predominant isolates during that 14-year period were (in decreasing order) echovirus 11; echovirus 9; coxsackievirus B5; echoviruses 30, 4, and 6; coxsackieviruses B2, B4, B3, and A9; echoviruses 3, 7, 5, and 24; and coxsackievirus B1 (113). The six serotypes most frequently isolated during each of the subsequent 6 years are shown in Table 2 (13–17, 19). Polioviruses, once major causes of aseptic meningitis (only occasionally followed by paralytic myelitis), are now rarely recovered from patients with aseptic meningitis (Table 1). Vaccine strains have occasionally caused meningitis in healthy children (72, 97) and children with CNS shunts (50); in the United States, vaccine strains are also recovered annually from as many as 10 persons who contract poliomyelitis following vaccination of themselves or of a close household contact (18, 20; see chapter 9).

While coxsackievirus B5 and several of the echoviruses (serotypes 4, 6, 9, 11, and 30) are the most common causes of aseptic meningitis in the United States (13–17, 19, 113), only a few EV serotypes have not been suspected (virus recovered from the stool or throat) or confirmed (virus recovered from the CSF or blood) to cause meningitis (23, 49, 76, 121). Those agents may indeed cause meningitis and may not have been recognized because of difficulty in viral isolation methods for certain serotypes or because most EV isolates are never specifically serotyped. It is clear, however, that neurotropism varies among the EV serotypes (see below). The observation that clinical stigmata do not differ significantly among the nonpolio EVs causing aseptic meningitis (53) coupled with the limited availability of typing serum pools (77) has made investigators increasingly content to identify individual cases or outbreaks as simply "an enterovirus" on the basis of the characteristic cytopathic effect in tissue culture (see chapter 17).

Host factors that predispose to EV meningitis, other than young age and immunodeficiency (see below), have been difficult to identify. Physical exercise, an established risk factor for paralytic poliomyelitis (52, 106, 107) and a hypothesized one for enteroviral myocarditis (45), may also predispose infected individuals to develop nonpolio EV aseptic meningitis. Attack rates for aseptic meningitis among athletes have been higher than those among other students during EV outbreaks (5, 82, 83). A male-to-female incidence ratio for EV infections of 1.3 to 1.5:1 has been reported (82). Individuals may develop more than one episode of EV meningitis (65, 86); however, the same EV serotype has not been implicated twice in any one immunocompetent patient (21). Immunization with poliovirus vaccines

TABLE 2 Most common EV isolates, 1984 through 1989[a]

Yr	Isolate[b]						% of total EV isolates[c]
	1	2	3	4	5	6	
1984	E9	E11	CB5	E30	CB2	CA9	58.4
1985	E11	E21	E6, E7[d]		CB2	CB4	58
1986	E11	E4	E7	E18	CB4, CB5[d]		66
1987	E6	E18	E11	CA9	CB2	E9	64
1988	E11	E9	CB4	CB2	E6	CB5	64
1989	CB5	E9	E11	CB2	E6	CA16	67

[a] Data are from references 13 through 17 and 19. Abbreviations: E, echovirus; CB, coxsackievirus B; CA, coxsackievirus A.
[b] 1, most common isolate; 2, second most common isolate; etc.
[c] Percentage attributable to the six most common isolates for that year.
[d] Isolates were equally common.

does not protect against nonpolio EV infections. Mixed infections involving EVs and other viruses (6, 72) or bacteria (36) are rare but have been described; in the latter cases, the clinical presentation and course are dominated by the bacterial pathogen.

PATHOGENESIS AND PATHOLOGY

The pathogenesis of EV infections has been studied at the molecular, cellular, and organ system levels (104; see chapters 2 through 8), and while much has been learned, much more remains unexplained. EVs are acquired by fecal-oral contamination and, less commonly, by respiratory droplet. Most of what is known about the subsequent viral pathway within the host was derived from experimental poliovirus infections in chimpanzees more than four decades ago (9, 10). While some replication occurs in the nasopharynx, with spread to upper respiratory tract lymphatics, most of the viral inoculum is swallowed. The EVs distinguish themselves from the rhinoviruses, another large genus of picornaviruses, by being stable at acid pH, the characteristic responsible for the ability of EVs to traverse the stomach en route to the site of primary infection in the lower gastrointestinal tract. There, EVs presumably bind to specific receptors on enterocytes; it is not known precisely which cells are susceptible and whether the so-called M cells responsible for reovirus uptake and penetration (128) are similarly involved during EV infection. The virus traverses the intestinal lining cells, perhaps with replication but without apparent cytopathogenicity, and reaches the Peyer's patches in the lamina propria, where significant viral replication occurs. A minor viremia that seeds numerous organ systems, including the CNS, liver, lungs, and heart, ensues. More significant replication at these sites results in a major viremia associated with the signs and symptoms of viral infection. If the CNS has not been seeded during the initial viremic episode, spread there may occur during the major viremia. Although fairly well established, viremia as the source of CNS infection has been long debated, with direct neural spread (35, 129) suggested as an alternate hypothesis. Indeed, both routes of spread may occur and may not be mutually exclusive (35). The mechanism by which EVs leave the blood and enter the CNS is entirely unknown; "leakiness" in the vessels of the choroid plexus (meningitis) and/or of the parenchyma (encephalitis) is likely responsible rather than active transport of viral particles across the blood-brain barrier. Endothelial cells may express EV receptors, in which case upregulation of those receptors, e.g., during systemic EV infection, may facilitate viral entry into the CNS. During clinical infections, EVs have been recovered from both the cellular and the plasma fractions of the blood (93; see chapter 11), and the more important of the blood compartments for establishing CNS infection is not known. Differences in susceptibilities of mononuclear cells to various EV serotypes have been demonstrated (28, 99a) and may have an impact on patterns of neurotropism if cell-associated transport into the CNS is important. In vitro, EVs are released into the medium by infected cells and can survive extracellularly for many days; hence, cell association (e.g., monocytes or lymphocytes) may not be as important for EV access to the CNS as it is for other viruses (92).

While all three serotypes of wild-type polioviruses are neurotropic and neurovirulent, those phenotypes vary widely among the nonpolio EV, with certain serotypes consistently reported as causes of meningitis and encephalitis and others only rarely infecting the CNS (4, 8, 23, 27, 113, 130) (Table 3). The presence or absence of specific cellular receptors is unlikely to explain all of this heterogeneity, however, as variations in neurotropism exist even within receptor families. Coxsackievirus B6, for example, is a rare cause of CNS infection, in contrast to the other five coxsackieviruses B, which are important causes of both meningitis and encephalitis (23, 76). The determinants of neurotropism and neurovirulence have been investigated extensively for the polioviruses (see chapters 2 and 3), and molecular neurovirulence determinants among the nonpolio EVs are now being studied in the hope of finding a genomic explanation for the increased frequency of aseptic meningitis and encephalitis observed with certain serotypes and the virtual absence of those diseases with others (Table 3). Studies of the echoviruses in our laboratory have identified specific base changes in the 5' nontranslated region of the EV genome that are unique to serotypes that rarely cause CNS disease; neurotropic echoviruses, in contrast, have base sequences identical to those of the polioviruses in these regions (99b). Coxsackievirus B4 strains with pancreatic tropism and virulence are distinguished from avirulent coxsackievirus B4 strains by a single amino acid residue in the VP1 capsid protein (12); it is not known whether the same locus determines neurotropism for coxsackievirus B4 or other serotypes.

The benign nature of EV meningitis has made human pathologic data for this disease sparse. A report of a child who died of coxsackievirus B5 myocarditis with concomitant meningitis (94) describes inflammation of the choroid plexus of the lateral and fourth ventricles, fibrosis of the vascular walls with focal destruction of the ependymal lining, and fibrotic basal leptomeninges. Parenchymal findings were limited to moderate, symmetric dilation of the ventricles and an increase in number and size of subependymal astrocytes. The inflammatory reaction at the choroid plexus supports the concept of viremic spread to the CNS. A second adolescent presenting with a similar constellation of findings died of systemic coxsackievirus B3 infection (115). The dura was grossly distended, with swelling also of the pia, arachnoid, and brain parenchyma. Microscopically, round cell infiltrates were noted in the meninges overlying the cerebellum; the brain parenchyma was congested with increased numbers of oligodendrocytes. Lymphocytic infiltration was most prominent around blood vessels in the cerebral white matter and the basal ganglia,

TABLE 3 Relative frequency of neurotropism and neurovirulence among nonpolio EVs

Nonpolio EV associated with CNS disease		
Most common	Common	Rare
Echovirus 30	Coxsackievirus B3	Coxsackievirus B6
Coxsackievirus B5	Coxsackievirus B4	Echovirus 12
Echovirus 11	Echovirus 6	Echovirus 2
Echovirus 7	Echovirus 4	Coxsackievirus B1
Echovirus 9	Coxsackievirus A9	Echovirus 22
EVs 70 and 71	Echovirus 18	Echovirus 3

again suggesting viremic access to the CNS; focal areas of necrosis and hemorrhage were also seen (115).

CLINICAL MANIFESTATIONS

The clinical disease observed during CNS EV infections varies with the host's age and immune status. Neonates are at risk for severe systemic illness, of which meningitis or meningoencephalitis is commonly a part (see chapter 10). In one study, group B coxsackieviruses were associated with aseptic meningitis in 62% of infants less than 3 months of age (61). Echoviruses identified in babies less than 2 weeks of age were associated with meningitis or meningoencephalitis in 27% of cases (80). In a recent prospective study of neonates (≤2 weeks of age) with proved EV infection, 75% had clinical and/or laboratory evidence of meningitis (1a). The infected neonate appears to be at greatest risk for severe morbidity and mortality when signs and symptoms develop in the first days of life, suggesting possible transplacental acquisition (61, 66, 80). Maternal illness has been reported in 59 to 68% of infected neonates (1a, 61, 66, 80); however, the degree to which maternal illness is associated with an additional risk to the neonate has been difficult to establish. Even in the youngest patients, fever is ubiquitous and is accompanied early by nonspecific signs such as vomiting, anorexia, rash, and/or upper respiratory tract findings (88). Neurologic involvement may or may not be associated with clinical signs of meningeal inflammation, including nuchal rigidity and bulging anterior fontanelle. As the neonatal disease progresses, major systemic manifestations such as hepatic necrosis, myocarditis, and necrotizing enterocolitis may develop (1a, 61, 66, 80, 84). Disseminated intravascular coagulation and other findings of sepsis result in patients with illness indistinguishable from that due to overwhelming bacterial infection. The CNS disease may progress to a more encephalitic picture with seizures and focal neurologic findings suggestive of herpes simplex virus infection. The incidences of morbidity and mortality due to perinatal EV infections are not precisely known, but they may be as high as 74 and 10%, respectively (61; see chapter 10). When death occurs, it is seldom if ever the result of CNS involvement but is, instead, the result of hepatic failure (echoviruses) or myocarditis (coxsackieviruses).

EV meningitis outside of the immediate neonatal period (<2 weeks of age) is rarely associated with severe disease or poor outcome. The natural history of typical EV meningitis is shown in Fig. 2 (53). Onset is usually sudden, and fever of 38 to 40°C is the most consistent clinical finding, occurring in 76 to 100% of patients (111, 126). The fever pattern may be biphasic, with the appearance first of nonspecific constitutional symptoms, which are followed by resolution and reappearance with the onset of meningeal signs. Nuchal rigidity occurs in more than half of the patients, particularly in children older than 1 to 2 years (111, 126). Headache is nearly always present in adults and children old enough to report it, and photophobia is also common. Nonspecific and constitutional signs and symptoms of viral infection, in decreasing order of occurrence, include vomiting, anorexia, rash, diarrhea, cough and upper respiratory tract findings (particularly pharyngitis), diarrhea, and myalgias (111, 126). Aseptic meningitis caused by certain EV serotypes is associated with particular clinical stigmata; e.g., hand-foot-mouth syndrome frequently occurs with EV 71 meningitis (4, 46, 55) and nonspecific rashes are especially common with echovirus 9 meningitis (112), although both incidental findings can occur with numerous other serotypes as well (23). Neurologic abnormalities are rare and, depending on the criteria used for identification of aseptic meningitis, may not occur at all. That is, because of the implicit benign clinical course associated with the diagnosis of aseptic meningitis, patients with abnormal neurologic findings are likely to be diagnosed with encephalitis or myelitis. Hence, the literature on EV meningitis rarely includes more than 5% of patients with abnormal neurologic examinations. Febrile seizures are

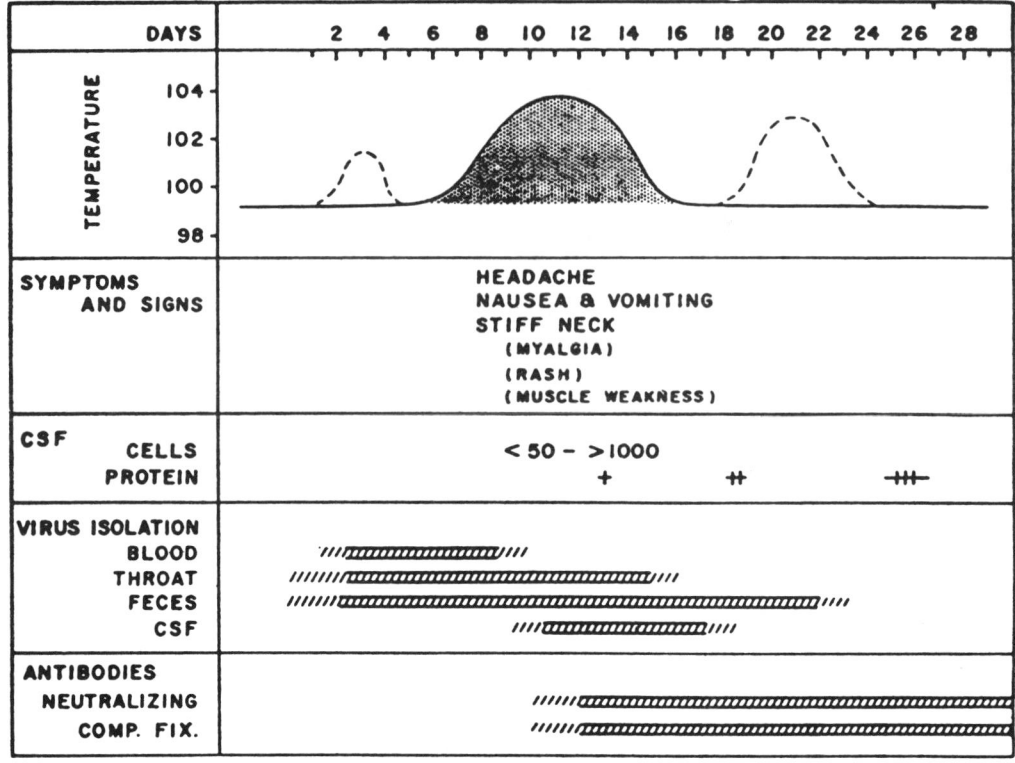

FIGURE 2 Clinical course of EV aseptic meningitis. Reprinted with permission (53).

among those neurologic abnormalities that may complicate aseptic meningitis in children without implying parenchymal brain involvement. The syndrome of inappropriate antidiuretic hormone was reported in 9 of 102 cases of EV meningitis in one study (22). A history of concomitant family illness, including rashes, upper respiratory or gastrointestinal tract symptoms, and occasionally meningitis, is often obtained (40). The duration of illness due to EV meningitis is usually less than 1 week, with some patients feeling better immediately after the lumbar puncture (56), presumably thanks to the reduction of intracranial pressure upon fluid removal. Occasional adult patients may have symptoms that persist for several weeks (69), not a frequent occurrence in children. The short-term prognosis for young children with EV meningitis early in life appears to be good, but there has been controversy regarding sequelae. Uncontrolled studies found numerous subtle long-term behavioral and neurologic abnormalities (63). Neurologic, cognitive, and developmental and/or language abnormalities have been reported in controlled studies of long-term outcome in children with EV meningitis during infancy (Table 4) (7, 39, 47, 58, 100, 109, 127). In the largest and most meticulously controlled study, however, no differences between patients and controls could be demonstrated in any of then eurodevelopmental parameters studied (Table 4) (100). Less well-studied are the ultimate outcomes of aseptic meningitis cases in older children and adolescents; preliminary data suggest possible school and learning difficulties, but no control patients were studied (38).

Unlike aseptic meningitis, encephalitis due to an EV may be a more severe acute disease and have more devastating long-term sequelae. In contrast to the typical focal disease seen

TABLE 4 Controlled long-term outcome studies of EV meningitis occurring in first year of life

Investigators (reference)	No. of patients	Controls	Abnormal findings[a]		
			Neurologic	Cognitive	Development and/or language
Sells et al. (109)	13	Age matched	+	+	+
Farmer et al. (39)	15	Matched	+	+	+
Wilfert et al. (127)	9	Matched	−	−	+
Jenista et al. (58)	71[b]	Matched	−	NS	+
Bergman et al. (7)	42	Siblings	−	−	−
Gonzalez-del-Ray et al. (47)	16	Matched	−	+	+
Rorabaugh et al. (100)	140[c]	Matched	−	−	−

[a] +, abnormalities found; −, abnormalities not found; NS, not stated.
[b] Neonatal patients with EV infections, not necessarily all meningitis.
[c] Patients with aseptic meningitis, not necessarily all caused by EVs.

with herpes simplex virus encephalitis, the EV have been more commonly associated with global encephalitis and generalized neurologic depression (29, 46, 54, 70, 116). The illness usually begins like aseptic meningitis, with a prodrome of fever, myalgias, and upper respiratory tract symptoms. Onset of CNS signs and symptoms is often abrupt, with confusion, weakness, lethargy, drowsiness, and/or irritability. Progression to coma and/or generalized seizures may occur. When meningeal signs and CSF pleocytosis accompany these findings, "meningoencephalitis" is the appropriate term for describing the illness. Unusual but occasional findings in patients with EV encephalitis include blurred optic discs and other signs of increased intracranial pressure, multifocal encephalomyelopathy, apnea, truncal ataxia, abnormalities of cranial nerves, and paralysis; the last sign is usually a manifestation of spinal cord involvement and, when it accompanies central signs and symptoms, is appropriately termed "encephalomyelitis."

Focal EV encephalitis is thought to be an unusual manifestation of CNS EV disease, but it may be underappreciated. As evidenced in antiviral studies by the National Institute of Allergy and Infectious Diseases, EVs are demonstrable by brain biopsy in 13% of patients suspected of having herpes simplex virus encephalitis, the most commonly identified cause of focal encephalitis (123, 124). Colleagues in Denver recently cared for an illustrative case. A 9-month-old male was admitted to the hospital for an afebrile seizure. One day prior to admission, the child developed gasping respiration, pallor, and a focal seizure of the left extremities and face. Except for a fall down the stairs 2 weeks prior to admission the child had an unremarkable history. The child had a normal physical examination and a neurologic examination that was nonfocal but notable for global depression. A CSF leukocyte count of 2/mm^3 on admission rose to 225/mm^3 by day 5, and the development of a maculopapular rash suggested EV infection; the child was empirically treated with antibiotics and acyclovir and required antiepileptic therapy as well. Computerized tomography revealed a focal area of low density in the right parietal area, with minimal contrast enhancement (Fig. 3). Viral culture of the child's CSF grew an EV; laboratory studies for other pathogens were negative. The child was well and seizure free at his 4-month follow-up examination. This case is similar to four that Modlin et al. reported recently and to an additional three from the literature that they reviewed (81). A variety of clinical focal neurologic findings and abnormalities in imaging studies were observed. Only two of the reported patients grew EV from cultures of the CSF; the remaining five cases were confirmed by serologic methods. Hence, EVs must be included in the differential diagnosis of both generalized and focal encephalitis.

Finally, the unique situation of a child or an adult with absent or deficient humoral immu-

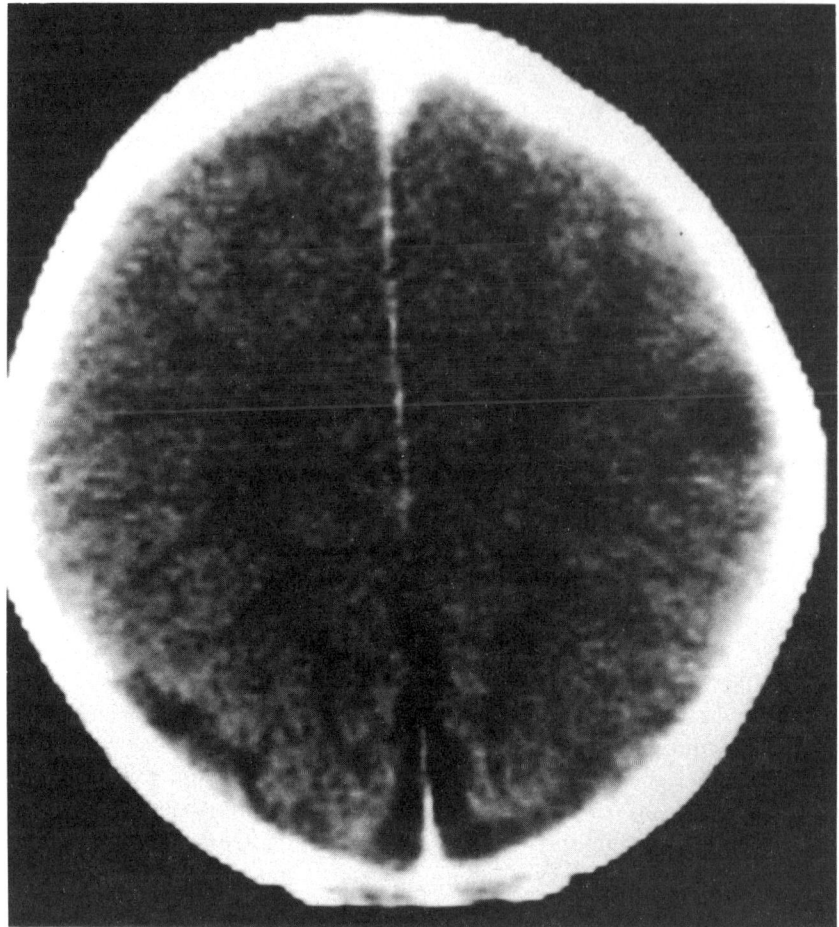

FIGURE 3 Computerized tomography scan of the brain of a 9-month-old infant with focal EV encephalitis (case described in the text). An area of low density consistent in location with the child's left-sided focal seizures can be seen in the right parietal lobe. Minimal enhancement was seen with dye injection. (Case and photo courtesy of John Ogle.)

nity illustrates an important experiment of nature with regard to EV infections of the CNS. Unlike other viruses, which are largely contained by cellular immune mechanisms, EVs are cleared from the host by antibody-mediated mechanisms. Agammaglobulinemic individuals infected with EV may develop chronic meningitis or meningoencephalitis lasting many years, often with a fatal outcome (74). Treatment with antibody preparations intravenously and intrathecally or intraventricularly has stabilized some of these patients. Although CSF culture-negative periods occur, PCR evidence of persistent virus despite ongoing antibody replacement therapy has been reported (103; Fig. 4). Alteration of the viral genome over time in the same individual has also been documented (90), as has the selection of a temperature-sensitive phenotype (51). With the availability of intravenous preparations of immunoglobulin and the early recognition of this illness, fewer patients appear to be progressing to the classic description of this disease, and atypical neurologic presentations have appeared. The expanded clinical spectrum of chronic EV

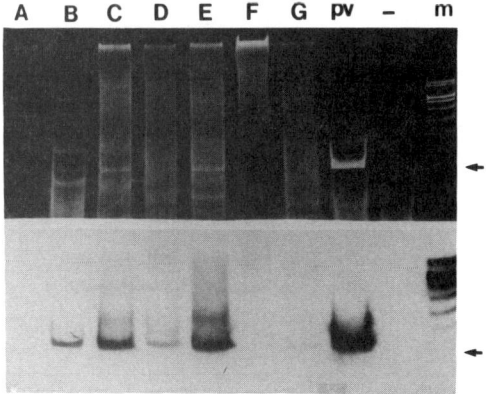

FIGURE 4 Serial results of PCR testing for EVs in CSF specimens from a patient with X-linked agammaglobulinemia. Polyacrylamide gel electrophoresis (top) and confirmatory Southern hybridization (bottom) PCR findings are for specimens collected over 18 months from an indwelling Ommaya reservoir or from lumbar punctures in a single patient (lanes A through G). Lanes B, C, D, E, and G were positive; lanes A and F were negative. Negative (lane −) and positive (lane pv) PCR controls and size markers (lane m) are also shown. The arrow indicates a band length of 154 nucleotides, the predicted length of the EV PCR-amplified products when our standard primers are used.

meningoencephalitis has been revealed by PCR studies of CSF from patients with these atypical manifestations (120). Our results for EV PCR testing of CSF specimens from 27 immunocompromised patients are shown in Table 5; EV infection was confirmed in 18 patients, only 2 of whom grew the virus in culture. More than half of the patients in our series who had chronic meningoencephalitis were already on intravenous immunoglobulin supplementation therapy at the time of diagnosis. This contrasts with 93% culture positivity in the classic review of this syndrome (74), in which only 5% of patients were receiving intravenous immunoglobulin at the time of diagnosis. The patients we studied were also more likely to have normal CSF protein (64%) and CSF cytology (27%) than were those patients previously reviewed (74), a further reflection of the alteration in the illness effected by intravenous antibody replacement. Five of six patients from whom we had serial CSF specimens were positive by PCR on more than one occasion (Fig. 4).

LABORATORY FINDINGS AND DIAGNOSIS

Of paramount importance in the diagnosis and management of meningitis and encephalitis is the establishment of etiology: specifically, bacteria (including partially treated meningitis and parameningeal infections), herpes simplex virus, and other causes for which specific therapies are available must be ruled out before EV infection can be assumed. Clues to the diagnosis of EV meningitis can be obtained from nonspecific CSF findings (62, 102). Pleocytosis is almost always present, although EVs have been isolated from the CSF of patients, usually young infants, with clinical evidence of meningitis but no cells (66, 131). CSF leukocyte counts may range as high as several thousand (79), but 100 to 1,000 cells are the rule (111). The higher the leukocyte count in the CSF, the greater the chance of isolating the causative EV (27). Polymorphonuclear cells may predominate early in meningeal infection, usually giving way to a lymphocytic profile over the first 8 to 48 h (41). Hypoglycorrhachia and elevated CSF protein, if they occur, are usually mild (111), but extreme degrees of both have been reported (71). When controlled for age of the patient, low CSF glucose was much more common than high CSF protein in one study (110). Wide variations in all parameters, however, are the rule, even during an epidemic involving a single serotype (54, 57). By definition, a Gram stain should be negative for bacteria; however, numerous cases of combined EV and bacterial infections have been reported (36), emphasizing the caution that must be used in determining viral etiology in a patient with meningitis, although combined EV and bacterial meningitis is dominated clinically by signs and symptoms attributable to the bacteria. Utility in distinguishing viral (usually EV) meningitis from that due to bacteria has been claimed by various groups studying CSF immunoglobulin levels (60), serum C-reactive protein (25,

TABLE 5 EV PCR: immunocompromised hosts

Underlying disease[a]	No. culture positive/ no. tested	PCR result for specimen (no. positive/no. tested)		
		Single CSF	Serial CSF	Single brain
XLA, XLA-like chronic ME	2/8	6/8[b]	3/4	0/2[b]
CVID/hypogammaglobulinemia				
Chronic ME	0/8	6/8[b]	1/1	1/2
Chronic myositis	0/1	1/1		
Status post AM	0/1	1/1		
Chronic GI shedding	0/2	0/2		
SCID	0/3	2/3		
ALL	0/2	2/2		
Unspecified	0/2	0/2		

[a]Abbreviations: XLA, X-linked agammaglobulinemia; ME, meningoencephalitis; CVID, common variable immunodeficiency; AM, aseptic meningitis (acute, self-limited); GI, gastrointestinal; SCID, severe combined immunodeficiency; ALL, acute lymphoblastic leukemia.

[b]One patient shown in this denominator is still under study but is shown here as negative pending the outcome of additional PCR investigations.

91), CSF lactic acid (26) and lactate dehydrogenase (87), and CSF interleukin-1B and tumor necrosis factor (67, 95). Of all these parameters, tumor necrosis factor may be the most specific for bacterial (versus aseptic) meningitis. In three reports studying CSF tumor necrosis factor detection in patients with meningitis (5a, 67, 95), none of 50 cumulative patients with aseptic meningitis or 19 patients without meningitis had detectable levels of CSF tumor necrosis factor. This compared with 107 (74%) of 145 cumulative patients with detectable CSF tumor necrosis factor accompanying bacterial meningitis (5a, 67, 95). In contrast, while interleukin-1B concentrations were much higher in the CSF of patients with bacterial meningitis, detectable levels were still present in the majority of patients with aseptic meningitis and in occasional patients without meningitis (95).

Specific virologic diagnosis of EV meningitis depends on the detection of virus from CSF in tissue culture (24, 125). Although a nonpolio EV isolated from the throat or rectum of a patient with aseptic meningitis is suggestive, the mean shedding periods from those sites following infection are 1 week and several weeks, respectively (see chapter 17). Hence, shedding from a past infection cannot be ruled out unless the virus is detected in nonpermissive sites, specifically the CSF or blood. Tissue culture has been the mainstay of EV diagnosis since Enders et al. first reported success in growing poliovirus in vitro (37). However, as a diagnostic modality, the technique has limitations (see chapter 17), prominent among which is a delay of several days in detecting viral growth. Investigators report 3.7 to 8.2 days as the mean time for CSF EVs to be detected in tissue culture (57, 96), so by the time results are available, they are often moot in distinguishing viral from bacterial infection, since final bacterial culture results are usually available by 72 h. PCR is the most promising alternative to viral culture for EV diagnosis (see chapter 17). Results from clinical studies using PCR to detect EVs in CSF are summarized in Table 6. Sensitivity ranges from 95 to 100%, with specificity approaching 100% in most studies. PCR of serum and urine samples may also be a sensitive way to diagnose certain patients with EV meningitis (2), but more experience with those types of samples is necessary.

Specific diagnosis of encephalitis due to any virus is much more problematic than diagnosis of viral meningitis, because CSF is much less likely to yield cultivable virus from patients with encephalitis (122). Brain biopsy is the most sensitive technique, but it is rarely per-

TABLE 6 EV PCR: clinical CSF specimens

Yr (reference)	Disease	No. of specimens	Sensitivity (%)	Specificity (%)
1990 (101)	Meningitis	20	100	100
1990 (103)	Encephalitis	8	100	NA[a]
1990 (89)	Meningitis	11	100	100
1993 (108)	Meningitis	257	≥97	≤100
1994 (92a)	Meningitis	54	95	60[b]
1994 (105)	Meningitis	114	95	97
1994 (70a)	Meningitis	504	96	99

[a] NA, not applicable.
[b] Six patients without meningitis were CSF culture negative and PCR positive; all six had positive stool cultures for EVs, and four of the six had positive throat cultures.

formed anymore with the widespread availability of acyclovir, a therapy effective only for encephalitis due to the herpes family viruses (122–124). PCR of CSF from patients with encephalitis appears to offer an attractive alternative for diagnosis of both herpes virus and EV encephalitis (see chapter 17).

TREATMENT AND PREVENTION

Specific antiviral therapy for the EVs is not currently available for clinical use, although a number of drugs that have efficacy in vitro and in animal studies have been developed (see chapter 18). One of these drugs, disoxaril, protects mice from developing meningoencephalitis due to echoviruses (73) and cured mice of chronic EV meningitis in another experimental model (59). Administered orally to infected mice, the drug reduced the incidence of paralysis due to echovirus 9 (73) and cleared persistent poliovirus type 2 CNS infection from cyclophosphamide-treated mice (59), both with minimal to no observed toxicity.

As noted above, clearance of EVs by the host is antibody mediated, and as might be expected, exogenously administered antibody has been useful in certain EV infections. Certain patients with agammaglobulinemia and chronic EV meningitis or meningoencephalitis have shown stabilization and improvement during therapy with gamma globulin, which is often administered by multiple routes, including directly into the CNS (74); other patients are less responsive to this therapy. Neonates with overwhelming EV sepsis, including meningitis, have received intravenous gamma globulin, maternal plasma, and exchange transfusions in occasionally successful attempts to reverse their otherwise bleak course (61, 80). A single randomized trial of intravenous gamma globulin plus standard therapy versus standard therapy alone in neonates suspected of having EV infection in the first 2 weeks of life has been undertaken, but too few patients have thus far been enrolled for a definitive conclusion to be reached (1). Among these patients, 75% had clinical and/or laboratory evidence of meningitis.

Supportive care for the patient with EV meningitis is usually adequate to ensure complete recovery. Attention to fluid balance is necessary to avoid or ameliorate the syndrome of inappropriate antidiuretic hormone and/or brain edema. Electrolytes and, on occasion, urine and serum osmolality may require monitoring. In patients with meningoencephalitis or encephalitis, brain edema is a rare complication and is readily managed with mannitol. Seizures may result from fever alone or may reflect direct viral or indirect inflammatory damage of brain parenchyma. Phenytoin or phenobarbital is the preferred agent for managing this complication. A rapidly progressive, downhill course requiring more-intensive support speaks strongly against an EV etiology, and other potentially treatable causes must immediately be considered. Involvement of the brain stem may require ventilatory support, and impairment of the gag response requires airway protection. Motor weakness or paralysis indicative of myelitis should be managed as with poliovirus infections (see chapter 9).

Poliovirus vaccines afford no protection against CNS or other disease caused by the nonpolio EVs. Vaccines for the nonpolio EVs are not available, and the literature contains only sparse evidence to suggest active ongoing research in this area (44).

SUMMARY

Like the polioviruses, the nonpolio EVs are neurotropic and neurovirulent. The most common CNS manifestations of the nonpolio EVs, meningitis and encephalitis, result in significant morbidity for tens of thousands of people in the United States each year. Recent advances in our understanding of the pathogenesis of these infections at the molecular, cellular, and organ system levels have led to important progress in our ability to diagnose and manage infected patients. Many enigmas remain to be resolved, including the precise route that EVs take to the CNS, host and viral determinants of neurovirulence, and the mechanism of persistence in humorally immunodeficient patients. The potential of the nonpolio EVs to cause paralytic myelitis, encephalitis, and severe nonneurologic disease should provide the necessary impetus to develop vaccines, but efforts in this area have been limited. Development of specific antiviral therapy for the EVs, now under way by several pharmaceutical companies, will allow us to reduce the clinical and financial impact of these pathogens even further.

REFERENCES

1. Abzug, M. J., H. L. Keyserling, M. L. Lee, M. J. Levin, and H. A. Rotbart. Neonatal enterovirus infection: virology, serology, and effects of intravenous immune globulin. *Clin. Infect. Dis.*, in press.
1a. Abzug, M. J., M. J. Levin, and H. A. Rotbart. 1993. Profile of enterovirus disease in the first two weeks of life. *Pediatr. Infect. Dis. J.* **12**:820–824.
2. Abzug, M. J., M. Loeffelholz, and H. A. Rotbart. 1994. Rapid diagnosis of neonatal enterovirus infection by polymerase chain reaction of serum and urine, abstr. H102, p. 239. *Program Abstr. 34th Intersci. Conf. Antimicrob. Agents Chemother.*
3. Adair, C. V., R. L. Gauld, and J. E. Smadel. 1953. Aseptic meningitis, a disease of diverse etiology: clinical and etiologic studies on 854 cases. *Ann. Intern. Med.* **39**:675–704.
4. Alexander, J. P., L. Baden, M. A. Pallansch, and L. J. Anderson. 1994. Enterovirus 71 infections and neurologic disease—United States, 1977–1991. *J. Infect. Dis.* **169**:905–908.
5. Alexander, J. P., Jr., L. E. Chapman, M. A. Pallansch, W. T. Stephenson, T. J. Torok, and L. J. Anderson. 1993. Coxsackievirus B2 infection and aseptic meningitis: a focal outbreak among members of a high school football team. *J. Infect. Dis.* **167**:1201–1205.
5a. Arditi, M., K. R. Nanogue, and R. Yogev. 1989. CSF cachectin (TNF-alpha) activity in children with bacterial and aseptic meningitis. *Pediatr. Res.* **25**:117a.
6. Balfour, H. H., Jr., G. L. Seifert, M. H. Seifert, Jr., P. G. Quie, C. K. Edelman, H. Bauer, and R. A. Siem. 1973. Meningoencephalitis and laboratory evidence of triple infection with California encephalitis virus, echovirus 11 and mumps. *Pediatrics* **51**:680–684.
7. Bergman, I., M. J. Painter, E. R. Wald, D. Chiponis, A. L. Holland, and H. G. Taylor. 1987. Outcome in children with enteroviral meningitis during the first year of life. *J. Pediatr.* **110**:705–709.
8. Berlin, L. E., M. L. Rorabaugh, F. Heldrich, K. Roberts, T. Doran, and J. F. Modlin. 1993. Aseptic meningitis in infants <2 years of age: diagnosis and etiology. *J. Infect. Dis.* **168**:888–892.
9. Bodian, D. 1954. Poliomyelitis: pathogenesis and histopathology, p. 479–518. In T. M. Rivers and F. L. Horsfall, Jr. (ed.), *Viral and Rickettsial Infections of Man*, 3rd ed. Lippincott, Philadelphia.
10. Bodian, D. 1955. Emerging concept of poliomyelitis infection. *Science* **122**:105–108.
11. Buescher, E. L., M. S. Artenstein, and L. C. Olson. 1968. Central nervous system infections of viral etiology: the changing pattern. *Res. Public Assoc. Res. Nerv. Ment. Dis.* **44**:147–163.
12. Caggana, M., P. Chan, and A. Ramsingh. 1993. Identification of a single amino acid residue in the capsid protein VP1 of coxsackievirus B4 that determines the virulent phenotype. *J. Virol.* **67**:4797–4803.
13. Centers for Disease Control. 1984. Enterovi-

rus surveillance—United States, 1984. *Morbid. Mortal. Weekly Rep.* **33**:388.
14. **Centers for Disease Control.** 1985. Enterovirus surveillance—United States, 1985. *Morbid. Mortal. Weekly Rep.* **34**:494–495.
15. **Centers for Disease Control.** 1986. Enterovirus surveillance—United States, 1986. *Morbid. Mortal. Weekly Rep.* **35**:503.
16. **Centers for Disease Control.** 1987. Enterovirus surveillance—United States, 1987. *Morbid. Mortal. Weekly Rep.* **36**:570–575.
17. **Centers for Disease Control.** 1988. Enterovirus surveillance—United States, 1988. *Morbid. Mortal. Weekly Rep.* **37**:516.
18. **Centers for Disease Control.** 1989. Summary of notifiable diseases, United States, 1989. *Morbid. Mortal. Weekly Rep.* **37**:1–57.
19. **Centers for Disease Control.** 1990. Enterovirus surveillance—United States, 1990. *Morbid. Mortal. Weekly Rep.* **39**:788–789.
20. **Centers for Disease Control.** 1992. Summary of notifiable diseases, United States, 1992. *Morbid. Mortal. Weekly Rep.* **41**:23.
21. **Chang, T. W.** 1971. Recurrent viral infection (reinfection). *N. Engl. J. Med.* **284**:765–773.
22. **Chemtob, S., E. R. Reece, and E. L. Mills.** 1985. Syndrome of inappropriate secretion of antidiuretic hormone in enteroviral meningitis. *Am. J. Dis. Child.* **139**:292–294.
23. **Cherry, J. D.** 1992. Enteroviruses: polioviruses (poliomyelitis), coxsackieviruses, echoviruses, and enteroviruses, p. 1705–1753. *In* R. D. Feigin and J. D. Cherry (ed.), *Textbook of Pediatric Infectious Diseases*, 3rd ed. The W. B. Saunders Co., Philadelphia.
24. **Chonmaitree, T., C. D. Baldwin, and H. L. Lucia.** 1989. Role of the virology laboratory in diagnosis and management of patients with central nervous system disease. *Clin. Microbiol. Rev.* **2**:1–14.
25. **Clarke, D., and K. Cost.** 1983. Use of serum C-reactive protein in differentiating septic from aseptic meningitis in children. *J. Pediatr.* **102**:718–720.
26. **Controni, G., W. J. Rodriguez, J. M. Hicks, M. Ficke, S. Ross, G. Friedman, and W. Khan.** 1977. Cerebrospinal fluid lactic acid levels in meningitis. *J. Pediatr.* **91**:379–384.
27. **Dagan, R., J. A. Jenista, and M. A. Menegus.** 1988. Association of clinical presentation, laboratory findings, and virus serotypes with the presence of meningitis in hospitalized infants with enterovirus infections. *J. Pediatr.* **113**:975–978.
28. **Dagan, R., and M. A. Menegus.** 1992. Replication of enteroviruses in human mononuclear cells. *Isr. J. Med. Sci.* **28**:369–372.
29. **Dai-ming, W., Z. Guo-chang, Z. Shi-mei, and Z. Yu-cai.** 1993. An epidemic of encephalitis and meningoencephalitis in children caused by echovirus type 30 in Shanghai. *Chin. Med. J.* **106**:767–769.
30. **Dalldorf, G., and G. M. Sickles.** 1948. An unidentified, filtrable agent isolated from the feces of children with paralysis. *Science* **108**:61–62.
31. **Deibel, R., A. Barron, S. Millian, and V. Smith.** 1974. Central nervous system infections in New York State: Etiologic and epidemiologic observations, 1972. *N.Y. State J. Med.* **74**:1929–1935.
32. **Deibel, R., and T. D. Flanagan.** 1979. Central nervous system infections: etiologic and epidemiologic observations in New York State, 1976–1977. *N.Y. State J. Med.* **79**:689–695.
33. **Deibel, R., T. D. Flanagan, and V. Smith.** 1975. Central nervous system infections in New York State: etiologic and epidemiologic observations, 1974. *N.Y. State J. Med.* **75**:2337–2342.
34. **Deibel, R., T. D. Flanagan, and V. Smith.** 1977. Central nervous system infections: etiologic and epidemiologic observations in New York State, 1975. *N.Y. State J. Med.* **77**:1398–1404.
35. **Eggers, H. J.** 1993. Considerations and experiments on the pathogenesis of enterovirus disease, p. 499–515. *In* W. Doerfler and P. Boehm (ed.), *Virus Strategies*. VCH, Weinheim, Germany.
36. **Eglin, R. P., R. A. Swann, D. Isaacs, and E. R. Moxon.** 1984. Simultaneous bacterial and viral meningitis. *Lancet* **ii**:984.
37. **Enders, J. R., T. H. Weller, and F. C. Robbins.** 1949. Cultivation of the Lansing strain of poliomyelitis virus in cultures of various human embryonic tissues. *Science* **109**:85–87.
38. **Etter, C. G., J. Wedgwood, and U. B. Schaad.** 1991. Aseptische Meningitiden in der Padiatrie. *Schweiz Med. Wochenschr.* **121**:1120–1126.
39. **Farmer, K., G. A. MacArthur, and M. M. Clay.** 1975. A follow-up study of 15 cases of neonatal meningoencephalitis due to coxsackie virus B5. *J. Pediatr.* **87**:568–571.
40. **Faulkner, R. S., A. J. MacLeod, and C. E. Van Rooyen.** 1957. Virus meningitis—seven cases in one family. *Can. Med. Assoc. J.* **77**:439–444.
41. **Feigin, R. D., and P. G. Shackelford.** 1973. Value of repeat lumbar puncture in the differential diagnosis of meningitis. *N. Engl. J. Med.* **289**:571–574.
42. **Figueroa, J. P., D. Ashley, D. King, and B.**

Hull. 1989. An outbreak of acute flaccid paralysis in Jamaica associated with echovirus type 22. *J. Med. Virol.* **29**:315–319.
43. Flanagan, T. D., and R. Deibel. 1981. Central nervous system infections: etiologic and epidemiologic observations in New York State, 1978–1979. *N.Y. State J. Med.* **81**:1346–1353.
44. Fohlman, J., K. Pauksen, B. Morein, U. Bjare, N. Ilback, and G. Friman. 1993. High yield production of an inactivated coxsackie B3 adjuvant vaccine with protective effect against experimental myocarditis. *Scand. J. Infect. Dis.* **88**:103–108.
45. Gatmaitan, B. G., J. L. Chason, and A. M. Lerner. 1970. Augmentation of the virulence of murine coxsackievirus B-3 myocardiopathy by exercise. *J. Exp. Med.* **131**:1121–1136.
46. Gilbert, G. L., K. E. Dickson, M. Waters, M. L. Kennett, S. A. Land, and M. Sneddon. 1988. Outbreak of enterovirus 71 infection in Victoria, Australia, with a high incidence of neurologic involvement. *Pediatr. Infect. Dis. J.* **7**:484–488.
47. Gonzalez-del-Rey, J. A., R. C. Baker, A. W. Kummer, J. R. Schultz, Jr., and M. Ho. 1991. Neurodevelopmental outcome of infants with enteroviral meningitis in the first three months of life. *Pediatr. Res.* **29**(2):172A.
48. Grist, N. R., and E. J. Bell. 1984. Paralytic poliomyelitis and nonpolio enteroviruses: studies in Scotland. *Rev. Infect. Dis.* **6**:S385–S386.
49. Grist, N. R., E. J. Bell, and F. Assaad. 1978. Enteroviruses in human disease. *Prog. Med. Virol.* **24**:114–157.
50. Gutierrez, K., and M. J. Abzug. 1990. Vaccine-associated poliovirus meningitis in children with ventriculoperitoneal shunts. *J. Pediatr.* **117**:424–427.
51. Hodes, D. S., and D. V. Espinoza. 1981. Temperature sensitivity of isolates of echovirus type 11 causing chronic meningoencephalitis in an agammaglobulinemic patient. *J. Infect. Dis.* **144**:377.
52. Horstmann, D. M. 1950. Acute poliomyelitis: relation of physical activity at the time of onset to the course of the disease. *JAMA* **142**:236–241.
53. Horstmann, D. M., and N. Yamada. 1968. Enterovirus infections of the central nervous system. *Res. Publ. Assoc. Res. Nerv. Ment. Dis.* **44**:236–253.
54. Howden, C. W., W. R. Lang, and J. Laws. 1966. An epidemic of ECHO 9 virus meningitis in Auckland. *N.Z. Med. J.* **65**:673–684.
55. Ishimaru, Y., S. Nakano, K. Yamaoka, and S. Takami. 1980. Outbreaks of hand, foot, and mouth disease by enterovirus 71. High incidence of complication disorders of central nervous system. *Arch. Dis. Child.* **55**:583–588.
56. Jaffe, M., I. Srugo, E. Tirosh, A. A. Collin, and Y. Tal. 1989. The ameliorating effect of lumbar puncture in viral meningitis. *Am. J. Dis. Child.* **143**:682–685.
57. Jarvis, W. R., and G. Tucker. 1981. Echovirus type 7 meningitis in young children. *Am. J. Dis. Child.* **135**:1009–1012.
58. Jenista, J. A., L. E. Daizell, P. W. Davidson, and M. A. Menegus. 1984. Outcome studies of neonatal enterovirus infection. *Pediatr. Res.* **18**(2):230A.
59. Jubelt, B., A. K. Wilson, R. L. Ropka, P. L. Guidinger, and M. A. McKinlay. 1989. Clearance of a persistent human enterovirus infection of the mouse central nervous system by the antiviral agent disoxaril. *J. Infect. Dis.* **159**:866–871.
60. Kaldor, J., and A. A. Ferris. 1969. Immunoglobin levels in cerebro-spinal fluid in viral and bacterial meningitis. *Med. J. Aust.* **2**:1206–1209.
61. Kaplan, M. H., S. W. Klein, J. McPhee, and R. G. Harper. 1983. Group B coxsackievirus infections in infants younger than three months of age: a serious childhood illness. *Rev. Infect. Dis.* **5**:1019–1032.
62. Karandanis, D., and J. A. Shulman. 1976. Recent survey of infectious meningitis in adults: review of laboratory findings in bacterial, tuberculous, and aseptic meningitis. *South. Med. J.* **69**:449–457.
63. King, D. L., and D. T. Karzon. 1962. An epidemic of aseptic meningitis syndrome due to echo virus type 6. *Pediatrics* **29**:432–437.
64. Kinnunen, E., T. Hovi, M. Stenvik, O. Hellstrom, J. Porras, M. Kleemola, and M.-L. Kantanen. 1987. Localized outbreak of enteroviral meningitis in adults. *Acta Neurol. Scand.* **74**:346–351.
65. Klemola, E., and K. Lapinleimu. 1964. Multiple attacks of aseptic meningitis in the same individual. *Br. Med. J.* **1**:1087–1090.
66. Lake, A. M., B. A. Lauer, J. C. Clark, R. L. Wesenberg, and K. McIntosh. 1976. Enterovirus infections in neonates. *J. Pediatr.* **89**:787–791.
67. Leist, T. P., K. Frei, S. Kam-Hansen, R. M. Zinkernagel, and A. Fontana. 1988. Tumor necrosis factor-α in cerebrospinal fluid during bacterial, but not viral, meningitis: evaluation in murine model infections and in patients. *J. Exp. Med.* **167**:1743–1748.
68. Lennette, E. H., R. L. Magoffin, and E. G. Knouf. 1962. Viral central nervous system disease; an etiologic study conducted at the Los

Angeles County General Hospital. *JAMA* **179:**687–695.
69. **Lepow, M. L., D. H. Carver, H. T. Wright, W. A. Woods, and F. C. Robbins.** 1962. A clinical, epidemiologic and laboratory investigation of aseptic meningitis during the four-year period, 1955–1958. I. *N. Engl. J. Med.* **266:**1181–1187.
70. **Lepow, M. L., N. Coyne, L. B. Thompson, D. H. Carver, and F. C. Robbins.** 1962. A clinical, epidemiologic and laboratory investigation of aseptic meningitis during the four-year period, 1955–1958. II. *N. Engl. J. Med.* **266:**1188–1193.
70a. **Loeffelholz, M., S. Fast, C. Lewinski, G. H. McCracken, M. Sawyer, and S. Young.** 1994. Detection of enteroviruses in cerebrospinal fluid using PCR, p. 62. *Proc. 6th Annu. Prog. Clin. Virol. Meet.*
71. **Malcom, B. S., J. J. Eiden, and J. O. Hendley.** 1980. ECHO virus type 9 meningitis simulating tuberculous meningitis. *Pediatrics* **65:**725–726.
72. **Martin, G. J., J. L. Malone, and E. V. Ross.** 1993. Poliovirus in cerebrospinal fluid from an infant with adenovirus infection. *Clin. Infect. Dis.* **16:**342–343.
73. **McKinlay, M. A., J. A. Frank, Jr., D. P. Benziger, and B. A. Steinberg.** 1986. Use of WIN 51711 to prevent echovirus type 9-induced paralysis in suckling mice. *J. Infect. Dis.* **154:**676–681.
74. **McKinney, R. E., Jr., S. L. Katz, and C. M. Wilfert.** 1987. Chronic enteroviral meningoencephalitis in agammaglobulinemic patients. *Rev. Infect. Dis.* **9:**334–356.
75. **McLean, D. M., M. A. Coleman, R. P. B. Larke, and G. A. McNaughton.** 1966. Viral infections of Toronto children during 1965. I. Enteroviral disease. *Can. Med. Assoc. J.* **94:**839–843.
76. **Melnick, J. L.** 1990. Enteroviruses: polioviruses, coxsackieviruses, echoviruses, and newer enteroviruses, p. 549–605. *In* B. N. Fields and D. M. Knipe (ed.), *Virology.* Raven Press, New York.
77. **Melnick, J. L., and I. L. Wimberly.** 1985. Lyophilized combination pools of enterovirus equine antisera: new LBM pools prepared from reserves of antisera stored frozen for two decades. *Bull. W.H.O.* **63:**543–550.
78. **Meyer, H. M., Jr., R. T. Johnson, I. P. Crawford, H. E. Dascomb, and N. G. Rogers.** 1960. Central nervous system syndromes of "viral" etiology. *Am. J. Med.* **29:**334–347.
79. **Miller, S. A., E. R. Wald, I. Bergman, and R. DeBiasio.** 1986. Enteroviral meningitis in January with marked cerebrospinal fluid pleocytosis. *Pediatr. Infect. Dis.* **5:**706–707.
80. **Modlin, J. F.** 1986. Perinatal echovirus infection: insights from a literature review of 61 cases of serious infection and 16 outbreaks in nurseries. *Rev. Infect. Dis.* **8:**918–926.
81. **Modlin, J. F., R. Dagan, L. E. Berlin, D. M. Virshup, R. H. Yolken, and M. Menegus.** 1991. Focal encephalitis with enterovirus infections. *Pediatrics* **88:**841–845.
82. **Moore, M.** 1992. Enteroviral disease in the United States, 1970–1979. *J. Infect. Dis.* **146:**103–108.
83. **Moore, M., R. C. Baron, M. R. Filstein, J. P. Lofgren, D. L. Rowley, B. Schonberger, and M. H. Hatch.** 1983. Aseptic meningitis and high school football players, 1978–1980. *JAMA* **249:**2039–2042.
84. **Morens, D. M.** 1978. Enteroviral disease in early infancy. *J. Pediatr.* **92:**374–377.
85. **Moses, E. B., A. G. Dean, M. H. Hatch, and A. L. Barron.** 1977. An outbreak of aseptic meningitis in the area of Fort Smith, Arkansas, 1975, due to echovirus type 4. **74:**121–125.
86. **Nakao, T., and R. Miura.** 1971. Recurrent virus meningitis. *Pediatrics* **47:**773–776.
87. **Neches, W., and M. Platt.** 1968. Cerebrospinal fluid LDH in 287 children, including 53 cases of meningitis of bacterial and nonbacterial etiology. *Pediatrics* **41:**1097–1103.
88. **Nogen, A. G., and M. L. Lepow.** 1967. Enteroviral meningitis in very young infants. *Pediatrics* **40:**617–627.
89. **Olive, D. M., S. Al-Mufti, W. Al-Mulla, M. A. Khan, A. Pasca, and G. Stanway.** 1990. Detection and differentiation picornaviruses in clinical samples following genomic amplification. *J. Gen. Virol.* **71:**2141–2147.
90. **O'Neil, K. M., M. A. Pallansch, J. A. Winkelstein, T. M. Lock, and J. F. Modlin.** 1988. Chronic group A coxsackievirus infection in agammaglobulinemia: demonstration of genomic variation of serotypically identical isolates persistently excreted by the same patient. *J. Infect. Dis.* **157:**183–186.
91. **Peltola, H. O.** 1982. C-reactive protein for rapid monitoring of infections of the central nervous system. *Lancet* **i:**980–983.
92. **Peluso, R., A. Haase, L. Stowring, M. Edwards, and P. Ventura.** 1985. A Trojan horse mechanism for the spread of visna virus in monocytes. *Virology* **147:**231–236.
92a. **Petitjean, J., F. Freymuth, H. Kopecka, J. Brouard, P. Boutard, and P. Lebon.** 1994. Detection of enteroviruses in cerebrospinal fluids: enzymatic amplification and hybridization with a biotinylated riboprobe. *Mol. Cell. Probes* **8:**15–22.

93. Prather, S. L., R. Dagan, J. A. Jenista, and M. A. Menegus. 1984. The isolation of enteroviruses from blood: a comparison of four processing methods. *J. Med. Virol.* **14:**221–227.
94. Price, R. A., J. H. Garcia, and W. A. Rightsel. 1970. Choriomeningitis and myocarditis in an adolescent with isolation of coxsackie B-5 virus. *Am. J. Clin. Pathol.* **53:**825–831.
95. Ramilo, O., M. M. Mustafa, J. Porter, X. Saez-Llorens, J. Mertsola, K. D. Olsen, J. P. Luby, B. Beutler, and G. H. McCracken, Jr. 1990. Detection of interleukin 1β but not tumor necrosis factor in cerebrospinal fluid of children with aseptic meningitis. *Am. J. Dis. Child.* **144:**349–352.
96. Rantakallio, P., M. Leskinen, and L. von Wendt. 1986. Incidence and prognosis of central nervous system infections in a birth cohort of 12,000 children. *Scand. J. Infect. Dis.* **18:**287–294.
97. Rantala, H., M. Uhari, H. Tuokko, M. Stenvik, and L. Kennunen. 1989. Poliovaccine virus in the cerebrospinal fluid after oral polio vaccination. *J. Infect.* **19:**173–176.
98. Rassmussen, A. F., Jr. 1946. The laboratory diagnosis of lymphocytic choriomeningitis and mumps. Paper presented at the Rocky Mountain Conference on Poliomyelitis, Denver, Colo., 16 December 1946.
99. Ray, C. G., R. H. McCollough, I. L. Doto, J. C. Todd, W. P. Glezen, and T. D. Y. Chin. 1966. Echo 4 illness epidemiological, clinical and laboratory studies of an outbreak in a rural community. *Am. J. Epidemiol.* **84:**253–267.
99a. Romero, J. R., and H. A. Rotbart. 1990. Discriminant enteroviral replication in U937 cells: a candidate model for monocyte/enterovirus interactions, abstr. 1232, p. 291. *Program Abstr. 30th Intersci. Conf. Antimicrob. Agents Chemother.*
99b. Romero, J. R., and H. A. Rotbart. 1995. Sequence analysis of the downstream 5' nontranslated region of seven echoviruses with different neurovirulence phenotypes. *J. Virol.* **69:**1370–1375.
100. Rorabaugh, M. L., L. E. Berlin, L. Rosenberg, M. Rossman, M. Allen, and J. F. Modlin. 1992. Absence of neurodevelopmental sequelae from aseptic meningitis. *Pediatr. Res.* **30(2):**177A.
101. Rotbart, H. A. 1990. Diagnosis of enteroviral meningitis with the polymerase chain reaction. *J. Pediatr.* **117:**85–89.
102. Rotbart, H. A. 1991. Viral meningitis and the aseptic meningitis syndrome, p. 19–40. *In* W. M. Scheld, R. J. Whitley, and D. J. Durack (ed.), *Infections of the Central Nervous System.* Raven Press, New York.
103. Rotbart, H. A., J. P. Kinsella, and R. L. Wasserman. 1990. Persistent enterovirus infection in culture-negative meningoencephalitis—demonstration by enzymatic RNA amplification. *J. Infect. Dis.* **161:**787–791.
104. Rotbart, H. A., and K. Kirkegaard. 1992. Picornavirus pathogenesis: viral access, attachment, and entry into susceptible cells. *Semin. Virol.* **3:**483–499.
105. Rotbart, H. A., M. H. Sawyer, S. Fast, C. Lewinski, N. Murphy, E. F. Keyser, J. Spadoro, S. Y. Kao, and M. Loeffelholz. 1994. Diagnosis of enteroviral meningitis using the polymerase chain reaction with a colorimetric microwell detection assay. *J. Clin. Microbiol.* **32:**2590–2592.
106. Russell, W. R. 1947. Poliomyelitis; pre-paralytic stage and effect of physical activity on severity of paralysis. *Br. Med. J.* **2:**1023.
107. Russell, W. R. 1949. Paralytic poliomyelitis. The early symptoms and the effect of physical activity on symptoms and the course of disease. *Br. Med. J.* **1:**465.
108. Sawyer, M. H., D. Holland, and N. Aintablian. 1994. Diagnosis of enteroviral central nervous system infection by polymerase chain reaction during a large community outbreak. *J. Pediatr. Infect. Dis.* **13:**177–182.
109. Sells, C. J., R. L. Carpenter, and C. G. Ray. 1975. Sequelae of central-nervous-system enterovirus infections. *N. Engl. J. Med.* **293:**1–4.
110. Shohat, M., T. Lerman-Sagie, Y. Levy, and M. Nitzan. 1988. Cerebrospinal fluid findings in infants with nonpolio enteroviral meningitis. *Isr. J. Med. Sci.* **24:**233–236.
111. Singer, J. I., P. R. Maur, J. P. Riley, and P. B. Smith. 1980. Management of central nervous system infections during an epidemic of enteroviral aseptic meningitis. *J. Pediatr.* **96:**559–563.
112. Solomon, P., L. Weinstein, T. W. Chang, M. S. Artenstein, and C. T. Ambrose. 1959. Epidemiologic, clinical and laboratory features of an epidemic of type 9 echo virus meningitis. *J. Pediatr.* **55:**609–619.
113. Strikas, R. A., L. J. Anderson, and R. A. Parker. 1986. Temporal and geographic patterns of isolates of nonpolio enterovirus in the United States, 1970–1983. *J. Infect. Dis.* **153:**346–351.
114. Sumaya, C. V., and L. I. Corman. 1982. Enteroviral meningitis in early infancy: significance in community outbreaks. *Pediatr. Infect.*

Dis. 3:151–154.
115. Sutinen, S., J. L. Kalliomaki, R. Pohjonen, and R. Vastamaki. 1971. Fatal generalized coxsackie B3 virus infection in an adolescent with successful isolation of the virus from pericardial fluid. *Ann. Clin. Res.* 3:241–246.
116. Thivierge, B., and G. Delage. 1982. Infections du systeme nerveux central a enterovirus: 223 cas vus a un hopital pediatrique entre 1973 et 1981. *Can. Med. Assoc. J.* 127:1097–1102.
117. Wadia, N. H., S. M. Katrak, V. P. Misra, P. N. Wadia, K. Miyamura, K. Hashimoto, T. Ogino, T. Hikiji, and R. Kono. 1983. Polio-like motor paralysis associated with acute hemorrhagic conjunctivitis in an outbreak in 1981 in Bombay, India: clinical and serologic studies. *J. Infect. Dis.* 147:660–668.
118. Wallgren, A. 1925. Une nouvelle maladie infectieuse du systeme nerveus central? *Acta Paediatr. Scand.* 4(Suppl):158–182.
119. Wallgren, A. 1951. Die Atiologie der Enzephalomeningitis bei Kindern, besonders des Syndromes der akuten abakteriellen (aseptichen) Meningitis. *Acta Paediatr. Scand.* 40:541–565.
120. Webster, A. D. B., H. A. Rotbart, T. Warner, P. Rudge, and N. Hyman. 1993. Diagnosis of enterovirus brain disease in hypogammaglobulinemic patients by polymerase chain reaction. *Clin. Infect. Dis.* 17:657–661.
121. Wenner, H. A. 1972. The enteroviruses. *Am. J. Clin. Pathol.* 57:751–761.
122. Whitley, R. J. 1990. Viral encephalitis. *N. Engl. J. Med.* 323:242–250.
123. Whitley, R. J., C. G. Cobbs, C. A. Alford, S. Soong, M. S. Hirsch, J. D. Connor, L. Corey, D. F. Hanley, M. Levin, and D. A. Powell. 1989. Diseases that mimic herpes simplex encephalitis. *JAMA* 262:234–239.
124. Whitley, R. J., S. J. Soong, M. S. Hirsch, A. W. Karchmer, R. Dolin, G. Galasso, J. K. Dunnick, and C. A. Alford. 1981. Herpes simplex encephalitis. *N. Engl. J. Med.* 304:313–318.
125. Wildin, S., and T. Chonmaitree. 1987. The importance of the virology laboratory in the diagnosis and management of viral meningitis. *Am. J. Dis. Child.* 141:454–457.
126. Wilfert, C. M., S. N. Lehrman, and S. L. Katz. 1983. Enteroviruses and meningitis. *Pediatr. Infect. Dis.* 2:333–341.
127. Wilfert, C. M., T. R. Thompson, T. R. Sunder, A. O'Quinn, J. Zeller, and J. Blacharsh. 1981. Longitudinal assessment of children with enteroviral meningitis during the first three months of life. *Pediatrics* 67:811–815.
128. Wolf, J. L., R. H. Rubin, R. Finberg, R. S. Kauffman, A. H. Sharpe, J. S. Trier, and B. N. Fields. 1981. Intestinal M cells: a pathway for entry of reovirus into the host. *Science* 212:471–472.
129. Wyatt, H. V. 1976. Provocation poliomyelitis and entry of poliovirus to the CNS. *Med. Hypotheses* 2:269–274.
130. Yamashita, K., K. Miyamura, S. Yamadera, N. Kato, M. Akatsuka, S. Inouye, and S. Yamazaki. 1992. Enteroviral aseptic meningitis in Japan, 1981–1991. *Jpn. J. Med. Sci. Biol.* 45:151–161.
131. Yeager, A. S., F. W. Bruhn, and J. Clark. 1974. Cerebrospinal fluid; presence of virus unaccompanied by pleocytosis. *J. Pediatr.* 85:578.

ENTEROVIRAL MYOCARDITIS AND DILATED CARDIOMYOPATHY: A REVIEW OF CLINICAL AND EXPERIMENTAL STUDIES

Tamara A. Martino, Peter Liu, Martin Petric, and Michael J. Sole

14

Myocarditis is a clinical condition characterized by infiltration of the heart by inflammatory cells. There can be considerable destruction to the heart tissue, which in a significant number of patients may lead to persisting cardiac abnormalities or death. Dilated cardiomyopathy (DCM) may also occur as a late consequence of myocarditis. DCM is characterized by enlargement of the heart, severely impaired cardiac function, and clinical heart failure. Patients with cardiomyopathy (dilated and restrictive) have been reported to account for about half of all patients requiring heart transplants (127).

Over the past five decades, extensive investigative efforts have addressed the role of enteroviruses in these cardiac diseases. The association between enteroviruses and myocarditis is well recognized. There is also considerable evidence supporting an enterovirus etiology in a significant proportion of DCMs. In this chapter, we review the clinical and experimental evidence for enterovirus involvement in myocarditis and DCM. It should be noted that in this review, myocarditis and pericarditis (inflammation of the pericardium) are considered together, as myo(peri)carditis. Also, enterovirus involvement centers around the coxsackie group B viruses (CVB). Space limitations preclude a review of heart disease caused by other viral agents.

In the first section, epidemiologic data on the incidence of myocarditis and DCM and their associations with enteroviruses are presented. In the second section, the pathogenesis of enterovirus-induced heart disease is comprehensively reviewed, with particular attention given to experimental studies elucidating the viral and immunologic mechanisms of the disease process. The section is divided into eight parts; overview of pathology, viral replication in the heart, host defense mechanisms, cell-mediated destruction of myofibers, virus participation in chronic heart disease, autoimmunity, viral infection and cardiac dysfunction, and factors affecting disease severity. In the third section, the detection of enteroviral infection in patients with myocarditis and DCM is reviewed. In the fourth section, the clinical features of myocarditis and DCM are reviewed, and evidence that these diseases are two ends of the same disease spectrum is discussed. In the final section, conventional treatments for patients with myocarditis and DCM are re-

---

Tamara Martino, Peter Liu, and *Michael J. Sole,* The Center for Cardiovascular Research, EN-13-208 Toronto Hospital, 200 Elizabeth Street, Toronto, Ontario, Canada, M5G 2C4.   *Martin Petric,* The Virology Laboratory, Department of Microbiology, Elm Wing Room 7130, The Hospital for Sick Children, Toronto, Ontario, Canada, M5G 1X8.

viewed. In addition, the role of immunosuppression and future avenues of therapy are examined.

EPIDEMIOLOGY

The true incidence of viral heart disease in the general population remains unknown because of difficulties in (i) establishing a definitive clinical diagnosis, (ii) demonstrating viral infection of the heart, (iii) establishing an association between an infection and specific heart disease and because of (iv) sample biases and (v) the rarity of autopsies performed after sudden deaths.

In recent years, a number of important advances in defining heart disease have been made. The advent of the bioptome has allowed safe sampling of human myocardial tissue, and the establishment of histopathologic criteria (the Dallas Criteria) has resulted in a uniform definition of disease. In addition, there have been marked technologic improvements in the sensitivities of both noninvasive and invasive methods for detecting cardiac disease. Finally, newer and more sensitive molecular techniques for detecting virus-infected myocardium in patients with heart disease have been developed. Since these advances are relatively recent, they have not necessarily had an impact on the epidemiologic studies currently available as yet. With these considerations in mind, we discuss below studies that examined the incidence of myocarditis and DCM and the prevalence of viral infection associated with these two diseases.

Myocarditis

ESTIMATES OF MYOCARDITIS IN THE GENERAL POPULATION AS DETERMINED BY AUTOPSY

The incidence of myocarditis as determined by postmortem examination has been reviewed in a number of studies. In 1980, Woodruff predicted the overall incidence of myocarditis to be 2.3 to 5.0% (420). This estimate was based on unselected autopsy material submitted to the U.S. Army Institute of Pathology during World War II (110) and on autopsies of adult males (374) and children (19) who died sudden violent or accidental deaths. Similar figures have been reported more recently (89, 190). Nevertheless, these earlier studies have often been criticized for not being sufficiently strict in their definition of myocarditis. In 1987, newer and stricter histopathologic criteria were proposed; these have come to be termed the "Dallas Criteria" (14, 15). When these criteria were used to evaluate 12,747 autopsies done in Malmö, Sweden, from 1975 through 1984, a considerably lower incidence was reported: only 1.06% of cases fulfilled the criteria for myocarditis (114).

INCIDENCE OF CARDIOVASCULAR DISEASE ASSOCIATED WITH ENTEROVIRAL INFECTION IN THE GENERAL POPULATION

According to the World Health Organization, approximately 1.5% of all enteroviral infections are associated with cardiovascular signs and symptoms. This number rises to 3.2% when only CVB infections are considered (118). For coxsackievirus group A (CVA) and echovirus, 0.8 and 0.7% of infections, respectively, have been associated with cardiac symptoms (118). However, these data likely reflect a conservative estimate, as many cases of cardiac involvement may have been subclinical or unreported. Over a person's lifetime, repeated exposure to enteroviruses increases the likelihood of acquiring an enteroviral infection associated with cardiac symptoms. It has been suggested that overall, "at least 70% of the general population has been exposed to cardiotropic viruses, and no doubt half have had an episode of acute viral myocarditis, which was subclinical in the vast majority" (299).

INCIDENCE OF MYOCARDITIS ASSOCIATED WITH ENTEROVIRAL INFECTION IN PATIENTS PRESENTING WITH CLINICAL SYMPTOMS

Enteroviral infection in patients presenting with myocarditis has been diagnosed by a variety of methods. Although each method has weaknesses (which are discussed in the section on enterovirus diagnosis), an overall detection rate may be surmised from the studies listed in Table 1. By serologic analysis, 38 to 50% of myocarditis patients showed evidence of an enteroviral infection. In studies that specifically examined enteroviral RNA presence in the myocardium, enterovirus sequences were detected in 45% of the hearts by slot blot hybridization and in 25% by PCR or in situ hybridization. These rates are in close agreement with earlier estimates by Grist, who suggested that enteroviruses cause at least one-third of the cases classified as acute myocarditis (116). The most commonly distinguished viral agents in patients with myocarditis were CVB.

DCM

INCIDENCE OF DCM IN THE GENERAL POPULATION AS DETERMINED FROM POPULATION SURVEYS

The incidence of DCM in the general population has been reported to range from 0.73 to 10 cases per 100,000 inhabitants per year. In a study in Malmö, Sweden, that covered a 10-year period, 3.0 to 10 cases per 100,000 inhabitants per year were documented (383, 384). However, a more recent retrospective Scandinavian study reported 0.73 cases per 100,000 inhabitants, a figure considered to be a conservative minimum (17). A study in England found 8.3 cases per 100,000 population (409). A survey from Toyko demonstrated 2.6 cases of cardiomyopathy per 100,000 population, of which 38% were specifically attributed to DCM (reviewed in reference 3). In a population-based study in Minnesota, 6 cases per 100,000 population were reported (50).

INCIDENCE OF DCM AS A PROPORTION OF ALL HEART DISEASE

In a recent U.S. hospital discharge survey of 400 institutions and 18,346,000 patients with diseases of the circulatory system, approximately 0.67% (126,000 cases) were classified as cardiomyopathy (3). In a survey of the professional activities of American cardiologists, it was reported that cardiomyopathy accounts for 1.2 to 1.9% of all cardiologist-patient encounters (378). In the United States, DCM reportedly constitutes about 90% of all the cardiomyopathies (3).

INCIDENCE OF DCM ASSOCIATED WITH ENTEROVIRAL INFECTION IN PATIENTS PRESENTING WITH CLINICAL SYMPTOMS

Enterovirus detection rates are summarized in Table 1. By serologic analysis, 12 to 26% of DCM patients tested were positive for enteroviral infection. In studies that specifically examined the myocardium for the presence of enteroviruses, viral RNA was detected in 41% of the hearts by slot blot hybridization, in 15% by PCR, and in 23% by in situ hybridization. CVB were the most commonly identified viral pathogens in patients with DCM.

Factors Affecting Incidence

The incidence of enteroviral infection in the population is influenced by factors such as epidemics, institutional outbreaks, age and sex of the host, and pregnancy (100) (see chapter 1). Thus, it is not surprising that these factors also appear to influence the incidence of enterovirus-associated heart disease (420). The

TABLE 1 Prevalence of associated enteroviral infection in patients with myocarditis and DCM[a]

Method[b]	Prevalence (%)	
	Myocarditis	DCM
Serology	38–50	12–26
Slot blot	45	41
PCR	25	15
In situ	25	23

[a]These are summary data; the original data and references are given in Tables 2 and 3.
[b]Serology, serologic detection of enteroviral infection; slot blot, hybridization to heart tissue extracts using radiolabeled probes; PCR, PCR with endomyocardial biopsy samples; in situ, nucleotide probe hybridization to heart tissue.

effects of these factors on the incidence of viral myocarditis and DCM are discussed in more detail below.

INSTITUTIONAL OUTBREAKS AND EPIDEMICS

During epidemics and institutional outbreaks of enteroviral infection, the incidence of myocarditis rises. Approximately 5 to 12% of the infected general population may manifest acute cardiac disease. However, even higher estimates have been noted among select patient groups in the surrounding community. For example, during viral outbreaks, fatal myocarditis has been reported in up to 50% of infants with CVB infection (420).

HOST AGE (MYOCARDITIS)

The incidence of enterovirus-associated myocarditis varies with the age of the host. Children under 6 months of age are highly susceptible to coxsackievirus myocarditis (118, 420). Although most infants presumably contract infection during birth or shortly thereafter, there have also been reports of enterovirus-associated myocarditis acquired in utero (18, 45, 111, 183, 198) (see chapter 10).

The incidence of enterovirus-associated myocarditis beyond infancy has been summarized from four studies with a total of 98 patients (130, 339, 340, 366). Children 3 to 10 years of age constituted only 4% of the patient group. Although young children are very susceptible to infection (100, 118), they do not appear to be the age group most susceptible to cardiac conditions. During late childhood and adolescence, the incidence of viral myocarditis rises. Patients from 10 to 19 years of age account for approximately 10% of all cases. Young adults comprise the vast majority of cases. Patients from 20 to 39 years of age account for 52% of the cases. This finding is consistent with previous summary reports (108, 420), although in some cases the percentage varies slightly, possibly owing to influences from epidemic factors. In older adults from 40 to 49 years of age, the incidence of viral myocarditis decreases, accounting for only 14% of cases. For patients aged 50 to 59, the incidence is also 14%, but patients 60 years of age and older represent only 5% of cases. Overall, these studies show that the peak age for developing CVB-associated myocarditis is between 20 and 39 years, although the disease is not restricted to this age group.

HOST AGE (DCM)

The incidence of enterovirus-associated DCM also varies with age. A summary of four studies that included 78 patients (35, 197, 406, 407) revealed that children and adolescents less than 19 years of age compose only 3% of the patient group. For young adults, the incidence rises steadily. However, in contrast to the situation with myocarditis, the young-adult group is not the most susceptible group, and patients aged 20 to 39 composed only 28% of cases. Older adults represent the vast majority of cases, with patients aged 40 and older composing 69% of the cases. The mean age of the patients in these studies was approximately 45 years, which was consistent with 538 additional cases for which summary data (but not individual patient data) were reported (17, 50, 66, 92, 297). It is interesting that this older age distribution supports the theory that a significant proportion of DCMs may occur as long-term sequelae to myocarditis.

SEX OF THE HOST (MYOCARDITIS)

Coxsackievirus myo(peri)carditis is more prevalent among males. In a survey of four studies that included 98 cases, males composed 60% of the patient group (130, 339, 340, 366). Male-to-female ratios ranged from 1.1:1 to 2:1. A higher prevalence among males has been previously surmised (420).

SEX OF HOST (DCM)

The incidence of DCM is also significantly higher in males than in females. Male-to-female ratios range from 1.9:1 to 4.3:1 (17, 50, 66, 197, 297, 383, 384, 406, 425). In the United States, the mortality rate in males as a percentage of cardiovascular deaths is twice that of females; 0.94% of cardiovascular deaths in males and 0.48% in females are attributed to cardiomyopathy (3).

RACE AND GEOGRAPHY

In the United States, the mortality rate from cardiomyopathy for blacks is reported to be 2.4 times higher than that for whites: 1.5% of blacks versus 0.63% of whites (3). This observation is intriguing, since susceptibility to enteroviral infections is not considered to be influenced by race (100). However, neither is susceptibility to enteroviral infections influenced by geography (100), yet the incidence of DCM appears to be higher in underdeveloped and tropical countries (3). In Africa, DCM is reported to be responsible for 10% of acquired heart diseases in children and for 30% in adults (8). In South America, the Caribbean, India, and Japan, DCM accounts for about 5% of all cardiac conditions encountered at autopsy (8). In Cali, Colombia, cardiopathy (of undetermined origin) was found in approximately 30% of patients who died of cardiovascular disease, with about 3% of cases attributed to myo(peri)carditis (51). In Bahai, Brazil, lymphocytic heart disease was found in approximately 45% of all autopsied patients (3, 202). In some cases, particularly in underdeveloped countries, the higher incidence could be due to exposure to higher inocula of enteroviruses because of differing social conditions (i.e., occupation, housing, sanitation, eating habits, education, and interpersonal relations) (100). Endemic diseases such as Chagas' disease or dengue or chikungunya fever, which mimic the pathogenesis of enterovirus-associated myocarditis and DCM (reviewed in references 8, 51, 79, 82, 202, 298, 365) should also be considered.

PREGNANCY

The sudden onset of DCM during the final trimester of pregnancy or within 5 months of delivery has been termed peripartum cardiomyopathy (65). Peripartum cardiomyopathy is not common in Western countries, where the reported incidence is one case in 1,300 to 4,000 deliveries. However, in Africa, it may occur in up to 1% of deliveries. The great majority of cases have been observed among the black population, and the disease is rather rare among white women. Mortality is estimated to be in the range of 30 to 60% for the mother and approximately 10% for infants whose mothers had congestive heart failure (65, 144, 173, 391).

A high incidence of myocarditis is detected in patients with peripartum cardiomyopathy (277, 279, 300, 343). This observation, in combination with the increased sensitivity to enteroviral infection during pregnancy (420), makes it tempting to speculate on an enteroviral etiology in the pathogenesis of peripartum cardiomyopathy. However, at present, a number of possible causes in addition to viral infection have been suggested (65, 144, 173, 253, 277, 343, 391).

PATHOGENESIS

The role of CVB in the pathogenesis of myocarditis and DCM cannot be established by Koch's postulates in a clinical setting. However, CVB has been isolated from the myocardia of patients with suspected viral myocarditis (86, 100, 234, 376, 377), and in one particular case, it had been demonstrated that the isolated virus was cardiotropic when injected into mice (376). In many other studies, CVB has been isolated from stool specimens or pharyngeal secretions of patients with suspected viral myocarditis and proved to be cardiotropic when administered to mice (60, 100, 101, 272, 420).

Over the past five decades, animal models have provided a framework in which the general pathogenic mechanisms of CVB heart disease could be carefully studied. CVB infection in animals causes heart disease closely resembling human myocarditis and DCM (see references 53, 60, 101, 213, 251, 272, 327, 411, 420, and many others). The pathogenesis of viral heart disease has been studied most extensively in mice. Consequently, murine experiments constitute the bulk of the studies reviewed in this section. Nevertheless, responses to CVB infection also occur in other animals, including hamsters, ferrets, squirrels, bats, and higher primates such as monkeys and chimpanzees (60, 272, 274, 275, 276, 308, 404, 420).

Through experimental studies of CVB infection, two principal pathogenic mechanisms have come to light. The first is viral pathogenicity, in which the virus plays a direct role in engendering myocardial damage and triggering the immunologic response of the host. The second is immune-mediated pathogenicity, in which the heart disease is brought about by a host defense system gone awry (see chapter 8). In this section, we discuss studies on all aspects of viral heart disease to demonstrate the complementary relationship of the pathogenic mechanisms involved.

Overview of Pathology

Mice injected intraperitoneally with cardiotropic virus (e.g., CVB3), exhibit noticeable changes in the myocardium within 2 days of infection. The heart muscle cells, or myocytes, show evidence of cytopathology, including coarse granularity, pallor of the cytoplasm, and multivesicular vacuolation (269, 411). From days 3 to 5, large clusters of myocytes are affected. At this time, there is also early calcification of single cells (269). By day 7, numerous foci of necrotic and calcified myocardial cells are evident (269). From 7 to 14 days after infection, the characteristic lesions of acute myocarditis, namely, numerous foci of necrotic myocytes accompanied by mononuclear cells, are abundant throughout the myocardium (Fig. 1 and 2) (see references 48, 199, 232, 269, 411, 420, and others).

Studies in our laboratory and others have also demonstrated extensive microvascular abnormalities in the myocardia of virus-infected mice (Fig. 3). Casting with Microfil (liquid silicone rubber) revealed spasm or constriction of the coronary microvasculature (70, 363) similar to that seen in genetically myopathic hamsters (78, 370).

In murine strains susceptible to chronic myocarditis, there are extensive pathologic changes even beyond day 14. Histologic examination of the heart reveals continuing necrosis of myocardial muscle and inflammatory cell infiltrates, albeit at a lower intensity. This situation leads to replacement fibrosis, calcification, and hypertrophy in the remaining myocytes (90, 214, 232, 346, 411). Later still, DCM similar to that seen in humans becomes evident. An overview of the proposed pathogenic processes involved is presented in Fig. 4. The observed pathologic changes consist of myocardial scarring in the absence of inflammation, endocardial and subendocardial scarring, and dilation of the cardiac chambers (255, 327, 397).

Viral Replication in the Heart

In murine models of CVB infection, viremia is detected within 24 h of virus inoculation (321). The virus seeds and grows in target organs such as the heart, pancreas, liver, spleen, and brain. One initial factor determining viral cardiotropism is likely the presence of virus receptors on vascular endothelial cells of the heart (see chapter 3). This possibility is supported by the finding that cardiotropic CVB3 was capable of infecting heart-derived endothelial cells in culture (152, 159). The endothelial cells presumably act as foci of initial infection, in that virus infection of endothelial cells, replication, and subsequent cell lysis lead to virus entry into the underlying myocardial tissue.

During CVB infection, cytolytic T cells have often been viewed as the main cause of damage to myocardial tissue. However, there is considerable in vivo evidence that viral replication in the heart tissue can itself play an important role in myocytolysis. Necrotic myofibers, which are present at 3 days postinoculation, appear well before the inflammatory cell response appears (255, 269, 411). Histopathological examination of the hearts of CVB-infected mice also reveals cytolytic and necrotic changes associated with viral replication well beyond day 3 of infection, as was elegantly described by McManus and colleagues (269). Extensive cardiac damage has also been noted in severe combined immunodeficient (47), athymic (176, 332, 347), and

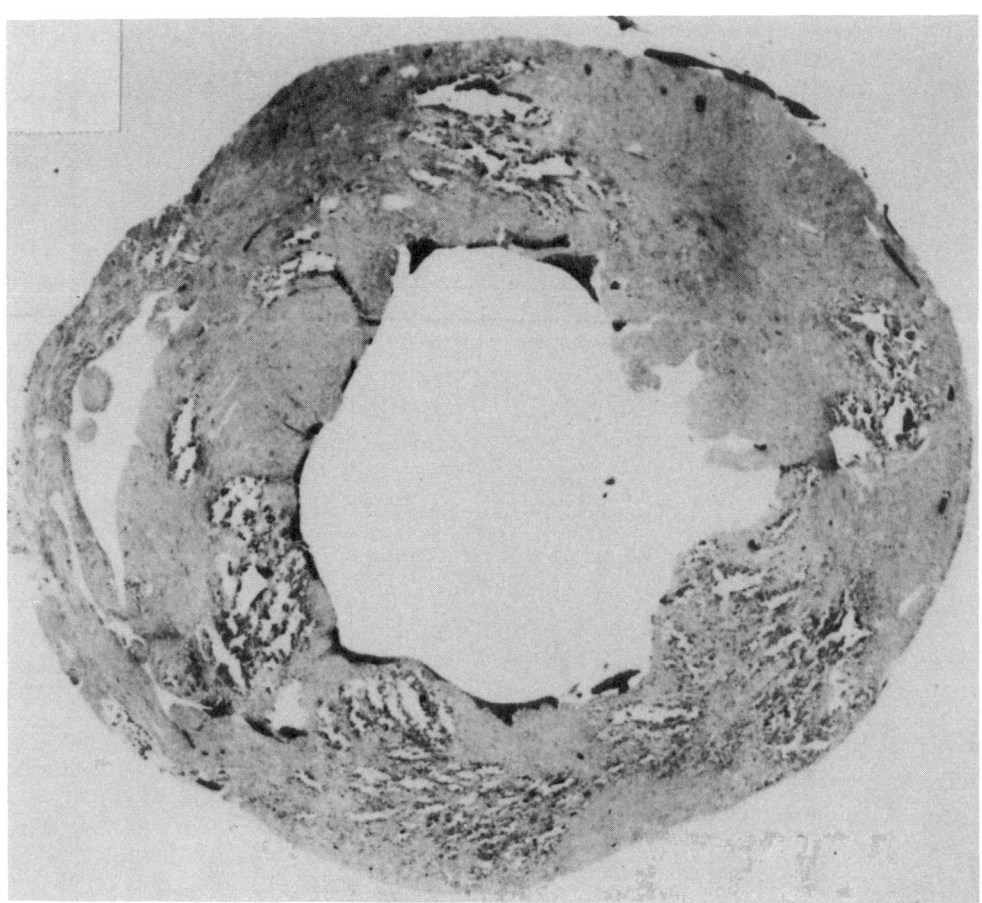

FIGURE 1 Transverse cross-sectional slice of representative heart from virus-infected mice. Note the multifocal nature of the myocardial lesions, which consist of necrotic myocardial cells and an inflammatory cell infiltrate. Hematoxylin and eosin stain. Magnification, ×15. Reproduced from the *Journal of Clinical Investigation* (70), by copyright permission of the American Society for Clinical Investigation.

marasmic (418, 421, 422) mice, in all of which the expected inflammatory cell infiltrate is genetically or experimentally suppressed. Finally, immunosuppressive therapy has no beneficial effect on the severity of myocarditis in several strains of inbred mice (reviewed below).

The mechanism by which CVB induces myocytolysis has been examined in vitro by use of cultured fetal human (177) and murine (428) heart cells. The virus is capable of infecting myocytes, as evidenced by the presence of viral particles in the cell cytoplasm on ultrastructural examination. Viral replication in the myocytes is indicated by the production of progeny virus. Damage to the myocytes occurs within 2 days of infection, by which time the majority have lost their contractile ability. Electron microscopy of affected myocytes reveals a pattern of classic cytopathic effect characterized by the destruction of myofibrils and filaments and the formation of vesicles and vacuoles throughout the cytoplasm.

Most recently, Kandolf and colleagues developed an electron microscopic in situ hybridization method that demonstrates that the same classic cytopathic effect occurs in vivo. Ultrastructural examination of myocardial tissue from CVB3-infected mice revealed virus

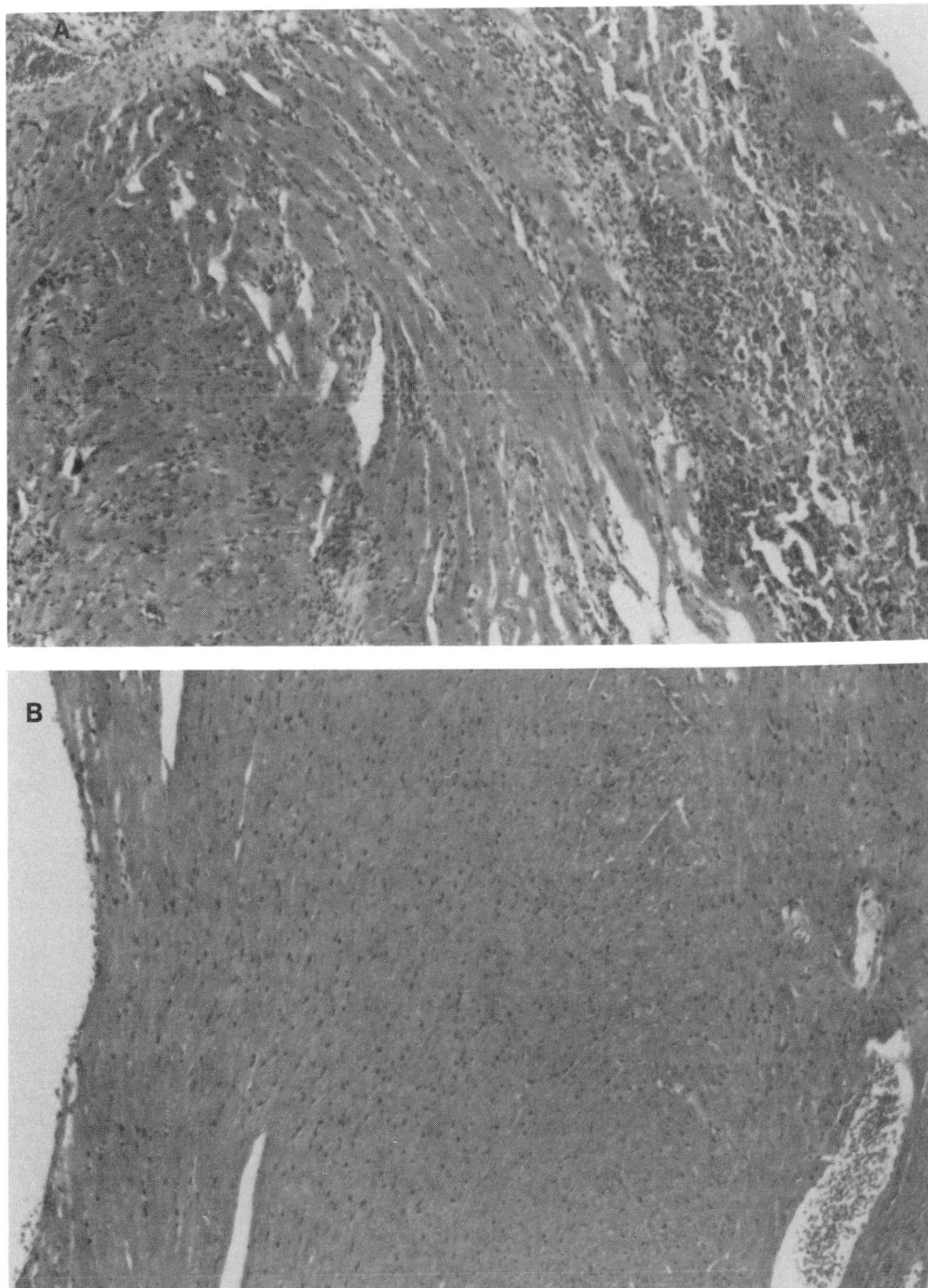

FIGURE 2 Light microscopic sections of representative murine hearts. (A) Pathologic changes in CVB3 murine myocarditis. Note the massive myocardial necrosis and inflammatory cell infiltrate in the ventricular

in the cytoplasm of infected myocytes, reorganization of cellular components essential for viral replication, cytoplasmic vesicles, and myofibril disintegration (140, 200, 247).

Host Defense Mechanisms

Approximately 4 days after inoculation with CVB, host reponses become evident. Neutralizing antibody as well as infiltrating macrophages and natural killer cells contribute to limiting viral dissemination in the heart and help clear the virus from the myocardium. There is also mounting evidence that interferon (IFN) enhances resistance to viral challenge. The individual mechanisms are described in more detail below (see also chapter 8).

NEUTRALIZING ANTIBODY

Circulating antibodies are believed to play a role in the resistance of mice to CVB3 infection. Serum antibodies are clearly capable of neutralizing the virus in vitro (see reference 420 and many others), and passive administration of very high doses of homologous antiserum before or shortly after viral inoculation protects mice in vivo (46, 322). Furthermore, the appearance of a rising antibody titer is closely related to the elimination of virus from the heart. In DBA/2 and BALB/c mice, a vigorous humoral response (presumably immunoglobulin M [IgM]) manifests itself between days 7 and 10, at which time maximal viral titers in the heart are noted. Thereafter, both anti-CVB3 antibodies and virus concentrations decrease to undetectable levels (232). In many murine A strains (i.e., A/J, A.BY/SnJ, and A.SW/SnJ), maximal antibody responses are delayed to the third or fourth week, which may correlate with the higher levels of viremia and greater disease severity noted in those strains (232, 413).

With the longer duration of viremia, one might expect to see an increase in CVB3 titers in target organs as well. However, Wolfgram et al. reported that this is not necessarily the case. Concentrations of CVB3 remain constant in the heart in different murine strains regardless of the duration and level of viremia and the onset of a neutralizing antibody response (413). Thus, neutralizing antibodies do not appear to be exclusively responsible for resistance to CVB infection. Further evidence comes from a study in which CD-1 mice were given cortisone acetate at the time of CVB3 inoculation. These mice exhibited abnormally high, persistent levels of virus in heart tissue even though a normal neutralizing antibody response was present. There was, however, a markedly reduced mononuclear cell infiltrate in these animals, indicating that inflammatory cells had also been important for suppressing the viral infection (419). Finally, malnourished mice exhibit enhanced susceptibility to CVB3 infection and an accompanying decrease in mononuclear cell response in the myocardium. Transfer of immune lymphoid cells to marasmic mice reverses the diminished myocardial inflammatory response, and resistance to CVB infection returns to normal (418, 421, 422). Thus, infiltrating mononuclear cells play a definite role in the resolution of CVB infection.

MACROPHAGES

Macrophages are the predominant cells in mononuclear infiltrates in the heart 5 to 10 days following CVB infection of mice, and they are believed to play a role in suppressing viral infection (420). This belief is indirectly supported by a number of studies. First, injection of silica particles, which are selectively taken up by macrophages and which impair their function, increases the mortality of mice infected with CVB3 (322). Second, cultured peritoneal macrophages from noninfected adult mice, especially after stimulation with protease-peptone, inactivate CVB3 infectivity (322). Third, when mice are pretreated with

---

myocardium of an A/J mouse at day 7 postinfection. (B) Control heart from an uninfected age-matched mouse. Hematoxylin and eosin stain. Magnification, ×40.

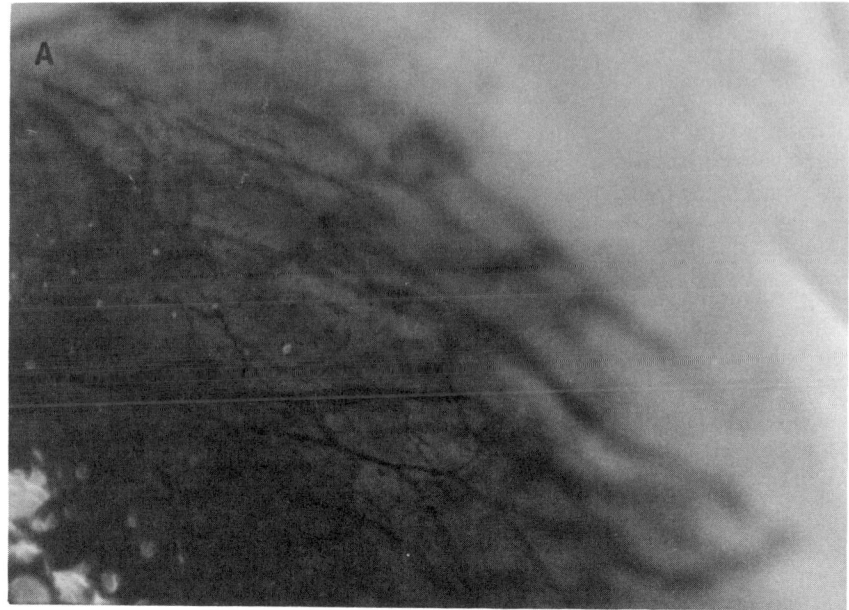

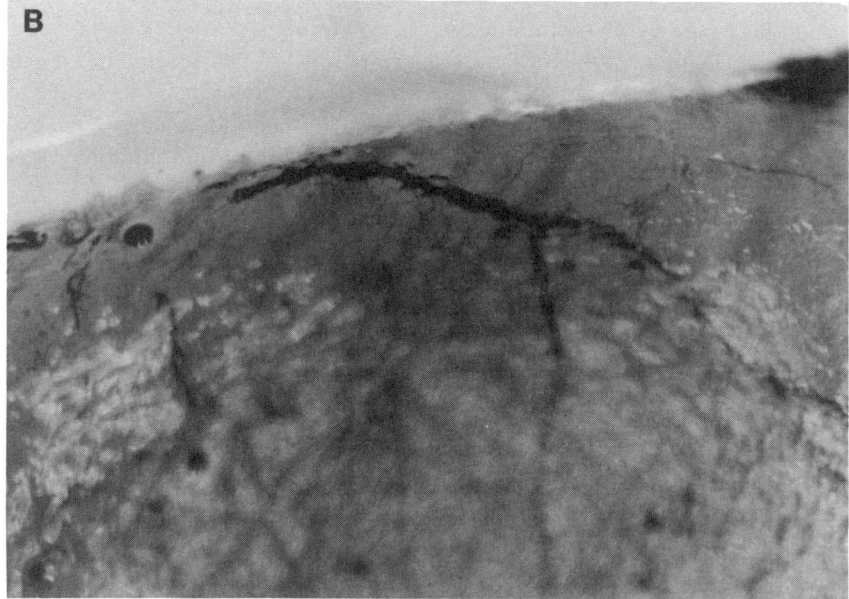

FIGURE 3 Microvascular perfusion from thick sections. Microfil (liquid silicone rubber) was perfused to cast the coronary vessels. (A) Control (verapamil treated) on day 14, with many smooth vessels. (B) Virus-infected heart on day 14. Vessels show multiple focal areas of constriction and narrowing. Magnification, ×100. The photograph was kindly contributed to our laboratory by Fayez Dawood and Wen-Hu Wen.

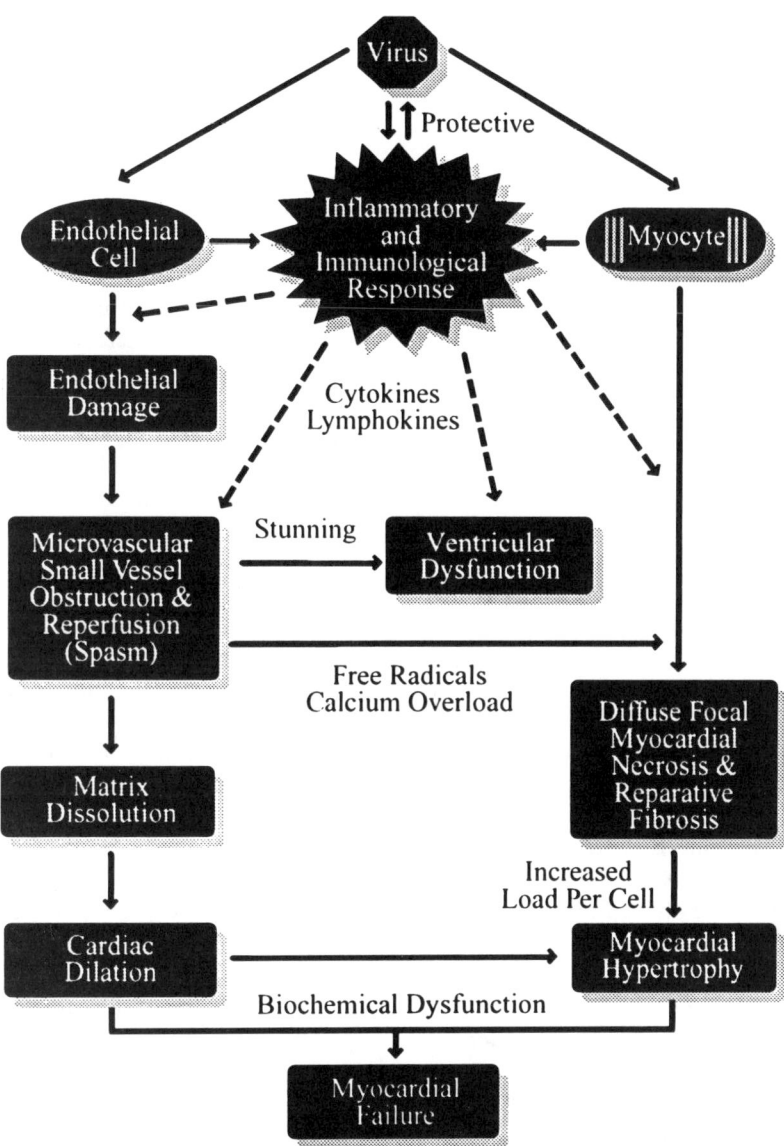

FIGURE 4 Proposed mechanisms involved in the pathogenesis of DCM following viral myocarditis. Reprinted with permission from the American College of Cardiology (370).

cortisone, myocardial necrosis and mortality are enhanced. This drug interferes with the release of monocytes from the bone marrow, although it also has a direct toxic effect on the heart (419).

Macrophages may protect against infection by their capacity to directly inactivate the virus. This is supported by a study in which suckling mice, which are presumed to possess immature macrophages, were protected from lethal CVB infection by transfer of adult syngeneic peritoneal exudate cells (322). Macrophages have receptors for IgM, IgG, and complement, which may also explain the increased protection noted when diluted antibody (which by itself is not protective) was transferred along with the peritoneal cell preparations (322). Finally, macrophages may be protective by attracting other immunocytes participating in viral clearance. This possibility is supported by a recent finding that CVB infects human monocytes in vitro, stimulating the release of cytokines (132–134), and the cytokines may in turn attract other immune cells (11).

NK CELLS

Natural killer (NK) cells infiltrating virus-infected tissues may also be involved in suppressing infection. Murine strains with decreased NK-cell responses (e.g., strain A mice) exhibit prolonged viral infection (232), whereas murine strains with high endogenous levels of NK-cell activity are less susceptible to infection (393), indirectly supporting this hypothesis. Also, a temporal relationship between virus-induced NK-cell activity in the spleen and CVB3 replication in the heart has been reported (105, 107).

Further support of a defensive role for NK cells during viral infection comes from depletion studies. Mice were treated with antiserum against the NK-cell glycosphingolipid marker asialo-GM_1; the antiserum was cytotoxic and eliminated NK activity in the spleen (188). The mice were then infected with CVB3. NK-cell-deficient mice exhibited increased viral titers in the heart and more severe myocarditis than did their "intact" littermates (105, 107). Moreover, splenic cells from CVB3-infected donor mice were protective when inoculated into CVB3-infected recipient mice, and transfer of asialo-GM_1^+ cells was required for the protection (106). However, since anti-asialo-GM_1 antibody may also eliminate T-lymphocyte precursor cells (91, 375), these results should be interpreted with some caution.

The observation that myocarditic CVB3 but not inactivated CVB3 elicits NK activity indicates that NK-cell activation depends on virus replication (105, 106). The activated NK cells then appear to provide some protection against CVB3-induced myocarditis, although the mechanism by which this occurs is not clear. Virus-induced cellular antigens have been described (99, 151, 238, 309, 314), and they may play a role in attracting NK cells (99, 106). Direct NK cytotoxicity may then occur. Perforin is a cell pore-forming protein elaborated by NK cells, and it may be involved in lysis of CVB-infected myocardial cells (359, 360). Since the NK cells would interact only with virus-infected myofibers, there would be no further contribution to lesion pathology, as expected (107). NK cells may also act through antibody-dependent cell-mediated cytotoxicity mechanisms (403). However, the addition of anti-CVB antibody to NK-cell cytotoxicity assays enhances reactivity only slightly (156), indicating only a minor role for antibody-dependent cell-mediated cytotoxicity. This is not surprising, since viral particles detectable by anti-CVB antibody are not significantly expressed on the surfaces of infected cells (272, 337, 420). Finally, NK cells and IFN frequently interact to control virus infections (403).

IFN

The mechanisms of IFN activity have been extensively reviewed elsewhere (68, 80). A role for IFN in ameliorating the early phase of enteroviral heart disease has long been speculated on. CVB myocarditis can be diminished in mice when the level of IFN is increased early in infection. If administered within 24 h of virus inoculation, IFN-β treatment reduces the number of CVB3-induced myocardial lesions in CD-1 mice (237). IFN- treatment of mice before or simultaneously with inoculation of encephalomyocarditis virus (EMCV) also protects against myocarditis (254, 256–259). The IFN inducer poly(I-C) prolongs survival time of CVB3-infected mice if it is administered before or shortly after infection (46, 237). Interestingly, protection is enhanced when poly(I-C) treatment is combined with antiviral-antibody administration, possibly indicating a synergistic protective effect (46).

The ability of IFN to suppress acute viral replication has been demonstrated in vitro. Pretreatment with IFN-β (129, 177, 180) or recombinant IFN-γ (129) reduced CVB3 titers in cultured human heart cells, and IFN-α reduced plaque formation caused by EMCV in FL (human amnion) cells (254, 258).

Note, however, that CVB-induced "native" IFN does not appear to be fully protective. This is not particularly surprising; it has been noted that CVB is generally considered a poor inducer of IFN both in vivo and in vitro (420). Thus, the role of native IFN in terminating viral growth early in infection remains an enigma.

In the studies discussed above, exogenous IFN treatment was beneficial in ameliorating myocarditis only when IFN was administered prior to or during the early stages of infection. Thus, it seems likely that IFN evokes other antiviral processes. Studies in our laboratory have indicated that IFN-mediated induction of nitric oxide is important for controlling enteroviral infection. Mice lacking both the IFN regulatory gene *IRF-1* (262) and the ability to produce nitric oxide (174) were infected with CVB3. The "knockout" mice rapidly succumbed to CVB3 myocarditis compared to normal infected mice carrying the IFN gene (unpublished data). The importance of IFN induction of nitric oxide for substantive antiviral activity in vitro and in vivo has also been noted for other viruses (80, 174, 187).

Cell-Mediated Destruction of Myofibers

T cells respond to virus infection in the context of molecules encoded by the major histocompatibility complex (MHC) (69). Foreign particles such as virus and/or virus antibody complexes are reduced to component peptides inside the cell, and the peptides are then placed in the groove of MHC molecules for presentation to the T-cell receptor ($\alpha\beta$TcR). At a basic level, murine T cells divide into two major subpopulations according to their recognition of class I or class II MHC molecules. Cytotoxic T cells ($CD8^+$) recognize virus-derived peptides presented by class I MHC and generally respond to the antigenic challenge by lysis of the target cells. Helper T cells ($CD4^+$) recognize peptides presented by class II MHC and play a role in the activation and/or proliferation of B cells, cytotoxic T lymphocytes, and macrophages. Note, however, that there is considerable plasticity and that both T-cell populations may exhibit characteristics of cytotoxic or helper cells.

The important role that T lymphocytes play in immunity has been observed for many viruses. Cytotoxic T lymphocytes are crucial for eliminating lymphocytic choriomeningitis virus (37, 429) and for controlling vaccinia virus primary infections (209). Infection with vesicular stomatitis virus is controlled by neutralizing antibodies, and helper T lymphocytes play a critical role in the immunoglobulin class switch from IgM to IgG (7, 103, 123). Thus, it is not particularly surprising that when T cells are incapacitated, the ability of the host to respond to viral infection is severely hampered.

$p56^{lck}$ is a small protein tyrosine kinase expressed predominantly in T lymphocytes (250). It is functionally and physically associated with the cytoplasmic domains of CD4 and CD8 antigens (392) and is crucial for normal thymic maturation of T cells (284, 316). Mutant mice lacking $p56^{lck}$ possess only an immature thymocyte population, which is not efficient in generating effective antiviral immune responses. Lck-deficient mice fail to generate cytotoxic-T-lymphocyte responses against lymphocytic choriomeningitis virus, vesicular stomatitis virus, and vaccinia virus or immunoglobulin class switching during vesicular stomatitis virus infection; these mice fail to clear virus effectively (283).

One might therefore find it surprising that Lck-deficient mice are resistant to CVB3 myocarditis (unpublished data). In these mice, virus replicates in the heart and is cleared from the myocardium at a rate comparable to that in immunologically intact littermates, yet there is only minimal damage to the cardiac tissue. It may be that NK cells or macrophages, which are unaffected by the Lck mutation, are primarily responsible for clearing the virus from the myocardium in both Lck-deficient and immunologically intact mice. The presence of functioning T cells, however, appears to be critical to producing substantive myofiber necrosis after CVB3 infection.

The original discovery that T cells play a major role in the pathogenesis of CVB infection was reported over two decades ago. Mice depleted of T cells by pretreatment with antithymocyte serum and then infected with CVB3 exhibit a marked reduction in myocardial disease. Antithymocyte serum suppresses the inflammatory response and tissue injury and reduces mortality. The reduction in myofiber damage is unrelated to impairment of viral replication, since viral titers were similar in both antithymocyte serum-treated and untreated mice (423). Furthermore, mice that have been thymectomized, irradiated, and reconstituted with bone marrow cells (TXBM mice) are also protected against lethal infection with CVB3. The degree of cardiac inflammation and necrosis is significantly less than that found in immunologically intact mice or in mice reconstituted with both bone marrow and thymus cells (423).

SPLENIC T LYMPHOCYTES REACTIVE AGAINST VIRUS-INFECTED MYOFIBERS IN VITRO

From day 4 postinoculation, male mice infected with CVB3 produce spleen cells that are capable of lysing virus-infected myofiber and fibroblast targets in culture (154, 156–158, 415, 416). Four studies have indicated that the reactive spleen cells are T lymphocytes. First, the reactive cells could not be removed by glass wool; macrophages and other adherent cells would be excluded by this procedure. Second, an MHC restricting element was indicated, in that the reactive spleen cells from male BALB/c mice of the $H-2^d$ haplotype infected with CVB3 could kill virally infected syngeneic targets (BALB/c mice, $H-2^d$ background) but not virally infected allogenic targets (CBA mice, $H-2^k$ background). Third, the response was antigen specific. When reciprocal assays using both CVB and vaccinia viruses were performed, the spleen cells obtained from mice infected with CVB lysed only target cells infected with CVB but not those infected with vaccinia virus. Conversely, vaccinia-immune cells lysed only vaccinia-infected target cells. Finally, treatment of the splenic cell preparations with antibodies against T cells (anti-Thy 1.2 serum) completely abolished all reactivity to virus-infected target cells. The discovery of T lymphocytes with cytolytic activity against virus-infected myofibers was very significant. It indicated a mechanism by which the T cells could contribute to cardiac inflammation and necrosis during CVB infection in vivo.

VIRUS-SPECIFIC CYTOLYTIC T LYMPHOCYTES

The reactive T cells have been termed cytolytic T lymphocytes (CTLs), and they are divided into two distinct populations. The first group contains the virus-specific CTLs, which recognize virus antigens on the surfaces of infected myocardial cells. Recognition of CVB3 antigens may explain why CTLs can distinguish between myofibers infected with different viruses (i.e., CVB3 and vaccinia) (415). Recently, it has been reported that T cells may recognize an enteroviral group-specific antigen(s). Sensitized T cells taken from mice infected with CVB2 or UV-inactivated CVB3 proliferated in vitro in response to CVB2, CVB3, CVB6, CVA16, and poliovirus 1 antigens but not to EMCV or influenza A virus (22) (see also chapter 8).

Virus-specific CTLs presumably belong to the CD4$^+$ T-cell subpopulation and are probably MHC class II restricted. This probability is supported by the observation that a monoclonal antibody (MAb) to the murine MHC class II IA^d antigen abrogates sensitization of the virus-specific CTLs in vitro (77).

The specific nature of CVB antigen to which the virus-specific CTLs respond remains unclear. It is not likely that this antigen is a virus capsid protein. CVB do not bud from infected cells (272, 337), nor do they express cell surface antigens on infected myocytes that could be recognized by antiserum directed against virus capsid proteins (157, 415, 416). However, it is possible that a presently unidentified component of the virus becomes localized on the cell membrane.

METABOLIC T LYMPHOCYTES

The second group of T lymphocytes has been designated metabolic CTLs. This group is said to react with de novo cellular antigens on the surface of myocytes infected with CVB3. Although the nature of such antigens has not been conclusively determined, there is mounting support for this hypothesis. Studies examining virus-induced antigens of cellular origin are described in more detail below.

It has been reported that heart extracts from CVB-infected mice contain newly synthesized cardiac cell antigens that are 50 to 80 kDa in size. Peritoneal exudate cells from mice infected with CVB3 are immunoreactive with this extract (309, 314). This finding is obviously significant, but for now, the ability of these neoantigens to elicit responses specifically from T-cell populations is still in question.

Murine neonatal skin fibroblasts also undergo cell membrane changes during CVB infection, expressing new surface residues of cellular origin (238). These findings may be particularly relevant for CTL destruction of CVB-infected myocardial fibroblasts in vivo.

Recently, it has been reported that myocardial cells treated with actinomycin D (an inhibitor of cellular metabolism) exhibit cell surface changes. Metabolic CTLs are capable of lysing these drug-treated cardiocytes, presumably reacting to neoantigens placed on the membrane of the cell. Similar alterations in the membranes of myocardial cells have also been noted following infection with CVB3 (153). In a subsequent experiment (151), it was hypothesized that the metabolic CTLs were responding to stress-related antigens such as heat shock proteins (HSP). Indirect evidence for this hypothesis came from Western blot (immunoblot) analysis, which revealed that HSP expression was enhanced on cardiocytes exposed to cellular injury from CVB3, transient heat shock, adriamycin, or myocarditic EMCV but not on cardiocytes exposed to UV-irradiated (nonreplicating) CVB3 or untreated cells. Furthermore, CTLs from mice infected with CVB3 were far more cytotoxic to all cardiocytes with enhanced HSP expression than to normal unstressed cells.

INFLUENCE OF HOST GENETIC BACKGROUND ON T-LYMPHOCYTE RESPONSES

Immunosuppressive treatment aimed at depressing the immunocyte response is not always effective. For example, prednisone has no therapeutic effect in CVB-infected BALB/c mice but is beneficial in CVB-infected A/J and DBA/2 mice. Moreover, cyclosporin treatment has proved deleterious in CVB-infected BALB/c mice but is slightly beneficial in CVB-infected A/J mice and is significantly useful for treating CVB-infected DBA/2 mice (76, 136, 245). In the studies discussed above that used mice of differing genetic backgrounds, T-cell populations appeared to respond differentially to CVB infection, influencing the outcome of the disease. Further studies examining the immunopathogenic roles of different T-cell subsets are described below.

The pathogenesis of CVB infection in BALB/c mice is mediated through cytotoxic T cells. Thus, when BALB/c mice are depleted of cytotoxic cells (Lyt 2^+) prior to virus infection, cardiac lesions are markedly fewer than in mice depleted of helper cells (L3T4$^+$) or in control littermates (232). Conversely, when BALB/c mice are depleted of T cells, reconstituted with cytotoxic lymphocytes (Lyt 2^+), and infected with CVB, there is an increased degree of myocarditis. In these animals, reconstitution with helper T cells (Lyt 1^+) has little effect (124). Interestingly, BALB/c mice treated with polyclonal immunoglobulin and then infected with CVB3 exhibit a reduction in myocarditis and a significant decrease in T helper cells but not cytotoxic cells, indicating that other pathogenic mechanisms may be involved as well (401).

Helper T cells are important in the pathogenesis of CVB infection in DBA/2 mice. CVB-infected DBA/2 mice depleted of helper cells (L3T4$^+$) are resistant to viral myocarditis (32, 232). Moreover, TXBM DBA/2 mice given helper T cells (CD4$^+$) prior to virus infection develop severe myocarditis, compared with TXBM mice not given T lymphocytes or TXBM mice given cytotoxic T cells (CD8$^+$) (32). Complement depletion also prevents myocardial disease in CVB-infected DBA/2 mice (161).

In CVB-infected A/J mice, elimination of only helper cells (L3T4$^+$) has little effect on the development of myocarditis, whereas elimination of only cytotoxic cells (Lyt 2$^+$) dramatically aggravates the myocarditis. Elimination of both helper and cytotoxic cells is necessary for preventing myocardial disease. In A/J mice, it has been proposed that "T suppressor cells might have been present which incompletely regulated T cell autoimmunity" (232).

Recently, it has been discovered that the T-cell mechanisms responsible for CVB myocarditis are not necessarily particular to specific inbred strains of mice but, rather, depend on the expression of specific genetic loci. As mentioned above, in BALB/c mice depleted of helper T cells, no effect on disease severity is noted, whereas depletion of cytotoxic T cells protects the animals from CVB myocarditis (232). However, this occurs only in the BALB/c CUM subline. BALB/c AnPt mice depleted of helper T cells are protected, and depletion of cytotoxic T cells has no effect, results similar to those obtained with DBA/2 mice (390). Congenic loci between BALB/c AnPt and DBA/2 mice may help explain this finding. In matrix studies of BALB/c CUM and DBA/2 mice, it was further discovered that the cellular responses in CVB myocarditis appear to be "inherent in the genetic repertoire of the animal, and not due to thymic selection during T cell ontogeny" (390).

INFLUENCE OF SEX ON CELL-MEDIATED CYTOTOXICITY

CVB-infected female mice show less inflammation of myocardial tissue, less necrosis, and lower mortality than males. Production and expression of cytolytic cells appear to play a role in the varied susceptibilities of female and male mice to CVB myocardial disease.

In female mice, reactive spleen cells produced during the first 3 days after CVB inoculation have the characteristics of NK cells (156, 158, 415). They do not appear to be MHC restricted, since they can kill both syngeneic and allogenic myofiber targets in vitro; they are not antigen specific, since they can kill both CVB-infected and uninfected cardiocytes; and they are not susceptible to lysis by anti-Thy 1.2 serum and complement. Moreover, the majority of reactive spleen cells obtained from female mice 3 to 7 days after infection retain these NK-cell characteristics.

In male mice, there is also an early NK-cell response, but it is weaker and more sporadic than that in female mice. Starting on day 4, however, the reactive NK cells of male mice are gradually replaced by T lymphocytes, with peak CTL reactivity noted on day 7 (156–158, 415–417). One possible explanation for these differences in cellular immune response in vivo is that in females there is a strong NK cell response and a weaker CTL response which may in turn reduce disease severity. Males, however, appear to have a biphasic cellular immune response culminating in the generation of CTLs, which may enhance disease severity in vivo.

INFLUENCE OF SEX HORMONES ON CELL-MEDIATED CYTOTOXICITY

The differing cellular immune responses observed in male and female mice may be partly due to the influence of sex hormones. When the effects of castration, testosterone, or estrone were examined in young (6- to 9-week-old) male and female mice infected with CVB3, the following observations were made (155). Mortality rates 2 weeks after infection were highest in uncastrated males (80%) and decreased slightly in castrated males given testosterone, whereas castrated males without hormonal treatment or given estrone had mortality levels in the same range as that of all groups of female mice (less than 9%). Inflammation and necrosis were greatest in uncastrated males and castrated males given testosterone and were reduced in untreated castrated males or males given estrone. Castrated females exhibited enhanced myocardial inflammation and necrosis, and estrone treatments reduced the myocarditis. In cytotoxicity assays on splenic cells, the treatments discussed above did not influence the type of cytolytic cell produced; T lymphocytes were generated in males, and NK-like cells were generated in females. However, in males, castration or castration plus estrone did reduce the amount of cytolytic activity against virus-infected myofibers, and testosterone treatment restored activity to the level of uncastrated males. In females, castration decreased cytolytic activity, and estrone treatment caused further reduction. Thus, in young male mice, it could be said that testosterone enhanced CVB heart disease, but in males and females, estrogen was protective.

The influence of sex hormones on cellular immune responses has also been noted in other model systems. Pregnant mice (which show a rise in progesterone concentrations during pregnancy) and castrated male and virgin female mice treated with progesterone are more susceptible to CVB3-induced myocarditis than are untreated virgin females or intact male controls (241). Also, as mice age, they become more susceptible to CVB infection (119, 120) and elicit stronger T-lymphocyte responses (240). In older female mice (32 to 40 weeks old), estrogen treatment prior to CVB infection reduces cardiac injury compared to that in infected but untreated age-matched controls (240).

The mechanisms by which sex hormones modulate cellular responses in male and female mice are not clear. One possible explanation is that sex hormones influence the generation of suppressor T cells, which in turn protect the animals from severe CVB infection (171). Alternatively, sex hormones such as estrone may stimulate antibody production, thereby indirectly lowering cytolytic T-cell responses (155).

Virus Participation in Chronic Heart Disease

Virus-specific and metabolic CTLs are reactive against virus-infected myofibers in vitro. If a similar mechanism operated during the first 2 weeks of CVB myocarditis (the acute phase), then the immunocytes would also be directed against virus-infected myocardial cells in vivo. However, 2 weeks after infection (the start of the chronic phase), culturable virus is eliminated, yet cytolytic immune cells are still directed to the myocardium. How can this paradox be reconciled? In recent years, it has been demonstrated both in vitro and in vivo that CVB infection can persist beyond 2 weeks, albeit in some altered form. Virus persistence may explain the ongoing attraction of CTLs to the myocardium. Studies examining the mechanisms of virus persistence are described in more detail below.

PERSISTING VIRAL RNA

Viral RNA persistence is a relatively recent and highly attractive hypothesis for explaining how virus or virus-immunity collaboration can cause cardiac damage, particularly in the chronic phase of CVB heart disease. This mechanism was discovered by using highly sensitive molecular techniques and was best demonstrated in a study by Klingel and colleagues (199). During the acute and chronic stages of infection, murine hearts were examined by in situ hybridization for the presence of CVB3 RNA. The sites where viral RNA was detected were then further studied for the extent of myocardial damage and inflammatory cell response. In the first 3 days after infection, myocytes containing CVB3 RNA were randomly distributed throughout the myocardium, presumably indicating hematogenous infection during viremia. By day 6, infected myocytes were adjacent to foci of inflammatory cells. The greatest numbers of CVB3 RNA-infected myocardial cells were noted from days 6 to 9, and this correlated with a significant increase in myocardial injury. From days 15 to 30 after infection, after infectious virus could no longer be detected, CVB3 RNA-infected myocardial cells were still present. These infected cells were found primarily within foci of myocardial lesions containing persistent mononuclear cell infiltrates. Thus, the presence of viral RNA appeared to be associated with the development of myocardial lesions.

To date, the persistence of viral RNA has been repeatedly demonstrated by in situ hybridization in many murine models of CVB infection. CVB3 RNA has been detected in the myocardium up to 56 days after infection in athymic mice (176) and up to 1 month in A.CA/SnJ *(H-2^f)* (199, 247), A.BY/SnJ *(H-2^b)*, SWR/J *(H-2^q)* (199), and C3H/He (203) mice. In EMCV-infected mice, in situ hybridization has detected viral RNA in the heart for up to 3 weeks and in the brain for up to 4 weeks (54).

The quantity of viral RNA present diminishes during the chronic phase of the disease; consequently, the RNA becomes progressively more difficult to detect by in situ hybridization. PCR, however, allows the detection of viral sequences from whole heart tissue, thus providing a more sensitive method for detecting viral RNA in the latter stages of disease. In our laboratory, we used PCR to demonstrate that EMCV RNA could be detected in the myocardium up to day 42 postinfection (397). Other studies have used PCR to show that the EMCV RNA signals were detectable even beyond 90 days (205). Similar findings have been noted when CVB-infected A/J mice were used (unpublished data).

These observations lead to the hypothesis that in the chronic phase, the T lymphocytes infiltrate the myocardium in response to viral-RNA-containing myofibers. Further evidence supporting this hypothesis comes from the observation that viral RNA persists in three different immunocompetent strains of mice, all of which progress to chronic myocarditis. In contrast, DBA/1J mice, which are capable of terminating the inflammatory processes through elimination of virus from the heart, show no evidence of viral RNA persisting in the myocardium (199). Moreover, during the chronic stage, it was reported that "up to 30 cardiac cells were infected in 1 mm^3 of heart tissue, and that this would clearly be sufficient to sustain myocardial inflammation" (199). Thus, the development of chronic myocarditis, in which there is ongoing inflammatory responses, appears to be dependent on the presence of viral RNA in the myocardium.

The mechanism by which persisting viral RNA is involved in pathogenesis (i.e., myocytolysis or attraction of cytolytic lymphocytes) remains to be elucidated. It is interesting, however, that the persisting viral RNA appears to be capable of replication. This is indirectly supported by strand-specific in situ hybridization. Serial sections of heart tissue from CVB-infected mice contained both plus- and minus-strand viral RNA in the acute (142, 199) and chronic (199) phases of the disease. In the absence of detectable virus titers, it seems likely that replication occurs in a restricted or altered manner (199); nevertheless, even such replication could be enough to induce metabolic or antigenic changes that do not occur in uninfected cells.

PERSISTING INFECTIOUS VIRUS

Persistence of infectious CVB3 for at least 6 months has been demonstrated in human myocardial fibroblasts in culture (129, 177, 180). The cytolytic viral infection is ongoing but in only a small proportion of the cells in the culture population. In recent years, CVB has been repeatedly shown to establish persistent infections in other cell cultures as well, namely, human lymphoid cell lines (26, 263), human rhabdomyosarcoma cells (16, 267, 427), human fetal aortic organ cultures (31), rat pancreatic cells (88), HeLa human cervical epithelial carcinoma cells (55), YAC-1 mouse lymphocytes, BGMK monkey kidney cells, and mouse fibroblasts (427).

It has been postulated that these infections may occur in murine CVB heart disease, particularly under conditions in which host defense mechanisms are depressed (177, 420). It is not known whether they also occur in noncompromised hosts or whether they could sustain myocytolysis or be involved in attracting immunocytes to the heart. Certainly, some of the means by which persistence has been established in culture (which include the presence of human serum [56], IFN [333], and defective interfering particles [64, 427]; the continuous replenishment of a small population of susceptible cells among intrinsically resistant cells [26, 263, 427]; and virus evolution [267]) may also occur in vivo. However, only very low levels of infectious virus must be generated in vivo, since the virus escapes detection in conventional culture assays.

Immune and Autoimmune Mechanisms

The hypothesis that CVB infection induces autoimmunity in the host is controversial. Recent studies with murine models of CVB infection have demonstrated the presence of cytolytic cellular responses to uninfected myocardial cells, the production of heart-reactive autoantibodies, and the presence of "self" antigens capable of inducing myocardial heart disease. Experimental animal studies elucidating the autoimmune mechanisms associated with viral heart disease are discussed in more detail below.

AUTOREACTIVE CYTOLYTIC CELLS

In cytotoxicity assays, it is frequently noted that some cytolytic cells from CVB-infected mice exhibit reactivity to uninfected myocardial cells in culture. Some autoreactive cells appear to have the characteristics of NK cells, since they are generated very soon after infection and a more vigorous in vitro autoreactive response is noted in females than in males (156, 158, 415). Treatment of the autoreactive cells with anti-Thy 1.2 and complement reduces cytolytic activity toward uninfected myofibers, indicating that NK cells are indeed present. However, since treatment with anti-Thy 1.2 did not abolish cytolytic activity, it seems that autoimmune T cells were present as well (160).

To demonstrate the potential of autoimmune CTLs in vivo, T cells from DBA/2 donor animals infected 7 days earlier with CVB3 are mixed with uninfected myocardial cells in culture. CTLs that selectively adsorbed to the cardiocytes are retrieved and then adoptively transferred into uninfected DBA/2 mice. Severe myocarditis occurs. A $CD4^+$ lymphocyte population is presumed to be responsible for causing the myocarditis in the DBA/2 mice, since selective adsorption of autotoxic T cells by uninfected cardiocytes can be inhibited by MAb to MHC class II (IA^d) but not to MHC class I (K^dD^d) antigens (32). Autoimmune CTLs may also occur in BALB/c mice (160), although these presumably belong to the $CD8^+$ phenotype (153, 213).

REGULATION OF IMMUNE AND AUTOIMMUNE T-CELL RESPONSES

The complements to autoimmune CTLs that promote myocarditis are immunoregulatory cells that inhibit autoimmune myocarditis. This phenomenon has been demonstrated in murine models of CVB3m (myocarditic) and CVB3ϕ (amyocarditic) infection. The mechanisms that limit viral replication (e.g., neutralizing antibody titer) are often equivalent in mice infected with CVB3m or CVB3ϕ (154, 235). However, mice infected with CVB3ϕ exhibit significantly less cardiac inflammation, necrosis, and permanent cardiac injury (fibrosis and calcification) than mice infected with CVB3m (154, 214, 235). Moreover, mice infected with CVB3ϕ do not produce autoimmune CTLs capable of lysing uninfected myocardial cells in vitro (154, 156, 235). Thus, it is postulated that CVB3ϕ-infected mice produce immunoregulatory cells that inhibit the genesis of autoimmune responses.

Further in vivo evidence supports the concept that immunoregulatory cells are involved during CVB3φ infection but not during CVB3m infection. Cyclophosphamide-treated mice infected with CVB3φ develop severe heart disease, and autoimmune CTLs similar to those produced by CVB3m-infected mice develop. The drug apparently alleviates T-cell-mediated suppression without inhibiting humoral or cell-mediated responses (235). Moreover, adoptive transfer of immune cells (presumably immunoregulators) from CVB3φ-infected mice into CVB3m-infected mice inhibits myocarditis, whereas transfer of CVB3m immune cells (presumably autoimmune CTLs) into CVB3φ-infected mice enhances myocarditis. $CD4^+$ lymphocytes constitute the population of cells that regulate autoimmunity in BALB/c mice, since selective elimination of these cells from the CVB3φ immune lymphocyte population reverses immunoregulation (235).

Recently, it has been reported that a helper-T-cell subset designated Th1 is predominantly produced by BALB/c mice infected with CVB3m. A second helper-T-cell subset designated Th2 is predominantly produced by BALB/c mice infected with CVB3φ. Lymphokines produced by Th2 cells (e.g., IL-10) can reportedly suppress Th1-cell responses. This finding of differential lymphokine induction may help explain the regulation of autoimmune T-cell responses observed in CVB3φ-infected mice (162).

Other factors that influence the immune system are also likely to be important. For example, it has been suggested that the poorly understood γ/δ TcR^+ lymphocytes may play a role in immune and autoimmune reactions (151, 286). These cells are reportedly capable of reversing the clonal anergy of α/β TcR^+ cells in immunocompetent hosts in vivo. Other possibilities include a decrease in immunologic tolerance of antigens expressed on the cell surface, clonal expansion of T cells that have escaped thymic education, and T-cell-mediated stimulation of other immunocytes.

The mechanism by which CVB3m and CVB3φ induce the differential T cell responses in vivo is not known. One possible explanation is that the variants use different surface receptors. It appears that CVB3 can bind to more than one cellular receptor in vitro (56, 148–150, 249, 324), and interestingly, CVB3m and CVB3φ apparently recognize different receptors. This finding was supported by studies with a MAb designated 10A1, which is presumably directed against one of the cell surface receptors. It inhibited CVB3m but not CVB3φ infection of murine myocardial cells in vitro and diminished CTL reactivity toward uninfected myocardial cells in culture. This antibody also abrogated myocarditis in CVB3m-infected mice, despite viral replication in the heart (402). Since the CVB receptors have not been identified, the mechanism by which the type of immune response is modulated is not known.

AUTOANTIBODIES

Wolfgram et al. reported that heart-specific autoantibodies are produced in suckling A.SW/SnJ mice infected with CVB3. Some were demonstrated to be antisarcolemma antibodies, while others are directed against contractile proteins (414). It was subsequently demonstrated that murine strains susceptible to chronic myocarditis are more likely than more resistant strains of mice to produce heart-specific autoantibodies. The presence or absence of heart-specific autoantibodies appears to be determined by non-MHC genes (413).

Since these experiments, autoantibodies have been demonstrated in many experimental models of viral myocarditis. They were generally termed heart-reactive autoantibodies (HRA), since specificity for heart tissue was not always determined. They can be divided into three categories: (i) HRA indicative of ongoing heart disease that are not pathogenic, for example, the IgM HRA in BALB/c mice (161, 232); (ii) HRA associated with cardiac injury but not disease progression, for example, the IgG HRA in DBA/2 mice (161, 232); and (iii) HRA associated with cardiac injury and ongoing heart disease, for example, IgG HRA in A/J mice (232).

ANTI-Ids

One mechanism by which HRA may arise is through anti-idiotype networks. For this, secondary antibodies directed against the antigenic determinant of a primary antibody molecule and also against antigens in heart tissue are produced. An example is the MAb designated MAb 10A1. This antibody is believed to be directed against anti-CVB antibodies. Indirect evidence for this is that the MAb could capture B cells apparently making virus-reactive antibody, and it reacts with virus-immune sera in a double-diffusion Ouchterlony assay (405). Theoretically, the binding site of this antibody retains a tertiary structure similar to that of CVB3, which allows it to also bind to a cell surface viral receptor (402). In another example of this phenomenon, splenic B cells from healthy mice were exposed in vitro to anti-idiotype antibodies (anti-Ids) and then transferred into syngeneic recipient mice. These mice produced anti-CVB3 antibodies, presumably through anti-idiotype networking, since they had never been exposed to the virus (313).

Some anti-Ids appear to be protective. For example, MAb 10A1 abrogates myocarditis when it is injected into CVB3-infected mice (405). Other anti-Ids capable of binding to myocyte antigens also abrogate CVB murine myocarditis (310–312). These responses are believed to result, in part, from anti-Id modulation of cellular immunity (310–313, 405).

The ability of anti-Ids to affect immune cells has been noted in several studies. They can stimulate secondary B-cell responses in anti-Id-primed or CVB3-infected animals, increase the in vitro migration of macrophages from immunized animals, and suppress the proliferation of T cells (310–312).

There is also evidence to suggest that some anti-Ids are pathogenic. Splenic B cells pulsed with anti-Ids (presumably against CVB antibodies) are capable of causing myocarditis when transferred into syngeneic recipient mice. Control experiments that pulsed B cells with anti-Ids unrelated to CVB infection did not produce myocarditis (313). However, since in vitro stimulation of the B cells was required, it is possible that immunoregulatory events unrelated to idiotype involvement may have caused the myocarditis.

ANTIMYOSIN AUTOANTIBODIES AND ANTIGENIC MIMICRY

A second mechanism by which HRA may arise is through antigenic mimicry. That is, the antibodies are directed against shared epitopes on CVB and on myocardial cell molecules. At present, perhaps the most closely studied and hotly contested example is antimyosin autoantibody.

Indirect evidence for cross-reactivity between antimyosin antibodies and CVB comes from panels of MAbs to CVB. (i) From a panel of 66 anti-CVB4 MAbs, one IgG antibody, designated 356-1, neutralized virus in vitro and reacted with heart tissues from several animals by immunohistochemical analysis. Moreover, MAb 356-1 recognized the VP1 protein of CVB4 and murine alpha cardiac myosin heavy chain on Western blot analysis (23–25, 318, 319, 338, 371). (ii) Two MAbs were selected from a panel of antistreptococcal IgM antibodies. In cytotoxicity assays, MAbs 36.2.2 (strongly) and 54.2.8 (more weakly) reacted with epitopes on the surfaces of rat heart and fibroblast cell lines in culture. They also detected WB3 coat proteins and murine cardiac myosin on Western blot analysis (57). (iii) A panel of 23 hybridomas was generated from adult female BALB/c mice inoculated with CVB3 mixed with Freund's complete adjuvant. Three of the MAbs (MAbs 1, 5, and 13) bound to murine heart cells in culture, demonstrated CVB3 neutralizing capabilities, and detected rabbit myosin on immunoblot staining. In addition, antisera prepared in CD-1 mice against purified CVB3 also detected myosin by immunoblot (95).

It has been postulated that antimyosin antibodies may play an immunopathogenic role in viral heart disease. This possibility was indirectly supported by the finding that some MAbs that react with CVB and cardiac myosin demonstrate cell lysis capabilities in cytotoxicity assays (57) and elicit macrophage chemotactic activity in vitro (95). Induction of myocardial pathology has also been demonstrated when some cross-reacting MAbs are injected into mice (95, 97).

Nevertheless, it has also been reported that antimyosin antibodies from mice infected with CVB3 are not capable of neutralizing virus (291). It was demonstrated that viable cardiocytes do not appear to express myosin epitopes on the cell surface (293), suggesting that the cell-specific reactivity mentioned above may have resulted from permeabilization of the cell membrane or was potentially mitigated through other cross-reactive epitopes. In terms of pathogenic potential, murine strains most susceptible to CVB myocarditis produce antimyosin antibodies when they are immunized with myosin (290). However, antimyosin antibodies can be demonstrated in several strains of healthy mice even without prior immunization (293, 295). Moreover, passive transfer of high-titer myosin autoantibodies prepared from mice immunized with cardiac myosin (but not necessarily CVB) do not induce myocarditis (293).

Antimyosin antibodies probably do have practical importance, as they appear to be serologic markers for ongoing heart disease in CVB-infected mice. However, on most other issues, one wonders whether cross-reacting antimyosin antibodies are pathogenetically important or are a paraphenomenon generated through a diversity of technical methods. Their origin and the nature of their pathogenic potential seem to depend on the experimental system used, and it is difficult to know how closely these systems reflect viral myocarditis in vivo.

OTHER AUTOANTIBODIES

Panels of murine MAbs that react to a number of cardiac antigens, including tropomyosin, keratin, vimentin, laminin, actin, and other proteins with N-acetyl-β-D-glucosamine residues, have been described. In some cases, they also exhibit cross-reactivity to CVB3 capsid proteins (57, 58, 362). Indeed, future studies of these autoantibodies may be important for understanding autoimmune mechanisms in CVB heart disease.

ADP-ATP CARRIER AUTOANTIGEN

The ADP-ATP carrier is a transport protein located within the inner mitochondrial membrane that is essential for energy metabolism within eukaryotic cells. The ADP-ATP carrier can become an autoantigen. This hypothesis is supported by the finding that guinea pigs immunized with isolated ADP-ATP carrier produce antibodies that react against the transport protein on solid-phase radioimmunoassay and Western blot (355).

Recently, synthetic peptides have been used to map antigenic determinants that are shared between ADP-ATP carrier protein and CVB3 (357). Thus, during CVB infection, anticarrier antibodies may initially arise through antigenic mimicry. Release of carrier protein from necrotic myocytes may serve as a second source of antigen for antibody production.

Antibodies against the shared antigenic determinants (i.e., CVB and ADP-ATP carrier) occur in patients with myocarditis and DCM (357). This observation, combined with the finding that anticarrier antibodies could penetrate viable myocytes in culture and could affect cardiac energy metabolism by inhibiting nucleotide transport across the carrier in vitro (355), is suggestive of the pathogenic process at hand. Thus, during CVB3 infection, in vivo immune responses to the ADP-ATP carrier protein may induce metabolic changes in cardiac cells that could culminate in heart failure.

CARDIAC MYOSIN AUTOANTIGEN

It has been hypothesized that cardiac myosin also acts as an antigen that initiates autoimmune processes. Indirect support for this hypothesis comes from a study in which murine strains susceptible to chronic CVB-induced myocarditis developed myocarditis upon injection of cardiac myosin [i.e., A/J (H-2^a), A.BY/SnJ (H-2^b), A.SW/SnJ (H-2^s), and A.CA/SnJ (H-2^f) mice]. In contrast, when murine strains resistant to CVB heart disease were immunized with cardiac myosin, no myocarditis occurred [i.e., C57BL/6J ($H-2^b$), C57BL/10J ($H-2^b$), and B.10A/SgSnJ ($H-2^a$) mice] (295).

Understanding how an intracellular cardiac protein such as myosin can elicit immunologic responses may be important in our understanding of CVB heart disease. Nevertheless, while these studies suggest that some similar mechanisms may be involved in causing myocarditis in CVB- and myosin-induced murine models, it should be kept in mind that substantial differences also exist. (i) Very high doses (at least 0.1 mg) of cardiac myosin along with Freund's complete adjuvant are required to induce myocarditis (295). (ii) A/J mice depleted of T helper cells exhibit significantly reduced levels of myosin-induced myocarditis (364, 365); it was previously reported that depletion of helper cells in A/J mice had little effect on CVB-induced myocarditis (232), although subline variations in the animal strains used may have occurred. (iii) Myosin-reactive T cells are not believed to directly target the cardiac myocyte (292, 294), whereas T lymphocytes from CVB-infected mice are clearly reactive with cardiac myocytes. (iv) The proposed primary targets for T cells involved in antimyosin responses are myosin epitopes presented by dendritic cells (292, 294); such targeting has not been demonstrated as a direct cause of myocarditis in CVB-infected mice to date. However, the possibility that targeting of dendritic cells occurs as a secondary consequence of CVB infection cannot be excluded.

CVB Infection and Cardiac Dysfunction

The specific mechanisms leading to cardiac dysfunction in viral myocarditis and DCM are not well understood. Viral and immunologic damage is clearly involved. Recent discoveries of inflammatory mediators that can modulate cardiac function in vivo underline the complexities involved. The potential roles of cytokines and nitric oxide in CVB heart disease are discussed below. In addition, the multiple elements involved in viral heart disease are examined with respect to microvascular damage.

CYTOKINES

Cytokines are soluble mediators that include the tumor necrosis factors (TNF-α and -β), IFNs (IFN-α, -β, and -γ), and interleukins. By design, cytokines are presumably beneficial substances that help coordinate immune and inflammatory responses (11). Some cytokines also display antiviral activity (80, 187). However, exaggerated or prolonged production of cytokines may also have adverse effects on cells in the microenvironment in which they are released. These detrimental effects are discussed in the context of CVB heart disease.

Cytokine production appears to be related to the development of chronic myocarditis. For example, mice infected with CVB1 express elevated levels of TNF-α mRNA in the brain for up to 21 days after infection (102). Moreover, murine strains naturally resistant to the chronic phase of CVB myocarditis become susceptible if cytokine production is stimulated by administration of CVB3 and lipopolysaccharide, of CVB3 and IL-1, or of CVB3 and TNF. In all cases, levels of TNF and IL-1 in serum are sustained throughout the disease process (207, 208). A role for cytokines in murine viral heart disease is also indicated in other model systems. Administration of amyocarditic virus (CVB3ϕ) and IL-1 or IL-2 resulted in a marked increase in myocarditis compared to that in mice given CVB3ϕ only. Moreover, in mice given CVB3ϕ and IL-2, immunohistochemical staining showed high levels of IL-1 in the myocardium, comparable to those in mice infected with myocarditic (CVB3m) virus alone (162).

One source of cytokines elaborated during CVB heart disease is likely the immune cells that infiltrate the myocardium. A specific population of cells that may be present is CVB-infected monocytes. This possibility is supported by the finding that CVB3 infects human monocytes in vitro and induces TNF-α, IL-1β, IL-6, and IFN (probably

IFN-α) production. Interestingly, these infected monocytes exhibit no apparent cell damage or loss of viability (132–134). Cytokines may also be produced or elaborated (to various degrees) by macrophages, T lymphocytes, leukocytes, fibroblasts, and endothelial cells (11, 80, 162).

It is well known that cytokines are involved in the activation and/or attraction of other immunocytes and that they induce the expression of MHC antigens on immune cells and organ tissues (11, 80, 121). These activities may indirectly contribute to disease pathogenesis. Immunocytes summoned to the myocardium may participate in the destruction of myocardial tissue expressing cytokine-induced MHC antigens.

Some cytokines may also act directly on heart cells, resulting in a loss of cardiac function. This hypothesis is supported by the observation that cytokines such as TNF-α, IL-1, IL-2, and IL-6 alter myocyte contractility in cultured Girardi heart cells (132), cultured neonatal rat myocytes (122a; unpublished observations), isolated adult feline cardiac myocytes (427a), and isolated hamster papillary muscles (83). IL-1 also indirectly reduces RNA and protein synthesis in rat neonatal myocytes in culture (146). Moreover, TNF-α exerts a negative inotropic effect on the feline ventricle in Langendorff-perfused hearts (427a), while IL-1 and IL-2 affect myocardial function in isolated perfused rat heart models (145, 368). The negative effects of cytokines on myocardial cells may be mediated through alterations in intracellular calcium homeostasis (427a), induction of secondary mediators produced in cardiac nonmuscle cells (146) or lymphocytes (368), modulation of β-adrenergic responsiveness (122a), and/or induction of nitric oxide signaling pathways (18c, 83, 354).

NITRIC OXIDE

Nitric oxide (NO) is a radical gas recently found to be synthesized in mammalian cells. The importance of NO was underlined by the designation "Molecule of the Year 1992" by the American Association for the Advancement of Science. The biochemical reactivity of NO has been extensively reviewed elsewhere (135, 236, 289, 372).

Recent studies indicate that NO plays an important role in the killing of infectious agents, including viruses such as CVB. One mechanism by which this occurs is collaborative NO and IFN pathways. For example, in our laboratory, we have found that mice lacking the ability to produce NO (through gene-targeted disruption of the IFN regulatory gene *IRF-1*) (174, 262) are highly susceptible to the lethal effects of CVB3-induced myocarditis (unpublished data). Conversely, overexpression of *IFR-1* cDNA in mutant HeLa cell lines appears to induce an antiviral response to EMCV, vesicular stomatitis virus, and Newcastle disease virus (317). Finally, murine macrophages treated with IFN-α (which stimulates inducible nitric oxide synthase [NOS] and allows the synthesis of NO from L-arginine) inhibit the replication of ectromelia virus, vaccinia virus, and herpes simplex virus type 1. Epithelial cells transfected with cDNA coding for NO production are also capable of restricting virus replication. The antiviral effects are reversed when cultures are treated with competitive inhibitors of inducible NOS (187).

However, NO is also associated with detrimental effects, some of which may be involved in CVB heart disease. This finding is indirectly supported by the observations that cytokines can stimulate NO production in mammalian myocardial tissue (presumably through transcriptional upregulation or enhancement of NOS) (18c, 83, 354) and that cytokines enhance murine susceptibility to CVB heart disease (207, 208). LPS also induces NO production in macrophages (424) and exacerbates murine CVB myocarditis (207, 208; unpublished observations). Moreover, heart tissues from patients with DCM show significant activity of inducible NOS and minimal constitutive NOS activity, which is presumably indicative of a pathologic condition (61).

NO production can adversely affect the heart in many ways, although determining the applicability of this finding to CVB heart disease depends on future study. Possible pathologic roles for NO in the myocardium include increasing the signaling molecule cGMP, which in turn may affect the regulation of cardiovascular tone (359); modulating β-adrenergic responsiveness, as noted in rat cardiac myocyte cultures (18a, 18b); or causing direct cytotoxicity, as noted for porcine aortic endothelial cells (307).

MICROVASCULAR DAMAGE

As mentioned above, microvascular spasm has been observed in the hearts of virus-infected mice (Fig. 3) (70, 363). Treatment of virus-infected mice with the calcium channel blocker verapamil prevents the development of microvascular spasm as well as of myocarditis and DCM (70, 370). This finding suggests that a number of interconnected mechanisms may be involved (Fig. 4).

The most obvious mechanism for producing microvascular changes would be virus proliferation in the cardiac endothelial cells in vivo. CVB3 has been shown to infect and replicate in endothelial cells cultured from neonatal mouse heart (152, 159) and human fetal aorta (31), thus providing indirect support for this hypothesis. However, in our laboratory, we have noted that verapamil ameliorates the microvascular spasm without affecting virus titers in the heart (398), indicating that viral replication is not a primary cause of the microvascular abnormalities.

Cell-mediated immunologic responses may also be involved in microvascular damage. This possibility is supported by the observation that CTLs from CVB-infected mice lyse virus-infected endothelial cells of the heart in culture (159). Moreover, in patients with myocarditis, lymphocytic infiltration in the myocardium is often associated with enhanced HLA expression on endothelial cells (125, 131, 163, 204, 244), which could allow for CTL reactivity to endothelial cells in the appropriate context.

The role of autoantibodies in mediating vascular injury during CVB infection is presently unknown but appears to be a fruitful line of investigation. In Kawasaki's disease, serum autoantibodies from patients cause complement-mediated lysis of cytokine-stimulated endothelial cell cultures, indicating a possible mechanism for vascular injury in vivo (215). Vascular autoantibodies have also been reported in some patients with myocarditis and DCM (125, 244). Finally, as mentioned above, cytokines (11, 80, 121) and NO (289, 307, 354), as well as many other vasoactive mediators (75), may also be implicated in the generation of endothelial-cell injury in vivo.

Factors Affecting Disease Severity

Many factors affect the severity of murine viral heart disease. As mentioned above, the genetic background of the inbred mouse strain is critically important to the response to viral infection. A number of other viral, physiologic, and environmental factors can also come into play. These are discussed in more detail below. However, it should be remembered that these are experimental systems; CVB infection shows a wide range of expression in mice, and the importance of any given factor may vary considerably in patients with viral heart disease.

VIRAL FACTORS

Enterovirus type. In mice, the infecting enterovirus type influences the severity of disease. CVB generally demonstrates cardiotropicity, whereas only a few variants of CVA exhibit an affinity for the murine heart, and polioviruses and echoviruses generally fail to produce disease (60, 81, 101, 164, 210–212, 272, 410, 411). CVA, CVB, echoviruses, and polioviruses use distinct cellular receptors (28, 115, 233, 278, 373, 380), and receptor affinities are believed to be a major determinant for enterovirus tissue tropism (143, 335) (see chapter 3). Thus, variable receptor expression in the heart could help explain why these enteroviruses differ in their capacities to induce myocarditis.

Intratypic variants. The prototype stain of CVB3, termed Nancy, was isolated in 1949 in Connecticut from a patient with minor febrile illness (272, 275). Experimental passage of the Nancy strain of CVB3 has produced variants that are myocarditic in mice (119, 421). These variants (and their derivatives) are used by most laboratories studying viral heart disease, although other variants exist.

Chow and colleagues recently demonstrated that four commonly used myocarditic variants (including three Nancy derivatives) differ in their relative abilities to induce myocarditis in several inbred strains of mice. They also differ in replicative capacities (i.e., virus titer) in the heart and in their abilities to induce myocardial lesions (i.e., size, distribution, extent of calcification) within each murine strain (48). There are also, of course, many amyocarditic variants that replicate in the murine heart but induce little or no myocarditis (104, 105, 154, 214, 235, 388, 389, 402).

Conformational epitopes are probably important for determining CVB cardiovirulence. For example, a canyon pocket similar to those found on poliovirus (141) and rhinovirus (334) has been predicted for the CVB virion (220). The canyon contains amino acids that interact with the cellular receptor (see chapter 3). Alterations to this site could affect CVB binding to specific receptors on cardiac cells. The conformation of other virion epitopes is also likely to be important for presentation to T cells or for autoimmune responses, such as anti-idiotyping or mimicry, to cardiac antigens.

It is not known whether cardiovirulence phenotypes can be predicted from the genetic sequence of the virus. A few variants of CVB3 have been completely or partially sequenced (201, 229, 230, 385, 387), and mutations apparently occur throughout the genome, which seems to indicate that it is tertiary structures that are important. Nevertheless, most CVB variants have not been sequenced. Future comparisons of genetic drift sites could indicate nucleotide or amino acid substitutions that are important for the virus to cause heart disease.

Reinfection. Reinfection appears to be a factor in the development of viral heart disease in the mouse model. However, the severity of secondary enteroviral infection depends on the timing of reinfection, dose, infecting virus, and type of immunologic response. It has been noted that more severe disease occurs in C3H/HeJ mice infected with a low primary dose of CVB2 followed by a higher dose of myocarditic CVB3 28 days later than in mice infected with CVB3 alone (20). The ability of CVB2-primed T cells to recognize CVB3-infected cells via a conserved antigenic epitope is postulated to play a role in enhanced myocardial disease (20, 22). In another study, however, C3H/HeJ mice infected with a host range variant (CVB3W-RD) and then challenged up to 70 days later with CVB1 were resistant to lethal disease compared to mice infected with CVB1 only (206). Moreover, murine CD-1 neonates that survived infection with a temperature-sensitive mutant of CVB3 were protected from heart disease as adolescents upon challenge with myocarditic CVB3 (104).

Whether interference or potentiation of viral heart disease occurs as a result of repeated exposure to enteroviruses over a person's lifetime is not known. However, humans with preexisting conditions (e.g., aberrant immunologic function, underlying cardiac conditions) may be more susceptible to severe forms of heart disease upon subsequent viral infection.

PHYSIOLOGIC FACTORS

Exercise. Exercise exacerbates coxsackieviral myocarditis in weanling mice. When forced to swim after CVB3 inoculation, mice exhibit greater mortality, greater dilation of the heart, more extensive inflammation and necrosis, and markedly increased viral titers in the heart compared to rested or uninfected controls (94). When these observations were extended over 15 months, enduring cardiac damage was most extensive in the infected group that had been forced to swim (327). CVA-infected mice that are forced to swim also exhibit increased viral titers in the heart, although disease severity is not as markedly enhanced as for CVB-infected mice (379).

The timing of strenuous exercise appears to be important for exacerbation of viral heart disease. CVB-infected weanling mice forced to swim from day 9 of infection exhibit some increase in mortality, but the disease is not as severe as in mice forced to swim from the day of virus inoculation (94). In adult female mice forced to swim 48 h after CVB inoculation, myocardial damage is enhanced and the composition of inflammatory cell populations in the myocardium is modified compared to the situation in mice exercised at the time of virus infection (0 h) (165).

In humans, further evidence of the adverse affects of exercise is scarce, as exercise is generally contraindicated as a therapy. However, Sutton et al. did report that one adult patient with CVB4 myocarditis exercised in the last days of his illness in an effort to lose weight and died soon after. It was speculated that exercise had exacerbated the myocarditis, possibly by enhancing viral localization to the heart (376). If microvascular spasm is important in the pathogenesis of myocardial damage in humans, then the adverse effects of exercise may also be based partially on the increase in myocardial ischemia.

Nutrition. Susceptibility to CVB3 infection is also enhanced in malnourished young mice. As the degree of dietary deprivation increases, there is higher mortality, evidence of gross cardiac lesions, hepatic necrosis, and abnormally high and persistent levels of virus in the heart, spleen, liver, and pancreas. It is postulated that the enhanced severity of CVB infection in undernourished mice is related to immunologic defects (418, 421, 422).

Susceptibility to CVB3 myocarditis is also enhanced in vitamin E-deficient mice. The disease severity in vitamin E-deficient mice is also correlated with dietary fat intake. It is postulated that vitamin E deficiency is associated with oxidative stress and that such stress is a significant factor in the cardiotoxic effects of CVB infection (21). Interestingly, vitamin E deficiency also exacerbates myocarditis in mice infected with amyocarditic virus (CVB3φ). Moreover, both CVB3m and CVB3φ express a dramatic increase in the cardiovirulence phenotype when passaged from vitamin E-deficient to vitamin E-supplemented mice. The nature of the phenotypic (or genotypic) change(s) is unknown (21).

Sex of host. As mentioned previously, viral heart disease is more severe in male mice than in female mice. Differences in the elaboration of protective and destructive immunologic responses were noted; these responses may be influenced by the presence of different sex hormones.

Similarly, in humans, epidemiologic data presented above indicate that males are more susceptible than females to myocarditis and DCM. However, in humans, susceptibility to enteroviral infection is not influenced by the sex of the individual (100). Moreover, although enteroviruses constitute the principal virus type associated with heart diseases such as myocarditis (420), there may be many other etiologic causes of the disease (2, 4). Thus, until epidemiologic data on the sex of the host are sorted along etiologic lines, sex-based susceptibility to viral heart disease is in doubt, and extrapolation to murine models should be performed with caution.

Pregnancy: maternal and fetal infections. Female mice infected with CVB3 during pregnancy develop more severe myocarditis than female mice infected at other times (240). CVB may cross the placental barrier during pregnancy, although virus titers can generally be determined in murine fetuses for only a short time (281, 282, 361, 369) (see chapter 10). CVB isolation from murine fetuses over an extended period is often complicated by the increased rate of premature abortion. High mortality has also been noted among delivered pups (59, 281, 282, 361, 369). Maternal antibody to CVB3 does not protect against stillbirth but does protect neonates against postnatal mortality (281). Maternal antibodies transmitted to the offspring through milk also protect neonates against subsequent virus challenge (273). In contrast, CVA fail to replicate in the murine fetus under similar experimental conditions (361). In studies with the enterovirus Theiler's murine encephalomyelitis virus, it has been demonstrated that a placental barrier that impedes infection of the fetus with this virus can develop during pregnancy (5, 6) (see chapter 10).

In humans, there is a high frequency of myocarditis in peripartum cardiomyopathy (277, 279, 300, 343). This may suggest an underlying enteroviral infection, although it has not been conclusively demonstrated, and changes in hormonal and immunologic responses in pregnant women can not be excluded as important etiologic causes of peripartum heart disease (144, 173, 253, 277, 391). In pregnant women with evidence of enteroviral infection, transplacental transmission of the virus may occur, and cardiovascular anomalies or fatal heart disease has been noted in newborns (18, 45, 111, 183, 198).

ENVIRONMENTAL FACTORS

CVB heart disease is enhanced in adult mice persistently exposed to low temperatures (33) and in suckling animals exposed to whole-body irradiation (44) prior to virus infection. Host defense responses are presumably depressed in these animals (420).

In mice, the tissue distribution of environmental pollutants and lipids changes during CVB infection. Intravenously injected ^{109}Cd exhibits increased accumulation in the spleen and kidneys, ^{63}Ni levels in the pancreas and ventricular myocardium increase, and [^{14}C]cholesterol localized in the heart and pancreas increases. It has been postulated that heavy-metals can enhance myocardial disease, possibly through stimulation of autoimmune mechanisms, and that lipid accumulation can facilitate heavy metal deposition or may possibly act as an initiating factor for artherosclerosis in humans (166, 168).

ENTEROVIRUS DETECTION IN PATIENTS WITH MYOCARDITIS AND DCM

In experimental murine models, the specific etiologic agent causing heart disease is obviously the administered enterovirus. In humans, however, the etiology is not so evident. To date, there is no routine laboratory test for detecting enteroviral infection in heart disease, as there is considerable controversy over which viruses are most important, how important the viruses are compared with other etiologic causes (e.g., metabolic, hereditary, and drug causes), how patients should be assigned to a specific etiologic group, and how data on viral infection should be interpreted. Nevertheless, there is considerable evidence indicating that enteroviruses are highly significant etiologic agents of myocarditis and probably also of DCM. The serologic, virologic, and molecular evidence of enteroviral involvement in myocarditis and DCM is discussed below.

Serologic Diagnosis

Serologic studies have established a preliminary association of enteroviral infections with myo(peri)carditis, as summarized in Table 2. Although individual reports may vary, IgM antibodies to enteroviruses (primarily CVB) are present in approximately 38% of reported cases. Neutralizing antibody titers of at least 1:160 (the majority are significantly higher) are present in about 50% of tested patients. A four-fold or greater change in paired sera is noted in approximately 44% of patients. All measurements were markedly higher than for healthy control patients (Table 2). These findings are similar to earlier estimates (reviewed in reference 72).

The association of enteroviral infection with cardiomyopathy is less well established by serology, as shown in Table 2. By one interpretation, serologic studies seem to indicate that enteroviral infection is recent, and that it exacerbates a preexisting myocardial dysfunction. This interpretation is supported by the finding of high and/or rising serologic titers in patients with DCM, particularly those with a

TABLE 2 Serologic association of enteroviral infection with heart disease in humans[a]

Test[b]	Myo(peri)carditis		Idiopathic DCM		Other cardiac conditions		Healthy controls	
	% Positive (n)	Reference(s)	% Positive (n)	Reference(s)	% Positive (n)	Reference(s)	% Positive (n)	Reference(s)
IgM Ab to EV	38 (151/400)	74, 265, 288, 386	19 (44/230)	74, 189, 221, 242, 288, 407	19 (54/282)	189, 265, 386, 407	7 (30/442)	189, 265, 342
N Ab ≥ 1:160	50 (321/647)	112, 117, 130, 265, 287, 339, 366, 386	12 (14/116)	197	32 (201/621)	117, 242, 265, 287, 386	11 (29/275)	117, 197, 265
4-fold change	20 (98/499)	111, 130, 186, 246, 287, 339, 366	26 (5/19)	39, 242	0 (0/79)	287		

[a] These data are compiled data, and individual reports varied in positivity. In some cases, select patient groups were used.
[b] Abbreviations: Ab, antibody; EV, enteroviruses (mostly CVB); N Ab, neutralizing antibody; 4-fold change, change in antibody titer in paired sera.

more recent onset of symptoms (39, 74, 197, 242, 288, 407). An alternative interpretation, however, is that enterovirus-associated myocarditis progresses to DCM in some patient subsets. For example, high and persistent CVB antibody titers have been reported in patients with ongoing myo(peri)carditis and in DCM patients, some of whom had clinical evidence suggestive of previous myocarditis (39, 189, 242, 288).

The ability of serologic studies to resolve these concepts is limited, since diagnostically significant rises in antibody titer may not be detected in patients if DCM occurs as a distant sequela to viral myocarditis. Moreover, the presence of antibodies in DCM studies is not always significantly greater than their presence in the general population (Table 2), probably because of the high prevalence in the general population of enteroviral infections, most of which are not associated with cardiac complications. The heterogeneity of enteroviral antibody responses has led to complications in identifying the putative enteroviral serotypes most associated with cardiac conditions and in determining whether the antibodies are directed primarily against virus or against cross-reacting cardiac autoantigens. Thus, for now, serology provides only a presumptive association of enteroviral etiology in DCM.

Virus Isolation

In summary or case studies, there are numerous reports of virus isolation from blood, throat, or stool samples of patients with myocarditis or pericarditis (74, 86, 117, 130, 139, 147, 339, 340, 366). Nevertheless, although isolation provides unequivocal evidence of infection, it does not distinguish coincidental infection from an etiologically significant cardiac condition.

The definitive establishment of viral etiology in heart disease requires the demonstration of replicating virus in myocardial cells. Infectious CVB particles have been isolated from the heart muscle (147, 234, 376) and pericardial fluid (248, 344, 377) at autopsy of patients with fatal cases of myo(peri)carditis. CVB antigens have also been detected in autopsy heart specimens by indirect immunofluorescence (36, 86). CVB-like particles were observed postmortem by electron microscopy in the myocardium of one cardiomyopathy patient, but culture was not possible (138). Unfortunately, myocardial specimens are seldom available, and when they are, isolation of viral particles is rare except in very severe cases. Consequently, an enteroviral etiology in myocarditis and DCM is very difficult to establish by using these techniques.

Detection of Viral RNA

Most recently, studies that have applied molecular technology to the clinical diagnosis of enteroviral infection have shed a new light on the importance of viral involvement in myocarditis and DCM (reviewed in reference 251). By use of probe hybridization and PCR, enteroviral RNA has been detected in the myocardia of patients with myocarditis, chronic heart disease, and DCM. The technique of endomyocardial biopsy for sampling heart tissue is discussed in the next section under clinical diagnosis.

SLOT BLOT HYBRIDIZATION

The first use of the hybridization technique was reported by Bowles et al. in 1986. Those investigators used a slot blot method in which a radiolabeled probe complementary to the CVB genome was hybridized to RNA purified from endomyocardial biopsy samples (34). They initially reported a positive hybridization signal for coxsackievirus RNA in the hearts of 9 of 17 patients with myocarditis or DCM but in none of the controls. Recently, this group has detected enteroviral RNA in 21 (45%) of 47 cardiac biopsy samples from patients with myocarditis, 35 (43%) of 82 biopsy samples from patients with healed myocarditis or DCM, and 0 of 39 controls (12) (Table 3). The numbers may represent overestimates of the true incidence of enterovirus in the heart; nevertheless, these are landmark studies. This group was the first to report the detection of viral RNA in clinical heart tissue, and in doing so, they provided a new method for determining viral etiology in patients with heart disease.

PCR

Most recently, PCR has also been used to detect viral RNA in the myocardia of patients with myocarditis. This technique is considered more sensitive and specific than slot blot hybridization, since it allows for primer-mediated high-copy-number amplification of viral sequences, thus distinguishing them from the background nucleic acid in the tissue sample.

Our laboratory was the first to use PCR to detect enteroviral RNA in endomyocardial biopsy samples (170). When 48 patients with clinically suspected myocarditis or idiopathic DCM were tested, enteroviral RNA was detected in endomyocardial biopsy samples from 2 patients with myocarditis and 3 patients with DCM. It is particularly important that the three PCR-positive DCM patients had histories suggestive of myocarditis and that their biopsy specimens exhibited significant amounts of fibrosis and myocyte hypertrophy. These findings indicate resolved (healed) myocarditis, thus supporting the link between enteroviral infection, myocarditis, and progression to DCM in certain patient subsets. Since that report, numerous other reports have described the detection by PCR of enterovirus by PCR from patients with myocarditis and DCM (Table 3).

Reports on the frequency of PCR detection of enteroviral RNA in heart tissues of patients with myocarditis and DCM or other heart conditions vary widely, as shown in Table 3. There are a number of reasons for this. (i) In many cases, clinical or morphologic diagnosis of myocarditis or DCM is not clear, and the association of enteroviral diagnosis with a specific clinical condition cannot be accurately estimated. (ii) The inherent focal nature of myocardial heart disease and inadequate sampling through biopsy can lead to underdiagnosis and a further underestimate of the true incidence of enteroviral RNA. (iii) The enteroviral probes used in PCR amplification

TABLE 3 Molecular detection of enteroviral RNA in hearts of patients with myocarditis and DCM

Method[a]	Enterovirus detected (no. of patients positive/no. tested [%]) in patients with:			Reference(s)
	Myocarditis	DCM	Other cardiac conditions	
Slot blot	21/47 (45)	35/82 (43)	0/39 (0)	12, 13, 34, 35
		1/6 (17)	0/8 (0)	408
Avg	21/47 (45)	36/88 (41)	0/47 (0)	
PCR	2/25 (8)	3/23 (13)		170
	3/9 (33)	8/25 (32)		203
		0/21 (0)	0/19 (0)	113
		6/50 (12)	13/75 (17)	192
		0/35 (0)		221
		6/19 (32)	0/21 (0)	356
	1/5 (20)	0/11 (0)	0/21 (0)	400
		5/11 (45)	9/24 (38)	399
		1/5 (20)	0/8 (0)	430
	7/10 (70)[b]		7/10 (70)[b]	139
	2/10 (20)[b]		0/10 (0)[b]	139
Avg	15/59 (25)	29/200 (15)	29/188 (15)	
In situ	5/12 (42)		0/5 (0)	72
	2/10 (20)[b]		0/10 (0)[b]	139
	2/9 (22)		1/8 (13)[c]	386
	23/95 (24)	10/33 (30)[d]	0/53 (0)	175, 178, 179, 181, 182
		8/47 (17)[e]		
Avg	32/126 (25)	18/80 (23)	1/76 (1)	
Avg, all methods	68/232 (29)	83/368 (23)	30/311 (10)	

[a] Abbreviations: Slot blot, slot blot hybridization; In situ, in situ hybridization.
[b] These studies used two different hybridization probes with different sensitivities.
[c] Controls in this study had clinically suspected myocarditis but were negative according to the Dallas Criteria.
[d] Recent onset.
[e] Chronic.

on Southern blot analysis vary greatly between laboratories. Some use serotype-specific probes, whereas others use group-specific probes. Hence, not all results are comparable. Moreover, it is likely that only some genotypes are important in heart disease. (iv) Contamination is always a concern with PCR. For example, virus from a recent and unrelated enteroviral infection may be present in the blood, or infected immune cells could be trapped in the bioptome sample. Exogenous contamination in the laboratory (i.e., work areas or utilities contaminated through work with enteroviruses) is also a major risk in these studies. These concerns may be overcome by using another method, namely, in situ hybridization, which is discussed below. (v) Finally, the PCR technique varies greatly between laboratories. Since the high sensitivity of PCR is dependent on many technical factors, these variations can significantly affect the rate of detection of enteroviral RNA by PCR (see chapter 17).

To address these final issues, we have designed a control enteroviral RNA standard fragment that can be amplified along with clinical specimens (252). The final yield of the control product provides quantitative information that can be used to objectively monitor the efficacy of the PCR test. The quantitative assay may also have diagnostic and prognostic value, which we are in the process of evaluating.

IN SITU HYBRIDIZATION

In situ hybridization is technically more difficult than slot blot hybridization or PCR, but it offers the advantage of visualizing the specific cells infected with enteroviral RNA. As with slot blot hybridization, probes complementary to the viral RNA are used, but they are hybridized directly onto histologic sections cut from the biopsy samples.

Using in situ hybridization, Easton and Eglin detected enteroviral RNA in endomyocardial biopsy samples from patients with clinically suspected myocarditis and noted two patterns of infectivity (72). First, the viral RNA was detected in the adventitia of blood vessels, presumably indicating initial viremia and perivascular delivery of the virus. Second, viral RNA was detected in cardiac muscle cells, possibly indicating the subsequent spread of virus through the heart tissue. Kandolf et al. reported similar findings in patients with myocarditis and also noted that the viral RNA signals appeared to spread from the immediate areas of inflammation. This finding was significant, because it suggested that cell-to-cell spread of virus had occurred, which would indicate actively replicating virus in the infected heart tissue (181). Kandolf et al. further reported the presence of enteroviral RNA in biopsy specimens from patients with DCM (181). Recently, other groups have also reported in situ detection of enteroviral RNA from biopsy specimens (Table 3).

Summary and Possible Prognostic Significance

In summary, an enteroviral etiology has been difficult to establish in patients with heart disease. There are interpretational difficulties with serologic data. Infectious virus is not readily detectable in the myocardium. New molecular techniques have allowed us to detect viral RNA without completely understanding the processes that may occur in myocardial cells harboring the genetic material. Nevertheless, serologic, virologic, and molecular studies combined with experimental models of CVB infection (i.e., indicating mechanisms triggered by viral infection) strongly support the theory that enteroviruses play a highly significant role in the pathogenesis of myocarditis and DCM.

In terms of prognostic significance, it is interesting that in a 15-year follow-up study of myocarditis patients, 10 of 42 patients exhibiting a fourfold or greater rise in antibody titer to CVB died from subsequent chronic myocarditis or cardiomyopathy compared with 0 of 26 patients with negative viral serology (217). Moreover, the presence of enteroviral RNA in heart tissue has been associated with poorer patient prognosis. Enteroviral RNA was detected in the myocardia of a higher proportion of patients who underwent cardiac transplantation because of DCM than in the myocardia of control groups (35). Also, in a follow-up study of patients with myocarditis, DCM, or other specific heart muscle disease, 26% of patients with myocardial biopsy samples positive for enteroviral RNA died compared with only 3% of patients who were enterovirus negative (12).

In the future, when specific therapeutic strategies for altering the natural history of enteroviral heart disease become available, the precision of etiologic diagnosis will be of paramount importance (see chapter 18). Unfortunately, current therapy is not so specific, and at present, there is no clinical mandate for establishing an etiologic diagnosis in all cases of myocarditis or DCM.

CLINICAL PRESENTATIONS

Myocarditis

The term "myocarditis" was initially used by Sobernheim in 1837 to mean inflammation of the myocardium (367, 395). Despite its simplicity, this definition raised considerable controversy. Today, myocarditis is operationally defined in pathologic terms as cardiac disease in which there is inflammation of the myocardium with necrosis and/or degeneration of adjacent myocytes, that is not typical of ischaemic damage associated with coronary artery disease (14, 15). Note that the definition excludes etiologic causes. In this section, the clinical, pathologic, and prognostic aspects of myocarditis are discussed.

CLINICAL PRESENTATION AND DIAGNOSIS

Myocarditis presents in many ways, and its diagnosis can often be difficult to confirm. The clinical and diagnostic features of acute myocarditis have been extensively reviewed elsewhere (1, 108, 128, 184, 190, 358). Briefly, myocarditis is probably subclinical in the vast majority of patients. In those presenting with obvious cardiac symptoms, common complaints are of chest pains and palpitations. Common physical findings include a pericardial friction rub, a ventricular gallop, and possibly tachyarrhythmias. Sinus tachycardia disproportionate to the febrile response is often seen in children. Patients may present with heart failure, and the disease occasionally mimics a myocardial infarction.

Electrocardiographic changes can be used to support the diagnoses of acute myo(peri)-carditis (108, 184–186, 190). Serial recordings indicate ST-segment elevation in the first few days, and early T-wave inversion. In the intermediate stage, the electrocardiogram (ECG) is more or less normal. In the late stage, T-wave inversions may occur again, but the tracing usually normalizes after a few months. The degree of ST-segment elevation and the degree and duration of the late T-wave inversions correlate with myocardial enzyme release and thus with the amount of cell necrosis.

Blood tests can be used to determine myocardial enzyme release (184–186). When present, levels of creatine kinase, aspartate aminotransferase, and possibly troponin T in serum may be elevated and therefore useful in the diagnosis of myo(peri)carditis.

Imaging is also a valuable tool (108, 184). Chest X ray may reveal transient cardiac enlargement in some patients. Echocardiography can be used to monitor ventricular dilation, thickening of the myocardium, and lowered ejection fraction. In addition to global left ventricular dysfunction, regional wall motion abnormalities can also be appreciated. A pericardial effusion may also be found. In acute myocarditis, echocardiographic changes normalize in a few days.

Noninvasive nuclear imaging may be particularly useful. Recently, a number of radioisotopes that can detect myocardial necrosis or inflammation have been employed as aids in diagnosis. Technetium-99m pyrophosphate myocardial scintigrams may be positive in severe forms of myocarditis (306). Gallium-67 uptake occurs in only a few cases, indicating that these scans are of more limited clinical value (301, 302). Indium-111 antimyosin antibody imaging, on the other hand, is useful for recording the extent of myocardial necrosis and is more sensitive than myocardial biopsies for monitoring the course of the disease (41, 42, 62, 426). Preliminary studies indicate that magnetic resonance imaging may also be useful in detecting tissue alterations caused by myocardial inflammation during the acute stage of the disease (43, 93). However, none of these methods are specific for myocardial damage secondary to viral myocarditis.

HISTOMORPHOLOGIC PRESENTATION AND DIAGNOSIS

Endomyocardial biopsy was first performed more than 32 years ago (341) and is currently the acceptable "gold standard" for the pathologic diagnosis of myocarditis. Initially, nonuniform approaches in the histologic definition of myocarditis caused problems in accuracy and consistency (14, 15, 49, 264, 304, 395). However, the meeting of a panel of cardiovascular pathologists in 1984 in Dallas, Tex., led to the establishment of the Dallas Criteria, a set of standardized pathologic definitions for use in the histomorphologic diagnosis of myocarditis (14, 15).

Application of the Dallas Criteria to the diagnosis of myocarditis is summarized in Table 4. The categories are defined as follows (14, 15, 304, 305). (i) Active (acute) myocarditis is intense inflammatory cell infiltration, usually in the interstitium, that is associated with widespread myocardial necrosis. (ii) Resolving (healing) myocarditis is a less severe inflammation that is only occasionally associated with myocardial lesions. (iii) In resolved (healed) myocarditis, the inflammatory cell infiltrate has largely subsided,

TABLE 4 Morphologic classification of myocarditis[a]

Biopsy	Possible classification[b]
First	Active myocarditis Borderline myocarditis No myocarditis
Second	Ongoing or persistent myocarditis Resolving or healing myocarditis Resolved or healed myocarditis

[a]See references 14 and 15.
[b]See text for definition of categories.

although some inflammatory cells might still be noted within regions of fibrosis. (iv) For ongoing (persistent) myocarditis, findings are worse on subsequent biopsies. (v) Borderline myocarditis shows sparse inflammation, often without myocyte damage. (vi) No myocarditis is indicated by lack of inflammatory cell infiltrate and myocyte damage. Borderline myocarditis or myocarditis may require repeat biopsy.

Endomyocardial biopsy is often performed through the right ventricle, with samples taken from the interventricular septum. This is now an established procedure and is associated with very low morbidity or mortality (<1%). However, since myocarditis is focal in nature and since the total volume of tissue obtained is very small (i.e., a piece 2 to 3 mm in diameter or 2 to 5 mg in mass), there is a significant risk of sampling error. Consequently, it has been recommended that more than one biopsy sample be taken, although the actual number of samples required remains controversial. It has been recommended that a minimum of three separate biopsy specimens be obtained, although five are preferable (14, 15, 253, 305). However, it has been noted that some sampling error may occur even when 17 biopsies are taken (49).

Even with the Dallas Criteria, the incidence of biopsy-positive myocarditis in patients with cardiac dysfunction ranges from 0 to approximately 60%, depending on the patient series (30, 49, 126, 218, 219, 268, 270, 299). This may be partly explained by differences in the population studied, since biopsy-positive myocarditis has also been noted in other cardiac conditions, including DCM (reviewed in reference 299). In light of these observations, endomyocardial sampling probably serves best as an adjunct to the clinical diagnosis of myocarditis. Recently, a second set of criteria that encompasses both histomorphologic findings and clinical symptoms has been proposed (Table 5) (218, 219).

PROGNOSIS

The prognosis for acute myocarditis is good, and the majority of patients recover completely without evidence of cardiac sequelae. Acute congestive cardiac failure, probably stemming from severe inflammation, occurs in approximately 10% of cases. In the remainder, residual abnormalities may occur, indicating progression of cardiac disease.

Ongoing cardiac disease in patients with myocarditis has been examined in a number of studies. In a follow-up study of 42 patients with evidence of acute CVB myocarditis, 6 patients (15%) had persistently abnormal ECGs for 6 months to 6 years, and 2 of these patients subsequently died (366). In a series of 18 adults with CVB heart disease, 5 patients (28%) had ECG abnormalities and chronic heart failure on follow-up, and 3 patients (17%) reported a persistence of vague precordial pain and malaise (340). In a study of 90 consecutive cases of acute infectious myocarditis followed up after 5 years, approximately 25% of patients reported subjective symptoms; suspect phonocardiographic findings were recorded in 23%; rest and exercise ECGs were abnormal in 19 and 30%, respectively; work capacity was abnormally low in 41%; and heart volume was enlarged in 20% (27). In a report on 15 adult patients with acute nonrheumatic myo(peri)carditis examined 1 to 4 years after the onset of heart disease, ECG abnormalities were found in 11 patients (73%), although physical work capacity of the heart was within normal limits in 13 (87%) of the patients (29). In a study of 154 patients with myocarditis of various etiologies who were monitored for an average

TABLE 5 Proposed clinicopathologic classification of myocarditis[a]

Parameter	Fulminant	Acute	Chronic active	Chronic persistent
Cardiac symptoms (onset)	Distinct	Indistinct	Indistinct	Indistinct
Clinical presentation (initial)	Cardiogenic shock	Modestly advanced cardiac dysfunction	Modest cardiac dysfunction	Limited symptoms
First-biopsy diagnosis	Active myocarditis	Active or borderline	Active or borderline	Active or borderline
Clinical course	Complete recovery or death	Incomplete recovery or DCM	DCM	Limited symptoms
Follow-up biopsy diagnosis	Resolved	Resolved	Ongoing or resolving; fibrosis; giant cells	Ongoing or resolving
Benefits of immunosuppressive therapy	None	Sometimes	None	None

[a]See references 218 and 219.

of 7.3 years, rest and exercise ECG abnormalities were found in 30 and 22% of them, respectively; a slightly lowered physical work capacity occurred in 24%; and cardiac enlargement occurred in 8.5%, although clinically significant incapacity occurred in only 8% of the cases (216). Preliminary results from 16 patients with acute viral myocarditis monitored for a mean of 16.4 months showed that approximately half of the patients had evidence of persistent or new cardiac abnormalities (2, 280). In more recent studies, Quigley et al. reported that 8 (47%) of 17 patients had impaired left ventricular function after 6 to 8 months, and 7 of these patients had abnormal ejection fractions in response to exercise. Overall, a progression to DCM was observed in 12 patients, 4 of whom died (320). Remes et al. reported that of 18 patients evaluated 23 years after an outbreak of CVB myocarditis, the majority had fully recovered, although 2 had abnormal left ventricular ejection fraction responses to exercise, and 2 had died of heart failure (326). Finally, 42 patients with myocarditis and a fourfold or greater rise in antibody titer to CVB were examined after a follow-up period of 15 years. Ten (24%) of them had died from subsequent chronic myocarditis or cardiomyopathy, compared with 0 of 26 patients who were seronegative (217).

EVIDENCE LINKING MYOCARDITIS TO DCM

It has been suggested that for some patients, DCM occurs as a sequela to acute viral myocarditis. This hypothesis is supported by long-term follow-up studies that show progressive cardiac disease in a proportion of patients with myocarditis, some of whom develop DCM. Retrospective studies of patients with DCM have also indicated prior myocarditis in certain patient subsets. The high incidence of biopsy-proven myocarditis in patients with cardiomyopathy and the evidence of prior enteroviral infection or viral RNA persistence in patients with DCM further contribute to this hypothesis. An overall estimate of the number of patients with myocarditis who appear to subsequently develop DCM is estimated to be in the range of 10 to 20% (299, 370). This incidence is greater by several orders of magnitude than the incidence of DCM in the general population (0.73 to 10 cases per 100,000 population).

DCM

According to the World Health Organization, DCM is defined as "heart muscle disease of unknown origin" (407a). DCM is characterized by dilation and impaired function of one or both cardiac ventricles. The clinical features have been extensively reviewed elsewhere (2, 92, 184, 190, 191,

193, 301, 303, 304, 406, 425, 426) and are summarized below.

CLINICAL PRESENTATION AND DIAGNOSIS

The initial presentation of DCM in patients varies, ranging from asymptomatic status with an abnormal ECG to chest pain, arrhythmias, or symptoms of heart failure. Physical findings may indicate mitral insufficiency, ventricular dilation, and/or cardiac failure. Chest X ray often reveals an enlarged heart. Echocardiograph abnormalities are frequent and may indicate an enlarged left ventricle and poor systolic function. Ventricular thrombi are noted in up to one-third of patients. Many of these features are similar to those seen in patients with coronary-induced heart failure; thus, imaging studies may be employed to help differentiate between the two disease etiologies. For patients with recent symptoms, endomyocardial biopsy is helpful in determining whether active myocarditis is present.

IMMUNOLOGIC ABNORMALITIES IN PATIENTS WITH MYOCARDITIS OR DCM

Defective in vitro suppressor cell function (9, 73, 87) is noted in a significant number of patients with DCM. It is not known whether this defect is acquired or genetically determined. In terms of disease pathogenesis, deficiencies in immunoregulation could lead to lymphocyte overreaction to stimuli (such as viral infection), possibly resulting in the development of chronic inflammatory reactions and autoimmunity.

Decreased in vitro NK-cell activity is also observed for some patients with myocarditis and up to 50% of patients with DCM (9, 271). The pathogenetic significance of this finding is unclear, but it is tempting to speculate that the NK deficiency predisposes patients to enteroviral-associated heart disease or plays a role in disease progression.

It has also been reported that patients with myocarditis and DCM produce autoantibodies directed against the cardiac-cell ADP-ATP carrier. The antibodies may develop through antigenic mimicry with CVB, and/or may arise in response to carrier autoantigen released from necrotic myocardial cells. These autoantibodies may play a contributory role in the impairment of cardiac function (348–353, 355, 357).

Autoantibodies against the cardiac β-adrenoceptor have been detected in the sera of 30 to 40% of patients with DCM but in only 12% of healthy controls. β-receptor dysfunction is common in the failing myocardium, and autoantibodies may further contribute to this process (222–228, 243, 396).

Antilaminin antibody levels are reported to be elevated in patients with myocarditis and DCM. It has been proposed that the antibodies induce cytoskeletal changes that could contribute to cardiac impairment (412). A potential diagnostic or pathogenic role for antibodies against other β-helical coiled-coil molecules (i.e., myosin, tropomyosin, and vimentin) as well as other structural proteins (i.e., keratin and actin) or yet-unidentified cardiac antigens has also been indicated but awaits further study (38, 57, 58, 71, 246, 362).

HOST GENETICS

The MHC in humans (HLA) consists of three loci (HLA-A, HLA-B, and HLA-C) for class I antigens and three (HLA-DP, HLA-DQ, and HLA-DR) for class II antigens. No single HLA type accounts for all cases of DCM. However, uneven HLA distributions have been noted in these patients. Since immune responses are regulated through HLA-encoded antigens and may contribute to the pathogenesis of DCM, the expression of specific genetic loci may affect the outcome of the disease.

HLA-DR4 antigens are overrepresented in patients with DCM compared to controls (51 to 54% versus 27 to 32%, respectively) (10, 40). Interestingly, the occurrence of autoantibodies to β-adrenoceptor is also strongly linked to the HLA-DR4 phenotype (228). In certain patient subsets, a positive association between some HLA-DQB1 alleles (297, 407), HLA-DQw4 alleles (40), or HLA-B27 alleles

(10), and the occurrence of DCM has been indicated. Moreover, a combined DR4-DQw4 haplotype was found in 12% of DCM patients and 0% of controls (40). Potential links between HLA-A2 alleles and the development of persisting enteroviral IgM antibodies have also been indicated (288). In contrast, HLA-DR6Y (10) and HLA-DRw6 (40) are underrepresented in patients with DCM (9 versus 26% and 9 versus 24%, respectively).

PROGNOSIS

The prognosis for patients with DCM is usually poor. In a 20-year follow-up study of 104 patients diagnosed with DCM, the Mayo Clinic found that "77% of patients had an accelerated course to death, with two thirds of the deaths occurring within the first two years" (92). This is in agreement with the more recent suggestion that approximately 50% of patients with DCM die within 2 years of diagnosis (109).

TREATMENT

Conventional Treatment

At present, treatment for patients with viral myocarditis and DCM remains primarily supportive. Bed rest is recommended by most physicians. Depending on the severity of the disease, a treatment regimen may consist of vasodilators (i.e., angiotensin-converting enzyme inhibitors) and diuretics. Additional treatment to control ventricular arrhythmias, atrial fibrillation, or embolisms may be used for some patients.

Future Therapeutic Outlook

Experimental studies with animal models of CVB infection have indicated new avenues for the treatment of viral heart disease, as discussed below. We have discussed a fair sampling of studies that show either favorable or unfavorable treatment results for use as a general reference. Applicability to a clinical setting is noted where appropriate. Sole and Liu review the clinical significance of many of these treatments in more depth (370).

Briefly, although peak efficacy (or even contraindication) depends on the stage of the disease, very exciting experimental results have been noted for doxazosin (alpha$_1$-adrenergic antagonist), captopril (angiotensin-converting enzyme inhibitor), cytokine inhibitors, IFN (natural antiviral), ribavarin and other synthetic antiviral agents, carteolol (β-blocker), verapamil (calcium channel blocker), interleukin inhibitors (immunomodulators), and heparin (thrombolytic agent). Immunization is not likely to be of clinical use at present. Immunosuppressive treatments tend to have variable effects and are probably dependent on the type of immune response mounted by the host. On the basis of experimental studies, the following are not recommended for use in a clinical setting: adriamycin, anti-T-cell antibodies, corticosteroids, cyclophosphamide, interleukin, levamisole, nonsteroidal anti-inflammatory drugs, and TNF.

Alpha$_1$-Adrenergic Antagonists

DOXAZOSIN

Doxazosin is promising. It is effective at ameliorating microvascular spasm and myocarditis in a murine model of EMCV infection. Treatment up to 4 days after virus inoculation was effective (370).

PRAZOSIN

Prazosin is promising. It ameliorates microvascular spasm in hamster cardiomyopathy but has not yet been examined in enteroviral heart disease (reviewed in reference 370).

Angiotensin-Converting Enzyme Inhibitor: Captopril

Captopril is promising. Treatment has a beneficial effect on CVB3-induced murine myocarditis. Treatment beginning 1 to 3 days after infection reduces heart weight, myocardial necrosis, and calcification compared with those in infected untreated controls (329, 330). Later treatment reduces heart weight in CVB-infected mice (329).

Antiviral Agents (Natural and Synthetic)

See chapter 18 also.

DISOXARIL

Disoxaril is a promising synthetic antipicornavirus drug that effectively prevents poliovirus persistence in the central nervous system and late paralysis in mice in vivo (172). It has not yet been evaluated in murine or human viral myocarditis.

IFN TREATMENTS

IFN is a very promising natural antiviral cytokine. Although still in the experimental stages, IFN is a promising new avenue for the treatment of enterovirus-associated heart disease. For experiments performed to date, two considerations should be kept in mind. (i) In vitro, different viral mechanisms appear to occur in newly and persistently infected cultures. In newly infected cultures, IFN treatment manifests an antiviral effect only before viral replication has begun, whereas in persistently infected cultures, it is always effective. (ii) In murine models, experiments performed to date indicate that fairly high doses are required around the time of viral inoculation. However, lower doses and later treatment are expected to be effective in the future, when combinations of IFNs or of IFNs and other agents are used.

Acute infected cells in culture. In cultures of human fetal myocytes, IFN-β treatment prior to virus exposure protects heart cells from the cytotoxic action of CVB and significantly reduces progeny yields compared to those in infected untreated controls. IFN-β does not appear to have a direct cardiotoxic effect on myocardial cells (177, 180). An in vitro protective effect for IFN-β has also been noted for murine skin fibroblasts (99, 237).

In FL (human amnion) cells, recombinant IFN-α A/D reduced EMCV plaque formation in a dose-dependent manner (254, 258). IFN-α A/D plus ribavarin inhibited virus replication in vitro in a synergistic manner (257, 258).

Persistently infected cells in culture. In persistently CVB3-infected cultures of human myocardial fibroblasts, IFN-β or IFN-γ treatment virtually eliminates infectious virus from the culture in a dose-dependent manner (129, 177, 180).

Combined treatment with IFN-β plus recombinant IFN-γ markedly reduces progeny titers in persistently infected myocardial fibroblasts. The IFN's act in a synergistic manner, allowing low doses of IFN to be used, but an early antagonistic effect has been noted at some doses. In some cases, recovery of infectious virus is again noted after the cessation of IFN treatment (reactivation). Thus, if IFN is used as treatment in vivo, the dose and term of therapy must be carefully considered (129). It has also been reported that a mixture of IFN-α, -β, and -γ completely abolishes persistent infection of CVB3 in the MOLT-4 T-cell line within two passages (26).

Murine models of CVB or EMCV infection. In CVB3- or EMCV-infected mice, IFN-α A/D administered subcutaneously 1 day before or on the day of viral inoculation reduces viral titers in heart, inflammatory cell response, and myocardial damage (254, 257–259). IFN-β treatment shortly before or along with CVB3 infection reduces the number of myocardial lesions but does not substantially reduce viral titers in the heart (237). Interestingly, antiserum to IFN-β administered 72 h after virus infection also reduces myocarditic lesion numbers but not cardiac viral titers (237). One possible explanation for this is that the antibodies inactivate virus-induced IFN-β, which may reduce the activity of T suppressor cells early in infection (98). In other studies, the IFN inducer poly(I-C) prolonged survival in CVB3-infected mice (46, 237), particularly when antiviral antibody treatment was given as well (46). Treatment with IFN-α A/D plus ribavirin beginning at the time of EMCV inoculation is more effective at reducing myocardial disease than treatment with ribavarin or IFN alone. The synergistic activity allows some reduction in the effective dose (258).

MISCELLANEOUS PROMISING AGENTS

Some antiviral agents presently being developed are reportedly highly effective in inhibiting CVB replication in vitro (63) and preventing CVB-induced myocarditis in murine models (266).

RIBAVIRIN

Pretreatment with ribavirin (a promising synthetic antiviral agent) reduces EMCV replication in FL (human amnion) cells in culture (257, 258, 260). In DBA/2 mice, daily ribavirin treatment starting at the time of EMCV inoculation inhibits viral replication in the heart, reduces myocarditis, and decreases mortality in a dose-dependent manner (260). Treatment 1 day after virus infection results in an initial reduction in mortality but only over the short term. Inflammatory responses and myocardial necrosis are substantially reduced. C3H/He mice treated with ribavirin at the time of CVB3 infection exhibit decreased viral titers in the heart and reduced inflammation of the myocardium on day 7 in a dose-dependent manner (258). See the section above on IFN for a discussion of combination therapy.

WIN 54954

Results with the synthetic antiviral agent WIN 54954 have been variable. The drug has a protective effect on CVB3-induced murine myocarditis if treatment is started by 4 days after virus inoculation (169, 315). However, others have reported that WIN 54954 is completely inactive in preventing CVB3-induced death in mice (266). One possible explanation for these conflicting results is differences in the tertiary structures of the WIN-binding sites in the CVB3 variants used.

β-Blockers

Several investigators have reported the effectiveness of long-term β-blocker therapy in patients with congestive heart failure from DCM (reviewed in references 231, 381, 394, 425). Experimental studies in animal models have also indicated that some β-blocker therapies may be useful in the treatment of viral heart disease.

CARTEOLOL

Carteolol is a promising nonselective β-adrenergic receptor blocker with some vasodilatory properties. Carteolol markedly reduces the development of myocardial lesions and DCM in EMCV-infected DBA/2 mice (381).

METOPROLOL

Metoprolol is an unfavorable selective β-blocker with no vasodilatory properties. Metoprolol treatment does not cause any significant changes in the hearts of EMCV-infected mice (381) but exerts deleterious effects on acute CVB3-induced murine heart disease (331).

Calcium Channel Blocker: Verapamil

Verapamil treatment of EMCV-infected mice reverses microvascular spasm and markedly ameliorates myocarditis. Effective treatment has been demonstrated up to 4 days after viral inoculation (70) (Fig. 3). Verapamil has also been demonstrated to ameliorate hamster cardiomyopathy and cardiomyopathy associated with Chagas' disease (370).

Corticosteroid Therapy

CORTISONE

Cortisone acetate treatment of mice prior to viral infection markedly enhances CVB replication in the heart and the severity of myocarditis and increases mortality (194, 195, 419).

PREDNISOLONE

Early treatment with prednisolone adversely affects CVB and EMCV myocarditis in mice (190, 382). Later administration has no effect on EMCV-induced myocarditis (382).

PREDNISONE

Prednisone treatment has no beneficial effect in CVB-infected BALB/c mice. In CVB-infected A/J mice, a marked dose-dependent decrease in cardiac inflammation and necrosis has been noted. CVB-infected DBA/2 mice given a high dose of prednisone show reduced inflammatory lesions in the heart by day 7 postinfection (136, 245).

Immunization (Passive and Active)
Inactivated virus or subunit vaccines prevent the development of murine myocarditis upon subsequent challenge with an antigenically similar virus (84, 85, 257). However, the clinical utility is probably limited, because several antigenically distinct viruses may be involved in viral heart disease. Immunization in an effort to induce heterotypic virus resistance is contraindicated, since potentiating effects have been reported in murine models of CVB infection (20).

Normal polyclonal immunoglobulin serum for passive use is effective in murine models of CVB and EMCV infection (256, 401). Anti-CVB antibodies are not recommended for use, because in animal models, they were capable of enhancing myocardial injury through immunomodulation, anti-idiotyping, or shared epitopes on cardiac antigens (i.e., molecular mimicry).

Immunomodulating Therapy

ANTI-T-CELL ANTIBODIES
In mice, depletion of specific T-cell populations is used to examine cellular pathogenic mechanisms (232). T-cell depletion could prevent CVB-induced murine myocarditis. However, since the depletion must be achieved prior to virus infection, the required T-cell population varies with the genetic background of the host, and depletion of the "wrong" population could exacerbate the disease, this therapy is not suitable in a clinical setting.

BIOPLF-70
In mice, prophylactic administration of the drug BIOPLF-70 reduces the number of myocardial lesions induced by CVB3, possibly through modulation of T-cell and NK-cell responses. BIOPLF-70 does not alter the production of anti-CVB3 neutralizing antibodies or the titers of CVB3 measured in the heart at day 8 postinfection (96).

INTERLEUKINS
Exposure of normally resistant strains of mice to CVB3 and IL-1 promotes myocarditis (207, 208). Administration of CVB3ϕ and IL-1 or IL-2 results in a marked increase in myocarditis compared to that in mice given amyocarditic virus only (162). In a murine model of EMCV infection, treatment with IL-2 or treatment with anti-IL-2 receptor MAbs had no discernible effect on the disease pathogenesis (261). IL-1 and IL-2 have also been shown to affect the function of myocardial cells in culture and in perfused mammalian heart models (122a, 145, 146, 368).

IL-1 RECEPTOR ANTAGONIST
A/J mice were implanted with osmotic pumps containing IL-1 receptor antagonist and then were infected 12 h later with CVB. The treatment inhibited the development of interstitial lesions but not of focal myocardial lesions. The level of circulating antimyosin IgG antibody was reduced (296). This indicates possible new avenues for therapy.

LEVAMISOLE
Levamisole administration to several strains of mice at the time of or up to 4 days post-viral inoculation exacerbates CVB3-induced myocarditis. It is hypothesized that the increased number of myocardial lesions results from altered T-cell reactivities. Viral titers in the heart and the production of neutralizing antibody to CVB3 are unchanged compared to those in untreated CVB-infected littermates (122).

MISCELLANEOUS AGENTS
The drug FK-506 is reportedly effective in inhibiting autoimmune diseases but has not yet been tested for viral myocarditis (reviewed in reference 245).

QUINOLINE-3-CARBOXAMIDE (LS 2616)

Pretreatment with the immunomodulating drug quinoline-3-carboxamide (LS 2616) is effective at reducing murine viral myocarditis (167, 169).

TNF

An antiviral effect of TNF against EMCV infection has been reported in vitro. However, in vivo, TNF exacerbates EMCV-induced murine myocarditis (261). TNF also promotes CVB3 myocarditis in normally resistant strains of mice (207, 208). The difference between TNF efficacy in vitro and in vivo may be explained in part by the observation that TNF can exert an effect on myocardial cells (83, 122a, 132, 427a; unpublished observations).

Immunosuppressive Therapy

ADRIAMYCIN

In mice, adriamycin may induce autoimmune responses synergistic with those induced by CVB3m. It is also cardiotoxic (151).

CYCLOPHOSPHAMIDE

Cyclophosphamide selectively alleviates T-cell-mediated immunosuppression, with an unfavorable effect on murine enteroviral heart disease. Pretreatment with cyclophosphamide exacerbates the acute and chronic stages of CVB3-induced murine myocarditis (336). Treatment around the time of CVB3 infection is associated with deleterious effects: higher mortality (196, 323) and persistent viremia and severe lesions in target organs (323). Late treatment has no effect (196). Cyclophosphamide also markedly enhances myocarditis induced by CVB3φ variants (235, 239).

CYCLOSPORIN A

Cyclosporin A is a fungal metabolite whose mechanisms of action have been reviewed elsewhere (137, 325). Cyclosporin has been successfully used in the therapy of autoimmune diseases and the suppression of transplant rejection.

In murine models of CVB infection, cyclosporin treatment has had variable success. BALB/c mice treated with cyclosporin A shortly after CVB infection exhibit significantly decreased necrosis but slightly increased cardiac inflammation. In A/J mice, cyclosporin treatment slightly reduces necrosis and the inflammatory response. In DBA/2 mice, treatment significantly reduces both necrosis and inflammation (76, 136, 245). The variable success of cyclosporin A treatment probably depends on the different pathogenic mechanisms involved in the inbred strains of mice.

If cyclosporin is administered 1 week after EMCV infection (acute period), it is associated with greater mortality than that in controls. When administered 3 weeks after virus infection (early recovery period), it is associated with a greater degree of myocardial failure (285).

Immunosuppressive Therapy in Clinical Trials

The place of immunosuppressive therapy is still under investigation. The overall efficacy of immunosuppressive treatment summarized from studies of patients with biopsy-proven myocarditis and DCM is 56 to 64%. However, 48% of patients with myocarditis who are not immunosuppressed improve spontaneously (231, 299).

In an effort to determine whether immunosuppressive therapy has a significant beneficial effect, a recent National Institutes of Health-sponsored multicenter controlled trial was conducted. Over 2,000 patients were enrolled at 23 centers throughout Canada and the United States. Approximately 200 patients exhibited Dallas Criteria—positive myocarditis, and 111 of these had severely impaired left ventricular function. Patients in this final group were randomized into one of three categories: (i) conventional therapy, (ii) conventional therapy plus prednisone and cyclosporin A, or (iii) conventional therapy plus prednisone and azathioprine. The third category was discontinued at 14 months to reduce sample size requirements (67).

The multicenter trial was recently concluded. Although the final results have not yet been published, preliminary reports indicate that for patients receiving immunosuppressive treatment, there is no significant beneficial effect. "Many patients in categories 1 and 2 showed an improvement in left ventricular function but this was not significantly different between those treated with immunosuppression and those who were not. Death rates at one and two years were not significantly different" (67).

It is possible, however, that substantial benefit may still occur in some patient subsets, especially those with early presentation, with the danger of viremia already past. In another controlled study, patients without evidence of viral involvement (cytomegalovirus or enteroviruses) were treated with conventional therapy or were immunosuppressed with azathioprine plus prednisone. The immunosuppressed group exhibited a significant decrease in IgG levels and complement binding in biopsy samples and a marked improvement in hemodynamic status compared with patients given conventional therapy only (245). In other studies, the efficacy of prednisone or prednisone plus azathioprine ranged from no response to a markedly beneficial effect (reviewed in reference 264). Treatment with prednisone plus azathioprine may also have been effective for some patients with postpartum cardiomyopathy (279) but probably not for those with end-stage DCM.

Nonsteroidal Anti-Inflammatory Drugs

IBUPROFEN
Ibuprofen has a deleterious effect on the acute phase of CVB3-induced murine myocarditis (52).

INDOMETHACIN
Indomethacin has a deleterious effect on CVB3-induced murine myocarditis (328).

SALICYLATES
Sodium salicylate adversely affects CVB3-induced murine myocarditis (328).

Thrombolytic Agent: Heparin

Heparin treatment has a promising effect on murine viral heart disease. In CVB3-infected A/J mice, heparin treatment reduces mortality and significantly decreases fibrosis of the heart (collagen deposition). Heparin has no effect on viral replication. Treatment prior to virus infection is most favorable. Treatment on day 14 enhances myocarditis on day 28 but still reduces mortality and collagen deposition by day 58 (90).

ACKNOWLEDGMENTS

M. J. Sole is a Distinguished Research Professor, P. Liu is a Career Investigator, and T. Martino is a Research Trainee of the Heart and Stroke Foundation of Ontario. This work has been supported by grants from the Heart and Stroke Foundation of Ontario; the Medical Research Council of Canada; Knoll Pharmaceuticals, Markham, Ontario, Canada; and Searle Canada Inc., Oakville, Ontario, Canada.

We express sincere thanks to Lily Wee, Fayez Dawood, Wen-Hu Wen, Jack Liew, and Karen Aitken for their assistance.

REFERENCES

1. **Abelmann, W. H.** 1971. Virus and the heart. *Circulation* **44**:950–956.
2. **Abelmann, W. H.** 1984. Classification and natural history of primary myocardial disease. *Prog. Cardiovasc. Dis.* **27**:73–94.
3. **Abelmann, W. H.** 1985. Incidence of dilated cardiomyopathy. *Postgrad. Med. J.* **61**:1123–1124.
4. **Abelmann, W. H.** 1988. Etiology, pathogenesis, and pathophysiology of dilated cardiomyopathy, p. 3–22. *In* H.-P. Schultheiss (ed.), *New Concepts in Viral Heart Disease*. Springer-Verlag, Berlin.
5. **Abzug, M. J., H. A. Rotbart, and M. J. Levin.** 1989. Demonstration of a barrier to transplacental passage of murine enteroviruses in late gestation. *J. Infect. Dis.* **159**:761–765.
6. **Abzug, M. J., H. A. Rotbart, S. A. Magliato, and M. J. Levin.** 1991. Evolution of the placental barrier to fetal infection by murine enteroviruses. *J. Infect. Dis.* **163**:1336–1341.

7. Ahmed, R., L. D. Butler, and L. Bhatti. 1988. T4+ T helper cell function in vivo: differential requirement for induction of antiviral cytotoxic T-cell and antibody responses. *J. Virol.* **62:**2102–2106.
8. Akinkugbe, O. O., G. D. Nicholson, and J. K. Cruickshank. 1991. Heart disease in blacks of Africa and the Caribbean. *Cardiovasc. Clin.* **2**(3):377–391.
9. Anderson, J. L., J. F. Carlquist, and E. H. Hammond. 1982. Deficient natural killer cell activity in patients with idiopathic dilated cardiomyopathy. *Lancet* **ii:**1124–1127.
10. Anderson, J. L., J. F. Carlquist, J. R. Lutz, C. W. DeWitt, and E. H. Hammond. 1984. HLA A, B and DR typing in idiopathic dilated cardiomyopathy: a search for immune response factors. *Am. J. Cardiol.* **53:**1326–1330.
11. Arai, K., F. Lee, A. Miyajima, S. Miyatake, N. Arai, and T. Yokota. 1990. Cytokines: coordinators of immune and inflammatory responses. *Annu. Rev. Biochem.* **59:**783–836.
12. Archard, L. C., N. E. Bowles, L. Cunningham, C. A. Freeke, E. G. J. Olsen, M. L. Rose, B. Meany, H. J. F. Why, and P. J. Richardson. 1991. Molecular probes for detection of persisting enterovirus infection of human heart and their prognostic value. *Eur. Heart J. Suppl. D* **12:**56–59.
13. Archard, L. C., N. E. Bowles, E. G. J. Olsen, and P. J. Richardson. 1987. Detection of persistent coxsackie B virus RNA in dilated cardiomyopathy and myocarditis. *Eur. Heart J. Suppl. J* **8:**437–440.
14. Aretz, H. T. 1987. Myocarditis: the Dallas criteria. *Hum. Pathol.* **18:**619–624.
15. Aretz, H. T., M. E. Billingham, W. D. Edwards, S. M. Factor, J. T. Fallon, J. J. Fenoglio Jr., E. G. J. Olsen, and F. J. Schoen. 1987. Myocarditis. A histopathologic definition and classification. *Am. J. Cardiovasc. Pathol.* **1:**3–14.
16. Argo, E., B. Gimenez, and P. Cash. 1992. Non-cytopathic infection of rhabdomyosarcoma cells by coxsackie B5 virus. *Arch. Virol.* **126:**215–229.
17. Bagger, J. P., U. Baandrup, K. Rasmussen, M. Møeller, and T. Vesterlund. 1984. Cardiomyopathy in western Denmark. *Br. Heart J.* **52:**327–331.
18. Baker, D. A., and C. A. Phillips. 1980. Maternal and neonatal infection with coxsackievirus. *Obstet. Gynecol.* **55**(Suppl.):12S-15S.
18a. Ballingand, J.-L., R. A. Kelly, P. A. Marsden, T. W. Smith, and T. Michel. 1993. Control of cardiac muscle cell function by an endogenous nitric oxide signaling system. *Proc. Natl. Acad. Sci. USA* **90:**347–351.
18b. Balligand, J.-L., D. Ungureanu, R. A. Kelly, L. Kobzik, D. Pimental, T. Michel, and T. W. Smith. 1993. Abnormal contractile function due to induction of nitric oxide synthesis in rat cardiac myocytes follows exposure to activated macrophage-conditioned medium. *J. Clin. Invest.* **91:**2314–2319.
18c. Balligand, J.-L., D. Ungureanu, D. Pimental, R. A. Kelly, T. W. Smith, and T. Michel. 1993. Detection of transcripts for a cytokine inducible nitric oxide synthase isoform in adult rat ventricular myocytes. *Circulation* **88:**1–384.
19. Bandt, C. M., N. A. Staley, and G. R. Noren. 1979. Acute viral myocarditis: clinical and histologic changes. *Minn. Med.* **62:**234–237.
20. Beck, M. A., N. M. Chapman, B. M. McManus, J. C. Mullican, and S. Tracy. 1990. Secondary enterovirus infection in the murine model of myocarditis. *Am. J. Pathol.* **136:**669–681.
21. Beck, M. A., P. C. Kolbeck, L. H. Rohr, Q. Shi, V. C. Morris, and O. A. Levander. 1994. Vitamin E deficiency intensifies the myocardial injury of coxsackievirus B3 infection of mice. *J. Nutr.* **124:**345–358.
22. Beck, M. A., and S. M. Tracy. 1989. Murine cell-mediated immune response recognizes an enterovirus group-specific antigen(s). *J. Virol.* **63:**4148–4156.
23. Beisel, K. W., J. Srinivasappa, M. R. Olsen, A. C. Stiff, K. Essani, and B. S. Prabhakar. 1990. A neutralizing monoclonal antibody against coxsackievirus B4 cross-reacts with contractile muscle proteins. *Microb. Pathog.* **8:**151–156.
24. Beisel, K. W., J. Srinivasappa, and B. S. Prabhakar. 1991. Identification of a putative shared epitope between coxsackie virus B4 and alpha cardiac myosin heavy chain. *Clin. Exp. Immunol.* **86:**49–55.
25. Beisel, K. W., J. Srinivasappa, and B. S. Prabhakar. 1991. Molecular cloning of a heart antigen that cross-reacts with a neutralizing antibody to coxsackievirus B4. *Eur. Heart J. Suppl. D* **12:**60–64.
26. Bendinelli, M., D. Matteucci, P. G. Conaldi, A. M. Giangregorio, M. R. Capobianchi, and F. Dianzani. 1987. Mechanisms of group B coxsackie virus persistence in human cells. *Eur. Heart J. Suppl. J* **8:**441–444.
27. Bengtsson, E., and B. Lamberger. 1966. Five-year follow-up study of cases suggestive of acute myocarditis. *Am. Heart J.* **72:**751–763.
28. Bergelson, J. M., M. P. Shepley, B. M. C.

Chan, M. E. Hemler, and R. W. Finberg. 1992. Identification of the integrin VLA-2 as a receptor for echovirus 1. *Science* **255**:1718–1720.

29. Bergström, K., U. Erikson, F. Nordbring, B. Nordgren, and A. Parrow. 1970. Acute non-rheumatic myopericarditis: a follow-up study. *Scand. J. Infect. Dis.* **2**:7–16.

30. Billingham, M. E. 1989. Myocarditis and endomyocardial biopsy. *Ann. Intern. Med.* **110**:165–166.

31. Blacklow, N. R., F. B. Rose, and R. A. Whalen. 1975. Organ culture of human aorta: prolonged survival with support of viral replication. *J. Infect. Dis.* **131**:575–578.

32. Blay, R., K. Simpson, K. Leslie, and S. A. Huber. 1989. Coxsackievirus-induced disease. $CD4^+$ cell initiate both myocarditis and pancreatitis in DBA/2 mice. *Am. J. Pathol.* **135**:899–907.

33. Boring, W. D., G. M. ZuRhein, and D. L. Walker. 1956. Factors influencing host-virus interactions. II. Alteration of coxsackie virus infection in adult mice by cold. *Proc. Soc. Exp. Biol. Med.* **93**:273–277.

34. Bowles, N. E., P. J. Richardson, E. G. J. Olsen, and L. C. Archard. 1986. Detection of coxsackie-B-virus-specific RNA sequences in myocardial biopsy samples from patients with myocarditis and dilated cardiomyopathy. *Lancet* **i**:1120–1123.

35. Bowles, N. E., M. L. Rose, P. Taylor, N. R. Banner, P. Morgan-Capner, L. Cunningham, L. C. Archard, and M. H. Yacoub. 1989. End-stage dilated cardiomyopathy. Persistence of enterovirus RNA in myocardium at cardiac transplantation and lack of immune response. *Circulation* **80**:1128–1136.

36. Burch, G. E., S. C. Sun, H. L. Colcolough, R. S. Sohal, and N. P. DePasquale. 1967. Coxsackie B viral myocarditis and valvulitis identified in routine autopsy specimens by immunoflourescent techniques. *Am. Heart J.* **74**:13–23.

37. Byrne, J. A., and M. B. A. Oldstone. 1984. Biology of cloned cytotoxic T lymphocytes specific for lymphocytic choriomeningitis virus: clearance of virus in vivo. *J. Virol.* **51**:682–686.

38. Cafario, A. L. P., E. Bonifacio, J. T. Stewart, D. Neglia, O. Parodi, G. F. Bottazzo, and W. J. McKenna. 1990. Novel organ-specific circulating autoantibodies in dilated cardiomyopathy. *J. Am. Coll. Cardiol.* **15**:1527–1534.

39. Cambridge, C., C. G. C. MacArthur, A. P. Waterson, J. F. Goodwin, and C. M. Oakley. 1979. Antibodies to coxsackie B viruses in congestive cardiomyopathy. *Br. Heart J.* **41**:692–696.

40. Carlquist, J. F., R. L. Menlove, M. B. Murray, J. B. O'Connell, and J. L. Anderson. 1991. HLA class II (DR and DQ) antigen associations in idiopathic dilated cardiomyopathy. Validation study and meta-analysis of published HLA association studies. *Circulation* **83**:515–522.

41. Carrio, I., L. Berna, M. Ballester, M. Estorch, D. Obrador, M. Cladellas, L. Abadal, and M. Ginjaume. 1988. Indium-111 antimyosin scintigraphy to assess myocardial damage in patients with suspected myocarditis and cardiac rejection. *J. Nucl. Med.* **29**:1893–1900.

42. Casans, I., A. Villar, V. Almenar, and A. Blanes. 1989. Lyme myocarditis diagnosed by indium-111 antimyosin scintigraphy. *Eur. J. Nucl. Med.* **15**:330–331.

43. Chandraranta, P. A., W. G. Bradley, K. E. Korman, S. Minagoe, M. Delvicario, and S. H. Rahimtoola. 1987. Detection of acute myocarditis using nuclear magnetic resonance imaging. *Am. J. Med.* **83**:1144–1146.

44. Cheever, F. S. 1953. Multiplication of coxsackie virus in adult mice exposed to Roentgen radiation. *J. Immunol.* **71**:431–435.

45. Cherry, J. D. 1990. Enteroviruses, p. 325–366. *In* J. S. Remington and J. O. Klein (ed.), *Infectious Diseases of the Fetus and Newborn Infant*. The W. B. Saunders Co., Philadelphia.

46. Cho, C. T., K. K. Feng, V. P. McCarthy, and M. F. Lenahan. 1982. Role of antiviral antibodies in resistance against coxsackievirus B3 infection: interaction between preexisiting antibodies and an interferon inducer. *Infect. Immun.* **37**:720–727.

47. Chow, L. H., K. W. Beisel, and B. M. McManus. 1992. Enteroviral infection of mice with severe combined immunodeficiency: evidence for direct viral pathogenesis of myocardial injury. *Lab. Invest.* **66**:24–31.

48. Chow, L. H., C. J. Gauntt, and B. M. McManus. 1991. Differential effects of myocarditic variants of coxsackievirus B3 in inbred mice. A pathological characterization of heart tissue damage. *Lab. Invest.* **64**:55–64.

49. Chow, L. H., S. J. Radio, T. D. Sears, and B. M. McManus. 1989. Insensitivity of right ventricular endomyocardial biopsy in the diagnosis of myocarditis. *J. Am. Coll. Cardiol.* **14**:915–920.

50. Codd, M. B., D. D. Sugrue, B. J. Gersh, and L. J. Melton. 1989. Epidemiology of idiopathic dilated and hypertrophic cardiomyopathy. *Circulation* **80**:564–572.

51. Correa, P., C. Restrepo, C. Garcia, and A. C. Quiroz. 1963. Pathology of heart disease of undetermined etiology which occur in Cali, Colombia. *Am. Heart J.* **66:**584–596.
52. Costanzo-Nordin, M. R., E. A. Reap, J. B. O'Connell, J. A. Robinson, and P. J. Scanlon. 1985. A nonsteroid anti-inflammatory drug exacerbates coxsackie B3 murine myocarditis. *J. Am. Coll. Cardiol.* **6:**1078–1082.
53. Craighead, J. E., S. A. Huber, and S. Sriram. 1990. Biology of disease. Animal models of picornavirus-induced autoimmune disease: their possible relevance to human disease. *Lab. Invest.* **63:**432–446.
54. Cronin, M. E., L. A. Love, F. W. Miller, P. R. McClintock, and P. H. Plotz. 1988. The natural history of encephalomyocarditis virus-induced myositis and myocarditis in mice. Viral persistence demonstrated by *in situ* hybridization. *J. Exp. Med.* **168:**1639–1648.
55. Crowell, R. L. 1963. Specific viral interference in HeLa cell cultures chronically infected with coxsackie B5 virus. *J. Bacteriol.* **86:**517–526.
56. Crowell, R. L., A. K. Field, W. A. Schleif, W. L. Long, R. J. Colonno, J. E. Mapoles, and E. A. Emini. 1986. Monoclonal antibody that inhibits infection of HeLa and rhabdomyosarcoma cells by selected enteroviruses through receptor blockade. *J. Virol.* **57:**438–445.
57. Cunningham, M. W., S. M. Antone, J. M. Gulizia, B. M. McManus, V. A. Fischetti, and C. J. Gauntt. 1992. Cytotoxic and viral neutralizing antibodies crossreact with streptococcal M protein, enteroviruses, and human cardiac myosin. *Proc. Natl. Acad. Sci. USA* **89:**1320–1324.
58. Cunningham, M. W., S. M. Antone, J. M. Gulizia, B. A. McManus, and C. J. Gauntt. 1993. β-Helical coiled-coil molecules: a role in autoimmunity against the heart. *Clin. Immunol. Immunopathol.* **68:**118–123.
59. Dalldorf, G., and R. Gifford. 1954. Susceptibility of gravid mice to coxsackie virus infection. *J. Exp. Med.* **99:**21–27.
60. Dalldorf, G., and J. L. Melnick. 1965. Coxsackie viruses, p. 474–512. *In* F. L. Horsfall, Jr., and I. Tamm (ed.), *Viral and Rickettsial Infections of Man,* 4th ed. L. B. Lippincott Co., Philadelphia.
61. De Belder, A. J., M. W. Radomski, H. J. F. Why, P. J. Richardson, C. A. Bucknall, E. Salas, J. F. Martin, and S. Moncada. 1993. Nitric oxide synthase activities in human myocardium. *Lancet* **341:**84–85.
62. Dec, W. G., I. Palacios, T. Yasuda, J. T. Fallon, B. A. Khaw, H. W. Strauss, and E. Haber. 1990. Antimyosin antibody cardiac imaging: its role in the diagnosis of myocarditis. *J. Am. Coll. Cardiol.* **16:**97–104.
63. De Clerco, E., J. Murase, and V. E. Marquez. 1991. Broad-spectrum antiviral and cytocidal activity of cyclopentenylcytosine, a carbocyclic nucleoside targeted at CTP synthetase. *Biochem. Pharmacol.* **41:**1821–1829.
64. de la Torre, J. C., M. Dávila, F. Sobrino, J. Ortín, and E. Domingo. 1985. Establishment of cell lines persistently infected with foot-and-mouth disease virus. *Virology* **145:**24–35.
65. Demakis, J. G., and S. H. Rahimtoola. 1971. Peripartum cardiomyopathy. *Circulation* **44:**964–968.
66. De Maria, R., A. Gavazzi, F. Recalcati, G. Baroldi, C. De Vita, and F. Camerini. 1993. Comparison of clinical findings in idiopathic dilated cardiomyopathy in women versus men. *Am. J. Cardiol.* **72:**580–585.
67. De Ward, M. J. D. 1992. How can myocarditis be diagnosed and should it be treated? *Br. Heart J.* **68:**346–347 (Editorial).
68. Dianzani, F., M. R. Capobianchi, D. Matteucci, and M. Bendinelli. 1988. The role of interferon in picornavirus infections, p. 65–80. *In* M. Bendinelli and H. Friedman (ed.), *Coxsackieviruses: a General Update.* Plenum Press, New York.
69. Doherty, P. C., W. Allen, and M. Eichelberger. 1992. Roles of $\alpha\beta$ and $\gamma\delta$ T cell subsets in viral immunity. *Annu. Rev. Immunol.* **10:**123–151.
70. Dong, R., P. Liu, L. Wee, J. Butany, and M. J. Sole. 1992. Verapamil ameliorates the clinical and pathological course of murine myocarditis. *J. Clin. Invest.* **90:**2022–2030.
71. Drude, L., F. Wiemers, and B. Maisch. 1991. Impaired myocyte function in vitro incubated with sera from patients with myocarditis. *Eur. Heart J. Suppl. D* **12:**36–38.
72. Easton, A. J., and R. P. Eglin. 1988. The detection of coxsackievirus RNA in cardiac tissue by *in situ* hybridization. *J. Gen. Virol.* **69:**285–291.
73. Eckstein, R., W. Mempel, and H.-D. Bolte. 1982. Reduced suppressor cell activity in congestive cardiomyopathy and myocarditis. *Circulation* **65:**1224–1229.
74. El-Hagrassy, M. M. O., and J. E. Banatvala. 1980. Coxsackie-B-virus-specific IgM responses in patients with cardiac and other diseases. *Lancet* **ii:**1160–1162.
75. Ertl, G., B. Bauer, S. Neubauer, W. Schorb, and K. Kochsiek. 1991. Effect of mediators on coronary circulation. *Eur. Heart J.*

Suppl. D **12**:187–189.
76. **Estrin, M., M. Herzum, C. Buie, and S. A. Huber.** 1987. Immunosuppressives in murine myocarditis. *Eur. Heart J. Suppl. J* **8**:259–262.
77. **Estrin, M., and S. A. Huber.** 1987. Coxsackievirus B3 induced myocarditis: autoimmunity is L3T4⁺ T helper cell and IL-2 independent in Balb/c mice. *Am. J. Pathol.* **127**:335–341.
78. **Factor, S. M., T. Minase, S. Cho., R. Dominitz, and E. H. Sonnenblick.** 1982. Microvascular spasm in the cardiomyopathic Syrian hamster: a preventable cause of focal myocardial necrosis. *Circulation* **66**:342–354.
79. **Factor, S. M., H. Tanowitz, M. Wittner, and M. C. Ventura.** 1993. Interstitial connective tissue matrix alterations in acute murine Chagas' disease. *Clin. Immunol. Immunopathol.* **68**:147–152.
80. **Farrar, M. A., and R. D. Schreiber.** 1993. The molecular cell biology of interferon-g and its receptor. *Annu. Rev. Immunol.* **11**:571–611.
81. **Federici, E. E., A. M. Lerner, and W. H. Abelmann.** 1963. Observations on the course of coxsackie A-9 myocarditis in C3H mice. *Proc. Soc. Exp. Biol. Med.* **112**:672–676.
82. **Felix, J. C., B. F. von Kreuter, and C. A. Santos-Buch.** 1993. Mimicry of heart cell surface epitopes in primary anti-trypanosoma cruzi Lyt 2⁺ T lymphocytes. *Clin. Immunol. Immunopathol.* **68**:141–146.
83. **Finkel, M. S., C. V. Oddis, T. D. Jacob, S. C. Watkins, B. G. Hattler, and R. L. Simmons.** 1992. Negative inotropic effects of cytokines on the heart mediated by nitric oxide. *Science* **257**:387–389.
84. **Fohlman, J., N.-G. Ilbäck, G. Friman, and B. Morein.** 1990. Vaccination of Balb/c mice against enteroviral mediated myocarditis. *Vaccine* **8**:381–384.
85. **Fohlman, J., K. Pauksen, B. Morein, U. Bjare, N.-G. Ilbäck, and G. Friman.** 1993. High yield production of an inactivated coxsackie B3 adjuvant vaccine with protective effect against experimental myocarditis. *Scand. J. Infect. Dis. Suppl.* **88**:103–108.
86. **Foulis, A. K., M. A. Farquharson, S. O. Cameron, M. McGill, H. Schönke, and R. Kandolf.** 1990. A search for the presence of the enteroviral capsid protein VP1 in pancreases of patients with type 1 (insulin-dependent) diabetes and pancreases and hearts of infants who died of coxsackieviral myocarditis. *Diabetologia* **33**:290–298.
87. **Fowles, R. E., C. P. Bieber, and E. B. Stinson.** 1979. Defective in vitro suppressor cell function in idiopathic congestive cardiomyopathy. *Circulation* **59**:483–491.
88. **Frank, J. A., E. V. Shmidt, R. E. Smith, and C. M. Wilfert.** 1986. Persistent infection of rat insulinoma cells with coxsackie B4 virus. *Arch. Virol.* **87**:143–150.
89. **Friman, G., and J. Fohlman.** 1993. The epidemiology of viral heart disease. *Scand. J. Infect. Dis. Suppl.* **88**:7–10.
90. **Frizelle, S., J. Schwarz, S. A. Huber, and K. Leslie.** 1992. Evaluation of the effects of low molecular weight heparin on inflammation and collagen deposition in chronic coxsackievirus B3–induced myocarditis in A/J mice. *Am. J. Pathol.* **141**:203–209.
91. **Fujii, Y., F. Sendo, T. Kamiyama, and M. Naiki.** 1990. IgG antibodies to asialo GM1 are more sensitive than IgM antibodies to kill in vivo natural killer cells and premature cytotoxic T lymphocytes of mouse spleen. *Microbiol. Immunol.* **34**:533–542.
92. **Fuster, V., B. J. Gersh, E. R. Giuliani, A. J. Tajik, R. O. Brandenburg, and R. L. Frye.** 1981. The natural history of idiopathic dilated cardiomyopathy. *Am. J. Cardiol.* **47**:525–531.
93. **Gagliardi, M. G., M. Bevilacqua, P. Di Renzi, S. Picardo, R. Passariello, and C. Marcelletti.** 1991. Usefulness of magnetic resonance imaging for diagnosis of acute myocarditis in infants and children, and comparison with endomyocardial biopsy. *Am. J. Cardiol.* **68**:1089–1091.
94. **Gatmaitan, B. G., J. L. Chason, and M. Lerner.** 1970. Augmentation of the virulence of murine coxsackie-virus B-3 myocardiopathy by exercise. *J. Exp. Med.* **131**:1121–1136.
95. **Gauntt, C. J., H. M. Arizpe, A. L. Higdon, M. M. Rozek, R. Crawley, and M. W. Cunningham.** 1991. Anti-coxsackievirus B3 neutralizing antibodies with pathological potential. *Eur. Heart J. Suppl. D* **12**:124–129.
96. **Gauntt, C. J., H. M. Arzipe, J. T. Kung, K. K. Ogilvie, and U. O. Cheriyan.** 1985. Antimyocarditic activity of the guanine derivative BIOLF-70 in a coxsackievirus B3 murine model. *Antimicrob. Agents Chemother.* **27**:184–191.
97. **Gauntt, C. J., A. L. Higdon, H. M. Arizpe, M. R. Tamayo, R. Crawley, R. D. Henkel, M. E. A. Pereira, S. M. Tracy, and M. W. Cunningham.** 1993. Epitopes shared between coxsackievirus B3 (CVB3) and normal heart tissue contribute to CVB3–induced murine myocarditis. *Clin. Immunol. Immunopathol.* **68**:129–134.
98. **Gauntt, C. J., A. Higdon, D. Bowers, E.**

Maull, J. Wood, and R. Crawley. 1993. What lessons can be learned from animal model studies in viral heart disease? *Scand. J. Infect. Dis. Suppl.* **88:**49–65.

99. **Gauntt, C. J., W. C. Lutton, E. K. Godeny, S. M. Witherspoon, H. M. Arizpe, and R. E. Lanford.** 1987. Murine coxsackie virus B3 myocarditis. *Eur. Heart J. Suppl. J* **8:**393–397.

100. **Gelfand, H. M.** 1961. The occurrence in nature of the coxsackie and ECHO viruses. *Prog. Med. Virol.* **3:**193–244.

101. **Gifford, R., and G. Dalldorf.** 1951. The morbid anatomy of experimental coxsackie virus infection. *Am. J. Pathol.* **27:**1047–1056.

102. **Gillespie, J. S., H. M. A. Cavanagh, W. M. H. Behan, L. J. A. Morrison, F. McGarry, and P. O. Behan.** 1993. Increased transcription of interleukin-6 in the brains of mice with chronic enteroviral infection. *J. Gen. Virol.* **74:**741–743.

103. **Gobet, R., A. Cerny, E. Rüedi, H. Hengartner, and R. M. Zinkernagel.** 1988. The role of antibodies in natural and acquired resistance of mice to vesicular stomatitis virus. *Exp. Cell. Biol.* **56:**175–180.

104. **Godeny, E. K., R. S. Cassling, and C. J. Gauntt.** 1987. Studies on the mechanism(s) of resistance to coxsackie virus B3 (CVB3)-induced myocarditis at adolescence in mice vaccinated at birth with a temperature-sensitive mutant of CVB3. *Eur. Heart J. Suppl. J* **8:**403–405.

105. **Godeny, E. K., and C. J. Gauntt.** 1986. Involvement of natural killer cells in coxsackievirus B3 viral-induced myocarditis. *J. Immunol.* **137:**1695–1702.

106. **Godeny, E. K., and C. J. Gauntt.** 1987. Murine natural killer cells limit coxsackievirus B3 replication. *J. Immunol.* **139:**913–918.

107. **Godeny, E. K., and C. J. Gauntt.** 1987. Interferon and natural killer cell activity in coxsackie virus B3–induced murine myocarditis. *Eur. Heart J. Suppl. J* **8:**433–435.

108. **Goodwin, J. F.** 1987. Myocarditis and perimyocarditis. Histological survey, epidemiology and clinical features. *Eur. Heart J. Suppl. J* **8:**7–9.

109. **Goodwin, J. F.** 1992. Cardiomyopathies and specific heart muscle diseases. Definitions, terminology, classifications and new and old approaches. *Postgrad. Med. J. Suppl. I* **68:**S3–S6.

110. **Gore, I., and O. Saphir.** 1947. Myocarditis. A classification of 1402 cases. *Am. Heart J.* **34:**827–830.

111. **Goren, A., K. Kaplan, J. Glaser, and M. Isacsohn.** 1989. Chronic neonatal coxsackie myocarditis. *Arch. Dis. Child.* **64:**404–406.

112. **Goudevenos, J., G. Parry, and R. G. Gold.** 1990. Coxsackie B4 viral myocarditis causing ventricular aneurysm. *Int. J. Cardiol.* **27:**122–124.

113. **Grasso, M., E. Arbustini, E. Silini, M. Diegoli, E. Percivalle, G. Ratti, M. Bramerio, A. Gavazzi, M. Vigano, and G. Milanesi.** 1992. Search for coxsackievirus B3 RNA in idiopathic dilated cardiomyopathy using gene amplification by polymerase chain reaction. *Am. J. Cardiol.* **69:**658–664.

114. **Gravanis, M. G., and N. H. Sternby.** 1991. Incidence of myocarditis. *Arch. Pathol. Lab. Med.* **115:**390–392.

115. **Greve, J. M., G. Davis, A. M. Meyer, C. P. Forte, S. C. Yost, C. W. Marlor, M. E. Kamarck, and A. McClelland.** 1989. The major human rhinovirus receptor is ICAM-1. *Cell* **56:**839–847.

116. **Grist, N. R.** 1972. Viruses and myocarditis. *Postgrad. Med. J.* **48:**750–751.

117. **Grist, N. R., and E. J. Bell.** 1974. A six-year study of coxsackievirus B infections in heart disease. *J. Hyg. Camb.* **73:**165–172.

118. **Grist, N. R., E. J. Bell, and F. Assaad.** 1978. Enteroviruses in human disease. *Prog. Med. Virol.* **24:**114–157.

119. **Grodums, E. I., and G. Dempster.** 1959. The age factor in experimental coxsackie B-3 infection. *Can. J. Microbiol.* **5:**595–604.

120. **Grodums, E. I., and G. Dempster.** 1959. Myocarditis in experimental coxsackie B-3 infection. *Can. J. Microbiol.* **5:**605–615.

121. **Groenewegen, G., W. A. Buurman, and C. J. van der Linden.** 1985. Lymphokine dependence of in vivo expression of MHC class II antigens by endothelium. *Nature* (London) **316:**361–363.

122. **Gudvangen, R. J., P. S. Duffey, R. E. Paque, and C. J. Gauntt.** 1983. Levamisole exacerbates coxsackievirus B3–induced murine myocarditis. *Infect. Immun.* **41:**1157–1165.

122a. **Gulick, T., M. K. Chung, S. J. Pieper, L. G. Lange, and G. F. Schreiner.** 1989. Interleukin 1 and tumor necrosis factor inhibit cardiac myocyte β-adrenergic responsiveness. *Proc. Natl. Acad. Sci. USA* **86:**6753–6757.

123. **Gupta, S. C., H. Hengartner, and R. M. Zinkernagel.** 1986. Primary antibody responses to a well-defined and unique hapten are not enhanced by preimmunization with carrier: analysis in a viral model. *Proc. Natl. Acad. Sci. USA* **83:**2604–2608.

124. **Guthrie, M., P. A. Lodge, and S. A. Huber.** 1984. Cardiac injury in myocarditis induced by coxsackievirus group B, type 3 in

Balb/c mice is mediated by Lyt 2+ cytolytic lymphocytes. *Cell. Immunol.* **88**:558–567.
125. Hammond, R. H., R. L. Menlove, R. L. Yowell, and J. L. Anderson. 1993. Vascular HLA-DR expression correlates with pathological changes suggestive of ischemia in idiopathic dilated cardiomyopathy. *Clin. Immunol. Immunopathol.* **68**:197–203.
126. Hauck, A. J., D. L. Kearney, and W. D. Edwards. 1989. Evaluation of postmortem endomyocardial biopsy specimens from 38 patients with lymphocytic myocarditis: implications for the role of sampling error. *Mayo Clin. Proc.* **64**:1235–1245.
127. Heck, C. F., S. J. Shumway, and M. P. Kaye. 1989. The registry of the international society for heart transplantation: sixth official report—1989. *J. Heart Transplant.* **8**:271–276.
128. Heikkilä, J., and J. Karjalainen. 1982. Evaluation of mild acute infectious myocarditis. *Br. Heart J.* **47**:381–391.
129. Heim, A., A. Canu, P. Kirschner, T. Simon, G. Mall, P. H. Hofschneider, and R. Kandolf. 1992. Synergistic interaction of interferon-β and interferon-γ in coxsackievirus B3–infected carrier cultures of human myocardial fibroblasts. *J. Infect. Dis.* **166**:958–965.
130. Helin, M., J. Savola, and K. Lapinleimu. 1968. Cardiac manifestations during a coxsackie B5 epidemic. *Br. Med. J.* **3**:97–99.
131. Hengstenberg, C., G. Hufnagel, A. Haverich, E. G. J. Olsen, and B. Maisch. 1993. De novo expression of MHC class I and class II antigens on endomyocardial biopsies from patients with inflammatory heart disease and rejection following heart transplantation. *Eur. Heart J.* **14**:758–763.
132. Henke, A., C. Hohr, H. Sprenger, C. Graebner, A. Stelzner, M. Nain, and D. Gemsa. 1992. Coxsackievirus B3–induced production of tumor necrosis factor-α, IL-1β, and IL-6 in human monocytes. *J. Immunol.* **148**:2270–2277.
133. Henke, A., M. Nain, A. Stelzner, and D. Gemsa. 1991. Induction of cytokine release from human monocytes by coxsackievirus infection. *Eur. Heart J. Suppl. D* **12**:134–136.
134. Henke, A., H.-P. Spengler, A. Stelzner, M. Nain, and D. Gemsa. 1992. Lipopolysaccharide suppresses cytokine release from coxsackie virus-infected human monocytes. *Res. Immunol.* **143**:65–70.
135. Henry, Y., M. Lepoivre, J. C. Drapier, C. Ducrocq, J. L. Boucher, and A. Guissani. 1993. EPR characterization of molecular targets for NO in mammalian cells and organelles. *FASEB J.* **7**:1124–1134.
136. Herzum, M., S. A. Huber, R. Weller, R. Grebe, and B. Maisch. 1991. Treatment of experimental murine coxsackie B3 myocarditis. *Eur. Heart J. Suppl D* **12**:200–202.
137. Hess, A. D. 1993. Mechanisms of action of cyclosporine: considerations for the treatment of autoimmune diseases. *Clin. Immunol. Immunopathol.* **68**:220–228.
138. Hibbs, R. G., V. J. Ferrans, W. C. Black, J. J. Walsh, and G. E. Burch. 1965. Virus-like particles in the heart of a patient with cardiomyopathy. *Am. Heart J.* **69**:327–337.
139. Hilton, D. A., S. Variend, and J. H. Pringle. 1993. Demonstration of coxsackie virus RNA in formalin-fixed tissue sections from childhood myocarditis cases by *in situ* hybridization and the polymerase chain reaction. *J. Pathol.* **170**:45–51.
140. Hofschneider, P. H., K. Klingel, and R. Kandolf. 1990. Toward understanding the pathogenesis of enterovirus-induced cardiomyopathy: molecular and ultrastructural approaches. *J. Struct. Biol.* **104**:32–37.
141. Hogle, J. M., M. Chow, and D. J. Filman 1985. Three-dimensional structure of poliovirus at 2.9 Å resolution. *Science* **229**:1358–1365.
142. Hohenadl, C., K. Klingel, J. Mertsching, P. H. Hofschneider, and R. Kandolf. 1991. Strand-specific detection of enteroviral RNA in myocardial tissue by *in situ* hybridization. *Mol. Cell. Probes* **5**:11–20.
143. Holland, J. J. 1961. Receptor affinities as major determinants of enterovirus tissue tropisms in humans. *Virology* **15**:312–326.
144. Homans, D. C. 1985. Current concepts. Peripartum cardiomyopathy. *N. Engl. J. Med.* **312**:1432–1437.
145. Hosenpud, J. D., S. M. Campbell, and D. J. Mendelson. 1989. Interleukin-1 induced myocardial depression in an isolated beating heart preparation. *J. Heart Transplant.* **8**:460–464.
146. Hosenpud, J. D., S. M. Campbell, and G. Pan. 1990. Indirect inhibition of myocyte RNA and protein synthesis by interleukin-1. *J. Mol. Cell. Cardiol.* **22**:213–225.
147. Hosier, D. M., and W. A. Newton. 1958. Serious coxsackie infection in infants and children. *Am. J. Dis. Child.* **96**:251–267.
148. Hsu, K. H. L., and R. L. Crowell. 1989. Characterization of a YAC-1 mouse cell receptor for group B coxsackieviruses. *J. Virol.* **63**:3105–3108.
149. Hsu, K. H. L., K. Lonberg-Holm, B. Alstein, and R. L. Crowell. 1988. A monoclonal antibody specific for the cellular recep-

tor for the group B coxsackieviruses. *J. Virol.* **62:**1647–1652.
150. **Hsu, K. H. L., S. Paglini, B. Alstein, and R. L. Crowell.** 1990. Identification of a second cellular receptor for a coxsackievirus B3 variant, CB3-RD, p. 271–277. *In* M. A. Brinton and F. X. Heinz (ed.), *New Aspects of Positive-Strand RNA Viruses.* American Society for Microbiology, Washington D.C.
151. **Huber, S. A.** 1992. Heat-shock protein induction in adriamycin and picornavirus-infected cardiocytes. *Lab. Invest.* **67:**218–224.
152. **Huber, S. A., C. Haisch, and P. A. Lodge.** 1990. Functional diversity in vascular endothelial cells: role in coxsackievirus tropism. *J. Virol.* **64:**4516–4522.
153. **Huber, S. A., N. Heintz, and R. Tracy.** 1988. Coxsackievirus B-3 induced myocarditis. Virus and actinomycin D treatment of myocytes induces novel antigens recognized by cytolytic T lymphocytes. *J. Immunol.* **141:**3214–3219.
154. **Huber, S. A., and L. P. Job.** 1983. Differences in cytolytic T cell response of BALB/c mice infected with myocarditic and non-myocarditic strains of coxsackievirus group B, type 3. *Infect. Immun.* **39:**1419–1427.
155. **Huber, S. A., L. P. Job, and K. R. Auld.** 1982. Influence of sex hormones on coxsackie B-3 virus infection in Balb/c mice. *Cell. Immunol.* **67:**173–189.
156. **Huber, S. A., L. P. Job, K. R. Auld, and J. F. Woodruff.** 1981. Sex-related differences in the rapid production of cytotoxic spleen cells active against uninfected myofibers during coxsackievirus B-3 infection. *J. Immunol.* **126:**1336–1340.
157. **Huber, S. A., L. P. Job, and J. F. Woodruff.** 1980. Lysis of infected myofibers by coxsackievirus B-3-immune T lymphocytes. *Am. J. Pathol.* **98:**681–694.
158. **Huber, S. A., L. P. Job, and J. F. Woodruff.** 1981. Sex-related differences in the pattern of coxsackievirus B-3-induced immune spleen cell cytotoxicity against virus-infected myofibers. *Infect. Immun.* **32:**68–73.
159. **Huber, S. A., L. P. Job, and J. F. Woodruff.** 1984. In vitro culture of coxsackievirus group B, type 3 immune spleen cells on infected endothelial cells and biological activity of cultured cells in vivo. *Infect. Immun.* **43:**567–573.
160. **Huber, S. A., and P. A. Lodge.** 1984. Coxsackievirus B-3 myocarditis in Balb/c mice. Evidence for autoimmunity to myocyte antigens. *Am. J. Pathol.* **116:**21–29.
161. **Huber, S. A., and P. A. Lodge.** 1986. Coxsackievirus B-3 myocarditis. Identification of different pathogenic mechanisms in DBA/2 and Balb/c mice. *Am. J. Pathol.* **122:**284–291.
162. **Huber, S. A., J. Polgar, P. Schultheiss, and P. Schwimmbeck.** 1994. Augmentation of pathogenesis of coxsackievirus B3 infection in mice by exogenous administration of IL-1 and IL-2. *J. Virol.* **68:**195–206.
163. **Hufnagel, G., and B. Maisch.** 1991. Expression of MHC class I and II antigens and the Il-2 receptor in rejection, myocarditis and dilated cardiomyopathy. *Eur. Heart. J. Suppl. D* **12:**137–140.
164. **Hyypiä, T., M. Kallajoki, M. Maaronen, G. Stanway, R. Kandolf, P. Auvinen, and H. Kalimo.** 1993. Pathogenetic differences between coxsackie A and B virus infections in newborn mice. *Virus Res.* **27:**71–78.
165. **Ilbäck, N.-G., J. Fohlman, and G. Friman.** 1989. Exercise in coxsackie B3 myocarditis: effects on heart lymphocyte subpopulations and the inflammatory reaction. *Am. Heart J.* **117:**1298–1302.
166. **Ilbäck, N.-G., J. Fohlman, and G. Friman.** 1993. Altered distribution of heavy metals and lipids in coxsackievirus B3 infected mice. *Scand. J. Infect. Dis. Suppl.* **88:**93–98.
167. **Ilbäck, N.-G., J. Fohlman, S. Slorach, and G. Friman.** 1989. Effects of the immunomodulator LS 2616 on lymphocyte subpopulations in murine coxsackievirus B3 myocarditis. *J. Immunol.* **142:**3225–3228.
168. **Ilbäck, N.-G., A. Mohammed, J. Fohlman, and G. Friman.** 1990. Cardiovascular lipid accumulation with coxsackie B virus infection in mice. *Am. J. Pathol.* **136:**159–167.
169. **Ilbäck, N.-G., L. Wesslén, K. Pauksen, T. Stålhandske, G. Friman, and J. Fohlman.** 1993. Effects of the antiviral WIN 54954 and the immune modulator LS 2616 on cachectin/TNF and γ-interferon responses during viral heart disease. *Scand. J. Infect. Dis. Suppl.* **88:**117–123.
170. **Jin, O., M. J. Sole, J. W. Butany, W.-K. Chia, P. R. McLaughlin, P. Liu, and C.-C. Liew.** 1990. Detection of enterovirus RNA in myocardial biopsies from patients with myocarditis and cardiomyopathy using gene amplification by polymerase chain reaction. *Circulation* **82:**8–16.
171. **Job, L. P., D. C. Lyden, and S. A. Huber.** 1986. Demonstration of suppressor cells in coxsackievirus group B, type 3 infected female Balb/c mice which prevent myocarditis. *Cell. Immunol.* **98:**104–113.
172. **Jubelt, B., A. K. Wilson, S. L. Ropka, P.

L. Guidinger, and M. A. McKinlay. 1989. Clearance of a persistent human enterovirus infection of the mouse central nervous system by the antiviral agent disoxaril. *J. Infect. Dis.* **159**:866–871.
173. Julian, D. G., and P. Szekely. 1985. Peripartum cardiomyopathy. *Prog. Cardiovasc. Dis.* **27**:223–240.
174. Kamijo, R., H. Harada, T. Matsuyama, M. Bosland, J. Gerecitano, D. Shapiro, J. Le, S. I. Koh, T. Kimura, S. J. Green, T. W. Mak, T. Taniguchi, and J. Vilcek. 1994. Requirement for transcription factor IRF-1 in NO synthase induction in macrophages. *Science* **263**:1612–1615.
175. Kandolf, R. 1988. The impact of recombinant DNA technology on the study of enterovirus heart disease, p. 293–318. *In* M. Bendinelli and H. Friedman (ed.), *Coxsackieviruses: a General Update*. Plenum Press, New York.
176. Kandolf, R., D. Ameis, P. Kirschner, A. Canu, and P. H. Hofschneider. 1987. In situ detection of enteroviral genomes in myocardial cells by nucleic acid hybridization: an approach to the diagnosis of viral heart disease. *Proc. Natl. Acad. Sci. USA* **84**:6272–6276.
177. Kandolf, R., A. Canu, and P. H. Hofschneider. 1985. Coxsackie B3 virus can replicate in cultured human foetal heart cells and is inhibited by interferon. *J. Mol. Cell. Cardiol.* **17**:167–181.
178. Kandolf, R., A. Canu, K. Klingel, P. Kirschner, H. Schönke, J. Mertsching, R. Zell, and P. H. Hofschneider. 1990. Molecular studies on enteroviral heart disease, p. 340–348. *In* M. A. Brinton and F. X. Heinz (ed.), *New Aspects of Positive-Strand RNA Viruses*. American Society for Microbiology, Washington D.C.
179. Kandolf, R., and P. H. Hofschneider. 1989. Enteroviral heart disease. *Springer Semin. Immunopathol.* **11**:1–13.
180. Kandolf, R., P. Kirschner, D. Ameis, A. Canu, and P. H. Hofschneider. 1987. Cultured human heart cells: a model system for the study of the antiviral activity of interferons. *Eur. Heart J. Suppl. J* **8**:453–456.
181. Kandolf, R., K. Klingel, H. Mertsching, A. Canu, C. Hohenadl, R. Zell, B. Y. Reimann, A. Heim, B. M. McManus, A. K. Foulis, H. P. Schultheiss, E. Erdmann, and G. Riecker. 1991. Molecular studies on enteroviral heart disease: patterns of acute and persistent infections. *Eur. Heart J. Suppl. D* **12**:49–55.
182. Kandolf, R., K. Klingel, R. Zell, A. Canu, U. Fortmüller, C. Hohenadl, M. Albrecht, B.-Y. Reimann, W. M. Franz, A. Heim, U. Raab, and F. McPhee. 1993. Molecular mechanisms in the pathogenesis of enteroviral heart disease: acute and persistent infections. *Clin. Immunol. Immunopathol.* **68**:153–158.
183. Kaplan, M. H., S. W. Klein, J. McPhee, and R. G. Harper. 1983. Group B coxsackievirus infections in infants younger than three months of age: a serious childhood illness. *Rev. Infect. Dis.* **5**:1019–1032.
184. Karjalainen, J. 1993. Clinical diagnosis of myocarditis and dilated cardiomyopathy. *Scand. J. Infect. Dis. Suppl.* **88**:33–43.
185. Karjalainen, J., and J. Heikkilä. 1986. "Acute pericarditis": myocardial enzyme release as evidence for myocarditis. *Am. Heart J.* **111**:546–552.
186. Karjalainen, J., J. Heikkilä, M. S. Nieminen, H. Jalanko, M. Kleemola, K. Lapinleimu, and T. Sahi. 1983. Etiology of mild acute infectious myocarditis. Relation to clinical features. *Acta Med. Scand.* **213**:65–73.
187. Karupiah, G., Q.-W. Xie, R. M. L. Buller, C. Nathan, C. Duarte, and J. D. MacMicking. 1993. Inhibition of viral replication by interferon-γ-induced nitric oxide synthase. *Science* **261**:1445–1448.
188. Kasai, M., D. M. Iwamori, Y. Nagai, K. Okumura, and T. Tada. 1980. A glycolipid on the surface of mouse natural killer cells. *Eur. J. Immunol.* **10**:175–180.
189. Kawai, C. 1971. Idiopathic cardiomyopathy. A study on the infectious-immune theory as a cause of the disease. *Jpn. Circ. J.* **35**:765–770.
190. Kawai, C., A. Matsumori, Y. Kitaura, and T. Takatsu. 1978. Viruses and the heart: viral myocarditis and cardiomyopathy. *Prog. Cardiol.* **7**:141–162.
191. Kawai, C., and T. Takatsu. 1975. Clinical and experimental studies on cardiomyopathy. *N. Engl. J. Med.* **293**:592–597.
192. Keeling, P. J., S. Jeffery, A. Caforio, R. Taylor, G. F. Bottazzo, M. J. Davies, and W. J. McKenna. 1992. Similar prevalence of enteroviral genome within the myocardium from patients with idiopathic dilated cardiomyopathy and controls by the polymerase chain reaction. *Br. Heart J.* **68**:554–559.
193. Keren, A., and R. L. Popp. 1992. Assignment of patients into the classification of cardiomyopathies. *Circulation* **86**:1622–1633.
194. Kilbourne, E. D., and F. L. Horsfall, Jr. 1951. Lethal infection with coxsackie virus of adult mice given cortisone. *Proc. Soc. Exp. Biol. Med.* **77**:135–138.
195. Kilbourne, E. D., C. B. Wilson, and D.

Perrier. 1956. The induction of gross myocardial lesions by a coxsackie (pleurodynia) virus and cortisone. *J. Clin. Invest.* **35**:362–370.

196. **Kishimoto, C., K. A. Thorp, and W. H. Abelmann.** 1990. Immunosuppression with high doses of cyclophosphamide reduces the severity of myocarditis but increases the mortality in murine coxsackievirus B3 myocarditis. *Circulation* **82**:982–989.

197. **Kitaura, Y.** 1981. Virological study of idiopathic cardiomyopathy; serological study of virus antibodies and immunofluorescent study of myocardial biopsies. *Jpn. Circ. J.* **45**:279–294.

198. **Klein, J. O., and J. S. Remington.** 1990. Current concepts on infections of the fetus and newborn infant, p. 1–16. *In* J. S. Remington and J. O. Klein (ed.), *Infectious Diseases of the Fetus and Newborn Infant.* The W. B. Saunders Co., Philadelphia.

199. **Klingel, K., C. Hohenadl, A. Canu, M. Albrecht, M. Seemann, G. Mall, and R. Kandolf.** 1992. Ongoing enterovirus-induced myocarditis is associated with persistent heart muscle infection: quantitative analysis of virus replication, tissue damage, and inflammation. *Proc. Natl. Acad. Sci. USA* **89**:314–318.

200. **Klingel, K., and R. Kandolf.** 1993. The role of enterovirus replication in the development of acute and chronic heart muscle disease in different immunocompetent mouse strains. *Scand. J. Infect. Dis. Suppl.* **88**:79–85.

201. **Klump, W. M., I. Bergmann, B. C. Müller, D. Ameis, and R. Kandolf.** 1990. Complete nucleotide sequence of infectious coxsackievirus B3 cDNA: two initial 5' uridine residues are regained during plus-strand RNA synthesis. *J. Virol.* **64**:1573–1583.

202. **Köberle, F.** 1957. Die chronische Chagaskardiopathie. *Virchows Arch.* **330**:267–295.

203. **Koide, H., Y. Kitaura, H. Deguchi, A. Ukimura, K. Kawamura, and K. Hirai.** 1992. Genomic detection of enteroviruses in the myocardium. Studies on animal hearts with coxsackievirus B3 myocarditis and endomyocardial biopsies from patients with myocarditis and dilated cardiomyopathy. *Jpn. Circ. J.* **56**:1081–1093.

204. **Kuhl, U., M. Noutsias, B. Seeberg, M. Schannwell, L. B. Welp, H. P. Schultheiss, and B. E. Strauer.** 1994. Chronic inflammation in dilated cardiomyopathy. *Heart Failure* **9**:231–245.

205. **Kyu, B.-S., A. Matsumori, Y. Sato, I. Okada, N. M. Chapman, and S. Tracy.** 1992. Cardiac persistence of cardioviral RNA detected by polymerase chain reaction in a murine model of dilated cardiomyopathy. *Circulation* **86**:522–530.

206. **Landau, B. J., P. S. Whittier, S. D. Finkelstein, B. Alstein, J. B. Grun, M. Schultz, and R. L. Crowell.** 1990. Induction of heterotypic virus resistance in adult inbred mice immunized with a variant of coxsackievirus B3. *Microb. Pathog.* **8**:289–298.

207. **Lane, J. R., D. A. Neumann, A. Lafond-Walker, A. Herskowitz, and N. R. Rose.** 1992. Interleukin 1 or tumor necrosis factor can promote coxsackie B3–induced myocarditis in resistant B10.A mice. *J. Exp. Med.* **175**:1123–1129.

208. **Lane, J. R., D. A. Neumann, A. Lafond-Walker, A. Herskowitz, and N. R. Rose.** 1993. Role of IL-1 and tumor necrosis factor in coxsackie virus-induced autoimmune myocarditis. *J. Immunol.* **151**:1682–1690.

209. **Leist, T. P., S. P. Cobbold, H. Waldmann, M. Aguet, and R. M. Zinkernagel.** 1987. Functional analysis of T lymphocyte subsets in antiviral host defense. *J. Immunol.* **138**:2278–2281.

210. **Lerner, A. M.** 1965. An experimental approach to virus myocarditis. *Prog. Med. Virol.* **7**:97–115.

211. **Lerner, A. M., H. S. Levin, and M. Finland.** 1962. Age and susceptibility of mice to coxsackie A viruses. *J. Exp. Med.* **115**:745–762.

212. **Lerner, A. M., and J. A. Shaka.** 1962. Coxsackie A9 myocarditis in adult mice. *Proc. Soc. Exp. Biol. Med.* **111**:804–808.

213. **Leslie, K., R. Blay, C. Haisch, A. Lodge, A. Weller, and S. Huber.** 1989. Clinical and experimental aspects of viral myocarditis. *Clin. Microbiol. Rev.* **2**:191–203.

214. **Leslie, K. O., J. Schwarz, K. Simpson, and S. A. Huber.** 1990. Progressive interstitial collagen deposition in coxsackievirus B3-induced murine myocarditis. *Am. J. Pathol.* **136**:683–693.

215. **Leung, D. Y. M., R. S. Geha, J. W. Newburger, J. C. Burns, W. Fiers, L. A. Lapierre, and J. S. Pober.** 1986. Two monokines, interleukin 1 and tumor necrosis factor, render cultured vascular endothelial cells susceptible to lysis by antibodies circulating during Kawasaki syndrome. *J. Exp. Med.* **164**:1958–1972.

216. **Levander-Lindgren, M.** 1965. Studies in myocarditis. IV. Late prognosis. *Cardiologia* **47**:209–220.

217. **Levi, G., S. Scalvini, M. Volterrani, S. Marangoni, G. Arosio, and A. Quadri.** 1988. Coxsackie virus heart disease; 15 years after. *Eur. Heart J.* **9**:1303–1307.

218. **Lieberman, E. B., A. Herskowitz, N. R.**

Rose, and K. L. Baughman. 1993. A clinicopathologic description of myocarditis. *Clin. Immunol. Immunopathol.* **68:**191–196.
219. **Lieberman, E. B., G. M. Hutchins, A. Herskowitz, N. R. Rose, and K. L. Baughman.** 1991. Clinicopathologic description of myocarditis. *J. Am. Coll. Cardiol.* **18:**1617–1626.
220. **Liljas, L., A. M. Lindberg, and U. Pettersson.** 1993. Modelling of the tertiary structure of coxsackievirus B3 from the structure of poliovirus and rhinovirus. *Scand. J. Infect. Dis. Suppl.* **88:**15–24.
221. **Liljeqvist, J.-A., T. Bergström, S. Holmström, A. Samuelson, G. E. Yousef, F. Waagstein, and S. Jeansson.** 1993. Failure to demonstrate enterovirus aetiology in Swedish patients with dilated cardiomyopathy. *J. Med. Virol.* **39:**6–10.
222. **Limas, C. J., I. F. Goldenberg, and C. Limas.** 1989. Autoantibodies against β-adrenoceptors in human idiopathic dilated cardiomyopathy. *Circ. Res.* **64:**97–103.
223. **Limas, C. J., I. F. Goldenberg, and C. Limas.** 1989. Effect of cardiac transplantation on anti-beta-receptor antibodies in idiopathic dilated cardiomyopathy. *Am. J. Cardiol.* **63:**1134–1137.
224. **Limas, C. J., I. F. Goldenberg, and C. Limas.** 1990. Influence of anti-beta-receptor antibodies on cardiac adenylate cyclase in patients with idiopathic dilated cardiomyopathy. *Am. Heart J.* **119:**1322–1328.
225. **Limas, C. J., and C. Limas.** 1991. Beta-adrenoceptor antibodies and genetics in dilated cardiomyopathy—an overview and review. *Eur. Heart J. Suppl. D* **12:**175–177.
226. **Limas, C. J., and C. Limas.** 1993. Immune-mediated modulation of β-adrenoceptor function in human dilated cardiomyopathy. *Clin. Immunol. Immunopathol.* **68:**204–207.
227. **Limas, C. J., C. Limas, and I. F. Goldenberg.** 1991. Effect of antireceptor antibodies in dilated cardiomyopathy on cycling of cardiac beta receptors. *Am. Heart J.* **122:**108–114.
228. **Limas, C. J., C. Limas, S. H. Kubo, and M. T. Olivari.** 1990. Anti-beta-receptor antibodies in human dilated cardiomyopathy and correlation with HLA-DR antigens. *Am. J. Cardiol.* **65:**483–487.
229. **Lindberg, A. M., R. L. Crowell, R. Zell, R. Kandolf, and U. Pettersson.** 1992. Mapping of the RD phenotype of the Nancy strain of coxsackievirus B3. *Virus Res.* **24:**187–196.
230. **Lindberg, A. M., P. O. K. Stålhandske, and U. Pettersson.** 1987. Genome of coxsackievirus B3. *Virology* **156:**50–63.
231. **Liu, P., P. R. McLaughlin, and M. J. Sole.** 1992. Treatment of myocarditis: current recommendations and future approaches. *Heart Failure* **8:**33–40.
232. **Lodge, P. A., M. Herzum, J. Olszewski, and S. A. Huber.** 1987. Coxsackievirus B-3 myocarditis. Acute and chronic forms of the disease caused by different immunopathogenic mechanisms. *Am. J. Pathol.* **128:**455–463.
233. **Lonberg-Holm, K., R. L. Crowell, and L. Philipson.** 1976. Unrelated animal viruses share receptors. *Nature* (London) **259:**679–681.
234. **Longson, M., F. Cole, and D. Davies.** 1969. Isolation of a coxsackie virus group B, type 5, from the heart of a fatal case of myocarditis in an adult. *J. Clin. Pathol.* **22:**654–658.
235. **Loudon, R. P., A. F. Moraska, S. A. Huber, P. Schwimmbeck, and P. Schultheiss.** 1991. An attenuated variant of coxsackievirus B3 preferentially induces immunoregulatory T cells in vivo. *J. Virol.* **65:**5813–5819.
236. **Lowenstein, C. J., and S. H. Snyder.** 1992. Nitric oxide, a novel biologic messenger. *Cell* **70:**705–707.
237. **Lutton, C. W., and C. J. Gauntt.** 1985. Ameliorating effect of IFN-β and anti-IFN-β on coxsackievirus B3–induced myocarditis in mice. *J. Interferon Res.* **5:**137–146.
238. **Lutton, C. W., and C. J. Gauntt.** 1986. Coxsackie B3 infection alters plasma membrane of neonatal skin fibroblasts. *J. Virol.* **60:**294–296.
239. **Lutton, C. W., R. J. Gudvangen, T. J. Nealon, R. E. Paque, and C. J. Gauntt.** 1985. Cellular immune responses in mice challenged with an amyocarditic variant of coxsackievirus B3. *J. Med. Virol.* **17:**345–357.
240. **Lyden, D., J. Olszewski, and S. A. Huber.** 1987. Influence of sex hormones on coxsackie virus group B, type 3 induced myocarditis in Balb/c mice. *Eur. Heart J. Suppl. J* **8:**389–391.
241. **Lyden, D. C., and S. A. Huber.** 1984. Aggravation of coxsackievirus, group B, type 3-induced myocarditis and increase in cellular immunity to myocyte antigens in pregnant Balb/c mice and animals treated with progesterone. *Cell. Immunol.* **87:**462–472.
242. **MacArthur, C. G. C., D. Tarin, J. F. Goodwin, and K. A. Hallidie-Smith.** 1984. The relationship of myocarditis to dilated cardiomyopathy. *Eur. Heart J.* **5:**1023–1035.
243. **Magnusson, Y., S. Marullo, S. Hoyer, F. Waagstein, B. Andersson, A. Vahlne, J. G. Guillet, A. D. Strosberg, Å. Hjalmarson,**

and J. Hoebeke. 1990. Mapping of a functional autoimmune epitope on the β_1-adrenergic receptor in patients with idiopathic dilated cardiomyopathy. *J. Clin. Invest.* **86:**1658–1663.

244. Maisch, B., C. Hengstenberg, C. Bethge, M. Herzum, G. Hufnagel, and U. Schonian. 1994. Immunological factors in dilated cardiomyopathy. *Heart Failure* **9:**246–259.

245. Maisch, B., M. Herzum, and U. Schönian. 1993. Immunomodulating factors and immunosuppressive drugs in the therapy of myocarditis. *Scand. J. Infect. Dis. Suppl.* **88:**149–162.

246. Maisch, B., R. Trostel-Soeder, E. Stechemesser, P. A. Berg, and K. Kochsiek. 1982. Diagnostic relevance of humoral and cell-mediated immune reactions in patients with acute viral myocarditis. *Clin. Exp. Immunol.* **48:**533–545.

247. Mall, G., K. Klingel, M. Albrecht, M. Seemann, P. Rieger, and R. Kandolf. 1991. Natural history of coxsackievirus B3-induced myocarditis in ACA/Sn mice: viral persistence demonstrated by quantitative *in situ* hybridization histochemistry. *Eur. Heart. J. Suppl. D* **12:**121–123.

248. Mandin, J. M., and M. A. Mandin. 1963. Les péricarditis virales: considérations étiologiques à propos des virus coxsackie. *Montpellier Med.* **64:**20–22.

249. Mapoles, J. E., D. L. Krah, and R. L. Crowell. 1985. Purification of a HeLa cell receptor protein for group B coxsackieviruses. *J. Virol.* **55:**560–566.

250. Marth, J. D., R. Peet, E. G. Krebs, and R. M. Perlmutter. 1985. A lymphocyte-specific protein-tyrosine kinase gene is rearranged and overexpressed in the murine T cell lymphoma LSTRA. *Cell* **43:**393–404.

251. Martino, T. A., P. Liu, and M. J. Sole. 1994. Viral infection and the pathogenesis of dilated cardiomyopathy. *Circ. Res.* **74:**182–188.

252. Martino, T. A., M. J. Sole, L. Z. Penn, C. C. Liew, and P. Liu. 1993. Quantitation of enteroviral RNA by competitive polymerase chain reaction. *J. Clin. Microbiol.* **31:**2634–2640.

253. Mason, J. W., and J. B. O'Connell. 1990. A model of myocarditis in humans. *Circulation* **81:**1154–1156.

254. Matsumori, A., C. S. Crumpacker, and W. H. Abelmann. 1987. Prevention of viral myocarditis with recombinant human leukocyte interferon A/D in a murine model. *J. Am. Coll. Cardiol.* **9:**1320–1325.

255. Matsumori, A., and C. Kawai. 1982. An animal model of congestive (dilated) cardiomyopathy: dilation and hypertrophy of the heart in the chronic stage in DBA/2 mice with myocarditis caused by encephalomyocarditis virus. *Circulation* **66:**355–360.

256. Matsumori, A., and C. Kawai. 1987. Experimental animal models of viral myocarditis. *Eur. Heart J. Suppl. J* **8:**383–388.

257. Matsumori, A., C. Kawai, C. S. Crumpacker, and W. H. Abelmann. 1987. Pathogenesis and preventive and therapeutic trials in an animal model of dilated cardiomyopathy induced by a virus. *Jpn. Circ. J.* **51:**661–664.

258. Matsumori, A., I. Okada, C. Kawai, C. S. Crumpacker, and W. H. Abelmann. 1988. Animal models for therapeutic trials of viral myocarditis: effect of ribavirin and alpha interferon on coxsackievirus B3 and encephalomyocarditis virus myocarditis, p. 377–384. *In* H.-P. Schultheiss (ed.), *New Concepts in Viral Heart Disease.* Springer-Verlag, Berlin.

259. Matsumori, A., N. Tomioka, and C. Kawai. 1988. Protective effect of recombinant alpha interferon on coxsackievirus B3 myocarditis in mice. *Am. Heart J.* **115:**1229–1232.

260. Matsumori, A., H. Wang, W. H. Abelmann, and C. S. Crumpacker. 1985. Treatment of viral myocarditis with ribavirin in an animal preparation. *Circulation* **71:**834–839.

261. Matsumori, A., T. Yamada, and C. Kawai. 1991. Immunomodulating therapy in viral myocarditis: effects of tumour necrosis factor, interleukin 2 and anti-interleukin-2 receptor antibody in an animal model. *Eur. Heart J. Suppl. D* **12:**203–205.

262. Matsuyama, T., T. Kimura, M. Kitagawa, K. Pfeffer, T. Kawakami, N. Watanabe, T. M. Kündig, R. Amakawa, K. Kishihara, A. Wakeham, J. Potter, C. L. Furlonger, A. Narendran, H. Suzuki, P. S. Ohashi, C. J. Paige, T. Taniguchi, and T. W. Mak. 1993. Targeted disruption of IRF-1 or IRF-2 results in abnormal type 1 IFN gene induction and aberrant lymphocyte development. *Cell* **75:**83–97.

263. Matteucci, D., M. Paglianti, A. M. Giangregorio, M. R. Capobianchi, F. Dianzani, and M. Bendinelli. 1985. Group B coxsackieviruses readily establish persistent infections in human lymphoid cell lines. *J. Virol.* **56:**651–654.

264. Maze, S. S., and R. J. Adolph. 1990. Myocarditis: unresolved issues in diagnosis and

treatment. *Clin. Cardiol.* **13**:69–79.
265. **McCartney, R. A., J. E. Banatvala, and E. J. Bell.** 1986. Routine use of μ-antibody-capture ELISA for the serological diagnosis of coxsackie B virus infections. *J. Med. Virol.* **19**:205–212.
266. **McKinlay, M. A.** 1993. Discovery and development of antipicornaviral agents. *Scand. J. Infect. Dis. Suppl.* **88**:109–115.
267. **McLaren, J., E. Argo, and P. Cash.** 1993. Evolution of coxsackie B virus during in vitro persistent infection: detection of protein mutations using two-dimensional polyacrylamide gel electrophoresis. *Electrophoresis* **14**:137–147.
268. **McManus, B. M., L. H. Chow, S. J. Radio, S. M. Tracy, M. A. Beck, N. M. Chapman, K. Klingel, and R. Kandolf.** 1991. Progress and challenges in the pathological diagnosis of myocarditis. *Eur. Heart J. Suppl.* D **12**:18–21.
269. **McManus, B. M., L. H. Chow, J. E. Wilson, D. R. Anderson, J. M. Gulizia, C. J. Gauntt, K. E. Klingel, K. W. Beisel, and R. Kandolf.** 1993. Direct myocardial injury by enterovirus: a central role in the evolution of murine myocarditis. *Clin. Immunol. Immunopathol.* **68**:159–169.
270. **McManus, B. M., and R. Kandolf.** 1991. Evolving concepts of cause, consequence, and control myocarditis. *Cur. Opin. Cardiol.* **6**:418–427.
271. **McManus, B. M., B. L. Switzer, T. J. Kendall, J. B. O'Connell, and J. W. Mason.** 1989. Markedly diminished natural killing and antibody-dependent cell-mediated cytotoxicity in patients with idiopathic dilated cardiomyopathy and biopsy proven myocarditis. *Circulation* **80**(Suppl. II):II-666.
272. **Melnick, J. L.** 1990. Enteroviruses: polioviruses, coxsackieviruses, echoviruses, and new enteroviruses, p. 549–605. *In* B. N. Fields, D. M. Knipe, R. M. Chanock, J. L. Melnick, B. Roizman, and R. E. Shope (ed.), *Virology*, 2nd ed. Raven Press, Inc., New York.
273. **Melnick, J. L., N. A. Clarke, and L. M. Kraft.** 1950. Immunological reactions of the coxsackie viruses. III. Cross-protection tests in infant mice born of vaccinated mothers. Transfer of immunity through the milk. *J. Exp. Med.* **92**:499–505.
274. **Melnick, J. L., and A. S. Kaplan.** 1952. Quantitative studies on the virus-host relationship in chimpanzees after inapparent infection with coxsackie viruses. I. The virus carrier state and the development of neutralizing antibodies. *J. Exp. Med.* **97**:367–400.
275. **Melnick, J. L., and N. Ledinko.** 1950. Immunological reactions of the coxsackie viruses. I. The neutralization test: technic and application. *J. Exp. Med.* **92**:463–482.
276. **Melnick, J. L., and N. Ledinko.** 1950. Infection of cynomolgus monkeys with the Ohio type of coxsackie virus (C virus). *J. Immunol.* **64**:101–110.
277. **Melvin, K. R., P. J. Richardson, E. G. J. Olsen, K. Daly, and G. Jackson.** 1982. Peripartum cardiomyopathy due to myocarditis. *N. Engl. J. Med.* **307**:731–734.
278. **Mendelsohn, C. L., E. Wimmer, and V. R. Racaniello.** 1989. Cellular receptor for poliovirus: molecular cloning, nucleotide sequence, and expression of a new member of the immunoglobulin superfamily. *Cell* **56**:855–865.
279. **Midei, M. G., S. H. DeMent, A. M. Feldman, G. M. Hutchins, and K. L. Baughman.** 1990. Peripartum myocarditis and cardiomyopathy. *Circulation* **81**:922–928.
280. **Miklozek, C. L., P. C. Come, H. D. Royal, C. S. Crumpacker, and W. H. Abelmann.** 1984. Viral heart disease—a precursor of congestive cardiomyopathy, p. 95–98. *In* H. D. Bolte (ed.), *Viral Heart Disease*. Springer-Verlag, Heidelberg, Germany.
281. **Modlin, J. F., and M. Bowman.** 1987. Perinatal transmission of coxsackievirus B3 in mice. *J. Infect. Dis.* **156**:21–25.
282. **Modlin, J. F., and C. S. Crumpacker.** 1982. Coxsackievirus B infection in pregnant mice and transplacental infection of the fetus. *Infect. Immun.* **37**:222–226.
283. **Molina T. J., M. F. Bachmann, T. M. Kündig, R. M. Zinkernagel, and T. W. Mak.** 1993. Peripheral T cells in mice lacking p56lck do not express significant antiviral effector functions. *J. Immunol.* **151**:699–706.
284. **Molina, T. J., K. Kishihara, D. P. Siderovski, W. Van Ewijk, A. Narendran, E. Timms, A. Wakeham, C. J. Paige, K. U. Hartmann, A. Veillete, D. Davidson, and T. W. Mak.** 1992. Profound block in thymocyte development in mice lacking p56lck. *Nature* (London) **357**:161–164.
285. **Monrad, E. S., A. Matsumori, J. C. Murphy, J. G. Fox, C. S. Crumpacker, and W. H. Abelmann.** 1986. Therapy with cyclosporine in experimental murine myocarditis with encephalomyocarditis virus. *Circulation* **73**:1058–1064.
286. **Moraska, A., and S. A. Huber.** 1993. Synergism between adriamycin and coxsackie virus group B type 3 (CVB3) in induction of myocardial injury: potential role for γ/δ TcR+ T lymphocytes in pathogenesis. *Clin. Immunol. Immunopathol.* **68**:124–128.

287. Morgan-Capner, P., P. J. Richardson, C. McSorley, K. Daly, and J. R. Pattison. 1984. Virus investigations in heart muscle disease, p. 99–115. In H. D. Bolte (ed.), *Viral Heart Disease*. Springer-Verlag, Heidelberg, Germany.

288. Muir, P., F. Nicholson, A. J. Tilzey, M. Signy, T. A. H. English, and J. E. Banatvala. 1989. Chronic relapsing pericarditis and dilated cardiomyopathy: serological evidence of persistent enterovirus infection. *Lancet* **i**:804–807.

289. Nathan, C. 1992. Nitric oxide as a secretory product of mammalian cells. *FASEB J.* **6**:3051–3064.

290. Neu, N., K. W. Beisel, M. D. Traystman, N. R. Rose, and S. W. Craig. 1987. Autoantibodies specific for the cardiac myosin isoform are found in mice susceptible to coxsackievirus B3–induced myocarditis. *J. Immunol.* **138**:2488–2492.

291. Neu, N., S. W. Craig, N. R. Rose, F. Alvarez, and K. W. Beisel. 1987. Coxsackievirus induced myocarditis in mice: cardiac myosin autoantibodies do not cross-react with the virus. *Clin. Exp. Immunol.* **69**:566–574.

292. Neu, N., R. Kliever, M. Frühwirth, and P. Berger. 1991. Cardiac myosin-induced myocarditis as a model of postinfectious autoimmunity. *Eur. Heart J.* **12**:117–120.

293. Neu, N., B. Ploier, and C. Ofner. 1990. Cardiac myosin-induced myocarditis. Heart autoantibodies are not involved in the induction of the disease. *J. Immunol.* **145**:4094–4100.

294. Neu, N., C. Pummerer, T. Rieker, and P. Berger. 1993. T cells in cardiac myosin-induced myocarditis. *Clin. Immunol. Immunopathol.* **68**:107–110.

295. Neu, N., N. R. Rose, K. W. Beisel, A. Herskowitz, G. Gurri-Glass, and S. W. Craig. 1987. Cardiac myosin induces myocarditis in genetically predisposed mice. *J. Immunol.* **139**:3630–3636.

296. Neumann, D. A., J. R. Lane, G. S. Allen, A. Herskowitz, and N. R. Rose. 1993. Viral myocarditis leading to cardiomyopathy: do cytokines contribute to pathogenesis? *Clin. Immunol. Immunopathol.* **68**:181–190.

297. Nishi, H., A. Kimura, S. Fukuta, R. Kusukawa, K. Kawamura, Y. Nimura, M. Nagano, H. Yasuda, C. Kawai, T. Sugimoto, R. Okada, Y. Yazaki, H. Tanaka, K. Harumi, Y. Koga, T. Sasazuki, and H. Toshima. 1992. Genetic analysis of dilated cardiomyopathy—HLA and immunoglobulin genes may confer susceptibility. *Jpn. Circ. J.* **56**:1054–1061.

298. Obeyesekere, I., and Y. Hermon. 1972. Myocarditis and cardiomyopathy after arbovirus infections (dengue and chikungunya fever). *Br. Heart J.* **34**:821–827.

299. O'Connell, J. B. 1987. The role of myocarditis in end-stage dilated cardiomyopathy. *Tex. Heart Inst. J.* **14**:268–275.

300. O'Connell, J. B., M. R. Costanzo-Nordin, R. Subramanian, J. A. Robinson, D. E. Wallis, P. J. Scanlon, and R. M. Gunnar. 1986. Peripartum cardiomyopathy: clinical hemodynamic, histologic and prognostic characteristics. *J. Am. Coll. Cardiol.* **8**:52–56.

301. O'Connell, J. B., and R. E. Henkin. 1985. Myocardial gallium-67 imaging in dilated cardiomyopathy. *Postgrad. Med. J.* **61**:1132–1135.

302. O'Connell, J. B., R. E. Henkin, J. A. Robinson, R. Subramanian, B. J. Scanlon, and R. M. Gunnar. 1984. Gallium-67 imaging in patients with dilated cardiomyopathy and biopsy-proven myocarditis. *Circulation* **70**:58–62.

303. Olsen, E. G. J. 1984. Histomorphological relations between myocarditis and dilated cardiomyopathy, p. 5–12. In H. D. Bolte (ed.), *Viral Heart Disease*. Springer-Verlag, Heidelberg, Germany.

304. Olsen, E. G. J. 1991. The value of endomyocardial biopsies in myocarditis and dilated cardiomyopathy. *Eur. Heart J. Suppl. D* **12**:10–12.

305. Olsen, E. G. J. 1993. Morphological recognition of viral heart disease. *Scand. J. Infect. Dis. Suppl.* **88**:45–47.

306. Olsen, H. G., K. P. Lyons, W. S. Aronow, J. Kuperus, J. R. Orlando, and H. J. Waters. 1980. Technetium-99m pyrophosphate myocardial scintigrams and pericardial disease. *Am. Heart J.* **99**:459–467.

307. Palmer, R. M. J., L. Bridge, N. A. Foxwell, and S. Moncada. 1992. The role of nitric oxide in endothelial cell damage and its inhibition by glucocorticoids. *Br. J. Pharmacol.* **105**:11–12.

308. Paque, R. E., C. J. Gauntt, and T. J. Nealon. 1981. Assessment of cell-mediated immunity against coxsackievirus B3–induced myocarditis in a primate model *(Papio papio)*. *Infect. Immun.* **31**:470–479.

309. Paque, R. E., C. J. Gauntt, T. J. Nealon, and M. D. Trousdale. 1978. Assessment of cell-mediated hypersensitivity against coxsackievirus B3 viral-induced myocarditis utilizing hypertonic salt extracts of cardiac tissue. *J. Immunol.* **120**:1672–1678.

310. Paque, R. E., and R. Miller. 1988. Modulation of murine coxsackievirus-induced

myocarditis utilizing anti-idiotypes. *Viral Immunol.* **1**:207–224.
311. Paque, R. E., and R. Miller. 1989. Polyclonal anti-idiotypes influence macrophage chemotaxis in coxsackievirus-induced murine myocarditis. *J. Leucocyte Biol.* **45**:79–86.
312. Paque, R. E., and R. Miller. 1989. Monoclonal anti-idiotypic antibodies regulate the expression of virus-induced murine myocarditis. *Infect. Immun.* **57**:2864–2871.
313. Paque, R. E., and R. Miller. 1993. Antiidiotype-pulsed B cells in the induction and expression of autoimmune myocarditis. *Clin. Immunol. Immunopathol.* **68**:111–117.
314. Paque, R. E., D. C. Straus, T. J. Nealon, and C. J. Gauntt. 1979. Fractionation and immunologic assessment of KCl-extracted cardiac antigens in coxsackievirus B3 virus-induced myocarditis. *J. Immunol.* **123**:358–364.
315. Pauksen, K., N.-G. Ilbäck, G. Friman, and J. Fohlman. 1993. Therapy of coxsackie virus B3-induced myocarditis with WIN 54954 in different formulations. *Scand. J. Infect. Dis. Suppl.* **88**:125–130.
316. Penninger, J., K. Kishihara, T. Molina, V. A. Wallace, E. Timms, S. M. Hedrick, and T. W. Mak. 1993. Requirement for tyrosine kinase p56lck for thymic development of transgenic γδ T cells. *Science* **260**:358–361.
317. Pine, R. 1992. Constitutive expression of an ISGF2/IRF1 transgene leads to interferon-independent activation of interferon-inducible genes and resistance to virus infection. *J. Virol.* **66**:4470–4478.
318. Prabhakar, B. S., M. V. Haspel, P. R. McClintock, and A. L. Notkins. 1982. High frequency antigenic variants among naturally occurring human coxsackie B4 virus isolates identified by monoclonal antibodies. *Nature* (London) **300**:374–376.
319. Prabhakar, B. S., J. Srinivasappa, K. B. Beisel, and A. L. Notkins. 1988. Virus-induced autoimmunity: cross-reactivity of antiviral antibodies with self-components, p. 169–178. *In* H.-P. Schultheiss (ed.), *New Concepts in Viral Heart Disease*. Springer-Verlag, Berlin.
320. Quigley, P. J., P. J. Richardson, B. T. Meany, E. G. J. Olsen, M. J. Monaghan, G. Jackson, and D. E. Jewitt. 1987. Long-term follow-up of acute myocarditis. Correlation of ventricular function and outcome. *Eur. Heart J. Suppl. J* **8**:39–42.
321. Rabin, E. R., S. A. Hassan, A. B. Jenson, and J. L. Melnick. 1964. Coxsackie virus B3 myocarditis in mice. *Am. J. Pathol.* **44**:775–797.
322. Rager-Zisman, B., and A. C. Allison. 1973. The role of antibody and host cells in the resistance of mice against infection by coxsackie B-3 virus. *J. Gen. Virol.* **19**:329–338.
323. Rager-Zisman, B., and A. C. Allison. 1973. Effects of immunosuppression on coxsackie B-3 virus infection in mice, and passive protection by circulating antibody. *J. Gen. Virol.* **19**:339–351.
324. Reagan, K. J., B. Goldberg, and R. L. Crowell. 1984. Altered receptor specificity of coxsackievirus B3 after growth in rhabdomyosarcoma cells. *J. Virol.* **49**:635–640.
325. Reem, G. H., L. A. Cook, and J. Vilcek. 1983. Gamma interferon synthesis by human thymocytes and T lymphocytes inhibited by cyclosporin A. *Science* **221**:63–65.
326. Reines, J., M. Helin, P. Vaino, and P. Rautio. 1990. Clinical outcome and left ventricular function 23 years after coxsackie virus myopericarditis. *Eur. Heart J.* **11**:182–188.
327. Reyes, M. P., K.-L. Ho, F. Smith, and A. M. Lerner. 1981. A mouse model of dilated-type cardiomyopathy due to coxsackievirus B3. *J. Infect. Dis.* **144**:232–236.
328. Rezkalla, S., G. Khatib, and R. Khatib. 1986. Coxsackievirus B3 murine myocarditis: deleterious effects of nonsteroidal anti-inflammatory agents. *J. Lab. Clin. Med.* **107**:393–395.
329. Rezkalla, S., R. A. Kloner, G. Khatib, and R. Khatib. 1990. Beneficial effects of captopril in acute coxsackievirus B3 murine myocarditis. *Circulation* **81**:1039–1046.
330. Rezkalla, S., R. A. Kloner, G. Khatib, and R. Khatib. 1990. Effect of delayed captopril therapy on left ventricular mass and myonecrosis during acute coxsackievirus murine myocarditis. *Am. Heart J.* **120**:1377–1381.
331. Rezkalla, S., R. A. Kloner, G. Khatib, F. Smith, and R. Khatib. 1988. Effect of metoprolol in acute coxsackievirus B3 murine myocarditis. *J. Am. Coll. Cardiol.* **12**:412–414.
332. Robinson, J. A., J. B. O'Connell, L. M. Roeges, E. O. Major, and R. M. Gunnar. 1981. Coxsackie B3 myocarditis in athymic mice (41028). *Proc. Soc. Exp. Biol. Med.* **166**:80–91.
333. Roos, R. P., O. C. Richards, J. Green, and E. Ehrenfeld. 1982. Characterization of a cell culture persistently infected with the DA strain of Theiler's murine encephalomyelitis virus. *J. Virol.* **43**:1118–1122.
334. Rossmann, M. G., E. Arnold, J. W. Erickson, E. A. Frankenberger, J. P. Griffith, H.-J. Hecht, J. E. Johnson, G. Kamer, M. Luo, A. G. Mosser, R. R. Rueckert, B. Sherry, and G. Vriend. 1985. Structure of a human common cold virus and functional relationship to other picornaviruses.

Nature (London) **317**:145–153.

335. Rotbart, H. A., and K. Kirkegaard. 1992. Picornavirus pathogenesis: viral access, attachment and entry into susceptible cells. *Semin. Virol.* **3**:483–499.
336. Rozee, K. R., G. A. Klassen, A. Ahmad-Raza, and S. H. S. Lee. 1992. A mouse model of coxsackievirus myocarditis. *Can. J. Cardiol.* **8**:145–148.
337. Rueckert, R. R. 1990. Picornaviridae and their replication, p. 507–548. *In* B. N. Fields, D. M. Knipe, R. M. Chanock, J. L. Melnick, B. Roizman, and R. E. Shope (ed.), *Virology*, 2nd ed. Raven Press, Inc., New York.
338. Saegusa, J., B. S. Prabhakar, K. Esanni, P. R. McClintock, Y. Fukuda, V. J. Ferrans, and A. L. Notkins. 1986. Monoclonal antibody to coxsackievirus B4 reacts with myocardium. *J. Infect. Dis.* **153**:372–373.
339. Sainani, G. S., M. P. Dekate, and C. P. Rao. 1975. Heart disease caused by coxsackie virus B infection. *Br. Heart J.* **37**:819–823.
340. Sainani, G. S., E. Krompotic, and S. J. Slodki. 1968. Adult heart disease due to the coxsackie virus B infection. *Medicine* **47**:133–147.
341. Sakakibara, S., and S. Konno. 1962. Endomyocardial biopsy. *Jpn. Heart J.* **3**:537–543.
342. Samuelson, A., E. Skoog, and M. Forsgren. 1990. Aspects on the serodiagnosis of enteroviral infections by ELISA. *Serodiagn. Immunother. Infect. Dis.* **4**:395–406.
343. Sanderson, J. E., E. G. J. Olsen, and D. Gatei. 1986. Peripartum heart disease: an endomyocardial biopsy study. *Br. Heart. J.* **56**:285–291.
344. Sanyal, S. K., M. Mahdary, M. O. Gabrielson, R. A. Vidone, and M. J. Browne. 1965. Fatal myocarditis in an adolescent caused by coxsackie virus, group B, type 4. *Pediatrics* **35**:36–41.
345. Sasaki, O., T. Karaki, and J. Imanishi. 1986. Protective effect of interferons with hand, foot and mouse disease virus in newborn mice. *J. Infect. Dis.* **153**:498–502.
346. Schnitt, S. J., I. E. Stillman, D. V. Owings, C. Kishimoto, H. F. Dvorak, and W. H. Abelmann. 1993. Myocardial fibrin deposition in experimental viral myocarditis that progresses to dilated cardiomyopathy. *Circ. Res.* **72**:914–920.
347. Schnurr, D. P., Y. Cao, and N. J. Schmidt. 1984. Coxsackievirus B3 persistence and myocarditis in N:NIH(S) II nu/nu and +/nu mice. *J. Gen. Virol.* **65**:1197–1201.
348. Schultheiss, H.-P. 1987. The mitochondrium as antigen in inflammatory heart disease. *Eur. Heart J. Suppl. J* **8**:203–210.
349. Schultheiss, H.-P., and H.-D. Bolte. 1985. Immunological analysis of autoantibodies against the adenine nucleotide translocator in dilated cardiomyopathy. *J. Mol. Cell. Cardiol.* **17**:603–617.
350. Schultheiss, H.-P., and M. Klingenberg. 1984. Immunochemical characterization of the adenine nucleotide translocator: organ-and conformation-specificity. *Eur. J. Biochem.* **143**:599–605.
351. Schultheiss, H.-P., and P. Schwimmbeck. 1986. Autoantibodies to the adenine-nucleotide translocator (ANT) in myocarditis (MC)—prevalence, clinical correlates and diagnostic value. *Circulation* **74**(Suppl. II):II-142.
352. Schultheiss, H.-P., P. Schwimmbeck, and H.-D. Bolte. 1984. Autoantibodies against the adenine nucleotide translocator in myocarditis and dilated cardiomyopathy, p. 131–143. *In* H.-D. Bolte (ed.), *Viral Heart Disease*. Springer-Verlag, Berlin.
353. Schultheiss, H.-P., P. Schwimmbeck, H.-D. Bolte, and M. Klingenberg. 1985. The antigenic characteristics and the significance of the adenine nucleotide translocator as a major autoantigen to antimitochondrial antibodies in dilated cardiomyopathy. *Adv. Myocardiol.* **6**:311–327.
354. Schulz, R., E. Nava, and S. Moncada. 1992. Induction and potential biological relevance of a Ca^{2+}-independent nitric oxide synthase in the myocardium. *Br. J. Pharmacol.* **105**:575–580.
355. Schulze, K., B. F. Becker, and H. P. Schultheiss. 1989. Antibodies to the ADP-ATP carrier, an autoantigen in myocarditis and dilated cardiomyopathy, penetrate into myocardial cells and disturb energy metabolism in vivo. *Circ. Res.* **64**:179–192.
356. Schwaiger, A., F. Umlauft, K. Weyrer, C. Larcher, J. Lyons, V. Mühlberger, O. Dietze, and K. Grünewald. 1993. Detection of enteroviral ribonucleic acid in myocardial biopsies from patients with idiopathic dilated cardiomyopathy by polymerase chain reaction. *Am. Heart J.* **126**:406–410.
357. Schwimmbeck, P. L., N. K. Schwimmbeck, H. P. Schultheiss, and B. E. Strauer. 1993. Mapping of antigenic determinants of the adenine-nucleotide translocator and coxsackie B3 virus with synthetic peptides: use for the diagnosis of viral heart disease. *Clin. Immunol. Immunopathol.* **68**:135–140.
358. Sekiguchi, M., M. Hiroe, S. Hiramitusu,

and T. Izumi. 1988. Natural history of acute viral or idiopathic myocarditis: a clinical and endomyocardial biopsy follow-up, p. 33–50. In H.-P. Schultheiss (ed.), *New Concepts in Viral Heart Disease*. Springer-Verlag, Berlin.
359. Seko, Y., Y. Shinkai, A. Kawasaki, H. Yagita, K. Okumura, and Y. Yazaki. 1993. Evidence of perforin-mediated cardiac myocyte injury in acute murine myocarditis caused by coxsackie virus B3. *J. Pathol.* **170**:53–58.
360. Seko, Y., T. Yamazaki, Y. Shinkai, H. Yagita, K. Okumura, S. Naito, K. Imataka, J. Fujii, and Y. Yazaki. 1992. Cellular and molecular bases for the immunopathology of the myocardial cell damage involved in acute viral myocarditis with special reference to dilated cardiomyopathy. *Jpn. Circ. J.* **56**:1062–1072.
361. Selzer, G. 1969. Transplacental infection of the mouse fetus by coxsackie viruses. *Isr. J. Med. Sci.* **5**:125–127.
362. Shikhman, A. R., N. S. Greenspan, and M. W. Cunningham. 1993. A subset of mouse monoclonal antibodies cross-reactive with cytoskeletal proteins and group A streptococcal M proteins recognizes N-acetyl-β-D-glucosamine. *J. Immunol.* **151**:3902–3913.
363. Silver, M., and D. Kowalczyk. 1989. Coronary microvascular narrowing in acute murine coxsackie B3 myocarditis. *Am. Heart J.* **118**:173–174.
364. Smith, S. C., and P. M. Allen. 1991. Myosin-induced acute myocarditis is a T cell-mediated disease. *J. Immunol.* **147**:2141–2147.
365. Smith, S. C., and P. M. Allen. 1993. The role of T cells in myosin-induced autoimmune myocarditis. *Clin. Immunol. Immunopathol.* **68**:100–106.
366. Smith, W. G. 1970. Coxsackie B myopericarditis in adults. *Am. Heart J.* **80**:34–46.
367. Sobernheim, J. F. 1837. *Diagnostik der inneren Krankheiten mit vorzuegeleicher Ruecksicht auf pathologische Anatomie*, p. 1–43. Hirschwald, Berlin.
368. Sobotka, P. A., J. McMannis, R. I. Fisher, D. G. Stein, and J. X. Thomas, Jr. 1990. Effects of interleukin 2 on cardiac function in the isolated rat heart. *J. Clin. Invest.* **86**:845–850.
369. Soike, K. 1967. Coxsackie B-3 virus infection in the pregnant mouse. *J. Infect. Dis.* **117**:203–208.
370. Sole, M. J., and P. Liu. 1993. Viral myocarditis: a paradigm for understanding the pathogenesis and treatment of dilated cardiomyopathy. *J. Am. Coll. Cardiol. Suppl. A* **22**: 99A-105A.
371. Srinvasappa, J., J. Saegusa, B. S. Prabhakar, M. K. Gentry, M. J. Buchmeier, T. J. Wiktor, H. Koprowski, M. B. A. Oldstone, and A. L. Notkins. 1986. Molecular mimicry: frequency of reactivity of monoclonal antiviral antibodies with normal tissues. *J. Virol.* **57**:397–401.
372. Stamler, J. S., D. J. Singel, and J. Loscalzo. 1992. Biochemistry of nitric oxide and its redox-activated forms. *Science* **258**:1898–1902.
373. Stauton, D. E., V. J. Merluzzi, R. Rothlein, R. Barton, S. D. Marlin, and T. A. Springer. 1989. A cell adhesion molecule, ICAM-1, is the major surface receptor for rhinoviruses. *Cell* **56**:849–853.
374. Stevens, P. J., and K. E. Underwood-Ground. 1970. Occurrence and significance of myocarditis in trauma. *Aerospace Med.* **47**:776–780.
375. Stitz, L., J. Baenziger, H. Pircher, H. Hengartner, and R. M. Zinkernagel. 1986. Effect of rabbit anti-asialo GM1 treatment in vivo or with anti-asialo GM1 plus complement in vitro on cytotoxic T-cell activities. *J. Immunol.* **136**:4674–4680.
376. Sutton, G. C., H. B. Harding, R. P. Trueheart, and H. P. Clark. 1967. Coxsackie B4 myocarditis in an adult: successful isolation of virus from ventricular myocardium. *Clin. Aviation Aerospace Med.* **38**: 66–69.
377. Sutton, G. C., J. R. Tobin, R. T. Fox, R. J. Freeark, and J. F. Driscoll. 1963. Study of the pericardium and ventricular myocardium: exploratory mediastinotomy and biopsy in unexplained heart disease. *JAMA* **185**:786–788.
378. Swan, H. J. C., and R. W. Gifford. 1974. Current profile of the professional activities of the American cardiologist. *Am. J. Cardiol.* **34**:417–428.
379. Tilles, J. G., S. H. Elson, J. A. Shaka, W. H. Abelman, A. M. Lerner, and M. Finland. 1964. Effects of exercise on coxsackie A9 myocarditis in adult mice. *Proc. Soc. Exp. Biol. Med.* **117**:777–782.
380. Tomassini, J. E., D. Graham, C. M. DeWitt, D. W. Lineberger, J. A. Rodkey, and R. J. Colonno. 1989. cDNA cloning reveals that the major group rhinovirus receptor on HeLa cells is intercellular adhesion molecule 1. *Proc. Natl. Acad. Sci. USA* **86**:4907–4911.
381. Tominaga, M., A. Matsumori, I. Okada, T. Yamada, and C. Kawai. 1991. β-Blocker treatment of dilated cardiomyopathy. Beneficial effect of carteolol in mice. *Circulation* **83**:2121–

382. Tomioka, N., C. Kishimoto, A. Matsumori, and C. Kawai. 1986. Effects of prednisolone on acute viral myocarditis in mice. *J. Am. Coll. Cardiol.* **7:**868–872.
383. Torp, A. 1978. Incidence of congestive cardiomyopathy. *Postgrad. Med. J.* **54:**435–437.
384. Torp, A. 1981. Incidence of congestive cardiomyopathy, p. 18–26. *In* J. F. Goodwin, Å. Hjalmarson, and E. G. J. Olsen (ed.), *Congestive Cardiomyopathy*. A. B. Hässle, Mölndal, Sweden.
385. Tracy, S., N. M. Chapman, and H. L. Liu. 1985. Molecular cloning and partial characterization of the coxsackievirus B3 genome. *Arch. Virol.* **85:**157–163.
386. Tracy, S., N. M. Chapman, B. M. McManus, M. A. Pallansch, M. A. Beck, and J. Carstens. 1990. A molecular and serological evaluation of enteroviral involvement in human myocarditis. *J. Mol. Cell Cardiol.* **22:**403–414.
387. Tracy, S., N. M. Chapman, and Z. Tu. 1992. Coxsackievirus B3 from an infectious cDNA copy of the genome is cardiovirulent in mice. *Arch. Virol.* **122:**399–409.
388. Tracy, S. M., and C. J. Gauntt. 1987. Phenotypic and genotypic differences among naturally occurring coxsackie virus B3 variants. *Eur. Heart J. Suppl. J* **8:**445–448.
389. Van Houten, N., P. E. Bouchard, A. Moraska, and S. A. Huber. 1991. Selection of an attenuated coxsackie virus B3 variant using a monoclonal antibody reactive to myocyte antigen. *J. Virol.* **65:**1286–1290.
390. Van Houten, N., and S. A. Huber. 1991. Genetics of coxsackie B3 (CVB3) myocarditis. *Eur. Heart J. Suppl. D* **12:**108–112.
391. Veille, J. C. 1984. Peripartum cardiomyopathies: a review. *Am. J. Obstet. Gynecol.* **148:**805–818.
392. Veillette, A., M. A. Bookman, E. M. Horak, and J. B. Bolen. 1988. The CD4 and CD8 T-cell surface antigens are associated with the internal membrane tyrosine-protein kinase p56[lck]. *Cell* **55:**301–308.
393. Vella, C., and H. Festenstein. 1992. Coxsackievirus B4 infection of the mouse pancreas: the role of natural killer cells in the control of virus replication and resistance to infection. *J. Gen. Virol.* **73:**1379–1386.
394. Waagstein, F., K. Caidahl, I. Wallentin, C.-H. Bergh, and Å. Hjalmarson. 1989. Long-term β-blockade in dilated cardiomyopathy. Effects of short- and long-term metoprolol treatment followed by withdrawal and readministration of metoprolol. *Circulation* **80:**551–563.
395. Waller, B. F., J. D. Slack, C.D. Orr, J. H. Adlam, and V. M. Bournique. 1991. "Flaming," "smoldering" and "burned out": the fireside saga of myocarditis. *J. Am. Coll. Cardiol.* **18:**1627–1630. (Editorial comment.)
396. Wallukat, G., M. Morwinski, K. Kowal, A. Förster, V. Boewer, and A. Wollenberger. 1991. Autoantibodies against the β-adrenergic receptor in human myocarditis and dilated cardiomyopathy: β-adrenergic agonism without desensitization. *Eur. Heart J. Suppl. D* **12:**178–181.
397. Wee, L., P. Liu, L. Penn, J. W Butany, P. R. McLaughlin, M. J. Sole, and C. C. Liew. 1992. Persistence of viral genome into late stages of murine myocarditis detected by polymerase chain reaction. *Circulation* **86:**1605–1614.
398. Wee, L., T. Martino, M. J. Sole, and P. Liu. 1993. Mechanism of verapamil protection in myocarditis: does it attenuate viral proliferation? *Can. J. Cardiol.* **9**(Suppl. E):130E.
399. Weiss, L. M., X.-F. Liu, K. L. Chang, and M. E. Billingham. 1992. Detection of enteroviral RNA in idiopathic dilated cardiomyopathy and other human cardiac tissues. *J. Clin. Invest.* **90:**156–159.
400. Weiss, L. M., L. A. Movahed, M. E. Billingham, and M. L. Cleary. 1991. Detection of coxsackievirus B3 RNA in myocardial tissues by the polymerase chain reaction. *Am. J. Pathol.* **138:**497–503.
401. Weller, A. H., M. Hall, and S. A. Huber. 1992. Polyclonal immunoglobulin therapy protects against cardiac damage in experimental coxsackievirus-induced myocarditis. *Eur. Heart J.* **13:**115–119.
402. Weller, A. H., K. Simpson, M. Herzum, N. Van Houten, and S. A. Huber. 1989. Coxsackievirus-B3-induced myocarditis: virus receptor antibodies modulate myocarditis. *J. Immunol.* **143:**1843–1850.
403. Welsch, R. M., and M. Vargas-Cortes. 1992. Natural killer cells in viral infection, p. 107–150. *In* C. E. Lewis and J. O. McGee (ed.), *The Natural Killer Cell*. Oxford University Press, New York.
404. Wenner, H. A., T. Y. Lou, and P. S. Kamitsuka. 1960. Experimental infections with coxsackie viruses. I. Studies on virulence and pathogenesis in cynomolgus monkeys. *Arch. Gesamte Virusforsch.* **10:**426–450.
405. Weremeichik, H., A. Moraska, M. Herzum, A. Weller, and S. A. Huber. 1991. Naturally occurring anti-idiotypic antibodies— mechanisms for autoimmunity and immuno-

regulation? *Eur. Heart J. Suppl. D* **12:**154–157.
406. **Werner, G. S., H. R. Figulla, D. L. Munz, K. Klingel, R. Kandolf, D. Emrich, and H. Kreuzer.** 1993. Myocardial indium-111 antimyosin uptake in patients with idiopathic dilated cardiomyopathy: its relation to haemodynamics, histomorphometry, myocardial enteroviral infection, and clinical course. *Eur. Heart J.* **14:**175–184.
407. **Wesslén, L., A. Waldenström, B. Lindblom, S. Høyer, G. Friman, and J. Fohlman.** 1993. Genotypic and serotypic profile in dilated cardiomyopathy. *Scand. J. Infect. Dis. Suppl.* **88:**87–91.
407a. **WHO/ISFC Task Force.** 1980. Report on the definition and classification of cardiomyopathies. *Br. Heart J.* **44:**672–673.
408. **Wiegand, V., S. Tracy, N. Chapman, and C. Wucherpfennig.** 1990. Enteroviral infection in end stage dilated cardiomyopathy. *Klin. Wochenschr.* **68:**914–920.
409. **Williams, D. G., and E. G. J. Olsen.** 1985. Prevalence of overt dilated cardiomyopathy in two regions of England. *Br. Heart J.* **54:**153–155.
410. **Wilson, F. M., A. Hashimi, and A. M. Lerner.** 1965. Multiplication of Boston strains of coxsackievirus A9 in the adult mouse heart. *J. Bacteriol.* **90:**546–548.
411. **Wilson, F. M., Q. R. Miranda, J. L. Chason, and A. M. Lerner.** 1969. Residual pathologic changes following murine coxsackie A and B myocarditis. *Am. J. Pathol.* **55:**253–265.
412. **Wolff, P. G., U. Kühl, and H.-P. Schultheiss.** 1989. Laminin distribution and autoantibodies to laminin in dilated cardiomyopathy and myocarditis. *Am. Heart J.* **117:**1303–1309.
413. **Wolfgram, L. J., K. W. Beisel, A. Herskowitz, and N. R. Rose.** 1986. Variations in the susceptibility to coxsackievirus B3–induced myocarditis among different strains of mice. *J. Immunol.* **136:**1846–1852.
414. **Wolfgram, L. J., K. W. Beisel, and N. R. Rose.** 1985. Heart-specific autoantibodies following murine coxsackievirus B3 myocarditis. *J. Exp. Med.* **161:**1112–1121.
415. **Wong, C. Y., J. J. Woodruff, and J. F. Woodruff.** 1977. Generation of cytotoxic T lymphocytes during coxsackievirus B-3 infection. I. Model and viral specificity. *J. Immunol.* **118:**1159–1164.
416. **Wong, C. Y., J. J. Woodruff, and J. F. Woodruff.** 1977. Generation of cytotoxic T lymphocytes during coxsackievirus B-3 infection. II. Characterization of effector cells and demonstration of cytotoxicity against viral-infected myofibers. *J. Immunol.* **118:**1165–1169.
417. **Wong, C. Y., J. J. Woodruff, and J. F. Woodruff.** 1977. Generation of cytotoxic T lymphocytes during coxsackievirus B-3 infection. III. Role of sex. *J. Immunol.* **119:**591–597.
418. **Woodruff, J. F.** 1970. The influence of quantitated post-weaning undernutrition on coxsackievirus B3 infection of adult mice. II. Alteration of host defense mechanisms. *J. Infect. Dis.* **121:**164–181.
419. **Woodruff, J. F.** 1979. Lack of correlation between neutralizing antibody production and suppression of coxsackievirus B-3 replication in target organs: evidence for involvement of mononuclear inflammatory cells in host defense. *J. Immunol.* **123:**31–36.
420. **Woodruff, J. F.** 1980. Viral myocarditis. A review. *Am. J. Pathol.* **101:**425–484.
421. **Woodruff, J. F., and E. D. Kilbourne.** 1970. The influence of quantitated post-weaning undernutrition on coxsackievirus B3 infection of adult mice. I. Viral persistence and increased severity of lesions. *J. Infect. Dis.* **121:**137–163.
422. **Woodruff, J. F., and J. J. Woodruff.** 1971. Modification of severe coxsackievirus B3 infection in marasmic mice by transfer of immune lymphoid cells. *Proc. Natl. Acad. Sci. USA* **68:**2108–2111.
423. **Woodruff, J. F., and J. J. Woodruff.** 1974. Involvement of T lymphocytes in the pathogenesis of coxsackie virus B3 heart disease. *J. Immunol.* **113:**1726–1734.
424. **Xie, Q.-W., H. J. Cho, J. Calaycay, R. A. Mumford, K. M. Swiderek, T. D. Lee, A. Ding, T. Troso, and C. Nathan.** 1992. Cloning and characterization of inducible nitric oxide synthase from mouse macrophages. *Science* **256:**225–228.
425. **Yamada, T., M. Fukunami, M. Ohmori, K. Iwakura, K. Kumagai, N. Kondoh, E. Tsujimura, Y. Age, T. Nagareda, K. Kotoh, and N. Hoki.** 1993. New approach to the estimation of the extent of myocardial fibrosis in patients with dilated cardiomyopathy: use of signal-averaged electrocardiography. *Am. Heart J.* **126:**626–631.
426. **Yasuda, T., I. F. Palacios, W. Dec, J. T. Fallon, H. K. Gold, R. C. Leinbach, H. W. Strauss, B. A. Khaw, and E. Haber.** 1987. Indium 111-monoclonal antimyosin antibody imaging in the diagnosis of acute myocarditis. *Circulation* **76:**306–311.
427. **Yiyun, C., S. Yagi, and D. Schnurr.** 1989. Persistent infections by coxsackie virus B3, p. 105–112. *In* F. Auti (ed.), *Pathogenesis and Con-*

trol of Viral Infections. Sereno Symposia Publications, vol. 59, Raven Press, New York.

427a. **Yokoyama, T., L. Vaca, R. D. Rossen, W. Durante, P. Hazarika, and D. L. Mann.** 1993. Cellular basis for the negative inotropic effects of tumor necrosis factor-α in the adult mammalian heart. *J. Clin. Invest.* **92:**2303–2312.

428. **Yoneda, S., K. Senda, and K. Hayashi.** 1979. Experimental study of virus myocarditis in culture. *Jpn. Circ. J.* **43:**1048–1054.

429. **Zinkernagel, R. M., and R. M. Welsh.** 1976. H-2 compatibility requirement for virus-specific T-cell mediated effector functions in vivo. I. Specificity of T cells conferring antiviral protection against lymphocytic choriomeningitis virus is associated with H-2K and H-2D. *J. Immunol.* **117:**1495–1502.

430. **Zoll, G. J., W. J. G. Melchers, H. Kopecka, G. Jambroes, H. J. A. van der Poel, and J. M. D. Galama.** 1992. General primer-mediated polymerase chain reaction for detection of enteroviruses: application for diagnostic routine and persistent infections. *J. Clin. Microbiol.* **30:**160–165.

THE POSSIBLE ROLE OF ENTEROVIRUSES IN DIABETES MELLITUS

Marian Rewers and Mark Atkinson

15

INTRODUCTION

Epidemiology of IDDM

Insulin-dependent diabetes mellitus (IDDM) is the most common severe chronic childhood illness, affecting an estimated 123,000 children in the United States (121). Over 11,000 new cases are diagnosed annually. The disease is the leading cause of renal failure, blindness, and amputation and a major cause of cardiovascular disease and premature death in the industrialized countries (230). In the United States, medical care expenditures for IDDM total over $5 billion/year (193).

The occurrence of IDDM peaks at the ages of 2, 4 to 6, and 10 to 14 years, perhaps because of physiologic increases in sex hormone levels and insulin resistance or because of alterations in the pattern of infections. Incidence decreases in the third decade of life (102), only to increase again in the fifth to seventh decades of life (37, 131). There is no hard evidence, however, that childhood and adult insulin-dependent cases are etiologically similar.

The incidence of IDDM varies more than 30-fold worldwide, with the highest rates in Scandinavia and the lowest in Japan and Korea (177). Geographic variation in risk may reflect either different population pools of susceptibility genes or different prevalences of causative environmental factors or a combination of the two. Similar to the situation with multiple sclerosis (124), the risk of IDDM increases with latitude in the three major racial groups in the United States (46), suggesting that environmental rather than genetic factors underlie the north-to-south gradient in incidence.

The marked seasonal variation in the incidence of IDDM has been interpreted as evidence of infectious etiology (70). Incidence declines during the warm summer months in both the Northern and Southern hemispheres (51). This pattern occurs in children diagnosed after the age of 4 years (114) and differs by HLA-DR type (125, 228). Since the process leading to IDDM usually starts years before the diagnosis, the seasonality probably reflects promoting rather than initiating factors.

Many population-based registries have shown that the incidence of IDDM increases over time (47, 177), while other studies have shown no such trend (114). Most of these studies have observed periodic outbreaks superimposed on a steady secular increase. In-

---

Marian Rewers, Department of Preventive Medicine and Biometrics, School of Medicine, University of Colorado, Box C-245, 4200 East 9th Avenue, Denver, Colorado 80262.   *Mark Atkinson,* Department of Pathology, 100275 JHMHC, University of Florida, Gainesville, Florida 32610.

creasing rates of IDDM in some countries and epidemics of IDDM (178, 222) have been attributed to several candidate viruses. Herpesviruses (141, 161, 185), mumps virus (92, 175), rubella virus (76, 107), and retroviruses (197) have been implicated. However, picornaviruses have been most strongly linked to IDDM in humans and in animal models.

β-Cell Autoimmunity

In most cases, IDDM results from a chronic autoimmune destruction of the pancreatic β-cells that is probably initiated by exposure of a genetically susceptible host to an environmental agent. Several years prior to diagnosis of diabetes, islet cell antibodies (ICA) to various β-cell autoantigens can be detected in over 90% of patients (8, 166). However, these antibodies are not regarded as a direct cause of β-cell damage. β cells are selectively destroyed by cytotoxic T lymphocytes (CTLs) (188), with CD4 cells also playing an important role (87). HLA class I and II molecules as well as intercellular adhesion molecule-1 (ICAM-1) are expressed within the islets (31, 58).

Like most infectious and chronic diseases, clinical IDDM is just the tip of the iceberg of a broad spectrum of pathology. As much as 20 to 40% of the general population may be genetically susceptible; however, only a few people develop β-cell autoimmunity, and even fewer progress to diabetes. Evidence has accumulated that β-cell autoimmunity may remit without causing diabetes (101, 194, 204). Studies of schoolchildren with no family history of IDDM in the United States (126), Sweden (116), and Finland (106) have reported ICA remission rates between 10 and 78%. The prevalence of β-cell autoimmunity in these children was as high as 0.7 to 4.1%; however, only a minority of children with β-cell autoimmunity (one in three to eight) develop IDDM by the age of 15 years. In the remaining children, the penetrance, number of susceptibility genes, or environmental exposure is presumed to be insufficient.

It is likely that β-cell autoimmunity begins in early childhood in the majority of cases (167) and that the diabetes incubation period is as long as 9 to 13 years (21, 101). Although prevalence decreases with age (167, 181), 14 to 33% of adult-onset diabetics are ICA positive (82, 212). β-Cell autoimmunity may remit and reappear in the course of viral infections, and the cumulative insult, including increases in insulin resistance with obesity and physical inactivity, may eventually cause diabetes at a later age.

The amount of β-cell destruction necessary for IDDM manifestation appears to decrease with age, from an average of 80% in children younger than 7 years to 60% in those 7 to 14 years old, to 40% in those older than 14 years (60). Not all β cells are simultaneously destroyed: loss of β cells is complete within 1 to 2 years after diagnosis in the youngest patients but is much slower and often only partial in older patients (168). Histologic evidence of islet regeneration is modest (73).

Genetics of IDDM

In the general population, 1 in 400 children develops IDDM by the age of 15 years (177). The risk is increased to about 1 in 40 in offspring of IDDM fathers and to 1 in 66 in offspring of IDDM mothers (49a). The risk to siblings ranges from 1 in 12 to 1 in 35 (2, 217, 221, 224) and increases to 1 in 4 in HLA-identical siblings. A family history of IDDM may serve as a surrogate for susceptibility genes and probably for some of the shared environmental exposure(s). Familial cases represent less than 10% of IDDM cases and do not appear to be etiologically different from sporadic cases (154).

The primary loci of genetic susceptibility to IDDM have been mapped to the HLA-DR and HLA-DQ regions (17, 207), and new candidate genes outside the HLA region are being identified (16, 71, 159, 169). While 50% of non-Hispanic whites in the United States have the HLA-DR3 or HLA-DR4 allele, at least one of these alleles is present in 95% of patients with IDDM. These HLA alleles may increase the immune response to a β-cell autoantigen through efficient presentation of the antigen to the T cells. Alternatively, they may induce susceptibility to IDDM by presenting antigenic peptides that do not promote normal immunologic tolerance to self β-cell antigens. In contrast to the strong association with clinical diabetes, no particular HLA type seems to be associated with β-cell autoimmunity (20). However, persons who remain persistently and strongly ICA positive have HLA genotypes similar to those of IDDM patients (34, 120). In an animal model, specific major histocompatibility complex (MHC) class II alleles appear to control progression from subclinical to overt diabetes, rather than initiation of autoimmunity (128a), which is consistent with the human data. Thus, while β-cell autoimmunity may be triggered in anyone, the HLA genes may be crucial for progression from autoimmunity to IDDM.

PROPOSED PATHOPHYSIOLOGICAL MECHANISMS

Picornaviruses have long been examined for their role as the primary etiologic agent in the pathogenesis of IDDM. For earlier reviews, see references 12, 38, 67, 143, 176, 201, and 235. We review animal and in vitro models first and then relevant human studies. We propose to classify the existing evidence for picornaviral involvement in IDDM into the following six scenarios.

1. Acute lytic infection of pancreatic β cells leads to acute diabetes without autoimmunity.
2. Acute or chronic enteroviral infection of peri-insular tissue leads to β-cell destruction from abundance of free radicals, the "innocent bystander" theory.
3. An acute infection triggers the β-cell autoimmunity process, which persists even though the triggering agent is removed (the 'hit-and-run' theory).
4. A persistent infection triggers and sustains β-cell autoimmunity until destruction outweighs regeneration and overt diabetes ensues.
5. A persistent infection impairs insulin secretion from β cells without cell lysis or autoimmunity.
6. An infection protects from IDDM.

Acute Cytolytic Infection

Encephalomyocarditis virus (EMCV), a murine picornavirus, produces acute lytic infection of pancreatic β cells and diabetes whose severity correlates with the degree of β-cell lysis (39, 88). In this model, development of diabetes depends on the genetic makeup of both the host and the virus. The host genetic susceptibility is inherited as an autosomal recessive trait not associated with the MHC (23) but related instead to the virus attachment process. Susceptible SJL/J mice naturally express the receptor for EMCV on their β cells (but not on kidney cells), while resistant C57BL/6J mice do not (104). However, in cell culture, both β cells and kidney cells from the resistant animals can express the receptors and become susceptible to EMCV infection. In vivo, immunosuppression renders genetically resistant C3H/HeJ mice susceptible to EMCV-induced diabetes (80). However, it is not known whether this process occurs through induction of EMCV receptor expression.

The genetic variability of EMCV strains appears to define their tropism to β cells and their diabetogenicity. In genetically susceptible mice, the EMCV-D variant can infect and destroy pancreatic β cells, while the EMCV-B variant is generally nondiabetogenic (239). Analysis of additional EMCV variants has pinpointed their diabetogenicity to a single amino acid (Ala[GCC]-776) on the EMCV polyprotein that corresponds to amino acid 152 of VP1 (9). The diabetogenic protein variant probably allows the virus to attach to the pancreatic β cell (105, 183). In cell cultures, this single-point mutation has been observed to occur only to change a diabetogenic to a nondiabetogenic variant, i.e., from G to A (Ala to Thr).

EMCV rapidly destroys large numbers of β cells with little inflammatory response and T-cell involvement (238), although some controversy on this point remains (38). There is no indication that the EMCV triggers humoral β-cell autoimmunity, as evidenced by lack of ICA. This raises questions about the relevance of this animal model to human IDDM, which is associated in 70 to 90% of cases with the presence of ICA. A case report (158) demonstrated that human IDDM can develop rapidly without preceding autoimmunity. Such cases could account for 10 to 30% of human IDDM cases. Alternatively, in persons with ongoing β-cell autoimmunity induced by another mechanism, acute cytolytic infection could provide the final insult leading to overt diabetes (98). Chemical compounds, e.g., streptozotocin, can alone induce β-cell autoimmunity (53). The "multiple hits" concept that diabetes may result from repeated asymptomatic β-cell injury is based on the observation that a subdiabetogenic exposure to streptozotocin renders genetically resistant mice susceptible to diabetes induced by normally nondiabetogenic strains of coxsackie B virus (CVB) (210, 227). Streptozotocin is perhaps the best-characterized laboratory β-cell toxin, but many others, including nitrates and nitrosamines, occur naturally (176).

If an enterovirus causes IDDM in humans the same way that EMCV-D causes diabetes in mice, development of a live attenuated vaccine or a recombinant subunit vaccine could become a preventive strategy. Notkins and Yoon (144) were able to prevent EMCV-D-induced diabetes in SJL/J mice by immunization with the nondiabetogenic EMCV-B variant. This interference is independent of EMCV-B ability to induce interferon (77).

The simplicity of the model described above is illusory. Even within an inbred strain of mice, factors associated with insulin resistance appear to determine the severity of EMCV-induced diabetes, from normal or transiently impaired glucose tolerance through transient diabetes to fatal acute-onset diabetes (40). The extent of β-cell loss and the incidence of diabetes are higher at a younger age (41), in male animals (23), and at higher levels of androgens (138) and of corticosteroids and obesity (44). This pattern resembles the full spectrum of human diabetes, including its non-insulin-dependent form.

In addition, the paradigm that EMCV causes diabetes exclusively through an acute lytic infection has been recently questioned by the demonstration that EMCV-D can actually persist in a murine pancreas (evidenced by the presence of EMCV-D protein) long after the acute infection is resolved (208). In that study, both acinar and islet cells were initially infected; however, the persistent low-grade infection and insulitis with impairment of insulin production were limited to few islets. This observation is consistent with the concept of carrier culture persistence of CVB in the pancreas that is described later in this chapter.

Various strains of CVB cause glucose intolerance in laboratory animals (209, 237). Significant progress has been made in defining the genetic basis for β-cell tropism and the diabetogenicity of these CVB strains by using approaches similar to those that led to the identification of the EMCV-D (Ala[GCC]-776) variant (201). Candidate mutations have been identified in the coding sequences for VP1, VP4, P3-A, and P3-D CVB proteins, as well as in the 5' noncoding region (important for efficient translation and replication of the picornaviral genome). The mechanism of genetic susceptibility of mice to diabetogenic CVB appears to be similar to that for EMCV, and a candidate gene has been mapped to chromosome 4 (123). Thus, CVB-induced diabetes is likely to share some of the characteristics of the EMCV-induced diabetes model.

The Innocent Bystander Theory

CVB easily infects pancreatic acinar cells, but only a few strains infect β cells, usually causing only transient hyperglycemia (240). The innocent bystander theory hypothesizes that because of their low superoxide dismutase activity, β cells are particularly susceptible to a local excess of oxygen free radicals released, for instance, in the course of an infection in the surrounding tissue. This theory proposes that a viral infection occurs primarily in the periductal, acinar, or endothelial cells, leading to local release of interleukin-1α (IL-1α) and IL-1β. The selective loss of β cells would be due to the action of IL-1β on the IL-1 receptors of β cells, resulting in a rapid increase in cytosolic Na$^+$, free oxygen, and nitric oxide radicals, as well as impaired mitochondrial glucose oxidation, protease activation, and insulin release followed by inhibition of insulin secretion (3). Consequently, administration of free-radical scavengers, e.g., nicotinamide and N-acetylocysteine, has been proposed as a preventive measure. Ramshingh and collaborators (174) have established a mouse model of CVB4-induced pancreatitis with little involvement of endocrine cells. Mice infected with a virulent strain of CVB4 develop fatal acinar pancreatitis with hypoglycemia and hyperamylasemia but normal insulin concentrations. The severity of pancreatitis appears to be related to the MHC class II background of the host and to a point mutation (Thr-129) in the VP1 capsid protein of the virus. This model demonstrates tropism of some CVB strains to nonendocrine pancreatic tissue; however, the possible relationship of such an infection to β-cell autoimmunity and diabetes has not been tested. Even if the innocent bystander theory is correct, nonspecific inflammation and genetic susceptibility to IDDM are not sufficient to induce β-cell autoimmunity. Persons with HLA-DR3 and/or HLA-DR4 and chronic pancreatitis involving both exocrine and endocrine tissue do not develop β-cell autoantibodies, nor do they lose β-cell function faster than patients without these HLA risk markers (115).

An alternative innocent bystander theory (38) proposes that local inflammation in the peri-insular tissue may induce molecules on the surface of β cells that enteroviruses could use as cellular receptors. This, in turn, would render β cells more susceptible to enteroviral infection or superinfection. Some picornaviruses use as their cell surface receptor ICAM-1 (see chapter 3), which belongs to the immunoglobulin supergene family and, in response to cytokines, is expressed in pancreatic islets of IDDM subjects. ICAM-1 plays a role in the binding and activation of leukocytes, which may further promote its expression. Although ICAM-1 is used by picornaviruses not likely involved in IDDM, i.e., rhinoviruses (81, 196), and a similar member of the immunoglobulin superfamily is used by polioviruses (132), which are also unlikely IDDM triggers, it has been speculated that receptors for diabetogenic enteroviruses may also be hyperexpressed in β-cell autoimmunity. At least two cellular receptors for CVB, of about 50 and 60 kDa, have been identified (see chapter 3), but little is known concerning their physiologic role or a potential involvement in IDDM (241).

Acute Infection Triggering Autoimmunity

The actual mechanisms of self-tolerance and autoimmunity are still unclear despite intensive research. It has been proposed that the autoimmune process can be initiated by release of intracellular antigens against which self-tolerance is inadequate, expression of viral or inappropriate host antigens on the surfaces of infected cells, molecular mimicry, production of anti-idiotypic antibodies reacting with viral cell receptors, cytokine-induced overexpression of HLA class II molecules, or polyclonal activation of B and/or T lymphocytes as well as by virus-induced functional changes in antigen-presenting cells, effector or regulatory lymphocytes (176, 182, 235). The molecular mimicry model presented below provides the strongest evidence to date for an acute enteroviral infection initiating β-cell autoimmunity.

It has been postulated that IDDM may result from a misdirected immunologic attack on pancreatic β cells by lymphocytes responding to an acute (hit-and-run model) or chronic viral infection. In this process, termed molecular mimicry, sequence homologies between host and microbial antigens result in the generation of an antihost immune response (149). Evidence for molecular mimicry as a potential pathogenic mechanism underlying IDDM was enhanced by the finding of a sequence homology between human glutamate decarboxylase (GAD) and the CVB P2-C protein (109). In addition, the region of GAD showing homology with P2-C appears to contain a determinant(s) of anti-GAD cellular immunity in humans with IDDM (85) as well as an early target of cellular immunity in nonobese diabetic mice (108). Independently, Jones et al. (103) reported in IDDM patients an antibody cross-reactivity between a CVB nucleopeptide and GAD 65, which apparently share an identical sequence of 6 amino acids.

GAD catalyzes the formation of the inhibitory neurotransmitter γ-aminobutyric acid (GABA) from glutamine. The two forms of GAD are encoded by different genes located on human chromosomes 2 for GAD 65 and 10 for GAD 67 (27). In the rat, both forms of GAD have been identified within the GABA-nergic neurons of the brain and the pancreatic islet cells (54), whereas human islets express only GAD 65 (111, 165). Within the islet, GAD is predominantly observed in β cells and may have a role in the inhibition of somatostatin and glucagon secretion, as well as in regulation of proinsulin synthesis and insulin secretion (72).

Multiple studies utilizing crude 64-kDa extract (10, 11) and recombinant GADs (8, 166) have shown GAD 65 and GAD 67 autoantibodies in persons with or at risk for IDDM. The antibody response is primarily composed of anti-GAD 65 activity, and multiple epitopes are present within GAD (109). In the nonobese diabetic mouse, T-lymphocyte response to GAD is a key event in the induction and propagation of β-cell autoimmunity (108, 206). The cellular immune response in these animals appears to be confined initially to a limited region of GAD, but then, T-lymphocyte antigenicity spreads intramolecularly to additional GAD epitopes as well as to other autoantigens associated with IDDM (108).

To identify the T-lymphocyte-reactive determinants of GAD, an overlapping set of synthetic peptides was used to stimulate lymphocytes from individuals with anti-GAD antibodies (7). Proliferative responses were determined by using a standard [^{3}H]thymidine assay (stimulation index = cpm with antigen/cpm in antigen absence). Newly diagnosed IDDM subjects and those at high risk of IDDM showed elevated frequencies of lymphocyte responsiveness to GAD peptides, including amino acids 247 to 266 (peptide 17) and 260 to 279 (peptide 18). This region, i.e., amino acids 250 to 273, has significant sequence similarity to the P2-C protein of CVB (Fig. 1). The lymphocyte response to GAD peptide 17 and/or 18 was present in 47% (7 of 15) of persons at increased risk for IDDM, 25% (4 of 16) of newly diagnosed patients, and none of 13 healthy control subjects. The mean stimulation index ± standard error of the mean for GAD 247-266, GAD 260-279 and tetanus toxoid were 3.1 ± 1.3, 1.6 ± 0.3, and 49 ± 16 in persons at increased IDDM risk; 1.5 ± 0.5, 1.5 ± 0.3, and 31 ± 12 in newly diagnosed patients; and 1.0 ± 0.1, 0.9 ± 0.1, and 35 ± 9.4 in healthy controls. No correlation between reactivity to GAD peptides and subject age or sex was observed.

Anticoxsackievirus antibodies were analyzed in all subjects for indications of previous viral exposure. Antibody responses to at least one coxsackievirus strain were present in all persons tested (n = 9) whose lymphocytes were reactive to GAD peptides with coxsackievirus homology, with two-thirds (six of nine) positive for antibodies to CVB4. Antibodies against any coxsackievirus variant were not significantly more frequent in newly diagnosed patients (69%) or subjects at high risk for IDDM (81%) than in healthy controls (57%).

In a case-control study of CVB immunoglobulin M (IgM) in newly diagnosed patients and age- and sex-matched controls (43), 37 of 58 cases (64%) and 8 of 26 controls (31%) with CVB titers of ≥1:8 also had antibodies to GAD 65, compared with 55 of 104 cases (53%) and 5 of 66 controls (8%) with a CVB IgM titer of <1:8 (83). Thus, immunity to CVB and GAD 65 appeared to cluster even in persons without diabetes.

Critical information to support the mimicry hypothesis would involve the demonstra-

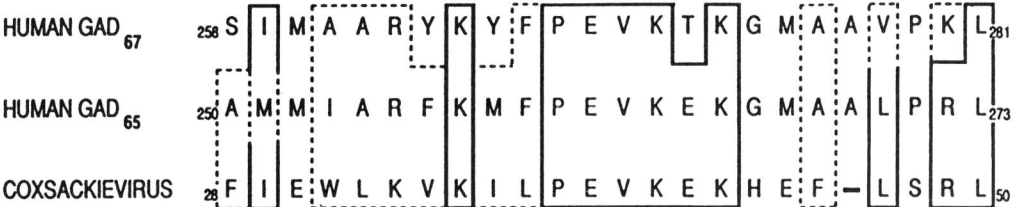

FIGURE 1 Molecular homology between GAD and coxsackievirus P2-C. Solid lines enclose identical amino acid residues. Dashed lines enclose residues with similar charges, polarities, or hydrophobicities. Reproduced from the *Journal of Clinical Investigation* (109), by copyright permission of the American Society for Clinical Investigation.

tion that peptides from the coxsackievirus sequence similarity region stimulate the cellular immune responses of IDDM patients or of those at increased risk for the disease. Toward this end, we measured the lymphocyte response to a peptide containing coxsackievirus P2-C amino acids 32 to 47 in three individuals who were previously identified as reactive to the GAD peptide with coxsackievirus homology. Strikingly, all three individuals were responsive to this coxsackievirus peptide in addition to showing continued reactivity to GAD peptide (stimulation indexes of 10.0 and 10.1, 2.9 and 7.0, and 4.3 and 3.6 for coxsackievirus and GAD peptide responses, respectively) (6a). Furthermore, we have observed that immunization of mice with coxsackievirus P2-C protein or the coxsackievirus peptide containing the region of sequence similarity with GAD 65 can induce T-cell immune responses that cross-react with GAD 65 or GAD 65 peptides corresponding to the region of sequence similarity (204a).

It must be emphasized that the data presented above, although indicative of a strong cross-reactivity between homologous epitopes on GAD and P2-C, are not uniformly accepted (180) and do not prove causality. P2-C is a highly conserved nonstructural protein that is likely to participate in RNA replication (see chapter 4) and, perhaps, in determination of virion structure (reviewed by Stanway [195]). It is unclear how cross-reactivity between P2-C and GAD, both primarily intracellular proteins, could lead to autoimmunity. The observed higher cross-reactivity in subjects at risk for IDDM than in newly diagnosed diabetics may be interpreted as evidence that molecular mimicry is more important in the early stages of β-cell autoimmunity than at the time of clinical presentation. However, it can also be interpreted as evidence for a protective effect of cross-reactivity. This dilemma can be resolved only through a prospective follow-up of high-risk subjects with and without GAD(p17/p18)-coxsackievirus P2-C cross-reactivity. Even better, subjects with no evidence of β-cell autoimmunity could be monitored for development of GAD autoimmunity as well as for evidence of concurrent infection with coxsackievirus or any enterovirus with homologous P2-C.

Persistent Infection as the Cause of β-Cell Autoimmunity

Because it is not known how autoimmunity could persist if the triggering agent is removed, it has been speculated that persistent viral infection is needed to sustain chronic autoimmunity. Well-established models of persistent viral infection leading to IDDM include reovirus type 1-induced diabetes (155) and lymphocytic choriomeningitis virus (LCMV)-induced diabetes in mice (153) as well as congenital rubella syndrome (CRS) in humans.

LCMV INFECTION

In the LCMV model, transgenic mice expressing a viral protein on β cells do not develop autoimmunity unless the host is exposed to the same virus later in life (152), even if CTLs specific to this viral antigen are present (147).

This may indicate that two episodes of viral infection are needed to initiate β-cell autoimmunity: the first results in persistent expression of a viral antigen in β cells, and the second, with an antigenically similar agent, initiates autoimmunity. Induction of diabetes in this model is influenced by the strain of LCMV, tumor necrosis factor alpha expression, MHC genotype, level of MHC class I expression, and induction of a threshold number of self-reactive CTLs (146).

CRS

After a 5- to 20-year-long incubation period, 12 to 40% of patients with CRS develop IDDM (56, 76, 133). In some cases of CRS (without IDDM), autopsy has demonstrated persistent infection of the pancreas with rubella virus (135). Autoantibodies to β-cell antigens are common, and molecular mimicry between an antigenic determinant on a rubella virus protein and a 52-kDa β-cell autoantigen has been found (107). CRS is responsible for only a minute proportion of IDDM cases. Of more importance may be the observation that persistent rubella virus infection and β-cell autoimmunity follow prenatal exposure only; postnatal rubella virus infection either with the wild strain (13, 19, 189) or after measles-mumps-rubella vaccination (18) is not associated with IDDM.

PERSISTENT ENTEROVIRAL INFECTION

Enteroviruses are generally not believed to establish persistent infection. However, they have been shown to persist in hypo- or agammaglobulinemic patients (130, 232, 233) (see chapter 13) and in subjects with postpolio syndrome (192) (see chapter 16) as well as in cultured cell lines (32, 136). CVB RNA has been detected by in situ hybridization in mouse (218) and human (5) pancreata in the absence of infective virus. Another picornavirus (foot-and-mouth disease virus) can cause persistent infection of cattle (29) with immature virions with deletions up to 3 kb (45). The murine enterovirus Theiler's virus causes persistent infection of the central nervous system in mice and demyelinating lesions similar to those seen in multiple sclerosis (62). Finally, persistent picornavirus infections have been associated with other chronic autoimmune diseases in humans such as myocarditis (see chapter 14), myositis (see chapter 16), and hepatitis (219).

Although convincing evidence for persistent enteroviral infection of human β cells is missing, it is plausible that persistent infection with a defective noncytopathic enterovirus may cause diabetes. Gerling et al. (75) studied acute and long-term effects of infection of genetically susceptible SJL/J and CD-1 mice with the E2 strain of CVB4. The animals showed elevated insulin release and high residual islet insulin content as well as high serum insulin and subnormal blood glucose levels 72 h postinfection (p.i.). These changes suggest that insulin synthesis and release of insulin were initially increased; however, they decreased to subnormal levels, and hyperglycemia ensued by 6 weeks p.i. and persisted until at least 8 weeks p.i. No infectious virus could be identified at 6 to 8 weeks p.i., but viral RNA could be detected, and the total protein synthesis was decreased by about 60%, suggesting viral persistence as the reason for impaired islet function. On the other hand, at 3 days p.i., infected islets contained two to three times more GAD 65 than control islets did, although normally detectable pancreatic GAD 67 was absent (75, 94). The infected mice subsequently developed 64-kDa (GAD 65) autoantibodies before becoming hyperglycemic late in infection (74). Insulitis and acinar necrosis following the infection were characterized by infiltration with mostly CD4$^+$ cells and major changes in the thymic, splenic, and peripheral lymphocyte repertoires (35). Thus, in this in vivo animal model, CVB was able to establish persistent infection of β cells associated with anti-GAD autoimmunity and impaired insulin secretion.

PATHOMECHANISM OF VIRAL PERSISTENCE

EMCV, CVB, and echovirus 4, classically associated with acute lytic infection, appear to have the potential to persist in β cells or peri-insular tissue, causing autoimmunity and impairment of insulin secretion without massive β-cell lysis. Both host factors (e.g., young age) and viral factors (e.g., ability to suppress expression of MHC class I antigens by infected cells or to suppress production of specific CTLs) determine viral persistence. Within an infected individual, selective pressure may lead to genotypic changes in the virus that favor persistent infection. This has been demonstrated for LCMV, which has a point mutation in the envelope glycoprotein (181), and for hepatitis A virus (118).

RNA viruses can persist through a steady-state or carrier culture mechanism. The latter mechanism, by which only a part of the susceptible cells is infected, is more likely to occur during picornaviral infections. β cells may be infected directly by diabetogenic variants of picornaviruses that develop in the community (86). However, a more likely site of initial infection is peri-insular tissue, where variants without β-cell tropism may give rise to β-cell-tropic mutants or may indirectly injure β cells through release of cytokines and free radicals.

PERINATAL TRANSMISSION
Much of what is known concerning tropism of enteroviruses to the human pancreas has been learned from autopsy studies of newborns and infants who died of fulminant enteroviral infection. Enteroviral infection of the human neonate is unusual but often fatal (see chapter 10). There are no reliable data to link in utero or early postnatal enteroviral infection to IDDM. Having said that, we add that this particular period in ontogenesis appears to be an ideal susceptibility window for acquiring persistent viral infection causing autoimmunity. CRS, described above, provides an excellent example.

Enteroviruses can cross the placenta, and if they do, the clinical outcome is usually abortion, stillbirth, or severe neonatal infection (134) (see chapter 10). It is not known, for animals or humans, whether in utero infection can lead to a persistent enteroviral infection associated with autoimmunity. On the basis of what is known concerning autoimmunity in mice postnatally infected with CVB4, one would expect GAD autoantibodies to be present very early p.i. (74), i.e., at birth. In the Diabetes Autoimmunity Study in the Young, 2 of 60 cord blood samples of children from the general Colorado population were positive for GAD (142a). The origin and meaning of these GAD autoantibodies are not known, but they may suggest in utero exposure to an enterovirus.

Two Scandinavian nested case-control studies have suggested that mothers whose children later became diabetic were two to four times more likely to have had an enteroviral infection during pregnancy than mothers of control children (42a, 95a). Clearly, this period of life deserves more attention in terms of testing the hypothesis that persistent enteroviral infection leads to β-cell autoimmunity.

Persistent Impairment of Insulin Secretion without β-Cell Lysis or Autoimmunity
A number of animal and in vitro studies have demonstrated that LCMV (153), EMCV (39, 91, 164, 223), CVB (170, 199, 200, 202, 209, 237), and echovirus 4 (203) can impair insulin synthesis and release of insulin from pancreatic islets without apparent cell lysis, autoreactive lymphocytes, or ICA. The exact course of events and the underlying mechanisms of the impairment of islet functions are controversial, and the postulated lack of autoimmunity may be spurious, owing to the imperfect techniques that have been used to detect it. While Gerling and colleagues (75) reported an initial increase in insulin synthesis and release followed by hypoinsulinemia, hyperglycemia, and GAD autoimmunity 6 to 8 weeks later, others (201, 202) suggested a selective decrease in insulin synthesis 2 to 48 h after infection. Szopa et al. (199) also reported increased insulin leakage from islets at the nonstimulatory glucose concentrations associated with fasting hyperinsulinemia and decreased glucose-stimulated insulin synthesis

late (6 months) p.i. These metabolic characteristics in the absence of autoimmunity are traditionally associated with human non-insulin-dependent diabetes rather than with IDDM. One study of humans found increased random insulin levels in the sera of 17 persons shortly after infection with echovirus 4 but normal levels at 18 months p.i. (50). One of the subjects was ICA positive at baseline and follow-up.

Changes in insulin synthesis and release following enteroviral pancreatitis appear to be well documented. However, such changes do not necessarily prove persistent β-cell infection, since they can be induced by cytokines released from peri-insular cells in response to acinar cell infection or they can be artifacts of islet preparation. Although no massive β-cell lysis was observed in these studies, a low-grade cytolysis cannot be excluded. Finally, in vivo studies with quantitative measurements of various β-cell antibodies and autoreactive T cells are needed before we exclude the presence of β-cell autoimmunity. Unless these conditions are met, the very existence of such a progressive, nonlytic, nonautoimmune β-cell dysfunction following enteroviral infection remains questionable.

Protective Effect of Viral Infection

Viral infection may protect the host from developing autoimmunity. Persistent infection with exogenous viruses prevents IDDM in mice (150, 151, 231) and rats (122). However, none of the picornaviruses has been associated with such a protective effect, and no evidence for a protective effect of viral infection in humans is available. Immunization with live measles virus appears to decrease the risk of IDDM (18), but the effect of current mass immunization programs on potentially diabetogenic viruses, e.g., mumps or rubella virus, is virtually unknown, because ICA have never been systematically measured following vaccination.

Seroepidemiologic data have usually been interpreted in favor of a positive association between CVB and IDDM. However, several case-control studies have reported a negative (protective) association (4, 157, 163). This may indicate that newly diagnosed IDDM patients have suppressed the production of antiviral immunoglobulins or have not been exposed to the virus or closely related viruses in the past or that infection with some of the enteroviruses may confer protection, as in the animal model, where EMCV-B can prevent EMCV-D-induced diabetes.

Summary

In summary, several distinct pathomechanisms related to picornaviral infections appear to have plausible roles in the etiology of IDDM in animal models. At present, it is not known, whether a single pathogenic mechanism is responsible for diabetes induced by various picornaviruses or whether diabetes can result from a spectrum of picornavirus-induced lesions, e.g., acute β-cell lysis, chronic autoimmunity, or insulin secretion defect. The rate of spontaneous mutation for enteroviruses is as high as 10^{-4} (172). Over 65 serotypes of enteroviruses have been characterized, but thousands of variants are indistinguishable by classic culture and serology. It is extremely difficult to accurately measure past exposure to agents that are so ubiquitous and cross-reactive and to differentiate causal from protective exposure, since prior infection with a related but nondiabetogenic strain of enterovirus may act as natural immunization against diabetogenic variants. These limitations must be kept in mind when we review data on humans.

HUMAN STUDIES

Autopsy Case Reports

Early case reports documented β-cell damage in fulminant CVB infection (1, 78, 198, 215, 236). Jenson et al. (100) studied 250 pancreata of newborns and young children who died in the course of fulminant viral infections. Insulitis was present in 4 of 7 cases of CVB infection, 20 of 45 cases of cytomegalovirus infection, 2 of 14 cases of varicella zoster virus infection, and 2 of 45 cases of congenital rubella infection.

Pancreatic findings in newly diagnosed IDDM patients have been inconsistent. In classic cases, CVB4 and CVB5 were isolated from the pancreata (78, 236) or feces (33) of newly diabetic patients. Several inbred strains of mice were inoculated with CVB4 isolated from a diabetic subject, but only SJL/J mice developed insulitis, β-cell necrosis, and diabetes, fulfilling Koch's postulates (236). In another study, SJL mice inoculated with CVB5 isolated from the feces of a diabetic child developed hyperglycemia and acinar cell necrosis but not β-cell necrosis (33). These results were consistent with autopsy results reported by Jenson et al. (100); i.e., in some newborns who died of fulminant coxsackievirus infection, β cells were predominantly affected, while in others, the damage was mostly to the acinar cells.

In one study of IDDM patients who died within 3 months of diagnosis, all 24 had residual β cells in their pancreata, and 89% of the insulin-containing islets stained for both HLA class I molecules and alpha interferon (59). Among 80 control pancreata, a similar pattern was observed in only 4 from patients with viral pancreatitis, which was shown by culture to be due to CVB in three cases. Thus, chronic enteroviral β-cell infection could result in release of alpha interferon, inducing HLA class I hyperexpression by adjacent endocrine cells and, in some cases, autoimmunity. Those authors were, however, unable to demonstrate acute enteroviral infection as the initial cause or final insult triggering IDDM in a larger series of 88 pancreata from IDDM patients who died at diagnosis (57). The diabetic pancreata and the pancreata from 20 persons who died of acute CVB myocarditis were stained with polyclonal rabbit antisera cross-reactive with the VP1 proteins of a wide variety of enteroviruses (229). None of the diabetic pancreata showed the presence of VP1, while among the myocarditis cases, VP1 was detected in 12 of 20 hearts and in all seven pancreata showing insulitis. This observation does not exclude the possibility that IDDM is caused by persistent infection of the β cells with a defective enterovirus not expressing VP1.

Coxsackievirus RNA could not be detected in pancreata from two HLA-DR3/4 toddlers who died at the diagnosis of diabetes ketoacidosis or in those from five control children (28). Reverse transcription of total RNA extracted from pancreatic samples was followed by PCR and Southern blot hybridization, which theoretically could detect as few as 5 to 10 genome copies. The primers used for CVB PCR were derived from a strongly conserved consensus sequence in the P2-C region of the CVB3 and CVB4 genomes. Mumps virus, rubella virus, or cytomegalovirus RNA also could not be detected. In summary, more recent autopsy studies have been generally unable to demonstrate enteroviral infection in patients with fatal IDDM.

It has been speculated that autoimmune responses may be associated with superantigen-induced activation of T-cell proliferation (148, 162, 211). Studies of nonobese diabetic mice have provided arguments against (127, 139, 225) and for (129) this hypothesis. Human data are extremely scarce and include a probable case reported by Foulis et al. (61) and two cases described by the Pittsburgh group (210a, 211). At present, there are important methodologic limitations to studying this hypothesis and no evidence that an enteroviral superantigen could be involved. Even if a superantigen reaction is involved in some cases of IDDM, it appears to be not a common finding but an exception limited to extremely rare cases when the patient dies with manifestations of diabetes and an overwhelming infection (187). Such rare fatal cases of IDDM appear to come in small epidemics, usually in spring, such as the one reported from Pittsburgh in 1974 (99).

IDDM or β-Cell Autoimmunity Following Enteroviral Infections

Hierholzer and Farris (93) found no diabetes among 109 children 4 years after the children had contracted CVB3 or/and CVB4 infection. Similarly, Dippe et al. (49) did not find anyone with glucose intolerance among 136 young residents of the isolated Pribilof Islands

5 years after an outbreak of CVB4. In contrast, 1 of 22 Swedish soldiers who contracted symptomatic CVB infection (most likely with CVB4) developed IDDM 10 weeks later (142). This subject was HLA-DR3/HLA-DR4, but ICA could not be demonstrated at the time of diabetes diagnosis. No long-term follow-up of the remaining 21 symptomatic soldiers and 228 healthy comrades has been reported.

Some authors have suggested that the estimated 10 to 30% of IDDM cases who are ICA negative at diagnosis could have diabetes due to an acute cytolytic enteroviral infection. In one prospective study of first-degree relatives of IDDM patients, seroconversion to ICA and CVB4 antibodies coincided with a relatively abrupt onset of IDDM in one case, while no CVB antibodies but persistent ICA preceded insidious onset of diabetes in a contrasting case (157). In another case report, CVB infection and ICA preceded IDDM by 3 years (6), but a concurrent ICA and CVB antibody seroconversion was not actually observed; titers of both antibodies were already high in the first sample available. Contrary to the hypothesis that enteroviral infection is associated with nonautoimmune IDDM, newly diagnosed IDDM patients positive for CVB IgM appear more likely than not to be ICA positive (190). A report from Cuba (216) suggested that ICA may be present in as many as 36% of children during echovirus 4 meningoencephalitis; however, no follow-up of these children for diabetes has been reported. Several years later, 17 patients from an echovirus 4 outbreak in Glasgow were studied (50). The group's mean insulin levels were transiently increased following infection, and one subject showed ICA positivity just after infection, with the ICA titer declining at follow-up. A preinfection ICA measurement for this subject was, however, not available.

In summary, there are conflicting case reports and small prospective studies. A large prospective study of young children monitored for concurrent development of enteroviral infections and β-cell autoimmunity is needed to test the hypothesis that symptomatic and/or serologically detectable enteroviral infection is associated with development of IDDM or β-cell autoimmunity. Such an investigation, the Diabetes Autoimmunity Study in the Young, is now in progress.

Ecological Studies

SEASONAL PATTERNS OF IDDM AND ENTEROVIRAL INFECTIONS

The seasonality of IDDM has prompted comparisons with the seasonal patterns of common childhood viral diseases (79, 178). The annual peak of enteroviral diseases (August through September) precedes the major peak of IDDM incidence (October through January). This difference could be interpreted in favor of the concept that enteroviral infections at least promote IDDM onset in persons with β-cell autoimmunity. However, a second peak of IDDM incidence (March through April in most of the populations studied) clearly does not fit into this scenario unless another seasonal triggering factor is hypothesized. In addition, the prevalence of neutralizing CVB antibodies is higher in IDDM patients diagnosed in winter (16 of 22) than in those diagnosed in fall (9 of 23) (42).

TEMPORAL TRENDS IN IDDM AND ENTEROVIRAL INFECTIONS

Gleason et al. (79) related temporal changes in the number of IDDM cases seen in the Joslin Clinic from 1964 through 1973 to the reported incidence of several infectious diseases, including enteroviral meningitis. The annual pattern of enteroviral meningitis (peaks in 1966 and 1970 through 1973) somewhat resembled that of IDDM in a selected group (11%) of young patients with rapid onset of diabetes. This hospital-based study suffered from underascertainment and case selection bias as well as from reporting of case counts rather than incidence rates. These limitations were avoided in a population-based study of IDDM and enteroviral meningitis incidence in 1970 through 1989 in Poland. During this observation period, an epidemic of IDDM coincided with an outbreak of enteroviral meningitis in 1984 through 1988. The age-specific incidence of IDDM and that of enteroviral meningitis displayed strikingly parallel temporal variation, especially in children aged 0 to 9 years (Fig. 2).

OUTBREAKS OF IDDM

In 1974, an outbreak of 12 cases of IDDM was reported from Florida. Three of 9 cases tested, compared to 2 of 36 controls, had elevated neutralizing antibodies to CVB3 (95). Such small clusters of IDDM cases are likely to occur by chance alone, and their in-depth investigation is rather futile.

CVB5 and echovirus 4 have been linked to larger outbreaks of childhood IDDM in populations covered by IDDM registries. During the 1984 epidemic of childhood IDDM in Poland, which was associated with a concurrent epidemic of aseptic meningitis, the incidence of IDDM almost doubled, from 3.5/100,000 in 1970 through 1981 to 6.6/100,000 in 1982 through 1984 (178). Figure 3 presents the 3-month moving average number of IDDM and enteroviral meningitis cases in the epidemic area, as well as the dominant enteroviral serotypes found in the meningitis cases by culture and traditional neutralizing assay. The four major peaks of IDDM (August 1982 through July 1983, January through July 1985, January 1986 through March 1987, and September 1987 through March 1988) appeared to be temporally linked with outbreaks of echovirus 4; echovirus 30; CVB5 and echovirus 9; and echoviruses 9, 6, and 7, respectively. It is noteworthy that at any time, the incidence of IDDM was approximately 10 times lower than that of enteroviral meningitis, which in turn was likely lower by another order of magnitude than the incidence of all enteroviral infections in that population. This incidence would be consistent with the view that IDDM is a very rare complication of enteroviral infection. These ecologic observations were evaluated in a case-control study conducted in cooperation with the Centers for Disease Control and Prevention in Atlanta

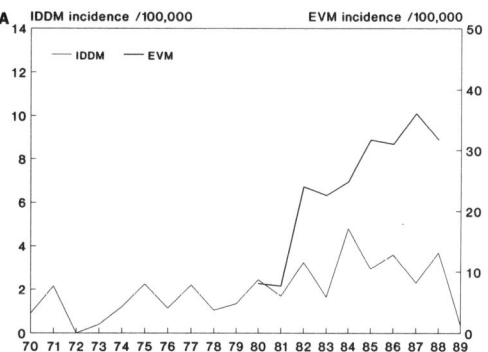

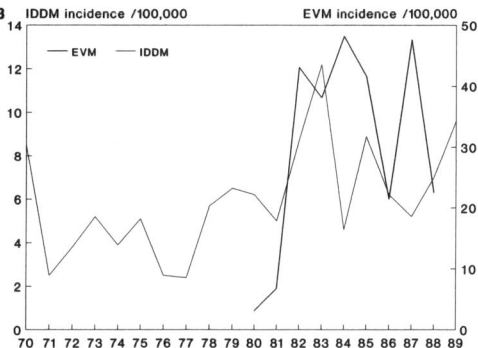

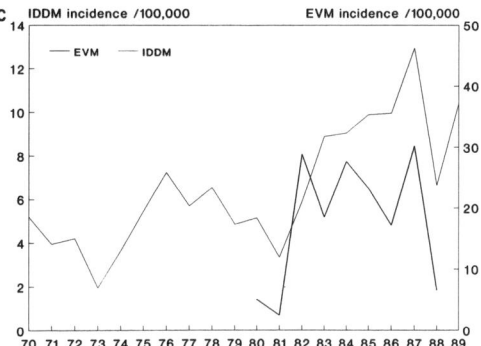

FIGURE 2 Incidences of IDDM (thin line) and enteroviral meningitis (EVM) (heavy line) in Wielkopolska, Poland. (a) Children aged 0 through 4 years; (b) children aged 5 through 9 years; (c) children aged 10 through 14 years.

(179). Using a novel monotypic detector system (89), we examined 98 IDDM patients and 66 control children for the presence of IgM and IgA antiviral antibodies against CVB1 through CVB6; CVA9; echoviruses 4, 6, 9, 11, 30, and 34; and enterovirus 71. Sera from these patients were collected within 1 month of the

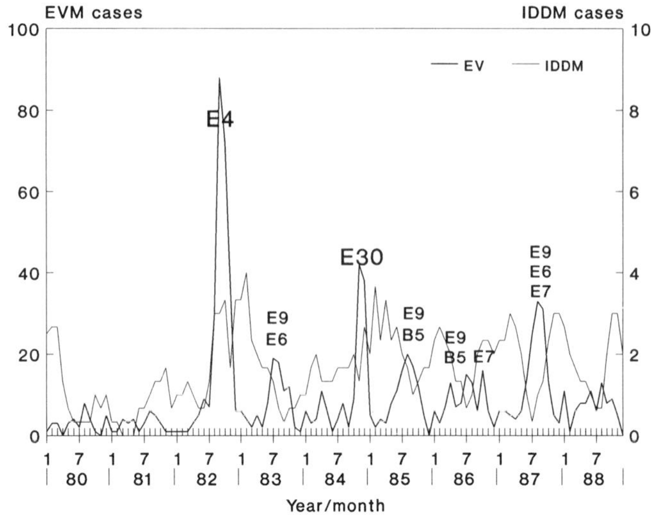

FIGURE 3 Incidence of IDDM (thin line) and enteroviral meningitis (EVM) (thick line) in Wielkopolska, Poland, 1980 through 1988. The IDDM curve reflects 3-month moving averages. The dominant serotypes of enteroviruses cultured from or determined serologically in the meningitis cases are shown. E, echovirus; B5, CVB5.

first insulin administration, and the analyses were stratified according to the date of blood collection. Several significant associations were found. In 1983 through 1984, IgM against CVB5 was more frequent in IDDM cases than controls (odds ratio = 3.2; P = 0.04). In 1984 through 1986, IgM against CVB3 was present in 41% of the cases and 17% of controls (odds ratio = 3.5; P = 0.017). These asociations were different from what was expected, because the predominant serotypes in 1983 through 1984 were echoviruses 9, 6, and 30 rather than CVB5, and those in 1984 through 1986 were echoviruses 30, 9, and 7 rather than CVB3 (Fig. 3).

The same assays were employed in a twin case-control study of 126 children diagnosed with IDDM in Pittsburgh, Pa., who were compared to 140 hospital controls group-matched by age, gender, and date of bleed (August 1983 through September 1985). This was a period of low, stable incidence of IDDM and enteroviral meningitis in the area. As in a Wisconsin study (43), older but not younger patients were more likely than controls to be IgM positive. IDDM was significantly associated with IgM to eight enteroviral serotypes in males older than 13 years and to nine serotypes in females older than 10 years (90). These data support a non-serotype-specific association between IDDM and enteroviral infection in children developing IDDM at or after puberty.

Observations strikingly similar to those made in Poland have been reported from Birmingham, Ala., where an epidemic of IDDM was also observed in 1983 through 1984 concurrently with an epidemic of CVB5 (222). The overall incidence in the year beginning July 1983, the month of the first isolation of CVB5, was 18.5/100,000, an excess of 6.7/100,000 over the average annual incidence for the previous 4 years.

In contrast to other CVB, CVB5 infections occur primarily in outbreaks, with comparatively few cases occurring during intervening years (84). Since a national surveillance system was established in 1961, there have been several outbreaks of CVB5 infections in the United States (major epidemics in 1961, 1972 through 1973, and 1983 through 1984 and minor ones in 1967 and 1977 through 1978). CVB5 isolates from the 1983 epidemic had fingerprints nearly identical to those of the 1967 strain but not to those of the 1972 through 1973 epidemic strain. Interestingly, several population-based IDDM registries have reported IDDM incidence increases in 1972 through 1973, 1977 through 1978, and 1983 through 1984 (47). These data suggest a role for CVB5 in some outbreaks of IDDM.

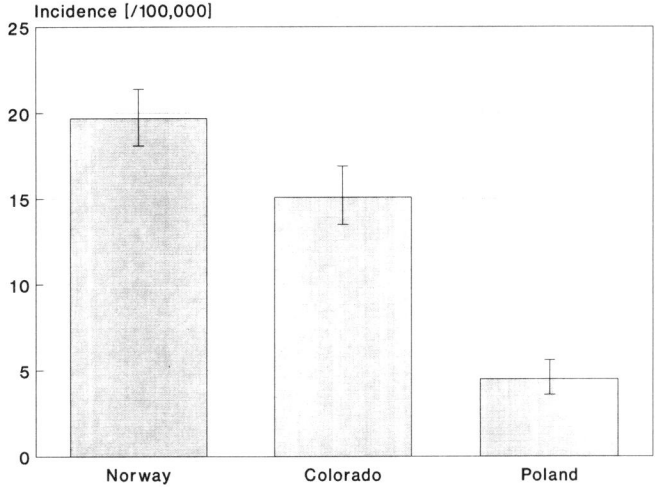

FIGURE 4 Incidence of IDDM in the age group 0 through 14 years in Norway, Colorado, and Poland in 1978 through 1980, showing significant geographic differences in incidence rates.

THE POLIO MODEL OF IDDM

It has been hypothesized that the pattern of IDDM follows the model of poliomyelitis, with children in areas of lower socioeconomic status acquiring the infection earlier in life but avoiding the more severe (i.e., paralytic) course associated with infection at older ages (see chapters 1 and 9). A population-based case-control study from Wisconsin (43) found that 60% of patients aged 0 to 9 years had no IgG antibody to any CVB serotype, indicating that these patients had never been exposed to those viruses. This result is consistent with the reported low prevalences of coxsackievirus in stool samples (0.1% [66]) and of neutralizing antibodies (2% [113]) in serum samples from U.S. children compared to those for children in developing countries (52% [160]).

In an ecologic analysis, we compared the age distribution of reported aseptic meningitis in three countries with comparable health care quality but different rates of IDDM and different per capita gross national products. The incidence of IDDM is highest in Norway, intermediate in the United States (Colorado), and lowest in Poland (Fig. 4). The per capita gross national product in 1991 was approximately $20,000 in the United States and Norway and $3,000 in Poland. According to the polio model, we expected the incidence of aseptic meningitis (a marker of enteroviral exposure) in the youngest children to be lowest in Norway, intermediate in Colorado, and highest in Poland. The observed rates generally confirmed these expectations (Fig. 5) except for a very high incidence of aseptic meningitis in Colorado infants compared to infants in the other two locations (perhaps because of more invasive rule-out-sepsis procedures practiced in the United States) (see chapter 11). The age distribution of aseptic meningitis in Poland, the area of high enteroviral exposure at younger ages, did not differ between low-incidence and epidemic years (Fig. 6). Interestingly, the temporal variation in aseptic meningitis incidence in Colorado appeared to be associated with the incidence of IDDM only in Hispanic children but not in higher-income non-Hispanic white children (Fig. 7). Together, these ecologic analyses suggest that IDDM may indeed follow the polio model of disease.

Cross-Sectional Seroepidemiologic Studies

CASE-CONTROL STUDIES OF ANTIVIRAL ANTIBODIES

Since the first report of higher frequency of CVB antibodies in newly diagnosed IDDM patients than in controls (69), at least 40 studies of similar design have been published from a number

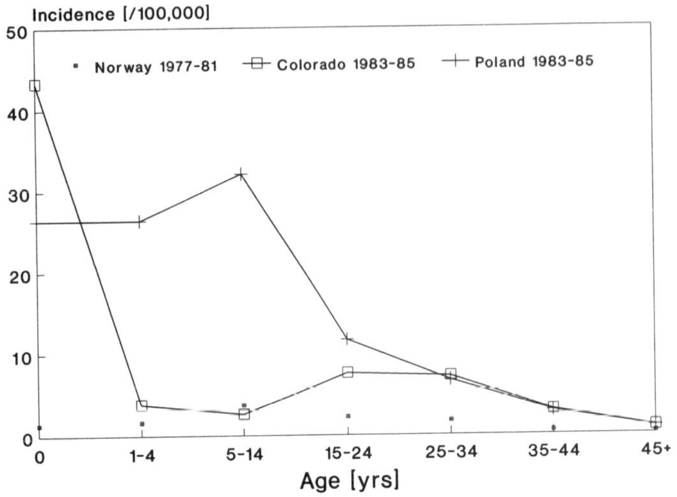

FIGURE 5 Age distribution of enteroviral meningitis in Norway, Colorado, and Poland. The high incidence of enteroviral meningitis in the age group 0 through 14 years in Poland (low IDDM risk) compared to those in Colorado (moderate IDDM risk) and Norway (high IDDM risk) supports the polio model of IDDM etiology.

of countries. A review of earlier cross-sectional studies (15) found that the reported odds ratios, ranging from 0.7 to 20, were inconclusive but weighed more for an association between CVB and IDDM than against it. Most of those studies used controls matched to IDDM patients for age and geographic area. Studies with sibling controls have generally found no association between CVB and IDDM, perhaps because of overmatching without taking into consideration genetic differences between siblings or perhaps because of virus mutation during household transmission (12).

Here, we summarize selected studies that were not included in two previous excellent reviews (12, 15), giving priority to studies that included controls whose ages, residences, and times of venipuncture closely resembled those of the IDDM patients. Gamble and Cumming (68) reported IgM capture enzyme-linked immunosorbent assay results for CVB1 through CVB5 in 589 children and with IDDM and 277 control children hospitalized for elective surgery. The two groups had similar age distributions in the range of 0 through 15 years. However, blood samples from cases and con-

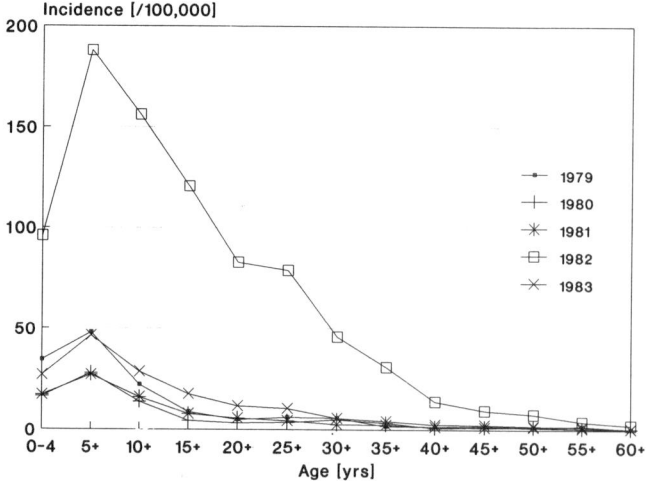

FIGURE 6 Age distribution of enteroviral meningitis in Wielkopolska, Poland. There was no evidence for a change in distribution during the epidemic year (1982) compared to that in the nonepidemic years (1979 through 1981 and 1983).

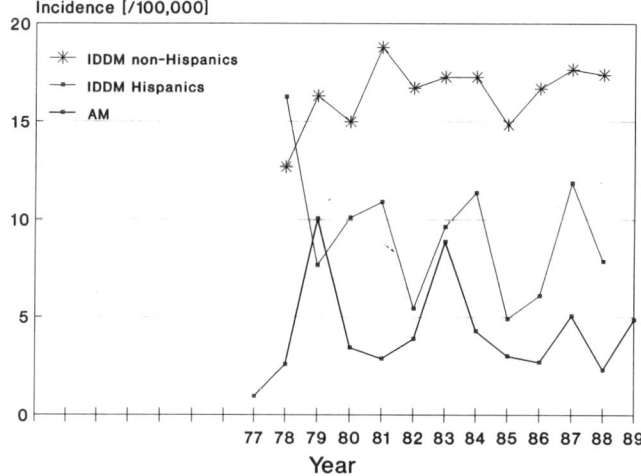

FIGURE 7 Incidence of IDDM and enteroviral meningitis (AM) in Colorado, 1978 through 1988. The incidence of IDDM paralleled that of enteroviral meningitis in lower-income Hispanics but not in higher-income non-Hispanic white children.

trols were not collected during the same periods (1979 through 1981 and 1981 through 1983, respectively), and the geographic distributions of the two groups were different. Moreover, duration of diabetes was <1 year in only 99 cases, 1 to 2 years in 183 cases, and >2 years in 307 cases. The authors made two observations that they interpreted as evidence against a role for CVB in IDDM. First, there was no decline in IgM levels with IDDM duration (consistent with studies reviewed by Barrett-Connor [15]). However, the presence of IgM does not necessarily indicate recent primary infection. IgM may result from reactivation of a latent infection, or it may indicate lack of viral clearance. Thus, persistently elevated IgM levels could also be interpreted as evidence of persistent CVB infection (205). Second, only in the youngest children, aged 6 months to 2 years, was there evidence of increased exposure to CVB (in 22 [39%] of 56 cases versus 4 [17%] of 24 controls). Interestingly, all 22 positive cases in this group had CVB5 IgM compared to only two controls. In our opinion, this second observation is consistent with the existence of a susceptibility window in early childhood, when an enteroviral infection is more likely to persist and lead to IDDM.

A Swedish group reported an extremely high prevalence of CVB IgM (16 of 24 [67%]) among children with IDDM diagnosed during an outbreak of IDDM in Uppsala in 1982 through 1984 but a complete absence of CVB IgM (0 of 24) in age-matched controls (63, 64). Among the IgM-positive patients, 11 of 16 were aged 4 to 8 years, and none was younger than 4 years. Neutralizing CVB antibodies, indicating an earlier infection, were detected in 11 of 16 of IgM-positive patients; however, in only 3 cases was there a significant rise in neutralizing antibody titer. The IgM antibodies were monotypic in 13 of 16 cases, but they were not specific to one serotype. The IgM antibodies persisted for 3 to 4 months, and their titers declined thereafter. The prevalence of CVB IgM was 2 of 6, 13 of 17, and 3 of 13 in 1982, 1983, and 1984, respectively (55). A retrospective study of 98 IDDM cases diagnosed in two regions of Sweden between 1978 and 1984 demonstrated the annual prevalence of CVB IgM to vary between 0 and 76% (214). Finally, a nationwide study of 98 children with IDDM who were diagnosed in Sweden in fall of 1985 and late spring 1986 and of 94 control children found no association between CVB IgM and IDDM (213). Although it has been argued that the incidence of IDDM decreased in Sweden during that period, this was a relatively modest decrease, perhaps most evident among children aged 5 to 9 years (145).

The frequency of CVB IgM and their serotype specificities are strikingly similar in IDDM patients and their nondiabetic siblings at the time of diagnosis (65, 157). This indicates that the IgM reflects recent or persistent infection rather than cross-reactivity with exogenous or endogenous antigens or nonspecific polyclonal activation of IgM-secreting cells. This also suggests that diabetogenic viral mutants are generated during intrafamilial spread of CVB or that other (genetic?) cofactors that produce IDDM must be present in the patients but not in their siblings. It is unlikely that IgM reflects just the first of a few infections needed to develop IDDM in the nondiabetic siblings and the final one in IDDM patients, because none of the control siblings developed IDDM during the subsequent 2 to 7 years (65).

If CVB infection initiates β-cell autoimmunity rather than provides the final insult that promotes diabetes onset, CVB IgM levels should be more strongly associated with the presence of ICA or GAD antibodies than with IDDM. Contrary to this hypothesis, fewer ICA-positive first-degree relatives of IDDM patients than of recent-onset IDDM patients had CVB IgG (88 versus 100%, respectively) or IgM (13 versus 67%, respectively) (220). The prevalence of CVB IgG and IgM in the ICA-positive relatives was no different from that in ICA-negative relatives or in unrelated controls; however, the study population was relatively small and included young adults rather than children. In contrast, a well-designed study of children aged 7 to 19 years who were screened for ICA (189) found CVB IgM in 14 (32%) of 44 ICA-positive children and in 7 (16%) of 44 age- and sex-matched ICA-negative classmate controls whose blood was collected on the same day as that of the patients. This difference was statistically not significant. More studies of prediabetic individuals defined by ICA and other β-cell autoantibodies that include well-selected control groups are needed to resolve the issue of whether enteroviral exposure is critical to initiation of β-cell autoimmunity or, rather, to its progression to overt diabetes.

Interpretation of the seroepidemiologic data is complicated by the capricious nature of antibody response to CVB infection. Early studies measured neutralizing CVB antibodies that if elevated on a single measurement might reflect a distant infection, a recent infection, or infection with another enterovirus (heterotypic response). Lennette et al. (119) showed that only 53% of patients with CVB4 infection confirmed by isolation exhibited homotypic antibody response, and 43% did not seroconvert for any CVB. Therefore, the earlier studies of neutralizing antibodies should be interpreted with caution. The IgM capture assay (112) was thought to overcome the problems with neutralizing antibodies because of its ability to reliably detect recent CVB infection; however, heterotypic IgM responses are also present. Newer monoclonal detection systems for IgM or IgA antibodies also have questionable specificities (234). Even if perfect type-specific detectors were available, there are multiple variants within each serotype, with few being diabetogenic and most being neutral or even protective. These serious limitations of the seroepidemiologic approach to studying past exposure to diabetogenic enteroviruses suggest two novel approaches: (i) a search for enteroviral RNA or proteins persistently present in the β cells or other tissues and (ii) a prospective virus watch, with serum samples tested at short intervals in the hope of detecting acute seroconversion to β-cell autoimmunity and concurrent infection evidenced by the presence of enteroviral nucleic acids.

The limitations of the first approach include obvious ethical problems with pancreatic biopsies in healthy subjects; the unrepresentativeness of autopsy in terms of studying early phases of the autoimmune process and even in terms of the general population of newly diagnosed IDDM cases; and the specificity of β-cell tropism, which may make testing of other tissues (e.g., lymphocytes) useless. Searching for persistently expressed viral proteins would require knowledge of the specific epitopes that are different from those of normal viral proteins. The search for viral RNA is complicated by the instability of uncoated RNA in biologic samples. One negative search for CVB RNA in the pancreata of toddlers who died at diagnosis of diabetes (28) is described above. Our negative studies summarized below likely resemble unsuccessful attempts in other laboratories.

Limitations of the virus watch approach are related to the patient population that needs to be studied. Since β-cell autoimmunity starts in early childhood, infants and toddlers should be studied. There are obvious problems with the participation of a large number of families with young children in such a demanding longitudinal protocol that would include multiple examinations, blood tests, and cultures. We have recently embarked on such an effort to monitor approximately 500 children with genetically increased risk of IDDM (Diabetes Autoimmunity Study in the Young). The examinations are spaced 6 to 12 months apart to ensure compliance. However, if an acute rather than a persistent enteroviral infection is associated with the onset of β-cell autoimmunity, many such events are likely to be missed.

CASE-CONTROL STUDIES OF VIRAL NUCLEIC ACIDS

Enteroviral nucleic acids can now be reliably detected in various body tissues to evaluate whether infection is present. We attempted to identify a persistent enteroviral infection in newly diagnosed IDDM subjects by using a reliable PCR-based technique (184) and peripheral blood mononuclear cells stored in liquid nitrogen. The results were disappointing, because only 1 in 12 samples was positive, and it was from a nondiabetic control. The circumstances surrounding blood sampling in that person, e.g., concurrent symptoms, were unknown. CVB readily establishes persistent infection in human lymphoid cell lines (128); however, enteroviruses are less likely to persist in peripheral blood mononuclear cells in vivo (173). Viral RNA is highly unstable when it is not protected by a viral capsid protein; freezing and thawing of samples may promote damage to the viral protein and loss of viral RNA. In future studies, nucleic acids for virus-specific PCR may need to be isolated in the presence of RNase inhibitors immediately after blood samples are obtained. Serum obtained at the same time should be tested for enteroviral IgM levels to assess whether the infection does elicit detectable IgM response or elicits a weak response, as suggested by some studies of newly diagnosed IDDM children (163).

PROSPECTIVE STUDIES

Case-control or cross-sectional comparisons conducted at the time of clinical IDDM onset are of little value in assessing the cause of β-cell autoimmunity, which might have begun several years earlier. Since IDDM onset is preceded by a long period of subclinical β-cell autoimmunity, it is necessary to measure antiviral IgM or nucleic acids close to the onset of autoimmunity rather than the onset of diabetes in order to fully assess the role of candidate viruses. Although there has been no report of a prospective study, such studies are in progress in several locations.

Gene-Environment Interaction

IDDM is likely caused by an interactive effect of genetic and environmental factors either within a limited age window of susceptibility or as a result of multiple insults to the β cells over a few decades of life. Although both the susceptibility genes and the candidate viruses appear to be quite common, the likelihood of these causal components meeting within the susceptibility age window may be fairly low (110).

In mice, the host gene or genes restrict the diabetogenic effect of EMCV (23) and of CVB (226) in a manner compatible with a recessive trait (156) not related to the MHC genes (238). The susceptibility locus is on murine chromosome 4 in a region conserved on human chromosome 1 (123). This locus may confer a state of immunodeficiency that is reversible in the murine model by an ad libitum diet (137). It is not known whether such immunodeficiency predisposes to or results from a diabetogenic infection.

A decreased immune responsiveness to viral antigens is a feature of human diabetes. For instance, 25 to 40% of diabetes patients fail to attain protective anti-hepatitis B virus antibody levels after three injections of hepatitis B virus vaccine (24, 171). IDDM patients also show impaired antibody production in response to influenza (48), mumps (96), and yellow fever vaccination (22) as well as to Epstein-Barr virus capsid antigen (97). This high nonresponse rate is unrelated to metabolic control of diabetes. In contrast, antibody response to pneumococcal polysaccharide, which is T-cell independent, appears to be normal (117). A putative gene (on human chromosome 1) responsible for this immunodeficiency has not yet been identified. Some of these low responses to viral antigens may be due to the higher frequency in IDDM patients, of the HLA-DR3 allele. HLA-DR3/3 persons are known to be at high risk for persistent viral infection and autoimmunity due to impaired virus clearance (e.g., hepatitis B virus), which is usually associated with low antibody response. It remains to be established whether DR3 or other gene products promote enteroviral persistence and β-cell autoimmunity in humans.

The available evidence for genetic susceptibility to virus-induced diabetes in humans is largely limited to studies of HLA-DR restriction. HLA-DR restriction of proliferative T-cell responses to viruses associated with IDDM (e.g., mumps virus, varicella-zoster virus, and CVB4) was compared in nine patients with long-standing IDDM and 44 healthy controls (26). Responses in patients were not significantly higher than those in controls. Among the controls, the highest responses to CVB were observed in persons with HLA-DR4, and the lowest responses were observed in those with HLA-DR2 (mostly DR2/DR3 heterozygotes). This and additional studies (25) suggest that HLA-DR3 and -DR4 molecules may restrict T-cell responses to CVB. However, the small number of IDDM subjects studied did not allow valid comparisons.

Reported associations between HLA-DR and CVB IgM are summarized in Table 1. Elevated CVB IgM levels in subjects with a specific HLA phenotype may reflect a greater ability to mount an immune response or a greater susceptibility to infection. Consistent with cellular studies, elevated CVB IgM levels were more strongly associated with HLA-DR4/x or HLA-DR4/3 than with HLA-DR3/x in children with IDDM studied in Pittsburgh, Pa., during a period of stable low incidence (1979 through 1982) (52). In contrast, a much stronger association with HLA-DR3/x than with HLA-DR4/x was reported from Uppsala, Sweden, during an IDDM epidemic in 1982 through 1984 (55). In the Swedish study, HLA-DR3 was associated with IgM responses to CVB4, while HLA-DR4 was associated with IgM responses to CVB2, CVB3, and CVB5. Newly diagnosed HLA-DR3-positive patients in Wisconsin also had more frequently elevated CVB IgM (26%) than did HLA-DR3-negative patients (11%) or age-matched controls (7%) (43). Finally, Austrian children with IDDM diagnosed in 1982 through 1983 showed similar associations of CVB IgM with HLA-DR4 and HLA-DR3 (190). It remains to be established whether these population differences in HLA associations reflect different dominant CVB serotypes.

IDDM Phenotype Associated with Enteroviral Infection

IDDM appears to be a heterogeneous condition. HLA-DR phenotype, season at onset, and age have been used in attempts to define different phenotypes of the disease. HLA-DR4-positive patients compared to HLA-DR4-negative patients more frequently have recent viral infection (62 versus 37%, respectively) and CVB antibodies (35 versus 18%, respectively) but lower total IgG levels, especially in males (52). The HLA-DR4-positive patients are more often diagnosed during peak season and have a more severe clinical manifestation and a lower residual β-cell function (125). On the other hand, the HLA-DR3 allele appears to be associated with a more insidious onset and less frequent CVB antibodies. Patients aged 0 to 6 years are more frequently HLA-DR3/4 and positive for β-cell autoantibodies; how-

TABLE 1 Associations between HLA phenotype and elevated CVB IgM levels in newly diagnosed IDDM patients

Study (reference)	CVB-specific IgM by HLA-DR type			
	DR4/DRx	DR4/DR3	DR3/DRx	DRx/DRx
	n (% IgM+)	n (% IgM+)	n (% IgM+)	n (% IgM+)
Pittsburgh, Pa. 1979–1982 (52)	62 (24)	52 (22)	39 (10)	19 (12)
Uppsala, Sweden, 1982–1984 (55)	18 (39)	11 (64)	5 (80)	2 (0)
Austria, 1982–1983 (190)	27 (26)	32 (34)	14 (29)	17 (6)

ever, they are less likely than older patients to be CVB antibody positive (106).

PERSPECTIVES OF PREVENTION

Notkins and Yoon (144) were able to prevent EMCV-D-induced diabetes in SJL/J mice by immunizing the mice with the nondiabetogenic EMCV-B variant. Current progress in identification of the genetic determinants of diabetogenicity of CVB suggests that recombinant subunit vaccines to protect against diabetogenic strains will be developed.

Information on the ultrastructure of the HLA peptide-binding grooves is rapidly becoming available, helping to disentangle the role of specific HLA alleles in susceptibility or resistance to infections and autoimmunity. It may become possible to design vaccine proteins that would provide optimal antigenic stimulus in the context of the host HLA phenotype, providing long-term protection and avoiding adverse effects. In addition to the HLA genes, several other IDDM susceptibility or resistance loci have been identified in human and animal models. The relevance of these genes to susceptibility to enteroviruses has not been studied.

An approach alternative to vaccination, antiviral agent WIN 54954 (see chapter 18), is effective when given orally on the day of infection to susceptible mice infected with the diabetogenic E2 strain of CVB4 (191). Seven weeks p.i. significantly fewer treated than control animals had persistent CVB4 infection, histologic islet abnormalities, and hyperglycemia.

Another approach in IDDM vaccine development uses recombinant GAD or insulin rather than known viral epitopes in order to induce self-tolerance to these β-cell autoantigens.

SUMMARY

Despite the extensive human and animal data reviewed above, the evidence for a causal relationship between enteroviruses and IDDM is still elusive. Attempts to identify such a relationship have been hampered by numerous factors (Table 2). Therefore, the unifying perspective presented here must be considered hypothetical.

Except for rare cases, human IDDM does not appear to result from an acute cytolytic enteroviral infection. Newer data indicate that in at least 90% of cases, IDDM is preceded by β-cell autoimmunity, a defect in forming peripheral tolerance to β-cell self antigens. Enteroviral infection could initiate β-cell autoimmunity in the following situations.

1. An immune response against a virus with molecular mimicry to a β-cell self protein (e.g., CVB P2-C protein and GAD) develops.

2. A wild-type β-cell-tropic enterovirus or a mutant produced in the course of peri-insular infection establishes persistent β-cell infection, with impairment of insulin secretion and expression of self antigens. Infection of the acinar cells or the vascular endothelium may render β cells susceptible to infection through induction of adhesion molecules used by enteroviruses as cellular receptors.

3. An environmental insult (e.g., acinar cell infection or exposure to a β-cell toxin) results in cytokine-induced impairment of insulin secretion and β-cell injury because of the limited capacity of β cells to neutralize free radicals. Self antigens released in this process may initiate β-cell autoimmunity.

In any of these scenarios, the autoimmune process would be amplified as self-reactive lymphocytes were recruited to the site of inflammation. The continued release of cytokines would result in overexpression of class I molecules on β cells, further potentiating β-cell destruction. Other effector mechanisms of immunologic destruction such as antibody-dependent cellular cytotoxicity, delayed-type hypersensitivity, complement, and cytotoxic concentrations of cytokines (e.g., gamma interferon, IL-1, etc.) could all play some role in β-cell destruction.

Factors regulating the speed at which these events occur include (i) the metabolic activity of the β cell, with the increased demands of puberty or obesity exacerbating the autoimmune process; (ii) the individual's HLA type, which restricts immune responsiveness; (iii) infection with non-β-cell-tropic agents that might restore some degree of immunosuppression or self-tolerance that could delay the progression of β-cell autoimmunity; and (iv) the age at which the inductive event occurs, with early age associated with more vigorous β-cell autoimmunity.

The investigation of the viral etiology of human IDDM will likely shift in the near future from cross-sectional and retrospective studies with diabetes as the endpoint to prospective studies with β-cell autoimmunity as the endpoint. Future studies must take into account the genetic susceptibility of the host and the genetic determinants of enteroviral diabetogenicity. If a causative role of enteroviruses in the etiology of IDDM is confirmed, a recombinant subunit vaccine will likely be the intervention of choice to prevent IDDM.

ACKNOWLEDGMENT

This work was supported by National Institutes of Health grant DK-32493.

REFERENCES

1. **Ahmad, N., and A. A. Abraham.** 1982. Pancreatic isleitis with coxsackie virus B5 infection. *Hum. Pathol.* **13:**661–662.
2. **Allen, C., M. Palta, and D. J. D'Alessio.** 1991. Risk of diabetes in siblings and other relatives of IDDM subjects. *Diabetes* **40:**831–836.
3. **Anderson, H. U., K. H. Jørgensen, J. Egeberg, T. Mandrup-Poulsen, and J. Nerup.** 1994. Nicotinamide prevents interleukin-1 effects on accumulated insulin release and nitric oxide production in rat islets of Langerhans. *Diabetes* **43:**770–777.
4. **Anderson, O. O., M. Christy, K. Arnung, K. Buschard, B. Christau, H. Kromann, J. Herup, P. Platz, L. P. Ryder, A. Svejgaard, and M. Thomsen.** 1977. Viruses and diabetes, p. 294–298. *In* J. S. Baja (ed.), *Diabetes.* Excerpta Medica, Amsterdam.
5. **Archard, L. C., N. E. Bowles, E. G. J. Olsen, and P. J. Richardson.** 1987. Detection of persistent coxsackie B virus RNA in dilated cardiomyopathy and myocarditis. *Eur. Heart. J.* **8**(Suppl. J):437–440.
6. **Asplin, C. M., M. K. Cooney, J. R. Crossley, T. L. Dornan, P. Raghu, and J. P. Palmer.** 1982. Coxsackie B4 infection and islet cell antibodies three years before overt diabetes. *J. Pediatr.* **101:**398–400.
6a. **Atkinson, M. A., et al.** Unpublished observations.
7. **Atkinson, M. A., M. Bowman, B. Darrow,**

TABLE 2 Problems in relating viruses to IDDM etiology

1. Long incubation period (in many but not all cases)
2. Ubiquitous nature of most candidate viruses and rarity of IDDM
3. Subclinical initial infection in many cases
4. Existence of cofactors
5. Heterogeneity of causes by age, race, and location
6. Variable diabetogenic virulence of viral strains
7. Variable host susceptibility determined by genetic, immunologic, and other age-related factors
8. Difference between humans and experimental animals in host susceptibility and disease manifestation
9. Serodiagnostics complicated by apparent immunodeficiency of diabetic subjects at onset (prior to onset?)

and D. Kaufman. 1994. Cellular immunity to an epitope common to glutamate decarboxylase (GAD) and coxsackie virus in insulin dependent diabetes (IDD). *Diabetes* **43**(Suppl. 1):93A.
8. Atkinson, M. A., D. L. Kaufman, L. Campbell, A. J. Tobin, and N. K. Maclaren. 1993. Islet cell cytoplasmic autoantibody reactivity to glutamate decarboxylase in insulin dependent diabetes. *J. Clin. Invest.* **91**:350–356.
9. Bae, Y.-S., and J.-W. Yoon. 1993. Determination of diabetogenicity attributable to a single amino acid Ala776, on the polyprotein of encephalomyocarditis virus. *Diabetes* **42**:435–443.
10. Baekkeskov, S., M. Landin, J. K. Kristensen, S. Srikanta, G. J. Bruining, T. Mandrup-Poulsen, C. De Beaufort, J. S. Soeldner, G. Eisenbarth, F. Lindgren, et al. 1987. Antibodies to a 64,000 Mr human islet cell antigen precede the clinical onset of insulin-dependent diabetes. *J. Clin. Invest.* **79**:926–934.
10a. Baekkeskov S., H. Jan-Aanstoot, S. Christgau, A. Reetz, M. Solimena, M. Cascalho, F. Folli, H. Richter-Olesen, and P. De-Camilli. 1990. Identification of the 64K autoantigen in insulin-dependent diabetes as the GABA-synthesizing enzyme glutamic acid decarboxylase. *Nature* (London) **347**:151–156.
11. Baekkeskov, S., J. H. Nielsen, B. T. Marner, J. Bilde, Ludvigsson, and A. Lernmark. 1982. Autoantibodies in newly diagnosed diabetic children immunoprecipitate human pancreatic islet cell proteins. *Nature* (London) **298**:167–169.
12. Banatvala, J. E. 1987. Insulin-dependent (juvenile-onset, type 1) diabetes mellitus coxsackie B viruses revisited. *Prog. Med. Virol.* **34**:33–54.
13. Banatvala, J. E., J. Bryant, G. Schernthaner, M. Borkenstein, E. Schober, D. Brown, L. M. De Silva, M. A. Menser, and M. Silink. 1985. Coxsackie B, mumps, rubella, and cytomegalovirus specific IgM responses in patients with juvenile-onset insulin-dependent diabetes mellitus in Britain, Austria, and Australia. *Lancet* **i**:1409–1412.
14. Barmeier H., D. K. McCulloch, J. L. Neifing, G. Warnock, R. V. Rajotte, J. P. Palmer, and A. Lernmark. 1991. Risk for developing type 1 (insulin-dependent) diabetes mellitus and the presence of islet 64K antibodies. *Diabetologia* **34**:727–733.
15. Barrett-Connor, E. 1985. Is insulin-dependent diabetes mellitus caused by coxsackie virus B infection? A review of the epidemiologic evidence. *Rev. Infect. Dis.* **7**:207–215.
16. Bell, G. I., S. Horita, and J. H. Karam. 1984. A polymorphic locus near the human insulin gene is associated with insulin-dependent diabetes mellitus. *Diabetes* **33**:176–183.
17. Bertrams, J., and M. P. Baur. 1984. Insulin-dependent diabetes mellitus, p. 348–358. In E. D. Albert (ed.), *Histocompatibility Testing 1984*. Springer-Verlag, Berlin.
18. Blom, L., L. Nystrom, and G. Dahlquist. 1991. The Swedish childhood diabetes study. Vaccinations and infections as risk determinants for diabetes in childhood. *Diabetologia* **34**:176–181.
19. Bodansky, H. J., P. J. Grant, B. M. Dean, J. McNally, G. F. Bottazzo, M. H. Hambling, and J. K. Wales. 1986. Islet-cell antibodies and insulin autoantibodies in association with common viral infections. *Lancet* **ii**:1351–1353.
20. Boehm, B. O., B. Manfras, J. Seissler, K. Schoffling, M. Gluck, G. Holzberger, S. Seidl, P. Kuhnl, M. Trucco, and W. A. Scherbaum. 1991. Epidemiology and immunogenetic background of islet cell antibody–positive nondiabetic schoolchildren. Ulm-Frankfurt population study. *Diabetes* **40**:1435–1439.
21. Bonifacio, E., P. J. Bingley, M. Shattock, B. M. Dean, D. Dunger, E. A. M. Gale, and G. F. Bottazzo. 1990. Quantification of islet-cell antibodies and prediction of insulin-dependent diabetes. *Lancet* **335**:147–149.
22. Bonnevie-Nielsen, V., M. L. Larsen, J. J. Frifelt, B. Michelsen, and A. Lernmark. 1989. Association of IDDM and attenuated response of 2',5'-oligoadenylate synthetase to yellow fever vaccine. *Diabetes* **38**:1636–1642.
23. Boucher, D. W., K. Hayashi, J. Rosenthal, and A. L. Notkins. 1975. Virus-induced diabetes mellitus. III. Influence of sex and strain of the host. *J. Infect. Dis.* **131**:462–466.
24. Bouter, K. P., R. J. A. Diepersloot, P. J. Wismans, et al. 1992. Humoral immune response to a yeast-derived hepatitis B vaccine in patients with type 1 diabetes mellitus. *Diabetic Med.* **9**:66–69.
25. Bruserud, O., J. Jervell, and E. Thorsby. 1985. HOLA-DR3 and -DR4 control T-lymphocyte responses to mumps and coxsackie B4 virus: studies on patients with type 1 (insulin-dependent) diabetes and healthy subjects. *Diabetologia* **28**:420–426.
26. Bruserud, O., and E. Thorsby. 1985. T lymphocyte responses to coxsackie B4 and mumps virus. I. Influence of HLA-DR restriction elements. *Tissue Antigens* **26**:41–50.
27. Bu, D. F., M. G. Erlander, B. C. Hitz, N. J. K. Tillakaratne, D. L. Kaufman, C. B. Wagner-McPherson, G. A. Evans, and A. J. Tobin. 1992. Two human glutamates decarboxylases, GAD 65 and GAD 67, are each en-

coded by a single gene. *Proc. Natl. Acad. Sci. USA* **89**:2115–2119.

28. **Buesa-Gomez, J., C. J. de la Torre, T. Dyrberger, M. Landin-Olsson, R. S. Mauseth, A. Lernmark, and M. B. A. Oldstone.** 1994. Failure to detect genomic viral sequences in pancreatic tissues from two children with acute-onset diabetes mellitus. *J. Med. Virol.* **42**:193–197.

29. **Burrows, R.** 1966. Studies on the carrier state of cattle exposed to foot-and-mouth disease virus. *J. Hyg. Camb.* **64**:81–90.

30. **Caggana, M., P. Chan, and A. Ramsingh.** 1993. Identification of a single amino acid residue in the capsid protein VP1 of coxsackievirus B4 that determines the virulent phenotype. *J. Virol.* **67**:4797–4803.

31. **Campbell, I. L., A. Cutri, D. Wilkinson, A. W. Boyd, and L. C. Harrison.** 1989. Intracellular adhesion molecule 1 is induced on isolated endocrine islet cells by cytokines but not by reovirus infection. *Proc. Natl. Acad. Sci. USA* **86**:4282.

32. **Cao, Y., and D. P. Schnurr.** 1988. Persistent infection of YAC-1 cells by coxsackie virus B3. *J. Gen. Virol.* **69**:59–65.

33. **Champsaur, H. F., G. F. Bottazzo, J. Bertrams, R. Assan, and C. Bach.** 1982. Virologic, immunologic, and genetic factors in insulin-dependent diabetes mellitus. *J. Pediatr.* **100**:15–20.

34. **Chase, H. P., M. A. Voss, N. Butler-Simon, S. Hoops, D. O'Brien, and M. J. Doberson.** 1987. Diagnosis of pre-type 1 diabetes. *J. Pediatr.* **111**:807–812.

35. **Chatterjee, N. K., J. Hou, P. Dockstader, and T. Charbonneau.** 1992. Coxsackievirus B4 infection alters thymic, splenic, and peripheral lymphocyte repertoire preceding onset of hyperglycemia in mice. *J. Med. Virol.* **38**:124–131.

36. **Chatterjee, N. K., C. Nejman, and I. Gerling.** 1988. Purification and characterization of a strain of coxsackievirus B4 of human origin that induces diabetes in mice. *J. Med. Virol.* **26**:57–69.

37. **Christau, B., and A. G. Molbak.** 1984. Further epidemiological evidence of a higher incidence level for the insulin-dependent diabetes mellitus in the older age groups. *Acta Endocrinol.* **95**(Suppl. 263):18.

38. **Craighead, J. E., S. A. Huber, and S. Sriram.** 1990. Animal models of picornavirus-induced autoimmune disease: their possible relevance to human disease. *Lab. Invest.* **63**:432–446.

39. **Craighead, J. E., and M. F. McLane.** 1968. Diabetes mellitus: induction in mice by encephalomyocarditis virus. *Science* **162**:913–915

40. **Craighead, J. E., and J. Steinke.** 1969. Temporary diabetes in mice caused by encephalomyocarditis virus. *Clin. Res.* **17**:380.

41. **Craighead, J. E., and J. Steinke.** 1971. Diabetes mellitus-like syndrome in mice infected with encephalomyocarditis virus. *Am. J. Pathol.* **63**:119–134.

42. **Cudworth, A. G., D. R. Gamble, G. B. B. White, R. Lendrum, J. C. Woodrow, and A. Bloom.** 1977. Aetiology of juvenile-onset diabetes: a prospective study. *Lancet* **i**:385–388.

42a. **Dahlquist, G., et al.** Unpublished data.

43. **D'Alessio, D. J.** 1992. A case control study of group B coxsackievirus immunoglobulin M antibody prevalence and HLA-DR antigens in newly diagnosed cases of insulin-dependent diabetes mellitus. *Am. J. Epidemiol.* **135**:1331–1338.

44. **D'Andrea, B. J., G. L. Wilson, and J. E. Craighead.** 1981. Effect of genetic obesity in mice on the induction of diabetes by encephalomyocarditis virus. *Diabetes* **30**:451.

45. **de la Torre, J. C., M. Davila, F. Sobrino, J. Ortin, and E. Domingo.** 1985. Establishment of cell lines persistently infected with foot-and-mouth disease virus. *Virology* **145**:24–35.

46. **Diabetes Epidemiology Research International Group.** 1988. Geographic patterns of childhood insulin-dependent diabetes mellitus. *Diabetes* **37**:1113–1119.

47. **Diabetes Epidemiology Research International Group.** 1990. Secular trends in incidence of childhood IDDM in 10 countries. *Diabetes* **39**:858–864.

48. **Diepersloot, R. J. A., K. P. Bouter, W. E. P. Beyer, J. L. B. Hoekstra, and N. Masurel.** 1987. Humoral immune response and delayed type hypersensitivity to influenza vaccine in patients with diabetes mellitus. *Diabetologia* **30**:97–100.

49. **Dippe, S. E., P. H. Bennett, M. Miller, J. E. Maynard, and K. R. Berquist.** 1975. Lack of causal association between coxsackie B4 virus infection and diabetes. *Lancet* **i**:1314–1317.

49a. **Dorman, J. S.** 1993. Personal communication.

50. **Dronfield, D. M.** 1993. Changes in serum insulin and islet cell antibodies following an outbreak of echovirus 4 in Glasgow. *Diabetic Med.* **10**(Suppl. 1):S41.

51. **Durruty, O., F. Ruiz, and M. Garcia de los Rios.** 1979. Age at diagnosis and seasonal variation in the onset of insulin-dependent diabetes in Chile (southern hemisphere). *Diabetologia* **17**:357–360.

52. **Eberhardt, M. S., D. K. Wagener, T. J. Orchard, R. E. LaPorte, D. E. Cavender,**

B. S. Rabin, R. W. Atchison, L. H. Kuller, A. L. Drash, and D. J. Becker. 1985. HLA heterogeneity of insulin-dependent diabetes mellitus at diagnosis. The Pittsburgh IDDM Study. *Diabetes* **34**:1247–1252.
53. Elias D., H. Prigozin, N. Polak, M. Rapoport, A. W. Lohse, and I. R. Cohen. 1994. Autoimmune diabetes induced by the β-cell toxin STZ. Immunity to the 60-kDa heat shock protein and to insulin. *Diabetes* **43**:992–998.
54. Erdo, S. L., and J. R. Wolff. 1990. Gamma-aminobutyric acid outside the mammalian brain. *J. Neurochem.* **54**:363–372.
55. Fohlman, J., J. Böhme, L. Rask, G. Frisk, H. Diderholm, G. Friman, and T. Tuvemo. 1987. Matching of host genotype and serotypes of coxsackie B virus in the development of juvenile diabetes. *Scand. J. Immunol.* **26**:105–110.
56. Forrest, J. M., M. A. Menser, and J. A. Burgess. 1971. High frequency of diabetes mellitus in young adults with congenital rubella. *Lancet* **ii**:332–334.
57. Foulis, A. K., M. A. Farquharson, S. O. Cameron, M. McGill, Schönke, and R. Kandolf. 1990. A search for the presence of the enteroviral capsid protein VP1 in pancreases of patients with type 1 (insulin-dependent) diabetes of coxsackieviral myocarditis. *Diabetologia* **33**:290–298.
58. Foulis, A. K., M. A. Farquharson, and R. Hardman. 1987. Aberrant expression of class II major histocompatibility complex molecules by B cells and hyperexpression of class I major histocompatibility complex molecules by insulin containing islets in type 1 (insulin-dependent) diabetes mellitus. *Diabetologia* **30**:333–343.
59. Foulis, A. K., M. A. Farquharson, and A. Meager. 1987. Immunoreactive α-interferon in insulin-secreting β cells in type 1 diabetes mellitus. *Lancet* **ii**:1423–1427.
60. Foulis, A. K., C. N. Liddle, M. A. Farquharson, J. A. Richmond, and R. S. Weir. 1986. The histopathology of the pancreas in type 1 (insulin-dependent) diabetes mellitus: a 25-year review of death in patients under 20 years of age in the United Kingdom. *Diabetologia* **20**:267–274.
61. Foulis, A. K., N. D. Francis, M. A. Farquharson, and A. Boylson. 1986. Massive synchronous B-cell necrosis causing type 1 (insulin-dependent) diabetes—a unique histopathological case report. *Diabetologia* **31**:46–50.
62. Friedman, A., and Y. Lorch. 1985. Theiler's virus infection: a model for multiple sclerosis. *Prog. Med. Virol.* **31**:43–48.
63. Friman, G., J. Fohlman, G. Frisk, H. Diderholm, U. Ewald, M. Kobbah, and T. Tuvemo. 1985. An incidence peak of juvenile diabetes. Relation to coxsackie B virus immune response. *Acta Paediatr. Scand.* (Suppl. 320):14–19.
64. Frisk, G., J. Fohlman, M. Kobbah, U. Ewald, T. Tuvemo, H. Diderholm, and G. Friman. 1985. High frequency of coxsackie-B-virus specific IgM in children developing type I diabetes during a period of high diabetes morbidity. *J. Med. Virol.* **17**:219–227.
65. Frisk, G., G. Friman, T. Tuvemo, J. Fohlman, and H. Diderholm. 1992. Coxsackie B virus IgM in children at onset of type 1 (insulin-dependent) diabetes mellitus: evidence for IgM induction by a recent or current infection. *Diabetologia* **35**:249–253.
66. Froeschle, J. E., P. M. Feorino, and H. M. Gelfand. 1966. A continuing surveillance of enterovirus infection in healthy children in six U.S. cities. II. Surveillance enterovirus isolates 1960–1963 and comparison with enterovirus isolates from cases of acute central nervous system disease. *Am. J. Epidemiol.* **83**:455–469.
67. Gamble, D. R. 1980. The epidemiology of insulin-dependent diabetes with particular reference to the relationship of virus infection to its etiology. *Epidemiol. Rev.* **2**:49–70.
68. Gamble, D.R., and H. Cumming. 1985. Coxsackie B virus and juvenile-onset insulin-dependent diabetes. *Lancet* **ii**:455–456.
69. Gamble, D. R., M. L. Kingsley, M. G. Fitzgerald, R. Bolton, and K. W. Taylor. 1969. Viral antibodies in diabetes mellitus. *Br. Med. J.* **3**:627–630.
70. Gamble, D. R., and K. W. Taylor. 1969. Seasonal incidence of diabetes mellitus. *Br. Med. J.* **3**:631–633.
71. Garchon, H.-J., P. Bedossa, L. Eloy, and J.-F. Bach. 1991. Identification and mapping to chromosome 1 of a susceptibility locus for periinsulitis in non-obese diabetic mice. *Nature* (London) **353**:260–262.
72. Garry, D. J., H. D. Coulter, M. G. Garry, and R. L. Sorenson. 1988. Immunoreactive immunolocalization of L-glutamate decarboxylase in rat pancreatic islets. *J. Histochem. Cytochem.* **36**:573–580.
73. Gepts, W. 1965. Pathologic anatomy of the pancreas in juvenile diabetes mellitus. *Diabetes* **14**:619–633.
74. Gerling, I., and N. K. Chatterjee. 1993. Lack of 64,000-M_r islet autoantigen overexpression and antibody development following coxsackievirus B4 infection in diabetes-resistant mice. *Autoimmunity* **14**:197–203.
75. Gerling, I., C. Nejman, and N. K.

Chatterjee. 1988. Effect of coxsackievirus B4 infection in mice on expression of 64,000-Mr autoantigen and glucose sensitivity of islets before development of hyperglycemia. *Diabetes* **37**:1419–1425.

76. **Ginsberg-Fellner, F., M. E. Witt, S. Yagihashi, M. J. Dobersen, F. Taub, B. Fedun, R. C. McEvoy, S. H. Roman, R. G. Davies, L. Z. Cooper, et al.** 1984. Congenital rubella syndrome as a model for type 1 (insulin-dependent) diabetes mellitus: increased prevalence of islet cell surface antibodies. *Diabetologia* **27**(Suppl. 1):87–89.

77. **Giron, D. J., and S. Yei.** 1993. Interference by a non-interferon-inducing subvariant of benign encephalomyelitis virus-B with the ability of EMCV-D to produce insulin-dependent diabetes mellitus in IRC Swiss male mice. *J. Interferon Res.* **13**:363–368.

78. **Gladish, R., W. Hofmann, and R. Waldherr.** 1976. Myocarditis and insulitis in coxsackievirus infection. *Z. Kardiol.* **65**:835–849.

79. **Gleason, R. E., C. B. Kahn, I. B. Funk, and J. E. Craighead.** 1982. Seasonal incidence of insulin-dependent diabetes in Massachusetts, 1964–1973. *Int. J. Epidemiol.* **11**:39–45.

80. **Gould, C. L., K. G. McMannama, N. J. Bigley, and D. J. Giron.** 1985. Virus-induced murine diabetes: enhancement by immunosuppression. *Diabetes* **34**:1217–1221.

81. **Greve, J. M., G. Davis, A. M. Meyer, C. P. Forte, S. C. Yost, C. W. Marlor, M. E. Kamarck, and A. McClelland.** 1989. The major human rhinovirus receptor is ICAM-1. *Cell* **56**:839.

82. **Groop, L. C., F. B. Bottazzo, and D. Doniach.** 1986. Islet cell antibodies identify latent type I diabetes in patients aged 35–75 at diagnosis. *Diabetes* **35**:237–241.

83. **Hagopian, W. A., S. McGrew, S. B. Kaliappan, A. E. Karlsen, and D. J. D'Allessio.** 1993. Recent coxsackie B virus infection associates with glutamic acid decarboxylase autoantibodies (GAD65 Ab) regardless of insulin-dependent diabetes (IDDM) status. *Am. Diabetes Assoc. 12th Int. Immunol. Diabetes Workshop.*

84. **Hamby, B. B., M. A. Pallansch, and O. M. Kew.** 1987. Reemergence of an epidemic coxsackievirus B5 genotype. *J. Infect. Dis.* **156**:288–292.

85. **Harrison, L. C., M. G. Honeymoon, H. J. DeAizpurua, R. S. Schmidli, P. G. Colman, B. D. Tait, and D. S. Cram.** 1993. Inverse relation between humoral and cellular immunity to glutamic acid decarboxylase in subjects at risk of insulin-dependent diabetes. *Lancet* **341**:1365–1369.

86. **Hartig, P. C., G. E. Madge, and S. R. Webb.** 1983. Diversity within a human isolate of coxsackie B4: relationship to viral-induced diabetes. *J. Med. Virol.* **11**:23–30.

87. **Haskins, K., and M. McDuffie.** 1990. Acceleration of diabetes in young NOD mice with a CD4$^+$ islet-specific T cell clone. *Science* **249**:1433–1436.

88. **Hayashi, K., D. W. Boucher, and A. L. Notkins.** 1974. Virus-induced diabetes mellitus. II. Relationship between β-cell damage and hyperglycemia in mice infected with encephalomyocarditis virus. *Am. J. Pathol.* **75**:91–102.

89. **Hayward, J. C., S. M. Gillespie, K. M. Kaplan, R. Packer, M. Pallansch, S. Plotkin, and L. B. Schonberger.** 1989. Outbreak of poliomyelitis-like paralysis associated with enterovirus 71. *Pediatr. Infect. Dis.* **8**:611–616.

90. **Helfand, R. F., H. Gary, C. Freeman, L. Anderson, Pittsburgh Diabetes Research Group, and M. Pallansch.** 1994. Association between enteroviruses and type 1 diabetes mellitus, Pittsburgh, Pennsylvania. *Colo. Dis. Bull.* **21**:4.

91. **Hellqvist, L. N. B., K. W. Taylor, and S. Zaluzny.** 1981. Selective disorganisation of biochemical function in B cells of islets of Langerhans infected by EMC-M virus in tissue culture. *FEBS Lett.* **132**:215–218.

92. **Helmke, K.** 1987. In Y. Becker (ed.), *Virus Infections and Diabetes Mellitus*, p. 127–142. Matinus Nijhoff Publishing, Boston.

93. **Hierholzer, J. C., and W. A. Farris.** 1974. Follow-up of children infected in a coxsackievirus B3 and B4 outbreak: no evidence of diabetes mellitus. *J. Infect. Dis.* **129**:741–746.

94. **Hou, J., S. Sheikh, D. L. Martin, and N. K. Chatterjee.** 1993. Coxsackie virus B4 alters pancreatic glutamate decarboxylase expression in mice soon after infection. *J. Autoimmun.* **6**:529–542.

95. **Huff, J. C., J. C. Hierholzer, and W. A. Farris.** 1974. An "outbreak" of juvenile diabetes mellitus: consideration of a viral etiology. *Am. J. Epidemiol.* **100**:277–287.

95a. **Hyöty, H., et al.** Unpublished data.

96. **Hyöty, H., M. Hiltunen, A. Reunanen, et al.** 1993. Decline of mumps antibodies in type 1 (insulin-dependent) diabetic children and a plateau in the rising incidence of type 1 diabetes after introduction of the mumps-measles-rubella vaccine in Finland. *Diabetologia* **36**:1303–1308.

97. **Hyöty, H., L. Räsänen, M. Hiltunen, M.**

Lehtinen, T. Huupponen, and P. Leinikki. 1991. Decreased antibody reactivity to Epstein-Barr virus capsid antigen in type 1 (insulin-dependent) diabetes mellitus. *APMIS* **99:**359–363.

98. **Ihm, S. H., K. U. Lee, R. G. McArthur, and J. W. Yoon.** 1990. Predisposing effect of anti-β-cell autoimmune process in NOD mice on the induction of diabetes by environmental insults. *Diabetologia* **33:**709–712.

99. **Japan, Poland, the Netherlands and Pittsburgh Childhood Diabetes Research Groups.** 1990. How frequently do children die at the onset of insulin-dependent diabetes? Analyses of registry data from Japan, Poland, the Netherlands and Allegheny County, Pennsylvania. *Diabetes Nutr. Metab.* **3:**57–62.

100. **Jenson, A. B., H. S. Rosenberg, and A. L. Notkins.** 1980. Pancreatic islet-cell damage in children with fatal viral infections. *Lancet* **ii:**354–358.

101. **Johnston, C., B. A. Millward, P. Hoskins, R. D. Leslie, G. F. Bottazzo, and D. A. Pyke.** 1989. Islet-cell antibodies as predictors of the later development of type 1 (insulin-dependent) diabetes. A study in identical twins. *Diabetologia* **32:**382–386.

102. **Joner, G., and O. Sovik.** 1991. The incidence of type 1 (insulin-dependent) diabetes mellitus 15–29 years in Norway 1978–1982. *Diabetologia* **34:**271–274.

103. **Jones, D. B., P. J. McLaughlin, N. Armstrong, M. Yeung, and A. Coulson.** 1992. Does coxsackie B4 virus infection induce GAD and HSP65 autoreactivity in type 1 diabetes? *Diabetic Med.* **9(Suppl. 2):**524A.

104. **Kang, Y., and J. W. Yoon.** 1993. A genetically determined host factor controlling susceptibility to encephalomyocarditis virus-induced diabetes in mice. *J. Gen. Virol.* **74:**1207–1213.

105. **Kaptur, P. E., D. C. Thomas, and D. J. Giron.** 1989. Differing attachment of diabetogenic and nondiabetogenic variants of encephalomyocarditis virus to β-cells. *Diabetes* **38:**1103–1108.

106. **Karjalainen, J. K.** 1990. Islet cell antibodies as predictive markers for IDDM in children with high background incidence of disease. *Diabetes* **39:**1144–1150.

107. **Karounos, D. G., J. S. Wolinsky, and J. W. Thomas.** 1993. Monoclonal antibody to rubella virus capsid protein recognizes a beta-cell antigen. *J. Immunol.* **150:**3080–3085.

108. **Kaufman, D. L., M. Clare-Salzler, J. Tian, T. Forsthuber, G. S. P. Ting, P. Robinson, M. A. Atkinson, E. E. Sercarz, A. J. Tobin, and P. V. Lehmann.** 1993. Spontaneous loss of T cell self tolerance to glutamate decarboxylase is a key event in the pathogenesis of murine insulin-dependent diabetes. *Nature* (London) **366:**69–72.

109. **Kaufman, D. L., M. G. Erlander, M. Clare-Salzler, M. A. Atkinson, N. K. Maclaren, and A. J. Tobin.** 1992. Autoimmunity to two forms of glutamate decarboxylase in insulin dependent diabetes mellitus. *J. Clin. Invest.* **89:**283–292.

110. **Khoury, M. J., W. D. Flanders, S. Greenland, and M. J. Adams.** 1989. On the measurement of susceptibility in epidemiologic studies. *Am. J. Epidemiol.* **129:**183–190.

111. **Kim, J. W., W. Richter, H. J. Aanstoot, Y. Shi, Q. Fu, R. Rajotte, G. Warnock, and S. Baekkeskov.** 1993. Differential expression of GAD65 and GAD67 in human, rat, and mouse pancreatic islets. *Diabetes* **42:**1799–1808.

112. **King, M. L., D. Bidwell, A. Voller, J. Bryant, and J. E. Banatvala.** 1983. Role of coxsackie B viruses in insulin-dependent diabetes mellitus. *Lancet* **ii:**915–916.

113. **Kogon, A., I. Spigland, T. E. Frothingham, L. Elveback, C. Williams, C. E. Hall, and J. P. Fox.** 1969. The virus watch program: a continuing surveillance of viral infections in metropolitan New York families. VII. Observations on viral excretion, seroimmunity, intrafamiliar spread and illness association in coxsackie and echovirus infections. *Am. J. Epidemiol.* **89:**51–61.

114. **Kostraba, J. N., E. C. Gay, Y. Cai, K. J. Cruickshanks, M. J. Rewers, G. J. Klingensmith, H. P. Chase, and R. F. Hamman.** 1992. Incidence of insulin-dependent diabetes mellitus in Colorado. *Epidemiology* **3:**232–238.

115. **Lampeter, E. F., I. Seifert, D. Lohmann, J. W. Heise, J. Bertrams, M. R. Christie, V. Kolb-Bachofen, and H. Kolb.** 1994. Inflammatory islet damage in patients bearing HLA-DR3 and/or DR4 haplotypes does not lead to islet autoimmunity. *Diabetologia* **37:**471–475.

116. **Landin-Olsson, M., A. Karlsson, G. Dahlquist, L. Blom, A. Lernmark, and G. Sundkvist.** 1989. Islet cell and other organ specific autoantibodies in all children developing type 1 (insulin-dependent) diabetes mellitus in Sweden during one year and in matched control children. *Diabetologia* **32:**387–395.

117. **Lederman, M. M., G. Schifman, and H. M. Rodman.** 1981. Pneumococcal immunisation in adult diabetics. *Diabetes* **30:**119–121.

118. **Lemon, S. M., P. C. Murphy, P. A. Shields, L. Ping, S. M. Feinstone, T. Cromeans,

and R. W. Jansen. 1991. Antigenic and genetic variation in cytopathic hepatitis A virus variants arising during persistent infection: Evidence for genetic recombination. *J. Virol.* **65**:2056–2065.
119. **Lennette, E. H., T. T. Shinomoto, N. J. Schmidt, and R. L. Magoffin.** 1960. Observations on the neutralizing antibody response to group B coxsackie viruses in patients with central nervous system disease. *J. Immunol.* **86**:257–266.
120. **Levy-Marchal, C., J. Tichet, I. Fajardy, F. Dubois, and P. Czernichow.** 1992. Follow-up of children from a background population with high ICA titres. *Diabetologia* **35**(Suppl. 1):A32.
121. **Libman, I., T. Songer, and R. LaPorte.** 1993. How many people in the U.S. have IDDM? *Diabetes Care* **16**:841–842.
122. **Like, A. A., D. L. Guberski, and L. Butler.** 1991. Influence of environmental viral agents on frequency and tempo of diabetes mellitus in BB/Wor rats. *Diabetes* **40**:259–262.
123. **Loria, R. M., L. B. Montgomery, L. Corey, and V. M. Chinchilli.** 1984. Influence of diabetes mellitus heredity on susceptibility to Coxsackie virus B4. *Arch. Virol.* **81**:251–262.
124. **Lowis, G. W.** 1988. Ethnic factors in multiple sclerosis: a review and critique of the epidemiological literature. *Int. J. Epidemiol.* **17**:14–20.
125. **Ludvigsson, J., and A. O. Afoke.** 1989. Seasonality of type 1 (insulin-dependent) diabetes mellitus: values of C-peptide, insulin antibodies and haemoglobin A_{1c} show evidence of a more rapid loss of insulin secretion in epidemic patients. *Diabetologia* **32**:84–91.
126. **Maclaren, N., G. Horne, R. Spillar, L. Brown, J. Silverstein, S. Shah, J. Malone, and W. Riley.** 1990. The feasibility of using ICA to predict IDD in U.S. school children. *Diabetes* **39**(Suppl. 1):122A.
127. **Maeda, T., T. Sumida, K. Kurosawa, H. Tomioka, I. Itoh, S. Yoshida, and T. Koike.** 1991. T-lymphocyte receptor repertoire of infiltrating T-lymphocytes into NOD mouse pancreas. *Diabetes* **40**:1580–1585.
128. **Matteucci, D., M. Paglianti, A. M. Giangregorio, M. R. Capobianchi, F. Dianzani, and M. Bendinelli.** 1985. Group B coxsackieviruses readily establish persistent infections in human lymphoid cell lines. *J. Virol.* **56**:651–654.
128a. **McDevitt, H., et al.** Unpublished observation.
129. **McDuffie, M., and A. Ostrowska.** 1993. Superantigen-like effects and incidence of diabetes in NOD mice. *Diabetes* **42**:1094–1098.
130. **McKinney, R. E., S. L. Katz, and C. M. Wilfert.** 1987. Chronic enteroviral meningoencephalitis in agammaglobulinemic patients. *Rev. Infect. Dis.* **9**:334–356.
131. **Melton, J. L., et al.** 1983. Incidence of diabetes mellitus by clinical type. *Diabetes Care* **6**:75–86.
132. **Mendelsohn, C. L., E. Wimmer, and V. R. Racaniello.** 1989. Cellular receptor for poliovirus: molecular cloning, nucleotide sequence, and expression of a new member of the immunoglobulin superfamily. *Cell* **56**:855.
133. **Menser, M. A., J. M. Forrest, and R.D. Bransby.** 1978. Rubella infection and diabetes mellitus. *Lancet* **i**:57–60.
134. **Modlin, J. F., and M. Bowman.** 1987. Perinatal transmission of coxsackievirus B3 in mice. *J. Infect. Dis.* **156**:21–25.
135. **Monif, G. R. G., G. B. Avery, S. B. Korones, and J. L. Sever.** 1965. Post-mortem isolation of rubella virus from three children with rubella-syndrome defects. *Lancet* **i**:723–724.
136. **Montgomery, L., D. Gordon, K. George, and E. Maratos-Flier.** 1991. Coxsackie infection of insulinoma cells leads to viral latency and altered insulin and class I MHC expression. *Diabetes* **40**(Suppl. 1):150A.
137. **Montgomery, L. B., R. M. Loria, and V. M. Chinchilli.** 1990. Immunodeficiency as primary phenotype of diabetes mutation db: studies with coxsackievirus B4. *Diabetes* **39**:675–682.
138. **Morrow, P. L., A. Freedman, and J. E. Craighead.** 1980. Testosterone effect on experimental mellitus in encephalomyocarditis (EMC) virus-infected mice. *Diabetologia* **18**:247.
139. **Nakano, N., H. Kikutani, H. Nishimoto, and T. Kishimoto.** 1991. T cell receptor V gene usage of islet β cell-reactive T cells is not restricted in non-obese diabetic mice. *J. Exp. Med.* **173**:1091–1097.
140. **Nathanson, N., and J. Martin.** 1979. The epidemiology of poliomyelitis: enigmas surrounding its appearance, epidemicity and disappearance. *Am. J. Epidemiol.* **110**:672–692.
141. **Nicoletti, F., G. Scalia, M. Lunetta, F. Concorelli, M. Di Mauro, W. Barcellini, S. Stracuzzi, M. Pagano, and P. L. Meroni.** 1990. Correlation between islet cell antibodies and anti-cytomegalovirus IgM and IgG antibodies in healthy first-degree relatives of type 1 (insulin-dependent) diabetic patients. *Clin. Immunol. Immunopathol.* **55**:139–147.
142. **Niklasson, B. S., M. J. Dobersen, C. J. Peters, W. H. Ennis, and E. Möller.** 1985. An outbreak of coxsackievirus B infection followed by one case of diabetes mellitus. *Scand.*

J. Infect. Dis. **17:**15-18.
142a. Norris, J. M., et al. Unpublished observations.
143. **Notkins, A. L., T. Onodera, and B. S. Prabhakar.** 1984. Virus-induced autoimmunity, p. 210-215. *In* A. L. Notkins (ed.), *Concepts in Viral Pathogenesis*. Springer, New York.
144. **Notkins, A. L., and J. W. Yoon.** 1982. Virus-induced diabetes in mice prevented by a live attenuated vaccine. *N. Engl. J. Med.* **1:**186.
145. **Nyström, L., G. Dahlquist, M. Rewers, and S. Wall.** 1990. The Swedish Childhood Diabetes Study: an analysis of the temporal variation in diabetes incidence 1978-1987. *Int. J. Epidemiol.* **19:**141-146.
146. **Ohashi, P. S., S. Oehen, P. Aichele, H. Pricher, B. Odermatt, P. Herrera, Y. Higuchi, K. Buerki, H. Hengartner, and R. M. Zinkernagel.** 1993. Induction of diabetes is influenced by the infectious virus and local expression of MHC class I and tumor necrosis factor-α. *J. Immunol.* **150:**5185-5194.
147. **Ohashi, P. S., S. Oehen, K. Buerki, H. Pircher, C. T. Ohashi, B. Odermatt, B. Malissen, R. M. Zinkernagel, and H. Hengartner.** 1991. Ablation of "tolerance" and induction of diabetes by virus infection in viral antigen transgenic mice. *Cell* **65:**305-317.
148. **Oksenberg, J. R., S. Stuart, A. B. Begovich, R. B. Bell, H. A. Erlich, L. Steinman, and C. C. A. Bernard.** 1990. Limited heterogeneity of rearranged T-cell receptor Vα transcripts in brains of multiple sclerosis patients. *Nature* (London) **345:**344-346.
149. **Oldstone, M. B. A.** 1987. Molecular mimicry and autoimmune disease. *Cell* **50:**819-820.
150. **Oldstone, M. B. A.** 1988. Prevention of type 1 diabetes in nonobese diabetic mice by virus infection. *Science* **239:**500-502.
151. **Oldstone, M. B. A.** 1990. Viruses as therapeutic agents. I. Treatment of nonobese insulin-dependent diabetes mice with virus prevents insulin-dependent diabetes mellitus while maintaining general immune competence. *J. Exp. Med.* **171:**2077-2089.
152. **Oldstone, M. B. A., M. Nerenberg, P. Southern, J. Price, and H. Lewicki.** 1991. Virus infection triggers insulin-dependent diabetes mellitus in a transgenic model: role of anti-self (virus) immune response. *Cell* **65:**319-331.
153. **Oldstone, M. B. A., P. Southern, M. Rodriguez, and P. W. Lampert.** 1984. Virus persists in beta-cells and islets of Langerhans and is associated with chemical manifestation of diabetes. *Science* **224:**1440-1444.
154. **O'Leary, L. A., J. S. Dorman, R. E. LaPorte, T. J. Orchard, D. J. Becker, L. H. Kuller, M. S. Eberhardt, D. E. Cavender, B. S. Rabin, and A. L. Drash.** 1991. Familial and sporadic insulin-dependent diabetes: evidence for heterogeneous etiologies? *Diabetes Res. Clin. Pract.* **14:**183-190.
155. **Onodera, T., A. Toniolo, U. R. Ray, A. A. Jenson, R. A. Knazek, and A. L. Notkins.** 1981. Virus-induced diabetes mellitus. XX. Polyendocrinopathy and autoimmunity. *J. Exp. Med.* **153:**1547-1573.
156. **Onodera, T., J. W. Yoon, K. K. Brown, and A. L. Notkins.** 1978. Evidence for a single locus controlling susceptibility to virus-induced diabetes mellitus. *Nature* (London) **274:**693-696.
157. **Orchard, T. J., R. W. Atchison, D. Becker, B. Rabin, M. Eberhardt, L. H. Kuller, R. E. LaPorte, and D. Cavender.** 1983. Coxsackie infection and diabetes. *Lancet* **ii:**631. (Letter.)
158. **Orchard, T. J., D. J. Becker, R. W. Atchison, R. E. LaPorte, D. K. Wagener, B. S. Rabin, L. H. Kuller, and A. L. Drash.** 1983. The development of type 1 (insulin-dependent) diabetes mellitus: two contrasting presentations. *Diabetologia* **25:**89-92.
159. **Owerbach, D., and K. H. Gabbay.** 1993. Localization of a type 1 diabetes susceptibility locus to the variable tandem repeat region flanking the insulin gene. *Diabetes* **42:**1708-1714.
160. **Pacsa, S., and J. Werblinska.** 1971. Natural immunity of Ghanaian children to polio and coxsackievirus: brief report. *Arch. Gesamte Virusforsch.* **33:**192-193.
161. **Pak, C. Y., E. Hyone-Myong, R. G. McArthur, and J. W. Yoon.** 1988. Association of cytomegalovirus infection with autoimmune type 1 diabetes. *Lancet* **ii:**1-3.
162. **Paliard, X., S. G. West, J. A. Lafferty, J. R. Clements, J. W. Kappler, P. Marrack, and B. L. Kotzin.** 1991. Evidence for the effects of a superantigen in rheumatoid arthritis. *Science* **253:**325-329.
163. **Palmer, J. P., M. K. Cooney, R. H. Ward, J. A. Hansen, J. B. Brodsky, C. G. Ray, J. R. Crossley, C. M. Asplin, and R. H. Williams.** 1982. Reduced coxsackie antibody titres in type I (insulin-dependent) diabetic patients presenting during an outbreak of coxsackie B3 and B4 infection. *Diabetologia* **22:**426-429.
164. **Petersen, K.-G., P. Heilmeyer, and L. Kerp.** 1975. Synthesis of proinsulin and large glucagon immunoreactivity in isolated islets of Langerhans from EMC virus infected mice. *Diabetologia* **11:**21-25.
165. **Peterson, J. S., S. Russel, M. O. Marshall, H. Kofod, K. Buschard, A. E. Cambon,**

A. E. Karlsen, E. Boel, W. A. Hagopian, K. R. Hejnaes, A. Moody, T. Dyrberg, A. E. Lernmark, O. D. Madsen, and B. K. Michelsen. 1993. Differential expression of glutamate decarboxylase in rat and human islets. *Diabetes* **42**:484–495.
166. Pietropaolo, M., and G. S. Eisenbarth. 1994. Biochemical determination of antibodies to three recombinant human autoantigens: high predictive value and stability of patterns. *Diabetes* **43**(Suppl. 1):153A.
167. Pilcher, C. C., K. Dickens, and R. B. Elliott. 1991. ICA only develop in early childhood. *Diabetes Res. Clin. Pract.* **14**(Suppl. 1):s82.
168. Pipeleers, D., and Z. Ling. 1992. Pancreatic beta cells in insulin-dependent diabetes. *Diabetes Metab. Rev.* **8**:209–227.
169. Pociot, F., R. Bergholdt, J. Johannsen, and J. Nerup. 1994. Genetic susceptibility to IDDM: chromosome 6p versus chromosome 2q. *Diabetologia* **37**(Suppl. 1):A6.
170. Portwood, N. D., and K. W. Taylor. 1990. Coxsackie B4 virus-induced changes in mouse pancreatic β-cell mRNAs. *Biochem. Soc. Trans.* **18**:1264.
171. Pozzilli, P., P. Arduini, N. Visalli, et al. 1987. Reduced protection against hepatitis B virus following vaccination in patients with type I (insulin dependent) diabetes. *Diabetologia* **30**:817–819.
172. Prabhakar, B. S., M. V. Haspel, P. R. McClintock, and A. L. Notkins. 1982. High frequency of antigenic variants among naturally occurring human coxsackie B4 virus isolates identified by monoclonal antibodies. *Nature* (London) **300**:374–376.
173. Prather, S. L., R. Dagan, J. A. Jenista, and M. A. Menegus. 1984. The isolation of enteroviruses from blood: a comparison of four processing methods. *J. Med. Virol.* **14**:221–227.
174. Ramsingh, A., J. Slack, J. Silkworth, and A. Hixson. 1989. Severity of disease induced by a pancreatropic coxsackie B4 virus correlates with the H-2Kq locus of the major histocompatibility complex. *Virus Res.* **14**:347–358.
175. Ratzmann, K. P., J. Strese, S. Witt, H. Berling, H. Kielacker, and D. Michaelis. 1984. Mumps infection and insulin-dependent diabetes mellitus (IDDM). *Diabetes Care* **7**:170–173.
176. Rayfield, E. J., and K. Ishimura. 1987. Environmental factors and insulin dependent diabetes mellitus. *Diabetes Metab. Rev.* **3**:925–957.
177. Rewers, M., R. E. LaPorte, H. King, and J. Tuomilehto. 1988. Trends in the prevalence and incidence of diabetes: insulin-dependent diabetes mellitus in childhood. *World Health Stat. Q.* **41**:179–189.
178. Rewers, M., R. LaPorte, M. Walczak, K. Dmochowski, and E. Bogaczynska. 1987. Apparent epidemic of insulin-dependent diabetes mellitus in midwestern Poland. *Diabetes* **36**:106–113.
179. Rewers, M., M. A. Pallansch, E. Bogaczynska, S. L. Patrick, L. A. Anderson, M. Walczak, and R. E. LaPorte. 1990. Conflicting evidence for enterovirus as the cause of childhood diabetes epidemic in Poland. *Diabetologia* **33**(Suppl. 1):A198.
180. Richter, W., T. Mertens, B. Schoel, S. Wolfahrt, P. Muir, W. A. Scherbaum, and B. O. Boehm. 1994. Autoantibodies to glutamate decarboxylase detect no molecular mimicry to viral antigens or heat shock protein 60. *Diabetologia* **37**(Suppl. 1):A63.
181. Riley, W. J., N. K. MacLaren, J. Krischer, R. P. Spillar, J. H. Silverstein, D. A. Schatz, S. Schwartz, J. Malone, S. Shah, C. Vadheim, and J. I. Rotter. 1990. A prospective study of the development of diabetes in relatives of patients with insulin-dependent diabetes. *N. Engl. J. Med.* **323**:1167–1172.
182. Rose, N. R., and D. E. Griffin. 1991. Virus-induced autoimmunity, p. 247–272. *In* N. Talal (ed.), *Molecular Autoimmunity*. Academic Press Ltd., London.
183. Rossmann, M. G., and A. C. Palmenberg. 1988. Conservation of the putative receptor attachment site in picornaviruses. *Virology* **164**:373–382.
184. Rotbart, H. A. 1991. Nucleic acid detection systems for enteroviruses. *Clin. Microbiol. Rev.* **4**:156–168.
185. Sairenji, T., M. Daibata, C. H. Sorli, et al. 1991. Relating homology between the Epstein-Barr virus BOLF1 and HLA-DQw8 beta chain to recent onset type 1-dependent diabetes mellitus. *Diabetologia* **34**:33–39.
186. Salvato, M., P. Borrow, E. Shimomaye, and M. B. A. Oldstone. 1991. Molecular basis of viral persistence: a single amino acid change in the glycoprotein of lymphocytic choriomeningitis virus is associated with suppression of the antiviral cytotoxic T-lymphocytep response and establishment of persistence. *J. Virol.* **65**:1863–1869.
187. Santamaria, P., C. Lewis, J. Jessurun, D. E. Sutherland, and J. J. Barbosa. 1994. Skewed T-cell receptor usage junctional and heterogeneity among isletitis αβ and γδ T-cells in human IDDM. *Diabetes* **43**:599–606.
188. Santamaria, P., R. E. Nakhleh, D. E. Sutherland, and J. J. Barbosa. 1992. Char-

acterization of T lymphocytes infiltrating human pancreas allograft affected by isletitis and recurrent diabetes. *Diabetes* **41**:53–61.
189. **Scherbaum, W. A., W. Hampl, P. Muir, M. Glück, J. Seißler, H. Egle, H. Hauner, B. O. Boehm, E. Heinze, J. E. Banatvala, and E. F. Pfeiffer.** 1991. No association between islet cell antibodies and coxsackie B, mumps, rubella and cytomegalovirus antibodies in non-diabetic individuals aged 7-19 years. *Diabetologia* **34**:835–838.
190. **Schernthaner, G., J. E. Banatvala, W. Scherbaum, J. Bryant, M. Borkenstein, E. Schober, and W. R. Mayr.** 1985. Coxsackie B virus specific IgM responses, complement-fixing islet cell antibodies, HLA DR antigens, and C-peptide secretion in insulin-dependent diabetes mellitus. *Lancet* **ii**:630–632.
191. **See, D. M., and J. G. Tilles.** 1993. WIN 54954 treatment of mice infected with a diabetogenic strain of group B coxsackievirus. *Antimicrob. Agents Chemother.* **37**:1593–1598.
192. **Sharief, M. K., R. Hentges, and M. Ciardi.** 1991. Intrathecal immune response in patients with the post-polio syndrome. *N. Engl. J. Med.* **325**:749–755.
193. **Songer, T. J.** 1990. Health services and costing in diabetes. *Med. J. Aust.* **152**:115–117.
194. **Spinas, G. A., L. Matter, T. Wilkin, O. Staffelbach, and W. Berger.** 1988. Islet-cell and insulin autoantibodies in first-degree relatives of type I diabetics: a 5-year follow-up study in a Swiss population. *Adv. Exp. Med. Biol.* **246**:209–214.
195. **Stanway, G.** 1990. Structure, function and evolution of picornaviruses. *J. Gen. Virol.* **71**:2483–2501.
196. **Staunton, D. E., V. J. Merluzzi, R. Rothlein, R. Barton, S. D. Marlin, and T. A. Springer.** 1989. A cell adhesion molecule, IAMC-1, is the major surface receptor for rhinoviruses. *Cell* **56**:849.
197. **Suenaga, K., and J. W. Yoon.** 1988. Association of beta-cell-specific expression of endogenous retrovirus with development of insulitis and diabetes in NOD mouse. *Diabetes* **37**:1722–1726.
198. **Sussman, M. L., L. Stauss, and U. L. Hodes.** 1959. Fatal coxsackie B virus infections in the newborn. Report of case with necropsy findings and brief review of the literature. *Am. J. Dis. Child.* **97**:483–492.
199. **Szopa, T. M., D. M. Dronfield, T. Ward, and K. W. Taylor.** 1989. In vivo infection of mice with coxsackie B4 virus induces long-term functional changes in pancreatic islets with minimal alteration in blood glucose. *Diabetic Med.* **6**:314–319.
200. **Szopa, T. M., D. R. Gamble, and K. W. Taylor.** 1986. Coxsackie B4 virus induces short-term changes in the metabolic functions of mouse pancreatic islets in vitro. *Cell Biochem. Funct.* **4**:181–189.
201. **Szopa, T. M., P. A. Titchener, N. D. Portwood, and K. W. Taylor.** 1993. Diabetes mellitus due to viruses—some recent developments. *Diabetologia* **36**:687–695.
202. **Szopa, T. M., T. Ward, D. M. Dronfield, N. D. Portwood, and K. W. Taylor.** 1990. Coxsackie B4 viruses with the potential to damage β-cells of the islets are present in clinical isolates. *Diabetologia* **33**:325–328.
203. **Szopa, T. M., T. Ward, and K. W. Taylor.** 1992. Disturbance of mouse pancreatic β-cell function following echo 4 virus infection. *Biochem. Soc. Trans.* **20**:3155.
204. **Thivolet, C., B. Beaufrere, H. Betuel, L. Gebuhrer, P. Chatelain, A. Durand, J. Tourniaire, and R. Francois.** 1988. Islet cell and insulin autoantibodies in subjects at high risk for development of type 1 (insulin-dependent) diabetes mellitus: the Lyon family study. *Diabetologia* **31**:741–746.
204a.**Tian, J., et al.** Submitted for publication.
205. **Tilzey, A. J., M. Signy, and J. E. Banatvala.** 1986. Persistent coxsackie B virus specific IgM response in patients with recurrent pericarditis. *Lancet* **i**:1491.
206. **Tisch, R., X. D. Yang, S. M. Singer, R. S. Liblau, L. Fugger, and H. McDevitt.** 1993. Immune response to glutamic acid decarboxylase correlates with insulitis in non-obese diabetic mice. *Nature* (London) **366**:72–75.
207. **Todd, J. A.** 1990. The role of MHC class II genes in susceptibility to insulin-dependent diabetes mellitus. *Curr. Top. Microbiol. Immunol.* **164**:17–40.
208. **Tolbert, M., and D. J. Giron.** 1994. Persistence of the D variant of encephalomyocarditis virus in the ICR-Swiss mouse. *Proc. Soc. Exp. Biol. Med.* **205**:124–131.
209. **Toniolo, A., T. Onodera, G. Jordan, J. W. Yoon, and A. L. Notkins.** 1982. Virus-induced diabetes mellitus. Glucose abnormalities produced in mice by the six members of the coxsackie B virus group. *Diabetes* **31**:496–499.
210. **Toniolo, A., T. Onodera, J. W. Yoon, and A. L. Notkins.** 1980. Induction of diabetes by cumulative environmental insults from viruses and chemicals. *Nature* (London) **288**:383–385.
210a.**Trucco, M.** Unpublished observations.
211. **Trucco, M., C. Ricordi, E. Weidmann, H. Rodriquez-Rio, G. Trucco, and D. Finegold.** 1993. Involvement of superantigens

in the etiology of IDDM. *Diabetes* **42**(Suppl. 1):4A.
212. Tuomi, T., L. C. Groop, P. Z. Zimmet, M. J. Rowley, W. Knowles, and I. R. Mackay. 1993. Antibodies to glutamic acid decarboxylase reveal latent autoimmune diabetes mellitus in adults with a non-insulin-dependent onset of disease. *Diabetes* **42**:359–362.
213. Tuvemo, T., G. Dahlquist, G. Frisk, L. Blom, G. Friman, M. Landin-Olsson, and H. Dierholm. 1989. The Swedish childhood diabetes study. III. IgM against coxsackie B viruses in newly diagnosed type 1 (insulin-dependent) diabetic children—no evidence of increased antibody frequency. *Diabetologia* **32**:745–747.
214. Tuvemo, T., G. Frisk, G. Friman, J. Ludvigsson, and H. Diderholm. 1988. IgM against coxsackie B viruses in children developing type I diabetes mellitus—a seven year retrospective study. *Diabetes Res.* **9**:125–129.
215. Ujevich, M. M., and R. Jaffe. 1980. Pancreatic cell damage. Its occurrence in neonatal coxsackie virus encephalomyocarditis. *Arch. Pathol. Lab. Med.* **104**:438–441.
216. Uriarte, A., E. Cabrera, R. Ventura, and J. Vargas. 1987. Islet cell antibodies and ECHO-4 virus infection. *Diabetologia* **30**(Suppl. 1):590A.
217. Vadheim, C. M., A. Zeidler, J. I. Rotter, M. Langbaum, I. A. Shulman, M. R. Spencer, G. Costin, W. J. Riley, and N. K. MacLaren. 1989. Different HLA haplotypes in Mexican Americans with IDDM. *Diabetes Care* **12**:497–500.
218. Vella, C., A. J. Easton, P. R. Eglin, C. L. Brown, and L. Perry. 1991. Coxsackie virus B4 infection of the mouse pancreas. I. Detection of virus-specific RNA in the pancreas by in situ hybridization. *J. Med. Virol.* **35**:46–49.
219. Vento, S., T. Garofano, G. DiPerri, L. Dolci, E. Concia, and D. Bassetti. 1991. Identification of hepatitis A virus as a trigger for autoimmune chronic hepatitis type 1 in susceptible individuals. *Lancet* **337**:1181–1187.
220. Vialettes, B., P. Demicco, C. Badier, J. Niccoline, and V. Lassmann-Vague. 1987. Anti-coxsackie B IgG and IgM antibodies in first degree relatives of type 1 (insulin-dependent) diabetic patients: lack of association with islet cell antibodies. *Diabetologia* **30**(Suppl. 1):594A.
221. Wagener, D. K., J. M. Sacks, R. E. LaPorte, and J. M. MacGregor. 1982. The Pittsburgh study of insulin-dependent diabetes mellitus. Risk for diabetes among relatives of IDDM. *Diabetes* **31**:136–144.
222. Wagenknecht, L. E., J. M. Roseman, and W. H. Herman. 1991. Increased incidence of insulin-dependent diabetes mellitus following an epidemic of coxsackievirus B5. *Am. J. Epidemiol.* **133**:1024–1031.
223. Ward, T., J. Clemens, and K. W. Taylor. 1990. Effects of a diabetogenic strain of encephalomyocarditis virus on protein synthesis in mouse islets of langerhans. *Biochem. J.* **270**:777–781.
224. Warram, J. H., B. C. Martin, and A. S. Krolewski. 1991. Risk of IDDM in children of diabetic mothers decreases with increasing maternal age at pregnancy. *Diabetes* **40**:1679–1984.
225. Waters, S. H., J. J. O'Neil, D. T. Melican, and M. C. Appel. 1992. Multiple TCR Vß usage by infiltrates of young NOD mouse islets of Langerhans. *Diabetes* **41**:308–312.
226. Webb, S. R., R. M. Loria, G. E. Madge, and S. Kibrick. 1976. Susceptibility of mice to group B coxsackie virus is influenced by diabetic gene. *J. Exp. Med.* **143**:1239–1248.
227. Wegner, V., A. Kewitsch, M. Madauss, L. Döhner, and H. Zühlke. 1985. Hyperglycemia in BALB/c mice after pretreatment with one subdiabetogenic dose of streptozotocin and subsequent infection with a coxsackie B4 strain. *Biomed. Biochem. Acta* **44**:21–27.
228. Weinberg, C. R., T. L. Dornan, J. A. Hansen, P. K. Raghu, and J. P. Palmer. 1984. HLA-related heterogeneity in seasonal patterns of diagnosis in type 1 (insulin-dependent) diabetes. *Diabetologia* **26**:199–202.
229. Werner, S., W. M. Klump, H. Schönke, P. H. Hofscheider, and R. Kandolf. 1988. Expression of coxsackievirus B 3 capsid proteins in Escherichia coli and generation of virus-specific antisera. *DNA* **7**:307–316.
230. WHO Study Group. 1985. *Diabetes Mellitus. Technical Report Series 727.* World Health Organization, Geneva.
231. Wilberz, S., H. J. Partke, F. Dagnaes-Hansen, and L. Herberg. 1991. Persistent MHV (mouse hepatitis virus) infection reduces the incidence of diabetes mellitus in non-obese diabetic mice. *Diabetologia* **34**:2–5.
232. Wilfert, C. M., R. H. Buckley, T. Mohanakumar, J. K. Griffiths, S. L. Katz, J. K. Whisnant, and P. A. Eggleston. 1977. Persistent and fatal central system echovirus infection in agammaglobulinaemia. *N. Engl. J. Med.* **296**:1485.
233. Wyatt, H. V. 1973. Poliomyelitis in hypogammaglobulinemics. *J. Infect. Dis.* **128**:802–806.
234. Yagi, S., D. Schnurr, and J. Lin. 1992. Spectrum of monoclonal antibodies to coxsack-

ievirus B-3 includes type- and group-specific antibodies. *J. Clin. Microbiol.* **30:**2498–2501.
235. **Yoon, J. W.** 1990. The role of viruses and environmental factors in the induction of diabetes. *Curr. Top. Microbiol. Immunol.* **164:**95–123.
236. **Yoon, J. W., M. Austin, T. Onodera, and A. L. Notkins.** 1979. Virus-induced diabetes mellitus: isolation of a virus from the pancreas of a child with diabetic ketoacidosis. *N. Engl. J. Med.* **300:**1173–1179.
237. **Yoon, J. W., T. L. London, L. Curfman, R. L. Brown, and A. L. Notkins.** 1986. Coxsackie virus B4 produces transient diabetes in nonhuman primates. *Diabetes* **35:**712–716.
238. **Yoon, J. W., P. R. McClintock, C. J. Bachurski, J. D. Longstreth, and A. L. Notkins.** 1985. Virus-induced diabetes mellitus: no evidence for immune mechanisms in the destruction of β-cells by the D-variant of encephalomyocarditis virus. *Diabetes* **34:**922–925.
239. **Yoon, J. W., P. R. McClintock, T. Onodera, and A. L. Notkins.** 1980. Virus-induced diabetes mellitus. XVIII. Inhibition by a nondiabetogenic variant of encephalomyocarditis virus. *J. Exp. Med.* **152:**878–892.
240. **Yoon, J. W., T. Onodera, and A. L. Notkins.** 1978. Virus-induced diabetes. XV. Beta-cell damage and insulin-dependent hyperglycemia in mice infected with coxsackie B4. *J. Exp. Med.* **148:**1060–1080.
241. **Zibert, A., and E. Wimmer.** 1993. Receptor for poliovirus and other picornaviruses, p. 325–345. *In* K. W. Adolph (ed.), *Genome Research in Molecular Medicine and Virology.* Academic Press, San Diego, Calif.

ENTEROVIRUSES AND HUMAN NEUROMUSCULAR DISEASES

Marinos C. Dalakas

16

Coxsackieviruses, echoviruses, and polioviruses have been implicated in the pathogenesis of human neuromuscular diseases because of their association with certain acute and chronic acquired myopathies and paralytic motor neuron syndromes (13, 14, 34, 39, 44, 64). The suspicion initially focused on the coxsackieviruses because of their association with an epidemic of pleurodynia on the Danish island of Bornholm (13, 38, 44, 64). In this epidemic, the patients developed acute, self-limited febrile illnesses characterized by pain in the lower thorax and diaphragmatic muscle without muscle weakness or elevation of muscle enzymes; muscle biopsy in two such patients showed endomysial inflammation. Because typical clinical and histologic features of inflammatory myopathy have not been documented, it is doubtful whether epidemic pleurodynia (also known as Bornholm disease) is actually a form of myositis.

A few years later, acute myositis with weakness and myoglobinuria was reported in connection with coxsackievirus infection (6, 28, 29, 31, 32, 58). Subsequently, data emerged from serologic, epidemiologic, and electron microscopic studies as well as from molecular mimicry determinations that implicated enteroviruses as possible agents of chronic inflammatory muscle diseases. The evidence supporting such an association, however, has been largely circumstantial or unconvincing. Viral serology does not prove a causative role, because healthy or asymptomatic individuals may have detectable antibody titers in the serum due to previous, unrelated enteroviral infections; everyone develops many separate infections throughout childhood and as adults. Serology cannot distinguish those occasional infections that may have triggered autoimmunity from the many that were transient and without long-term sequelae. The epidemiologic observation that polymyositis (PM) has a seasonal onset is based on patients' recollections of historical data and hence is subject to significant recall bias. Reports that these viruses have been seen by electron microscopy in the muscle biopsy samples of some patients (5, 9) are suspect, because enteroviruses are very small and form periodic arrays of crystals that are difficult to distinguish from ribosomes or glycogen aggregates. Finally, the proposed hypothesis of molecular mimicry, based on the observation that up to 10% of patients with inflammatory myopathies have antibodies against a histidyl-tRNA synthetase (Jo-1 anti-

Marinos C. Dalakas, Neuromuscular Diseases Section, Medical Neurology Branch, National Institute of Neurological Disorders and Stroke, Bethesda, Maryland, 20892-1428.

gen) that has structural homology to the genomic RNA of an animal picornavirus (47), has not yet been shown to be of pathogenetic significance (see below).

The strongest and most compelling evidence that enteroviruses can be myotoxic is derived from animal experiments in which infection with certain coxsackieviruses and other picornaviruses can cause myositis and myocarditis (13, 14; see below). Healthy human muscle in culture can be infected with these viruses, providing additional support for their myotoxic potential. The advent of new molecular techniques has added to both the capability of establishing and the controversy surrounding the role of enteroviruses in various acquired inflammatory muscle diseases and motor neuron syndromes such as PM, dermatomyositis (DM), chronic fatigue syndrome (CFS), postpolio syndrome (PPS), and amyotrophic lateral sclerosis (ALS), each of which is reviewed below.

MYOSITIS AND MYOCARDITIS IN MICE

In some strains of newborn mice, coxsackievirus A strains can cause myositis, while coxsackievirus B strains cause myositis and meningoencephalitis (11, 35, 53, 63, 74–76). Mice infected with coxsackievirus B1 develop proximal muscle weakness within 7 days after inoculation. Although the muscle weakness is progressive and active histologic abnormalities can persist for up to 16 weeks, the virus cannot be isolated from the muscle beyond week 2, and viral RNA cannot be detected for more than 4 weeks. These observations have been interpreted to suggest that the virus triggers myositis but that the ongoing inflammatory muscle disease is secondary to an autoimmune process rather than to viral persistence. This hypothesis was further supported by comparative experiments with T-cell-deficient (nude) mice and their T-cell-competent heterozygous cohorts (74). When inoculated with coxsackievirus B1, both groups of mice developed anticoxsackievirus antibodies and an acute myositis, but only the heterozygous mice developed a chronic (beyond 3 weeks) myopathy. Reconstitution of the nude mice with T cells from the healthy mice resulted in the development of chronic myopathy (75). These experiments provide evidence that normal T-cell function is required for the manifestation of chronic muscle disease in mice infected with coxsackievirus B1.

The encephalomyocarditis virus, a murine picornavirus similar to coxsackievirus, can also induce chronic myositis and myocarditis in mice (11). As in the model just discussed, viral cultures become negative by the second week of paralysis, and viral RNA can be detected in the muscles by in situ hybridization only up to weeks 3 to 4 of the infection.

Coxsackievirus B3 murine infections have also received extensive study as models of chronic inflammatory myopathy (33, 52). This virus causes myositis that also appears to have a strong immunopathologic component mediated by $CD8^+$ and $CD4^+$ cells. Animals develop autoantibodies that recognize epitopes on cardiac myosin, while their lymphocytes are sensitized to recognize epitopes on cardiac muscle and myotubes (33, 69).

On the basis of these observations, the following sequence of events may explain the development of coxsackievirus-induced chronic autoimmune muscle disease in mice. Viral infection is followed by development of antiviral antibodies that recognize muscle antigens and generate cytotoxic T cells sensitized to muscle autoantigens. These antibodies may initially clear the infection, but they subsequently bind to healthy muscle and, in conjunction with sensitized T cells, generate the self-sustaining chronic phase of an autoimmune myositis. It is not known whether a similar mechanism underlies human inflammatory muscle disease.

POSSIBLE SCENARIOS FOR ENTEROVIRAL PERSISTENCE IN HUMAN MUSCLE OR MOTOR NEURONS

The experimental data reviewed above suggest that coxsackieviruses can persist in the muscles of mice for up to 4 weeks. Following intracerebral inoculation of mice with poliovirus, the virus has persisted for up to 6 months. Similarly, in vitro infection of neuroblastoma cell lines with poliovirus results in persistent infection characterized by mutations in the viral genome (10). It is therefore possible that enteroviruses, although usually lytic, can under certain conditions cause persistent infection. Potential mechanisms of enteroviral persistence are extensively reviewed in the chapters on myocardial disease (chapter 14) and diabetes (chapter 15). Scenarios for enteroviral persistence in human muscle or motor neurons, in brief, include the following.

1. The immune system is defective and cannot clear the infection. This is clearly the mechanism for persistence of polioviruses and echoviruses in patients with humoral immunodeficiency. The latter syndrome, while usually manifesting as chronic respiratory or central nervous system infection (see chapter 13), is also associated with muscle disease (51, 64, 70; see below).

2. Lytic infection may be limited to a focal area, but expression of viral antigens may occur in both necrotic and surviving cells (68). Because of defective replication or a defective interfering viral genome, the virus can be trapped in a few cells that do not immediately lyse. Under these conditions, viral persistence may result in a low-level reinfection of new cells, with only a portion of them being eliminated by inflammatory cells during immune surveillance. If, during the initial phase of the active infection, the virus mutates, RNA synthesis may also be restrained, allowing persistence without replication (68). During periods of repair, division, cell stress, or metabolic alterations in response to cytokines (33), the virus can mutate and express new epitopes shared by host cell proteins that could trigger a slow, smoldering, inflammatory response. Alternatively, a persisting virus may affect only the luxury functions of the cells similar to those suggested by Oldstone in the chronic persistent lymphocytic choriomeningitis virus model (56).

3. Apoptotic cell death may be inhibited. In acute polio, we have evidence to suggest that neuronal cell death may be caused by apoptosis (22a). The same mechanism occurs in neurons infected with another RNA virus, the Sindbis virus. In the latter model, the virus causes acute encephalitis and death in young mice. In adult mice, however, because of the later expression of genes that inhibit apoptosis, it causes a nonfatal, persistent viral infection (46).

EVIDENCE FOR ENTEROVIRUSES IN CHRONIC HUMAN MUSCLE OR MOTOR NEURON DISEASES

PM and DM

The PM and DM complex encompasses a heterogeneous group of acquired muscle diseases called inflammatory myopathies because muscle weakness and inflammatory infiltrates within the skeletal muscles are the principal clinical and histologic findings (15, 17, 20, 21, 30). An autoimmune origin of the inflammatory myopathies is supported by their association with other putative or definite systemic autoimmune or connective tissue disorders, the presence of various autoantibodies, evidence of myocytotoxicity mediated by cytotoxic T cells in the case of PM or complement-mediated microangiopathy in the case of DM, and their response to immunotherapies (15, 17, 20, 21, 30).

Although there is circumstantial evidence implicating viruses as possible triggering factors in the inflammatory myopathies, viruses have not been isolated from the muscle except in rare, unconfirmed reports (65). Postviral PM may be a self-limiting illness (17). Occasionally, acute PM, a severe and difficult-to-treat inflammatory myopathy, can follow a viral illness (20, 21).

Picornaviruses have been proposed as possible triggering agents for some cases of PM or DM. This suggestion is based on a number of lines of evidence, including structural homology of the viruses with the Jo-1 antigen (47, 66). Jo-1, a histidyl-tRNA synthetase, is an enzyme that joins histidine to its cognate tRNA in the early stages of protein synthesis. This enzyme can interact with and join histidine not only to its native histidyl-tRNA but also to the genomic RNA of the encephalomyocarditis virus, whose tertiary structure has regions of homology with histidyl-tRNA synthetase of *Escherichia coli* and muscle proteins (47, 66). A theoretical interaction between this virus and the synthetase may result in a stable complex (such as that formed between the synthetase and its native tRNA substrate) that may be presented to the immune system as foreign, generating an autoimmune response. Alternatively, antibodies generated against a related picornavirus that a patient may be infected with could theoretically cross-react with both the histidyl-tRNA synthetase (Jo-1) and muscle proteins in a phenomenon of molecular mimicry. Anti-Jo-1 antibodies, however, occur in only the small subset of patients (10% of all patients with inflammatory myopathies) who have a coexisting interstitial lung disease, which suggests that Jo-1 antibodies may be more lung specific than muscle specific. There are no experimental data to support the theory that these reactions result in myositis or that these autoantibodies are directed against muscle-specific antigens triggered by these viruses. However, the potential association provides a reasonable basis to search for picornaviruses in the muscles of both PM and DM patients by using molecular virology tools, as discussed below. At present, the role of Jo-1 autoantibodies in the diagnosis, clinical description, and immunopathogenesis of the inflammatory myopathies is uncertain, and it would be premature to link them in any way to the fundamental disease process.

Human muscle myotubes and myoblasts express the poliovirus receptor and are susceptible to infection with poliovirus (41, 55), with dramatic cytopathic effect in culture. The virus is detected by electron microscopy in the submembrane regions of the myotubes and by PCR in the RNA extracted from the myotubes (41). Susceptibility of the human myotubes to infection does not, however, imply that the mature muscle fiber could also carry a productive or persistent poliovirus infection, as described above.

High neutralization antibody titers to coxsackievirus B are found in some patients with PM and DM (67). As noted above, however, high antibody titers can be found in asymptomatic persons previously infected with enteroviruses and do not necessarily provide a causal link with a chronic disease process. Enterovirus-like particles have been detected by electron microscopy in muscle biopsy specimens from some PM and DM patients (65). Because enteroviruses form periodic arrays of crystals similar or identical to glycogen and ribosomes, their exact identification by electron microscopy can be very difficult (43). Consequently, electron microscopic observations are difficult to interpret. In a single patient in whom electron microscopy of muscle biopsy specimen revealed suggestive particles, coxsackievirus A9 was grown from the affected muscle (65).

When slot blot hybridization was used, muscle biopsy preparations from five of nine patients with PM and DM gave positive results with a coxsackievirus B-derived probe (8). These hybridization signals were weak and similar to those observed with the control b-tubulin probe, making their distinction from background signal difficult. In situ hybridization experiments found positive signals in three of nine biopsy specimens from patients with DM (59). The meaning of those findings is, however, uncertain, because hybridization was observed only within the endomysial macrophages, not the muscle fibers, and only with a probe derived from a murine enterovirus (Theiler's virus), not with a cocktail of probes derived from human enteroviral serotypes. Coxsackievirus B mRNA was reportedly detected within the muscle fibers of 8 of 19 patients with PM or DM by using a poliovirus 1-derived probe and in situ hybridization (73). The detection of positive signals by any hybridization method that uses a large probe, such as the one used in that study, may reflect cross-reactivity with nonviral cellular nucleic acid. The specificity of the findings in this latter study was additionally clouded by the inability of the investigators to demonstrate viral antigens in the same specimens by immunocytochemistry.

In order to exclude the presence of enteroviruses in the muscles of patients with PM, DM, and inclusion body myositis, we used the sensitive PCR amplification technique and specific primers (positions 450 to 474 and 584 to 603 of the poliovirus 1 genome) that recognize a highly conserved region in the noncoding region at the 5' end of the viral RNA (45, 60) (see chapter 17 also). We studied muscle biopsy specimens from 39 patients (16 with PM, 12 with DM, and 11 with inclusion body myositis) who fulfilled the strict diagnostic clinicopathologic criteria of active inflammatory myopathy (20). Control specimens were obtained from 32 patients with noninflammatory myopathy, dystrophies, ALS, and normal muscle biopsy samples. Ten consecutive, 10-μm-thick, fresh-frozen sections totaling 50 mg of muscle tissue were studied for each patient. All specimens were coded and analyzed blindly. Mixtures of total RNA and DNA were extracted from each specimen. Proteins were digested with pronase, and DNA and RNA were precipitated with ethanol. A combined reverse transcription-PCR assay was performed twice on nucleic acids extracted from each specimen, using standard procedures and an RNA PCR kit (Cetus, Emeryville, Calif.) (42, 45, 49, 61). In each experiment, positive viral control specimens (polioviruses 1, 2, and 3 and coxsackievirus B3 [American Tissue Culture Collection, Rockville, Md.] grown in Vero cells) and nucleic acid-negative control samples containing only water were included. All specimens were analyzed by 10% polyacrylamide gel electrophoresis with ethidium bromide staining. Myosin primers 1 (5'GGCTTGAATGAGGAGTAGCT3') and 2 (5'CTGCTTCCTCCCAAGGAGCT3') were used in the PCR amplification to ensure the integrity of the nucleic acids extracted from the samples. The specificities of the viral sequences were confirmed by blot hybridizing the amplified PCR product at 50°C with a 21-oligonucleotide probe (positions 548 to 568 of the 5' end of poliovirus RNA) (60) labeled with ^{32}P by the T4 kinase method.

The predicted 106-bp fragment of myosin DNA was detected in all specimens, indicating that sufficient nucleic acids were extracted from the sections. With the viral primers, control poliovirus and coxsackievirus RNAs from infected cells were readily detected (Fig. 1). By contrast, with the same primers, no amplification bands of correct size were detected in the specimens from patients or controls (Fig. 1). The DNA fragments of low molecular weights observed in some of the amplified products (Fig. 1) were nonspecific, as they did not correspond to the expected sizes of amplified viral RNA sequences. Such nonspecific fragments, which were also observed in the control samples containing water instead of RNA (Fig. 1), were most likely caused by self-annealing of the primers. When the amplified products were hybridized to the enteroviral probe, only the control coxsackievirus- and poliovirus-infected cells gave positive hybridization signals (Fig. 2). None of the nonspecific amplified fragments hybridized with the probe, as previously described (45).

The PCR technique is sensitive enough to detect even low copy numbers of the viral genome, although viral particles sparsely distributed within the muscle biopsy specimens could theoretically escape detection if they happen to fall outside the 100-μm total length of the muscle tissue examined. Furthermore, this technique and the primers we used are broadly reactive for almost all known human enteroviral serotypes (60) and should detect even mutant or defective enteroviruses except those with alterations occurring within the sequences of the primers or those virions lacking part of the 5' noncoding conserved region. It is therefore unlikely, but not impossible, that persistent enteroviral infection plays a causative role in the pathogenesis of PM, DM, and inclusion body myositis. Whether an enterovirus has triggered the disease but cannot be detected in a chronic phase (analogous to the

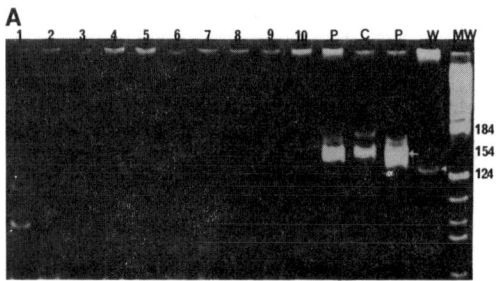

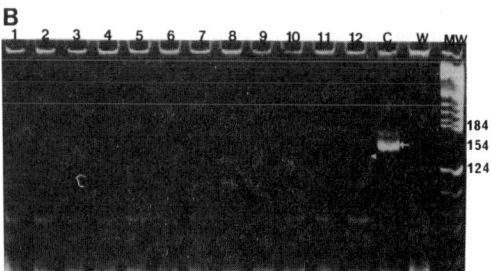

FIGURE 1 Polyacrylamide gel electrophoreses of enterovirus PCR performed on extracted RNA from muscle biopsy samples of patients with inflammatory myopathies and other neuromuscular diseases; also included are positive tissue culture and negative water controls subjected to the same amplification techniques. Lanes 1 through 4 (panel A) and 1 and 2 (panel B) are from patients with PM; lanes 5 through 8 (panel A) and 3 and 4 (panel B) are from patients with DM; lanes 5 through 7 (panel B) are from patients with inclusion body myositis; and lanes 9 and 10 (panel A) and 8 through 10 (panel B) are from patients with other neuromuscular diseases including PPS. Lane P, amplified RNA from poliovirus-infected cell cultures; lane C, amplified RNA from coxsackievirus-infected cultures; lane W, amplification products obtained from water alone; lane MW, molecular weight markers (in thousands). Specific amplification of the expected 154-bp fragment of enteroviral RNA is shown by arrows and was observed in virus-infected cells only; arrowheads indicate lower-molecular-weight bands that are nonspecific products. (45)

coxsackievirus B in mice described earlier) is unclear, but I believe that to be unlikely. The poliovirus receptor, a prerequisite for the infection of human muscle with poliovirus, is not present in healthy human muscle fibers (41). If human muscle similarly lacks receptors for the other enteroviruses, it is unlikely that muscle could be an important site of infection and replication of enteroviruses.

Muscle Disease with X-Linked Agammaglobulinemia

Approximately half of patients reported with X-linked (Bruton's) agammaglobulinemia and chronic central nervous system enteroviral infection (see chapter 13), including cases in which virus has been cultured from the muscle, have concomitant DM or PM (51). Based on experience with two muscle biopsy specimens, however, I believe that this form of myositis is not true muscle disease but rather a fasciitis with interstitial inflammation in the endomysial septae. Whether the echovirus causing the central nervous system infection is responsible for the histologic and clinical muscle abnormalities remains unknown. PCR for enteroviruses in one of our biopsy specimens gave negative results.

CFS

CFS, also known as postviral fatigue syndrome, includes a constellation of diverse symptoms of severe fatigue, myalgia, poor concentration, mild lymphadenopathy, and neurologic abnormalities that follow an acute viral illness. Although the early scientific investigations of CFS were limited by the lack of objective signs, recently imposed diagnostic criteria have defined CFS as a distinct clinical entity (40). Consequently, the search for possible viral pathogenesis in well-defined clinical groups can now be pursued. Enteroviruses have been considered as candidate viruses in the cause of CFS because enteroviruses have been isolated from stools in some patients (72), enteroviral VP1 antigen has been found in the sera of CFS patients (72), and serologic studies have shown patients with CFS to have a higher prevalence and/or higher titers of antienterovirus antibodies than control patients do (2, 50).

Molecular techniques have recently been applied to the search for viral RNA in muscle biopsy specimens of CFS patients. The search has focused on the muscle, because patients experience neuromuscular symptoms such as fatigue, myalgia, and weakness; there are reports of electrophysiologic abnormalities with single-fiber electromyography, suggesting impaired neuromuscular transmission; and histo-

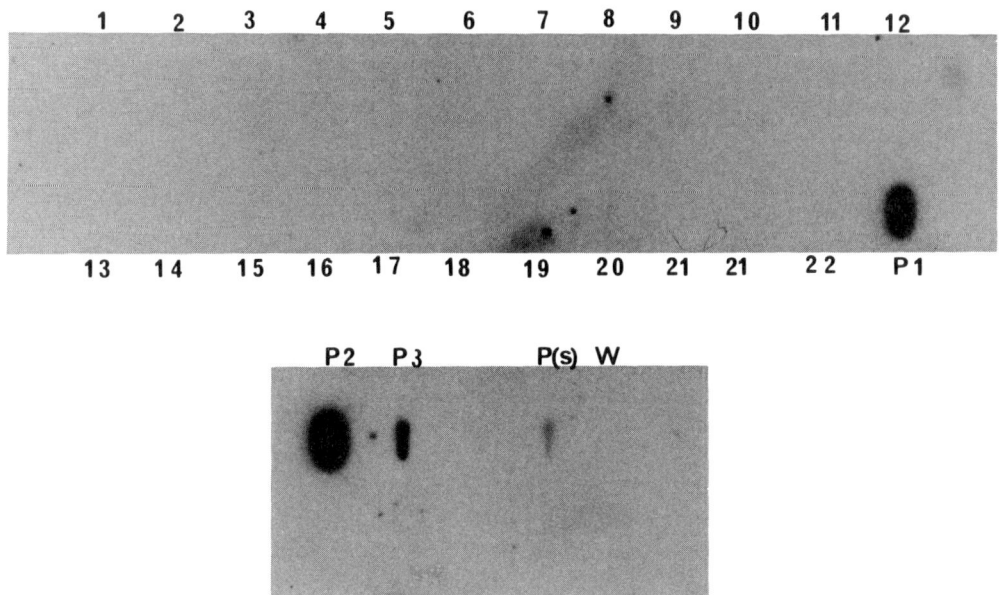

FIGURE 2 Slot blot hybridization of PCR products hybridized with a 23-mer 32P-labeled oligonucleotide probe. Slots 1 through 6, amplified product from patients with PM; slots 7 through 12, product from patients with DM; slots 13 through 17, product from patients with inclusion body myositis; slots 18 through 23, product from other disease controls including patients with PPS. P1, P2, and P3, amplified products from cell cultures infected with polioviruses 1, 2, and 3, respectively; W, amplified products of water alone; P(s), products from the supernatant of poliovirus-infected cells. Specific hybridization is noted only in virus-infected culture controls [P1, P2, P3, P(s)] but not in muscle biopsy specimens (45).

logic abnormalities consisting of abnormal muscle mitochondria have been observed by electron microscopy (3, 4). The results of hybridization and PCR studies have been conflicting, with strong associations to enteroviruses found by some (1, 12, 36) and no enteroviral evidence found by others (63a). Extended studies performed by one group that initially reported a positive association (36) led to the conclusion that evidence for enterovirus-induced CFS was lacking (37). The concern with these studies is the high incidence of positive results (by hybridization or PCR) in unaffected control patients, perhaps reflecting cross-reactivity of primers and/or probes with host nucleic acid.

Our own studies on several patients admitted to the National Institutes of Health by Stephen Straus have found normal electromyography studies (including single-fiber electromyography), normal neuromuscular transmission studies, and normal muscle biopsy by muscle enzyme histochemistry. In a few specimens, we have searched for enteroviruses by using the PCR technique outlined above and have been unable to amplify enteroviral RNA. Two recent studies using in situ hybridization, PCR, and sequence analysis of the amplified product have shown the presence of an enterovirus that differs from the typical strains in the 5' noncoding region, suggesting a virus defective or mutated in that region (4). These findings need confirmation and repeated experiments with many controls. My own laboratory is also pursuing this line of investigation with muscle biopsy specimens collected by Benjamin Natelson.

PPS

PPS consists of new muscle weakness and wasting, fatigue, and myalgia occurring 25 to 35 years following acute paralytic poliomyelitis due to infection with poliovirus (16, 23–26) (see chapter 9 also). In PPS, the new weakness usually affects the previously affected and (fully or partially) recovered muscles and, rarely, some previously unaffected muscles. The mechanism of PPS is believed to be the gradual attrition of the remaining motor neurons, healthy or previously scarred, that had compensated for the lost neurons by oversprouting to supply and maintain a larger-than-normal number of muscle fibers (16, 23–26). An ongoing denervation and reinnervation process continues from the time of the initial polio attack; new weakness (PPS) occurs when the remaining motor neurons can no longer maintain all of their distal sprouts, resulting in a denervation rate that exceeds the reinnervation rate, a loss of distal nerve terminals, and atrophy of muscle fibers (23, 24).

The ongoing nature of the denervating-reinnervating process from the time of the initial infection raises the possibility of slow, smoldering viral activity within the neuronal cell body (16, 23–26). The impetus to search for the presence of poliovirus in PPS patients was furthered by a number of tantalizing immunopathologic abnormalities, including signs of inflammation around motor neurons in the spinal cords of PPS patients as long as 30 years following acute disease (57), endomysial inflammation consisting of $CD8^+$ cells associated with focal major histocompatibility complex class I antigen expression in up to 40% of the muscle biopsy samples of PPS patients (18, 23–26), oligoclonal immunoglobulin G (IgG) bands (19), and increased levels of interleukin-2 and intrathecal IgM antipoliovirus antibody synthesis in the cerebrospinal fluid (62), and high IgM antipoliovirus antibody titers by enzyme-linked immunosorbent assay in the sera of up to 30% of PPS patients (22, 54).

If a mutated or defective interfering viral genome has escaped immune surveillance early in infection, the virus could theoretically have been trapped within some motor neurons. In that case, an immune process against motor neurons or axonal sprouts, triggered by viral proteins, could explain some of the immunopathologic phenomena of PPS.

Our efforts to find poliovirus in the muscles of PPS patients by using the PCR method described above have failed. Studies with in situ PCR of the spinal cord and amplification of poliovirus RNA in the cerebrospinal fluid are under way in my laboratory.

Acute Paralytic Poliomyelitis

I have also had the opportunity to examine muscle biopsy samples from patients with acute paralytic polio in a collaborative study with M. Agbotowballa from Pakistan. In these muscle biopsy specimens, removed during the first few months after the infection, we observed $CD8^+$ cells in proximity to the end plate region. Because human muscle end plates express the poliovirus receptor (41), we interpreted this finding of $CD8^+$ cells to suggest that during the viremic phase of acute infection, poliovirus may freely enter the end plate region, which lacks a blood-nerve barrier, and travel to the motor neuron via reverse axoplasmic flow. The endomysial inflammation may simply represent a reaction to the virus at the entry zone.

Our efforts to immunolocalize viral antigens by immunocytochemistry or to detect viral RNA by PCR in the muscle biopsy samples of 20 such patients have been unsuccessful. This failure could indicate either that by the time we examined the muscles it was too late to detect the virus or that virus binds only to the end plate and does not infect or replicate in the muscle. In support of the latter contention is our failure to identify the poliovirus receptor in healthy muscle. Since the presence of the poliovirus receptor is a prerequisite for binding of the virus to its target tissue, the absence of receptor from healthy muscle fiber may suggest that the mature muscle is not susceptible to poliovirus infection.

ALS

Since poliovirus is the prototype virus for causing motor neuron diseases and ALS is the prototypic acquired motor neuron disease, poliovirus has long been considered a leading candidate virus in the etiology of ALS. The search for such an association has included epidemiologic, serologic, histologic, and virologic investigations. All of these studies have provided mixed results and conflicting reports, with the majority finding no association. A recent report, however, reignited the interest and the controversy. Using PCR of wax-embedded material from spinal cords of patients with ALS and of age-matched controls, Woodall et al. amplified a 414-bp RNA sequence in the conserved 5' untranslated enterovirus regions from 8 of 11 patients with sporadic ALS but not in six control specimens (71). Sequence analysis of the amplified region showed a close relationship to coxsackievirus B but not to poliovirus. Concerns about this study include the detection of virus in patients with familial ALS (not expected to be of viral origin) and the ability of the authors to amplify RNA from paraffin-embedded tissue. Our own efforts to extract amplifiable RNA from such tissues have repeatedly failed. If spinal cord harbors these common enteroviruses, as the recent study suggests, their role in actually causing motor neuron diseases will need to be further documented by localizing the viral RNA to within the motor neurons. Studies using in situ PCR are now under way in my laboratory and others.

SUMMARY

Biologic plausibility coupled with preliminary laboratory data has focused much attention on the enteroviruses as causative agents in numerous acute and chronic human muscle diseases. The emergence of sensitive molecular tools has added to both the laboratory capability and the controversy regarding the role of these viruses. The coming years will surely lead to new and important information regarding the potential of the enteroviruses to trigger autoimmunity and/or cause chronic infection. At all times, caution must be taken to properly design and control clinical studies and to standardize laboratory procedures lest we perpetuate the current state of conflicting data and unresolved pathogenesis. With the advent of effective antiviral therapy (see chapter 18), it will be ever more important to define the role of infection in acute and chronic muscles diseases.

ACKNOWLEDGMENT

I thank M. Leon-Monzon for help with PCR studies.

REFERENCES

1. **Archard, L. C., N. E. Bowles, P. O. Behan, E. J. Bell, and D. Doyle.** 1988. Postviral fatigue syndrome: persistence of enterovirus RNA in muscle and elevated creatine kinase. *J. R. Soc. Med.* **81:**326–329.
2. **Behan, P. O., W. M. H. Behan, and E. J. Bell.** 1985. The postviral fatigue syndrome—an analysis of the findings in 50 cases. *J. Infect.* **10:**211–222.
3. **Behan, W. M. H., and P. O. Behan.** 1993. The role of viral infection in polymyositis, dermatomyositis and chronic fatigue syndrome. *Bailliere's Clin. Neurol.* **2:**637–657.
4. **Behan, W. M. H., and P. O. Behan.** 1994. Enteroviruses in chronic fatigue syndrome. *Ann. Intern. Med.* **120:**972–973.
5. **Ben-Bassat, M., and I. Machtey.** 1972. Picornavirus-like structures in acute dermatomyositis. *Am. J. Clin. Pathol.* **58:**245.
6. **Berlin, B. S., N. M. Simon, and R. N. Bovner.** 1974. Myoglobinuria precipitated by viral infection. *JAMA* **227:**1414.
7. **Bodensteiner, J. B., H. H. Morris, J. T. Howell, and S. S. Schochet.** 1979. Chronic Echo type 5 virus meningoencephalitis in X-linked hypogammaglobulinemia: treatment with immune plasma. *Neurology* **29:**815.
8. **Bowles, N. E., V. Dubowitz, C. A. Swery, and L. C. Archard.** 1987. Dermatomyositis, polymyositis and coxsackie B virus infections. *Lancet* **i:**1004–1007.
9. **Chou, S. M., and L. Gutmann.** 1970. Picornavirus-like crystals in subacute polymyositis. *Neurology* **10:**205.
10. **Colbere-Garpin, F., C. Christodoulou, R. Crainic, and T. Pelletier.** 1989. Persistent poliovirus infection of human neuroblastoma cells. *Proc. Natl. Acad. Sci. USA* **86:**7590–7594.
11. **Cronin, M. E., L. A. Love, F. W. Miller, P.**

R. McClintock, and P. H. Plotz. 1988. The natural history of encephalomyocarditis virus-induced myositis and myocarditis in mice: viral persistence demonstrated by in situ hybridization. *J. Exp. Med.* **168**:1639–1648.
12. Cunningham, L., N. E. Bowles, R. J. M. Lane, V. Dubowitz, and L. C. Archard. 1990. Persistence of enteroviral RNA in chronic fatigue syndrome is associated with the abnormal production of equal amounts of positive and negative strands of enteroviral RNA. *J. Gen. Virol.* **71**:1399–1402.
13. Curnen, E. D. 1960. The coxsackie viruses. *Pediatr. Clin. N. Am.* **7**:903.
14. Curnen, E. D., E. W. Shaw, and J. L. Melnick. 1949. Disease resembling nonparalytic poliomyelitis associated with a virus pathogenic for infant mice. *JAMA* **141**:894.
15. Dalakas, M. 1990. Inflammatory myopathies. *Curr. Opin. Neurol. Neurosurg.* **3**:689–696.
16. Dalakas, M. 1991. The post-polio syndrome. *Curr. Opin. Rheum.* **2**:901–907.
17. Dalakas, M. C. 1988. *Polymyositis and Dermatomyositis.* Butterworths Publications, Stoneham, Mass.
18. Dalakas, M. C. 1988. Morphological changes in the muscles of patients with post-poliomyelitis neuromuscular symptoms. *Neurology* **38**:99–104.
19. Dalakas, M. C. 1990. Oligoclonal bands in postpoliomyelitis muscular atrophy. *Ann. Neurol.* **3**:689–696.
20. Dalakas, M. C. 1991. Polymyositis, dermatomyositis and inclusion-body myositis. *N. Engl. J. Med.* **325**:1487–1498.
21. Dalakas, M. C. 1992. Inflammatory myopathies: pathogenesis and treatment. *Neuropharmacology* **5**:327–351.
22. Dalakas, M. C. Pathogenesis of postpolio syndrome: studies on electrophysiology, virology, pathology and immunopathology of muscle and spinal cord. *Ann. N.Y. Acad. Sci.*, in press.
22a. Dalakas, M.C. Unpublished observations.
23. Dalakas, M. C., G. Elder, M. Hallett, J. Ravitz, M. Baker, N. Papadoupolos, P. Albrecht, and J. L. Sever. 1986. A long term follow-up study of patients with postpoliomyelitis neuromuscular symptoms. *N. Engl. J. Med.* **314**:959–963.
24. Dalakas, M. C., and M. Hallett. 1988. The post-polio syndrome, p. 51–94. *In* F. Plum (ed.), *Advances in Contemporary Neurology.* F. A. Davis, Philadelphia.
25. Dalakas, M. C., and I. Illa. 1991. The postpolio syndrome: concepts in pathogenesis and etiologies, p. 495–511. *In* L. P. Rowland (ed.), *Advances in Neurology*, vol. 56. *Amyotrophic Lateral Sclerosis.* Raven Press, New York.
26. Dalakas, M. C., J. L. Sever, D. L. Madden, N. M. Papadopoulis, I. C. Shedarchi, P. Albrecht, and A. Krezlewicz. 1984. Late post-poliomyelitis muscular atrophy: clinical, virological, and immunological studies. *Rev. Infect. Dis.* **6**:S562–S567.
27. Davis, L. E., D. Bodian, D. Price, I. J. Butler, and J. H. Vickers. 1977. Chronic progressive poliomyelitis secondary to vaccination of an immunodeficient child. *N. Engl. J. Med.* **297**:241.
28. De Reuck, J., W. De Coster, and N. Indiradjapa. 1977. Acute viral polymyositis with predominant diaphragm involvement. *J. Neurol. Sci.* **33**:453.
29. Dunnet, J., J. Y. Paton, and C. E. Robertson. 1981. Acute renal failure and coxsackie viral infection. *Clin. Nephrol.* **16**:262.
30. Engel, A. G., R. Hohlfeld, and B. Q. Banker. 1994. The polymyositis and dermatomyositis syndromes, p. 1335–1383. *In* A. G. Engel and C. Franzini-Armstrong (ed.), *Myology.* McGraw Hill Book Co., New York.
31. Favara, B. E., G. F. Vawter, R. Wagner, et al. 1967. Familial paroxysmal rhabdomyolysis in children: a myoglobinuric syndrome. *Am. J. Med.* **42**:196.
32. Fukuyama, Y., T. Ando, and J. Yokota. 1977. Acute fulminant myoglobinuric polymyositis with picornavirus-like crystals. *J. Neurol. Neurosurg. Psychiatry* **40**:775.
33. Gauntt, C. J., A. L. Higdon, H. M. Aripze, M. R. Tamayo, R. Grawley, R. D. Henkel, M. E. A. Periera, S. M. Tracy, and M. W. Cunningham. 1993. Epitopes shared between coxsackievirus B3 (VB3) and normal heart tissue contribute to CVB3-induced murine myocarditis. *Clin. Immunol. Immunopathol.* **68**:129–134.
34. Ginsberg, H. S. 1990. Picornaviruses, p. 961–983. *In* B. D. David, R. Dulbecco, N. H. Eisen, and H. S. Ginsberg (ed.). *Microbiology*, 5th ed. Lippincott, Philadelphia.
35. Godman, G. C., H. Bunting, and J. L. Melnick. 1952. The histopathology of coxsackie virus infection in mice. I. Morphologic observations with four different viral types. *Am. J. Pathol.* **28**:223.
36. Gow, J., W. M. H. Behan, G. B. Clements, C. Woodall, M. Riding, and P. O. Behan. 1991. Enteroviral sequences detected by polymerase chain reaction in muscle biopsies of patients with the postviral fatigue syndrome. *Br. Med. J.* **302**:692–696.
37. Gow, J. W., W. M. H. Behan, K. Simpson, F. McGarry, S. Keir, and P. O. Behan. 1994.

Studies on enterovirus in patients with chronic fatigue syndrome. *Clin. Infect. Dis.* **18**(Suppl.): S126–S129.
38. **Grenier, B.** 1970. Epidemic myalgia (Bornholm disease): epidemiology and clinical description, p. 247. *In* R. Debre and J. Cellers (ed.), *Clinical Virology: the Evaluation and Management of Human Viral Infections.* The W. B. Saunders Co., Philadelphia.
39. **Hays, A. P., and E. T. Ganboa.** 1994. Acute viral myositis, p. 1308–1418. *In* A. G. Engel and C. Franzini-Armstrong (ed.), *Myology II.* McGraw Hill Book Co., New York.
40. **Holmes, G. P., J. E. Kaplan, N. M. Gantz, A. L. Komaroff, L. B. Schonberger, S. E. Strauss, J. F. Jones, R. E. Dubois, R. C. Cunningham, and S. Pahwa.** 1988. Chronic fatigue syndrome. A working case definition. *Ann. Intern. Med.* **108**:387–389.
41. **Illa, I., M. Monzon, and M. C. Dalakas.** The role of muscle in the acute polio infection. *Ann. N.Y. Acad. Sci.,* in press.
42. **Jenkins, O., J. D. Booth, P. D. Minor, and J. W. Almond.** 1987. The complete nucleotide sequence of coxsackievirus B4 and its comparison to other members of the picornaviridae. *J. Gen. Virol.* **68**:1835–1838.
43. **Katsuragi, S., H. Miyayama, and H. T. Takeuchi.** 1981. Picornavirus-like inclusions in polymyositis-aggregation of glucogen particles of the same size. *Neurology* **31**:1426–1480.
44. **Kibrick, S.** 1964. Current status of coxsackie and ECHO viruses in human disease. *Prog. Med. Virol.* **6**:27.
45. **Leon-Monzon, M., and M. C. Dalakas.** 1992. Absence of persistent infection with enteroviruses in muscles of patients with inflammatory myopathies. *Ann. Neurol.* **32**:219–222.
46. **Levine, B., A. Huang, J. T. Isaacs, et al.** 1993. Conversion of lytic to persistent alphavirus infection by the bcl-2 cellular oncogene. *Nature* (London) **361**:739–742.
47. **Love, L. A., R. L. Leff, D. D. Frazer, I. N. Targoft, M. Dalakas, P. Flotz, and F. W. Miller.** 1991. A new approach to the classification of idiopathic inflammatory myopathy: myositis-specific autoantibodies define useful homogenous patient groups. *Medicine* **70**:360–374.
48. **Maller, H. M., D. F. Poward, R. E. Horowitz, and B. Portnoy.** 1967. Fatal myocarditis associated with ECHO virus, type 22: infection in a child with apparent immunological deficiency. *J. Pediatr.* **7**:204.
49. **Maniatis, T., E. F. Fritsch, and J. Sambrook.** 1982. *Molecular Cloning: a Laboratory Manual.* Cold Spring Harbor Laboratory, Cold Spring Harbor, N.Y.
50. **McCartney, R. A., J. E. Banatavala, and E. J. Bell.** 1986. Routine use of M-antibody capture ELISA for the serological diagnosis of coxsackie B virus infection. *J. Med. Virol.* **19**:205–212.
51. **McKinney, R. E., S. L. Katz, and C. M. Wilfert.** 1987. Chronic enteroviral meningoencephalitis in agammaglobulinemic patients. *Rev. Infect. Dis.* **9**:334–356.
52. **McManus, B. M., L. H. Chow, J. E. Wilson, et al.** 1993. Direct myocardial injury by enteroviruses: a central role in the evolution of murine myocarditis. *Clin. Immunol. Immunopathol.* **68**:159–169.
53. **Melnick, J. L., and G. C. Godman.** 1951. Pathogenesis of coxsackie virus infection. Multiplication of virus and evolution of the muscle lesion in mice. *J. Exp. Med.* **93**:27.
54. **Monzon, M., and M. C. Dalakas.** Virological studies in blood, serum and spinal fluid in patients with post-polio syndrome. *Ann. N.Y. Acad. Sci.,* in press.
55. **Monzon, M., I. Illa, and M. C. Dalakas.** The expression of poliovirus receptor in normal and pathological muscle, nerve and spinal cord. *Ann. N.Y. Acad. Sci.,* in press.
56. **Oldstone, M. B. A.** 1989. Viruses can cause disease in the absence of morphological evidence of cell injury: implications for uncovering new diseases in the future. *J. Infect. Dis.* **139**:384.
57. **Pezeshkpour, G. H., and M. C. Dalakas.** 1988. Long term changes in the spinal cord of patients with old poliomyelitis: signs of continuous disease activity. *Arch. Neurol.* **45**:505–508.
58. **Porter, C. B., D. R. Hinthorn, G. Couchonnal, et al.** 1981. Simultaneous streptococcus and picornavirus infection. *JAMA* **245**:1545.
59. **Rosenberg, N. L., H. A. Rotbart, M. J. Abzug, S. P. Ringer, and M. J. Levin.** 1989. Evidence for a novel picornavirus in human dermatomyositis. *Ann. Neurol.* **26**:204–209.
60. **Rotbart, H. A.** 1990. PCR amplification of enteroviruses, p. 372–377. *In* M. A. Innis, D. H. Gelfand, J. J. Sninsky, and T. J. White (ed.), *PCR Protocols.* Academic Press, San Diego, Calif.
61. **Saiki, R. K., S. J. Scharf, F. Faloona, et al.** 1985. Enzymatic amplification of beta-globin genomic sequences and restriction site analysis for diagnosis of sickle cell anemia. *Science* **230**:1350–1354.
62. **Sharief, M. K., R. Hentges, and M. Crardi.** 1991. Intrathecal immune response in patients with the postpolio syndrome. *N. Engl. J. Med.* **325**:749–755.
63. **Strongwater, S. L., K. Dorovini-Zis, R. D.**

Ball, and T. J. Schnitzer. 1984. A murine model of polymyositis induced by coxsackievirus B1 (Tucson strain). *Arthritis Rheum.* **27**:433.

63a. Swanink, C. M. A., W. J. G. Melchers, J. W. M. van der Meer, J. H. M. M. Vercoulen, G. Bleijenberg, J. F. M. Fennis, and J. M. D. Galama. 1994. Enteroviruses and the chronic fatigue syndrome. *Clin. Infect. Dis.* **19**:860–864.

64. Sylvest, E. 1934. *Epidemic Myalgia: Bornholm Disease.* Oxford University Press, London.

65. Tang, T. T., G. V. Sedmak, K. A. Siegesmund, and S. R. McCreadie. 1975. Chronic myopathy associated with coxsackievirus type A. A combined electronmicroscopical and viral isolation study. *N. Engl. J. Med.* **292**:608–611.

66. Targoff, I. N., F. C. Arnett, and M. Reichlin. 1988. Antibody to threonyl-transfer RNA synthetase in myositis sera. *Arthritis Rheum.* **31**:515–524.

67. Travers, R. L., G. R. V. Hughes, G. Cambridge, and J. R. Sewell. 1977. Coxsackie B neutralization titers in polymyositis dermatomyositis. *Lancet* **i**:1268.

68. Vella, C., C. L. Brown, and D. A. McCarthy. 1992. Coxsackievirus B4 infection of the mouse pancreas: acute and persistent infection. *J. Gen. Virol.* **73**:1387–1394.

69. Weller, A. H., K. Simpson, M. Hersum, N. V. Hooten, and S. A. Huber. 1989. Coxsackievirus B3-induced myocarditis: virus receptor antibodies modulate myocarditis. *J. Immunol.* **143**:1843–1850.

70. Wilfert, C. M., R. H. Buckley, T. Mohanakumar, J. F. Griffith, S. L. Katz, J. K. Whisnant, P. A. Eggleston, M. Moore, E. Treadwell, M. N. Oxman, and F. N. Rosen. 1977. Persistent and fatal central nervous system echovirus infections in patients with agammaglobulinemia. *N. Engl. J. Med.* **296**:1485.

71. Woodall, C. J., M. H. Riding, D. I. Graham, and G. B. Clemens. 1994. Sequences specific for enteroviruses detected in spinal cord from patients with motor neuron diseases. *Br. Med. J.* **308**:1341–1343.

72. Yousef, G. E., E. J. Bell, G. F. Mann, V. Murugesan, D. G. Smith, R. A. McCartney, and J. F. Mowbray. 1988. Chronic enterovirus infection in patients with postviral fatigue syndrome. *Lancet* **i**:146–149.

73. Yousef, G. E., D. A. Isenberg, and J. F. Mowbray. 1990. Detection of enterovirus specific RNA sequences in muscle biopsy specimens from patients with adult onset myositis. *Ann. Rheum. Dis.* **49**:310–315.

74. Ytterberg, S. R., M. L. Mahowald, and R. P. Messner. 1987. Coxsackievirus B1-induced polymyositis: lack of disease expression in nu/nu mice. *J. Clin. Invest.* **80**:499.

75. Ytterberg, S. R., M. L. Mahowald, and R. P. Messner. 1988. T cells are required for coxsackie B1 induced murine polymyositis. *J. Rheumatol.* **15**:475.

76. Zoll, J., P. Jongen, J. Galama, F. V. Kuppeveld, and W. Melchers. 1993. Coxsackievirus B1-induced murine myositis: no evidence for viral persistence. *J. Gen. Virol.* **74**:2071–2076.

DIAGNOSIS AND TREATMENT

LABORATORY DIAGNOSIS OF ENTEROVIRAL INFECTIONS

Harley A. Rotbart and José R. Romero

17

In the United States alone, the enteroviruses (EVs) are estimated to cause 5 to 10 million symptomatic infections annually (78). In temperate climates, these infections occur during the summer and fall; young children are the most common victims, as both the incidence and severity of many EV infections vary inversely with the patient's age (see chapter 1). In addition to the actual diseases that they cause, the EVs are of great concern because they mimic other pathogens. Distinguishing EV infections from those due to common bacteria and other viruses is often difficult on clinical grounds alone (see chapters 10 through 14). Hence, unnecessary treatment for other infections is frequently instituted during EV infections.

As detailed in the preceding chapters, the EVs are responsible for a wide array of clinical diseases affecting many organ systems. From the perspective of laboratory diagnosis, it is important to reiterate a theme expressed many times in this volume: no disease is uniquely associated with any specific EV serotype, and no serotype is uniquely associated with any one disease (9, 46). This is true even of paralytic poliomyelitis, which has been associated with numerous nonpolio EV serotypes (18, 46). For that reason, in most circumstances it is sufficient to speak of diseases that "EVs cause" and to diagnose "an EV" in the laboratory without necessarily specifying or identifying the particular serotype. Certain clinical syndromes are indeed more likely to be caused by one or a few serotypes, but significant overlap exists among the serotypes and the diseases they cause.

CHARACTERISTICS OF THE VIRUSES

The chapters in Section I of this book describe the vast amount of recently accrued knowledge regarding the physical, chemical, and biological properties of the EVs. In the context of laboratory diagnosis, a few of those characteristics are worthy of brief review. The EVs comprise 67 distinct serotypes (54) within the family *Picornaviridae* (*pico* meaning small and *rna* for RNA). The traditional taxonomic subgroups of EVs (Table 1) are based on the patterns of replication of the individual serotypes in various host cells and tissues (see below and Table 2). Like other picornaviruses, EVs are small (27- to 30-nm diameter; 1.34

Harley A. Rotbart, Departments of Pediatrics and Microbiology, University of Colorado School of Medicine, 4200 East 9th Avenue, Box C227, Denver, Colorado 80262. *José R. Romero*, Combined Division of Pediatric Infectious Diseases, Creighton University/University of Nebraska Medical Center, 2500 California Plaza, Criss II Building, Room 409, Omaha, Nebraska 68178.

Human Enterovirus Infections, Edited by Harley A. Rotbart,
© 1995 American Society for Microbiology, Washington, DC 20005

TABLE 1 EV serotypes

Subgroup	Serotypes
Poliovirus	1–3
Coxsackieviruses A	1–22, 24[a]
Coxsackieviruses B	1–6
Echovirus	1–9, 11–27, 29–33[a]
Numbered EVs	68–71

[a] Coxsackievirus A23, echoviruses 10 and 28, and enterovirus 72 have been reclassified (54).

g/ml buoyant density); each virion consists of a simple viral capsid and a single strand of positive (message)-sense RNA (see chapter 7). EVs are acid and ether stable and grow optimally at core body temperature (36 to 37°C). The capsid contains four proteins, VP1 through VP4, arranged in 60 repeating protomeric units as an icosahedron (see chapters 3 and 7). Variations within capsid proteins VP1 through VP3 are responsible for the antigenic diversity among the EVs; neutralization sites are most densely clustered on VP1 (see chapter 3). VP4 is not present on the viral surface; rather, it is in close association with the RNA core, functioning as an anchor to the viral capsid. Destabilization of VP4 results in viral uncoating (see chapter 3). The atomic structures of two poliovirus serotypes, types 1 and 3, have recently been resolved by computerized crystallographic studies, which reveal a deep cleft or canyon in the center of each protomeric unit into which the specific cellular receptor for the EVs fits when virus encounters a susceptible host cell (see chapter 18).

The encapsidated RNA of the human EVs is approximately 7.4 kb long and serves as a template for both viral protein translation (see chapter 5) and RNA replication, the latter accomplished via a double-stranded replicative intermediate form of RNA (see chapter 4). A single reading frame begins at approximately nucleotide 740 from the 5' end and terminates at approximately nucleotide 7370, leaving 740 bases at the 5' end and 70 bases at the 3' end [just upstream from a poly (A) tail] untranslated; these untranslated sequences are felt to be involved in viral regulatory activities such as replication and translation (see chapters 2, 4, and 5). A single polyprotein is translated from the open reading frame. Posttranslational modification is accomplished by virus-encoded proteases and results in generation of the four capsid proteins as well as the enzymes necessary for replication and translation (see chapter 5).

Although genetic differences in the capsid coding regions result in the wide variety of EV serotypes, great similarities exist among the genomes of many of the EVs in a number of other regions along the RNA, including the untranslated sequences at the 5' and 3' ends (see chapter 2). Echoviruses 22 and 23 are genetically dissimilar from the other EVs and, like hepatitis A virus, require reclassification (26).

Laboratory diagnosis of the EVs has exploited many of the distinctive characteristics summarized above. The predictable and well-studied growth properties of the EVs in in vitro culture systems or animals have made viral culture the mainstay of diagnosis for the past four decades. Recent insights into the surface features of these agents have revitalized efforts to design immunoassays and serologic tests for both initial detection and subsequent serotyping. Recognition of genetic homology among all of the EVs spawned the development of sensitive and specific nucleic acid detections systems, particularly the PCR, which, as discussed in detail below, promises to revolutionize EV diagnosis.

COLLECTION AND STORAGE OF SPECIMENS

The EVs are quite stable in liquid environments, being able to survive for many weeks in water, body fluids, and sewage (see chapter 1). This characteristic results from a combination of thermostability in the presence of divalent cations, acid stability, and the absence of a lipid envelope. Cerebrospinal fluid, serum or whole blood, and urine may be submitted to the laboratory in their original collection tubes; rectal or throat swabs or nasal wash specimens are best transported and stored in a standard high-protein viral transport medium. Viral infectivity for cell culture is preserved for long periods (years) at −70°C and probably at −20°C as well. Stability is acceptable for shorter periods (weeks) at 4°C. Viral infectivity may decrease at room temperature over days to weeks. Hence, specimens suboptimally stored in refrigerators or freezers of other clinical laboratories prior to viral cultures being requested may still be adequate for EV isolation. Some small loss of viral titer occurs with each freeze-thaw; hence, multiple freeze-thaw cycles should be avoided, and original specimens should be aliquotted if repeat testing is anticipated.

Specimens for PCR detection of EV RNA (see below) should be handled in a way that preserves viral-capsid integrity, thus protecting the target EV RNA molecule from the ubiquitous nucleases in body fluids. Addition of RNase inhibitor substances such vanadyl ribonucleoside complex or placental RNase inhibitor to specimens prior to freezing may protect the RNAs of the relatively few virions that lyse during the freeze-thaw process.

Sera for antibody testing (see below) are best collected at both acute and convalescent stages of the infection (separated by 2 to 4 weeks), frozen at −20°C, and then thawed and tested simultaneously.

ISOLATION OF VIRUS

The original subclassification of the EVs was based on the abilities of individual serotypes to grow in various cell culture and animal systems (see chapters 1 and 3). Hence, coxsackievirus A serotypes were characteristically able to replicate in suckling mice, with resultant diffuse myositis and flaccid paralysis. However, these viruses were not readily grown in tissue culture cells derived from monkey or human tissues. In contrast, coxsackievirus B serotypes grow readily in tissue cultures of both simian and human origin as well as in suckling mice; the pathology in mice differs from that of the coxsackievirus A serotypes in that the myositis with B serotypes is more focal and direct infection of brain, myocardium, pancreas, and liver also occurs. Neither group of coxsackieviruses is pathogenic for monkeys. The echoviruses are defined by their ability to grow only in simian-derived tissue culture cells but not at all in animal systems. The polioviruses grow most prolifically in cells of human and simian origin and in monkeys, but they fail to grow in murine models. Since these original distinctions were observed, they have been significantly blurred by the identification of new strains and new tissue culture cell lines, resulting in crossover patterns of EV growth. For that reason, recent serotypes have simply been numbered (EVs 68 through 71) (50).

John Enders and his colleagues received the Nobel Prize in 1954 for successfully propagating poliovirus in a continuous cell culture system, thus paving the way for vaccine development (16). Isolation of EVs in cell culture remains the "gold standard" for diagnosis. The commercial availability of increasing numbers and types of continuous cell lines has provided numerous options for routine EV culturing. The general susceptibilities of commonly used cell lines for the EVs are summarized in Table 2; a quick glance at that table shows that no single cell line is optimal for all EV serotypes. Monkey kidney cell lines, the traditional first choice for EV isolation, have good sensitivity for the polioviruses, coxsackievirus B serotypes, and echoviruses, whereas human diploid fibroblasts like WI-38 and HELF (human embryonic lung fibroblasts) have higher yields for coxsackievirus A serotypes. RD cells, derived from a human rhabdomyosarcoma, are the most sensitive for detection of coxsackievirus A but fail with most coxsackievirus B serotypes; RD cells are notoriously difficult to work with in the laboratory, with rapid overgrowth and cell degeneration, and detection of EV growth frequently requires blind passages. For ease of use, most laboratories use a combination of a continuous monkey kidney cell line such as CMK (cynomolgous monkey kidney) and a human diploid fibroblast line such as WI-38, MRC-5, or HELF. Studies have shown improved yield and rapidity of EV detection with the

TABLE 2 Susceptibilities of commonly used cell lines to EVs

Cell line	Susceptibility to[a]:			
	Polioviruses	Coxsackieviruses		Echoviruses
		A	B	
Monkey kidney				
RhMK	+++	+	+++	+++
CMK	++++	+	+++	+++
BGM	+++	+	++++	++
Human cells				
HeLa	+++	+	+++	+
HK	+++	+	++	+++
WI-38	++	++	+	+++
HELF	+++	++	+	+++
MRC-5	+++	+	+	+++
RD	+++	+++	+	+++
HEp-2	+++	+	+++	+

[a]Relative susceptibilities of cell lines: +, minimally susceptible; ++++, very susceptible.

addition of BGM (Bavarian green monkey kidney) and RD cells, albeit their use is associated with greater cost and complexity (10, 13). Duplicate tubes of each cell line do not appear to significantly improve viral isolation except possibly with Rhesus monkey kidney cells (10). If enough cell lines are used, the patterns of growth in each by a single EV isolate may accurately predict the subclassification of the isolate (23, 33), although the clinical value of that information is limited. Primary human amnion cells have proven useful for isolation of many EV serotypes including the coxsackievirus A serotypes (85); the difficulty in preparing and maintaining these cells, however, has resulted in their disuse.

Preparation of clinical samples for inoculation into cell culture has been reviewed elsewhere (36, 51, 52, 61). Feces are suspended (10 to 20% final concentration) in a tube of sterile saline containing glass beads. Vigorous shaking and subsequent settling of the emulsified feces are followed by low-speed centrifugation of the supernatant for about 15 min. Antibiotics are added at concentrations comparable to those in viral transport media, and a longer low-speed (or shorter high-speed) centrifugation is performed. The resultant supernatant is inoculated directly onto cell cultures. An identical procedure may be performed for the following specimens: rectal swabs in viral transport media, throat swabs in viral transport media, and nasal or pharyngeal washes. Swabs should be squeezed out against the sides of the collection tube and discarded rather than broken off into the media, since swab components may be toxic to cells. Specimens already in transport media containing antibiotics need not be re-treated following the initial centrifugation. Cerebrospinal fluid, serum, and urine need no pretreatment and may be inoculated directly onto cell cultures. Serum and urine tend to be more toxic to cells and often require a change in the culture media within 24 h of inoculation. Occasionally, EVs may be antibody bound in serum or cerebrospinal fluid and detectable only following acid dissociation, procedures for which have been presented elsewhere in detail (47, 51). Preparation of body tissues from biopsy or autopsy for EV isolation is initiated by grinding the tissue into a fine slurry under sterile conditions, using mortar, pestle, and sterile sand or one of several commercially available homogenizers. The slurry is then centrifuged and the specimens are processed as described above for fecal specimens.

Although it is the most sensitive method for

laboratory diagnosis of some coxsackievirus A infections, isolation of EVs in suckling mice is rarely done any longer because of the difficulty of the technique and of animal maintenance. This method was recently reviewed elsewhere (53).

DIRECT DETECTION OF VIRAL COMPONENTS

There are numerous compelling reasons for seeking a rapid direct diagnostic assay for the EVs. Isolation of EVs in cell culture and recognition of cytopathic effect (see above) require a high level of expertise and may be quite labor intensive. Some EV serotypes, particularly within the coxsackievirus A group, do not grow at all in cell culture (23, 36, 41, 51, 52, 61, 85, 86). Of greater significance is the fact that 25 to 35% of specimens from patients with characteristic EV infections of any serotype are negative by cell culture (11) because of antibody neutralization in situ; inadequate collection, handling, and processing of the samples; or insensitivity intrinsic to the cell lines used. Suckling mouse inoculation improves the yield only modestly (23, 36, 51, 52–53). EVs that do grow in cell culture may do so slowly. Reported mean isolation times for EVs from cerebrospinal fluid range from 3.7 to 8.2 days (11, 30, 53, 86); EVs from other sites, where viral titers are higher, often grow more rapidly (20, 53, 56, 86).

Electron Microscopy

Electron microscopy for EV detection has found little to no application in clinical laboratory practice. The only clinical specimen that has a concentration of EVs high enough to reach detectability by electron microscopy is feces (86). The EVs are rarely causes of significant gastroenteritis; hence, fecal samples are usually solid, making detection difficult. Additionally, the presence of EVs in feces is in and of itself of little diagnostic import, as asymptomatic shedding may follow true infection for many weeks to months (see Evaluation and Interpretation of Results below). Other body fluids could be concentrated to enhance electron microscopic detection of the EVs, but this would contribute little to what can more easily be learned with other direct viral assays and viral isolation.

Immunoassays

The absence of a widely shared antigen has hampered the development of immunoassays for the EVs (21). The greatest success has been with assays limited to a particular subgroup of EV serotypes, e.g., the coxsackievirus B serotypes, which have an antigen in common (89). Recent reports of polyclonal (64) and monoclonal (77, 88, 90, 91) antibodies that cross-react with multiple EV serotypes are promising, but further testing is required to determine the clinical relevance of those observations. These reagents have been succesfully applied to serotyping of EV isolates (see below), but with the exception of a single report of a monoclonal antibody specific for echovirus 11 (55), the utility of these reagents for direct detection of EVs in clinical specimens has not been demonstrated.

Nucleic Acid Hybridization

In 1984, two laboratories reported the successful detection of multiple EV serotypes of different subclassifications with single molecular probes derived from a single serotype (28, 72). This accomplishment demonstrated that genetic homology among the EVs extended well beyond the few serotypes for which genomic sequence information was known at that time. In the ensuing 6 years, numerous investigators have extended those observations by using cDNA probes, RNA probes, and oligomeric probes (Table 3). Although EVs are readily detected in body fluids during reconstruction experiments (wherein EVs are "spiked" into body fluids obtained from uninfected patients) (73), the sensitivity in actual clinical specimens is only 33% or less. Generally, RNA probes are more sensitive but less specific than cDNA probes; oligomeric probes are more convenient and very specific but are the least sensitive of the probe types. The limiting variable in all of these hybridization-based assays is the low ti-

TABLE 3 Nucleic acid hybridization studies demonstrating sequence relationships among the EVs[a]

Probe and investigators (reference)	Yr	Probe serotype(s)	Target serotype(s) detected	Genomic region(s) of probes demonstrating homology
cDNA probes				
Tracy and Smith (82)	1981	PV1, PV2	PV1–PV3	Approx full length
Hyypiä et al. (28)	1984	CB3	PV3, CB2–CB4, CA9, E17	3' half
Rotbart et al. (72)	1984	PV1	PV1–PV3, CB1, CA9, E11	5' end; approx full length
Tracy (80)	1984	CB3	CB1–CB6	5' end; 3' half
Tracy (81)	1985	CB1–CB6	CB1–CB6	Approx full length
Rotbart et al. (73)	1985	PV1,[b] CB3[c]	PV1–PV3, CB1, CB6, CA9, CA16, E2, E4, E6, E11	5' end; 3' half
Hyypiä et al. (27)	1987	CB3,[d] CA21, PV3, EV70	45 serotypes	3' end; 3' half
Kandolf et al. (34)	1987	CB3	PV1, CB1–CB6, CA9, E11, E12	Approx full length
Easton and Eglin (15)	1988	CB4	PV3, CB1, CB2, CB4, CB6, CA1, CA7, E7, E11	Not specified
Zhang et al. (93)	1988	CB3[c]	PV1, CB1–CB6, CA7, CA9, E1, E7, E11	5' end; 3' half
Chatterjee et al. (8)	1988	CB4, E9	PV3, CB1–CB6, CA9, E3, E9, E11	5' end; 3' end
Newman et al. (58)	1989	CB3[c]	PV1–PV3, CB1, CB3, CA1–CA6, CA15, E7, E11, EV71	5' end; 3' end
Bruce et al. (5)	1989	CB4, CA21	28 serotypes	5' end; 3' end
RNA probes				
Cova et al. (12)	1988	PV1	PV1–PV3, CB1, CB3, CB4, CA7, CA9, CA21, E9, E11, E33	5' end; VP1
Rotbart et al. (69)	1988	PV1, CB3, E9, TMEV	PV1–PV3, CB1, CB6, CA4, CA9, CA14, CA16, CA17, CA24, E2, E4, E6, E11, E22	5' end; 3' half
Petitjean et al. (60)	1990	PV1[e]	PV1–PV3, CB2, CA16, E11, E14, E31	5' end; VP1
Synthetic oligomeric probes				
Rotbart et al. (70)	1988	CB3, E9	PV1, PV3, CB1, CB6, CA9, CA16, E2, E4, E6, E11, E22	5' end; protease gene
Bruce et al. (5)	1989	HRV14	PV1–PV3, CB1, CB2, CB4, CB6, CA1, CA16, CA21, E1–E4, E6, E19, E25	5' end
Alksnis et al. (3)	1989	CB3, CB4	CB3, CB4	VP1

[a] Abbreviations: PV, poliovirus; CB, coxsackievirus B; CA, coxsackievirus A; E, echovirus; EV, enterovirus; TMEV, Theiler's murine encephalomyocarditis virus; HRV, human rhinovirus.
[b] Same probes as used by Rotbart et al. (72).
[c] Same probes as used by Tracy (80).
[d] Same probe as used by Hyypiä et al. (28).
[e] Same probe as used by Cova et al. (12).

ter of EVs in many specimens, particularly cerebrospinal fluid from patients with aseptic meningitis, which may contain as few as 1 to 10 titratable virions per ml (86).

The experiences of many laboratories with nucleic acid probes derived from all regions of the EV genome have defined those areas of greatest conservation among the many EV serotypes that cause human disease (Table 3). This knowledge facilitated the design of primers and probes when PCR technology caught up with the field of EV diagnosis.

PCR

The most promising development in direct detection of the EVs has been the application of PCR (65, 66). Three general strategies have been employed: universal detection of many or all serotypes, serotype-specific or group-specific detection of a limited number of serotypes, and strain-specific detection of variations within a single serotype. Universal detection of EVs by PCR is discussed in this section. A potentially important application of group-specific EV PCR, namely, the discrimination of polioviruses from the nonpolio EVs in clinical specimens, is discussed below. Strain-specific PCR is of use mainly for the study of the genetic shifts and drifts of individual EV strains and the study of specific molecular virulence determinants (see chapters 1 and 2).

Three sets of universal PCR primers and probes for the EVs were reported between the end of 1989 and early 1990; each has a broad reactivity among many EV serotypes and a high specificity for the EVs (Fig. 1) (7, 25, 67). All are directed at highly conserved regions of the 5' noncoding region of the viral genome and are designed for reverse transcription (RT) combined with PCR (RT-PCR). One of these primer sets (67) has been tested against 66 (of the total 67) EV serotypes and found to amplify 60 of the serotypes tested (coxsackievirus A15 was not available for testing); only coxsackieviruses A11, A17, and A24 and echoviruses 16, 22, and 23 failed to amplify with these reagents (94). The last two serotypes, as noted above, are atypical of other EVs and may require reclassification (26). None of the six serotypes that failed to amplify with this primer set are among the commonly reported clinical isolates (78), which would predict successful application of these reagents in clinical testing. Since early 1990, numerous investigators have reported primers and probes from regions of the 5' nontranslated region of the EV genome that overlap or are near the three initially described sets of oligomers (Fig. 1); these reagents have various degrees of homology with the reported genomic sequences of the EVs (Table 4). EV RT-PCR with these and other primer-probe sets has now been tested in clinical settings by numerous investigators and found to be consistently more sensitive than culture and virtually 100% specific (57, 59, 68, 71, 76, 84).

Specimens to be studied by PCR must be treated to extract the target EV RNA and remove potentially inhibitive substances such as proteins and lipids. PCR testing of untreated body fluids is unsuccessful, as is PCR testing following simple heat treatment; this is true whether the fluids tested are relatively pristine, such as cerebrospinal fluid and serum, or more proteinaceous, like nasal washes or feces. The most commonly used extraction techniques employ either phenol-chloroform-sodium dodecyl sulfate or guanidinium thiocyanate (66). All solutions are prepared in diethyl pyrocarbonate-treated water (to minimize RNase contamination of water and glassware), and reactions are carried out in the presence of RNase inhibitors. Following extraction, RT of the EV RNA is accomplished with the downstream primer and any of several commercially available reverse transcriptases. PCR itself is performed with *Taq* polymerase in an automated thermal cycler for 30 to 35 cycles of denaturation, annealing, and extension. The amplified product can be detected by any of several conventional techniques that employ a confirmatory hybridization step that uses the oligomeric probe molecule, including ethidium bromide-stained agarose gels with confirmatory Southern hybridization or dot blot hybridization. The wide array of reported

PV1M 5'UUAAAACAGC UCUGGGGUUG UACCCACCCC AGAGGCCCAC GUGGCGGCUA GUACUCCGGU   60

        5'-CGGUAC CCUUGUACGC CUGU-3'(EP1)Gow→
AUUGCGGUAC CCUUGUACGC CUGUUUUAUA CUCCCUUCCC GUAACUUAGA CGCACAAAAC 120

                                     5'-CAAGCACTT CTGTTTCCCC
                         (PCR primer)5'-AAGCACTT CTGTTTCC-3'Hyypiä→
CAAGUUCAAU AGAAGGGGGU ACAAACCAGU ACCACCACGA ACAAGCACUU CUGUUUCCCC 180

GG-3'(Primer 1)Zoll→
GGUGAUGUCG UAUAGACUGC UUGCGUGGUU GAAAGCGACG GAUCCGUUAU CCGCUUAUGU 240

ACUUCGAGAA GCCCAGUACC ACCUCGGAAU CUUCGAUGCG UUGCGCUCAG CACUCAACCC 300

                                                   3'-CCGA
CAGAGUGUAG CUUAGGCUGA UGAGUCUGGA CAUCCCUCAC CGGUGACGGU GGUCCAGGCU 360

CGCAACCGCC GG-5'(Enterovirus probe)Hyypiä↓
GCGUUGGCGG CCUACCUAUG GCUAACGCCA UGGGACGCUA GUUGUGAACA AGGUGUGAAG 420

5'-TATTGA GCTAGTTGGT AGTCCTCCGG-3'(EP2)Gow↓
         5'-TCCTCCGG CCCCTGAATG CG-3'(Primer 2)Zoll→
           5'-TCCGG CCCCTGAATG-3'(E2)Chapman→
         5'-TCCTCCGG CCCCTGAATG CG-3'(C)Jin→
         5'-CCTCCGG CCCCTGAATG CGGCTAAT-3'(MD91)Rotbart→
AGCCUAUUGA GCUACAUAAG AAUCCUCCGG CCCCUGAAUG CGGCUAAUCC CAACCUCGGA 480
←Hyypiä(cDNA primer)3'-AGGAGGCC GGGGACTTAC-5'
                       ←Gow(EP4)3'-GACTTAC GCCGATTAGG ATT-5'

                             3'-C AGCATTGCCC GTTGAGACGT CGCCTTGGCT
                                                       3'-CCTTGGCT

GCAGGUGGUC ACAAACCAGU GAUUGGCCUG UCGUAACGCG CAAGUCCGUG GCGGAACCGA 540

GATGAAACCC ACAGGCACAA ATGAAAATA-5'(2)Jin↓
GATGAAACCC ACAGGCACA-5'(E3)Chapman↓
3'-ATGAAACCC ACAGGCACAA A-5'(Probe)Zoll↓
3'-ATGAAACCC ACAGGCACAA AG-5'(MD92)Rotbart↓
5'-CTACTTTGGG TGTCCG-3'(OL24)Olive→
CUACUUUGGG UGUCCGUGUU UCCUUUUAUU UUAUUGUGGC UGCUUAUGGU GACAAUCACA 600
                  ←Rotbart(MD90)3'-ACCG ACGAATACCA CTGTTA-5'
                     ←Jin(D)3'-ACCG ACGAATACCA CTGTTA-5'
             ←Zoll(Primer 3)3'-ACCG ACGAATACCA CTGTTA-5'

GAUUGUUAUC AUAAAGCGAA UUGGAUUGGC CAUCCGGUGA AAGUGAGACU CAUUAUCUAU 660
        ←Chapman(E1)3'-ACCTAACCG GTAGGCCAC-5'

CUGUUUGCUG GAUCCGCUCC AUUGAGUGUG UUUACUCUAA GUACAAUUUC AACAGUUAUU 720

UCAAUCAGAC AAUUGUAUCA UAAUGGGUGC UCAGGU.....GGGUGGUGGU GGAAGUUGCC 1197
                            ←Olive(OL68-1)3'-CCNACCACCA CCTTQAATGG-5

FIGURE 1 Sequences and locations of representative primers and probes for EVs superimposed on the genome of poliovirus type 1 Mahoney (PV1M) (underlined) (sequence obtained from reference 38). Homology of the primers and probes to a variety of sequenced enteroviruses is shown in Table 4. Primers are marked → for sense and ← for antisense relative to the viral genome. Probes are marked ↓. Investigators (first author) reporting the primers and probes are indicated; references follow the same investigators' names in Table 4. The names for each oligomeric sequence, as designated by the investigators, are shown in parentheses.

TABLE 4 Comparison of universal EV primers and probes with published EV genomic sequences

Investigator and sequence	Oligonucleotide[a]	% Homology with genomic sequence of[b]:									
		PV1	PV2	PV3	CA9	CA21	CB1	CB3	CB4	CB5	EV70
Chapman et al. (7)											
Antisense primer[c]	E1	100	100	94	100	89	100	100	94	94	94
Sense primer[c]	E2	100	100	100	100	100	100	100	100	100	100
Probe[c]	E3	100	100	100	100	100	100	100	96	100	100
Gow et al. (17)											
Antisense primer	EP4	95	100	100	95	100	100	100	100	100	95
Sense primer	EP1	90	95	95	95	90	100	100	100	90	90
Probe	EP2	81	81	73	96	81	96	100	100	96	85
Hyypiä et al. (25)											
Antisense primer	cDNA primer	100	100	100	100	100	100	100	100	100	100
Sense primer	PCR primer	100	100	94	94	100	94	94	88	94	88
Probe	EV	100	94	94	81	100	100	100	100	100	100
Jin et al. (32)											
Antisense primer	D	100	100	100	100	100	100	100	100	100	100
Sense primer	C	100	100	100	100	100	100	100	100	100	100
Probe	2	90	88	90	98	87	100	100	98	97	90
Olive et al. (59)											
Antisense primer	OL68-1	95	95	100	95	95	100	90	95	100	90
Sense primer	OL24	100	100	100	100	100	100	100	94	100	100
Rotbart (67)											
Antisense primer	MD90	100	100	100	100	100	100	100	100	100	100
Sense primer	MD91	100	100	100	100	100	100	100	100	100	100
Probe	MD92	100	100	100	100	100	100	100	100	100	100
Zoll et al. (94)											
Antisense primer	Primer 3	100	100	100	100	100	100	100	100	100	100
Sense primer	Primer 1	100	100	95	95	95	91	95	100	95	91
Probe	Probe	100	100	100	100	100	100	100	100	100	100

[a] See map for sequence and location of each oligonucleotide.
[b] As aligned with sequences from references 6, 24, 37, 75, 79, 79a, and 92. PV, poliovirus; CA, coxsackievirus A; CB, coxsackievirus B; EV, enterovirus.
[c] Investigators' nomenclature.

conditions for EV PCR extraction, RT, amplification, and detection have recently been reviewed (66). Each laboratory must derive its own optimal conditions, which will vary with the composition of primers and buffers, the enzymes used, and the specimens being tested. The nucleotide dUTP and the enzyme uracil N-glycosylase should be used in all PCR reactions (44), and other standardized precautions should be taken to minimize the risk of carryover contamination from one experiment to another (39).

The most dramatic development in PCR-based detection of the EVs has been the modification and adaptation of one of the original sets of primers and probe (67) to a single-buffer, microwell-based, colorimetric RT-PCR kit that is user-friendly enough that the procedure can be performed in 5 h by personnel in the routine diagnostic virology laboratory (35, 74). An accurate diagnosis of EV infections that is available in less than 1 day could have a significant impact on the quality and cost of patient management (11, 76a). As formatted in the prototypic kit that is currently undergoing clinical trials, EV RNA extraction is performed with a lysis solution containing guanidine thiocyanate, glycogen, and dithiothreitol in Tris buffer; precipitation is with isopropanol and 70% ethanol and is followed by resuspension in a diluent solution containing manganese acetate and potassium acetate in a bicine buffer. The resuspended specimen is added to a master mix containing uracil N-glycosylase, biotinylated primers, deoxynucleotide triphosphates (with dUTP in place of dTTP), and rTth enzyme, also in a bicine buffer. The rTth enzyme is capable of both RT and PCR in the same buffer solution, obviating the need to open the tube between steps; in additions to simplifying the procedure, this reduces the potential for aerosolization of the tube contents and subsequent carryover contamination (39). Following amplification in a thermal cycler, the sample is denatured, and amplification products are detected on microwell plates containing immobilized oligonucleotide probe specific for the EVs. Hybridization, incubation with conjugate, and addition of substrate are very similar to the detection steps of a typical microwell enzyme immunoassay, as previously reported (43). A yellow color appears in microwells containing positive specimens, and microwells are colorless for negative specimens (Fig. 2). Spectrophotometric measurement provides a numeric result; optical density of the wells is read at 450 nm, and results are scored as positive if the optical density exceeds a predetermined cutoff level.

Of 63 serotypes tested (coxsackieviruses A1, A2, A4, and A8 were unavailable for testing), the colorimetric RT-PCR assay described above detected all but echoviruses 22 and 23 (41a), which, as noted above, are genetically divergent from the other EVs and are pending reclassification as a separate genus of picornaviruses (26). The primers and probes used are either identical to or slightly modified from those previously reported (67); others found those reagents to "miss" coxsackieviruses A11, A17, and A24 and echovirus 16 (94), all of which are detected in this colorimetric format. The sensitivity of the assay is 1 50% tissue culture infective dose for most EV serotypes tested, and there is no cross-reactivity with any of the numerous non-EV viral, bacterial, or fungal causes of systemic or central nervous system infections (41a, 74). Of 22 rhinovirus serotypes tested, only 5 cross-reacted in this assay, all at titers generally thought to be higher than those seen clinically (66a). While of potential concern for diagnosing the etiology of viral respiratory tract infections, limited cross-reactivity of this EV RT-PCR assay with rhinoviruses will be of no significance in diagnosing EV-associated systemic infections, since rhinoviruses are not found in feces, blood, urine, or cerebrospinal fluid. The reproducibility of the colorimetric EV RT-PCR kit assay was determined by duplicate testing of 194 specimens (66a); only 5 of the paired specimens gave discordant results (i.e., one aliquot positive and the paired aliquot negative); confirmatory testing found 3 of those discordant specimens to be true positives and 2 to be negative (66a). Discordant results likely represent specimens with EV titers at the limit of the assay's sensitivity.

In two large clinical studies of cerebrospinal fluid specimens from a combined total of 658 patients with EV aseptic meningitis or other central nervous system infections and noninfected controls, the sensitivity of the colorimetric microwell RT-PCR assay com-

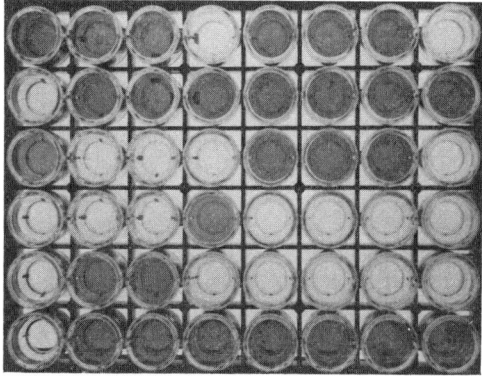

FIGURE 2 Colorimetric microwell plate assay format for detecting enteroviruses by RT-PCR. Colored wells (dark in this black and white photo, yellow in the actual assay) indicate a positive reaction; colorless wells are negative (see text for details).

pared to that of viral culture and clinical diagnosis was 94.7 to 96.3%, specificity was 94.7 to 99%, positive predictive value was 94.7 to 96.3%, and negative predictive value was 97.4 to 99% (42, 74). In a study of neonatal EV infections that used the same kit format, RT-PCR of serum and urine specimens was nearly three times as sensitive as culture of the same specimens and 100% specific (2).

A recent patient of ours illustrates the potential utility of this technique. A 1-month-old female infant who had been born prematurely at 32 weeks presented with sudden onset of respiratory deterioration, apnea, and bradycardia. Prior to this, although still hospitalized, the child had been thriving, nippling feeds, and requiring minimal supplemental oxygen. The child's mother had had a febrile viruslike illness 6 days previously. The mother had a history of recurrent genital herpes simplex virus infection, but no lesions were noted during labor or delivery (which was by cesarean section). The mother was also known to be colonized with group B streptococcus. The child's temperature rose to 99.9°F (ca. 37.7°C), and she was noted to be alternately irritable and lethargic. A sepsis workup was performed, and the baby was treated with ampicillin, cefotaxime, and acyclovir. A diffuse maculopapular rash developed the next day. Laboratory studies included a complete blood count, which showed 5,000 leukocytes per mm^3 (10% band forms, 49% neutrophils, and 33% lymphocytes) and 410,000 platelets per mm^3. Chest X ray and urinalysis were normal, and C-reactive protein was negative. Cerebrospinal fluid revealed 89 leukocytes per mm^3 (50% neutrophils, 50% lympohocytes), 6 erythrocytes per mm^3, 89 mg of protein per dl, and 51 mg of glucose per dl. Viral cultures of the nasopharynx, rectum, and cerebrospinal fluid were inoculated on September 8, and a colorimetric microwell PCR assay was performed on the cerebrospinal fluid on September 9. Results of the latter were positive for EV later that same day (September 9). Nasopharyngeal and rectal cultures were positive for EV on September 13, and cerebrospinal fluid was reported as positive for EV by viral culture on September 14. Hence, rapid colorimetric PCR can be expected to shorten the time to diagnosis of EV infections by many days, reducing unnecessary hospitalization and therapy with antibacterial and anti-herpes simplex medications.

Finally, a quantitative RT-PCR assay for the EVs has recently been reported (45). Such a test may become clinically important when antiviral therapy for these pathogens becomes available and monitoring of viral load in response to therapy becomes desirable.

SEROTYPE IDENTIFICATION

As noted above, the determination of the specific serotype of infecting EVs is often unnecessary, because the diseases caused by the EVs are not serotype specific. In most circumstances, therefore, it is adequate and useful for the diagnostic laboratory to report the presence of "an EV" without further detail. The most common exception to this principle is in pediatrics, where distinguishing between vaccine strain polioviruses and nonpolioviruses is critical to interpretation of viral culture results. During the first 2 years of life, children are repeatedly immunized with trivalent oral polio vaccine (Sabin strains), whose components, like all EVs, may be shed from the throat for 1 to 2 weeks and in the feces for several weeks to months. Hence, isolates from those two sites must be identified as either nonpolio or polio serotypes, with the latter presumed to be of vaccine origin unless unusual clinical circumstances suggest wild-type infection. Vaccine poliovirus has only rarely been recovered from cerebrospinal fluid or blood (19, 47); thus, further characterization of EV isolates from those sites is less important. Distinguishing between polioviruses and nonpolio EVs can be accomplished by two methods, one proven and one experimental. The standard method employs neutralization of the isolate with a pool of antisera directed against the three poliovirus serotypes (23). Successful inhibition of growth by the antisera confirms the poliovirus identity of the isolate, whereas failure to neutralize an isolate with typical cytopathic effect implies the presence of a nonpolio EV. The neutralization method, as previously detailed, utilizes a fixed titer of virus (typically 100 50% tissue culture infectious doses) and pooled antipoliovirus sera (each at a final dilution of 20 U) (23). The experimental method uses a set of PCR primers that is specific for the three poliovirus serotypes; the PCR assay is performed on the culture-passaged isolate and accurately discriminates between polioviruses and nonpolio EVs (1). This latter method has the potential for being simpler and more rapid than viral neutralization for distinguishing between vaccine strains of poliovirus and disease-causing nonpolio EVs, particularly as PCR assays become more user-friendly (see above).

Further identification of a nonpolio EV to specific serotype is useful under certain circumstances. Indeed, the very principle that most clinical manifestations of EV infections are not serotype specific was historically established by serotyping studies. Epidemiologic studies of patterns of EV infections require knowledge of specific serotypes (see chapter 1), as do descriptions of unusual clinical manifestations, such as poliomyelitis due to nonpolio EVs (18) and pandemic hemorrhagic conjunctivitis (see chapter 1) (83). Only via serotyping will new EVs be discovered, as happened most recently with the higher-numbered EVs (50). As noted above, an approximation as to subgroup of an isolate can be accomplished by analysis of the cell lines infected by an isolate (33); plaque morphology may give additional clues as to the serotype within a subgroup (23). The gold standard for EV serotype determination, however, continues to be the use of intersecting pools of lyophilized antisera, as established by Lim and Benyesh-Melnick (LBM pools) (48, 49). Each isolate can be screened against 16 antisera by using 8 pools or against 25 antisera by using 10 pools. A checkerboard analysis localizes the isolate to a single serotype designation based on the pattern of neutralization with the interesecting serum pools. Microtiter plate neutralization works equally well and saves significant quantities of serum reagents. The LBM pools are available in limited supplies from the World Health Organization.

Broadly reactive and serotype-specific EV monoclonal antibodies have been developed (77, 88, 90) and applied to tissue culture confirmation by immunofluorescence. Preliminary studies indicate that these reagents, used singly and in pools, may find an important role in serotype identification. Immunofluorescence is a more rapid, simpler procedure than traditional neutralization-based serotyping, and the supply of monoclonal antibodies is unlimited.

SEROLOGIC DIAGNOSIS

Serologic testing, like immunoassays, has had only a limited role in EV diagnosis because of the great diversity of EV serotypes and the lack of a single common antigen. If the specific serotype of an infecting EV is known or suspected, e.g., in community-wide outbreaks, confirmatory immunoglobulin G (IgG) serology can be performed on individual patients to document a rise in antibody titer from the acute to the convalescent phase of infection, thus providing useful epidemiologic information; little actual benefit accrues to the individual patient. In a situation where an EV is recovered from the feces or throat of a patient with unusual clinical manifestations, the etiologic role of the EV may be more firmly established by documenting a fourfold rise in antibody titer to that serotype in paired acute- and convalescent-phase sera. Serosurveys of populations for past exposure to specific EVs have been performed by testing for antibody in single serum specimens; such studies may be useful for retrospective disease associations, such as with EVs and diabetes mellitus (see chapter 15), dilated cardiomyopathy (see chapter 14), and chronic neuromuscular diseases (see chapter 16). Those types of studies are subject to many types of sampling bias and are therefore of limited value. In the usual scenario, when a patient presents with meningitis or other acute manifestations of illness and an EV is suspected, serology is not a practical option.

Three traditional types of antibody determinations have been applied to the EVs: neutralization, complement fixation, and hemagglutination inhibition. Neutralizing antibody levels rise early in infection with the EVs and persist for many years or for life. They may be assessed in standard tube dilutions or by microtiter plate; in either format, a fixed titer of a single serotype of EV is inoculated onto cells in the presence of serial dilutions of the patient's serum (36, 51, 52, 61); ideally, acute- and convalescent-phase sera are tested in parallel simultaneously. The rapid appearance of serum neutralizing antibodies following EV infection may make it difficult to document a fourfold rise in titer with convalescence. Complement fixation antibody assays are of much less utility, as these antibodies are transient (weeks to months) and broadly cross-reactive among EV serotypes, i.e., nonspecific. Historically, this assay was successfully applied only in testing for infection with the polioviruses. Only about a quarter to a third of all EV serotypes agglutinate erythrocytes, making hemagglutination inhibition of minimal usefulness; this type of antibody is also cross-reactive among EV serotypes, hence nonspecific.

More recently, coxsackievirus B IgM assays, which take advantage of the shared antigen among the six coxsackievirus B serotypes and the early appearance of the IgM class of antibodies, have seemed promising (4, 14, 62). Although the IgM response measured in these assays may be nonspecific, i.e., a response to a non-coxsackievirus B EV may result in a positive assay, the nonspecificity may actually make this test more broadly reflective of recent exposure to any of numerous EV serotypes; cross-reactivity with non-EV pathogens causing infection has not been thoroughly studied. Many patients in the reported studies had positive IgM assays but were negative for EV infection by culture, making the assay either more sensitive or less specific than traditional culture diagnosis. These tests are not yet widely available, and clinical experience with them remains limited. Attempts to use more broadly reactive EV antigens in IgM assays have met with technical shortcomings (62, 63).

EVALUATION AND INTERPRETATION OF RESULTS

The concept of permissive versus nonpermissive sites of infection is critical to the interpretation of EV assays. The nasopharynx and gastrointestinal tract are permissive sites of infection; i.e., EVs have ready access to these sites and may remain as colonizers for weeks to months. Detection of EVs by virus isolation or PCR of samples from these sites must be interpreted cautiously, because virus presence alone does not establish causality of the illness in question. The EV in the feces of a patient today may be left over from an infection of weeks ago and have nothing to do with the meningitis the patient presents with currently. Indeed, virtually 100% of patients with EV aseptic meningitis have detectable EV in feces (56), but most persons shedding EV in the feces at any particular time are asymptomatic. Feces are thus the most sensitive and least specific site for detecting true EV-associated illness. Since the shedding period in the nasopharynx after EV infection is shorter than that in the feces, the specificity of an EV isolate from the nasopharynx for true causation of current symptoms is better than with feces but far short of a definitive association. Further complicating the evaluation of results from these two body sites in young children is the frequent administration of live attenuated oral poliovirus vaccine in the first years of life. Most EV isolates that the diagnostic virology laboratory encounters in the feces and nasopharynges of young children are in fact vaccine strain polioviruses. Reporting an EV isolate in this setting without specifying poliovirus versus nonpolio EV can lead the physician to wrongly discontinue antibiotics or antiherpes therapy in the belief that an EV etiology has been established.

In contrast, the central nervous system, bloodstream, and genitourinary tract are nonpermissive sites of EV infection; i.e., detection of virus in specimens from these sites implies true invasive infection and a high likelihood of association with current illness. Rare reports of coinfections of the cerebrospinal fluid by bacteria and EVs have appeared (87). In these patients, the bacterium-associated clinical sequelae usually dominate; i.e., the patients are clinically suspected of having bacterial meningitis and the virus is isolated incidentally. The patients are sick enough that the identification of a virus before identification of the bacterium would have been unlikely to dissuade the clinician from continued use of antibiotics. In the much more common situation, where the clinical presentation is typical of viral meningitis, coinfection with a clinically "silent" bacteria would be extraordinarily unlikely. Hence, identification of an EV from a nonpermissive site in a patient with a clinically compatible illness is sufficient evidence for establishing EV causality. The distinction between polioviruses and nonpolio EVs in specimens from nonpermissive sites is less important, since vaccine strains of poliovirus have rarely been reported in such specimens and, in those rare instances, may actually have been causing the illness in question (19, 47).

The utilities and shortcomings of serologic assays are described above. In general, results of a single serologic assay are uninterpretable except perhaps for IgM tests, which remain to be standardized and more widely tested. Commercially available serologic or immunoassay panels for the EVs are, in general, derived from only limited numbers of serotypes and lack standardization or published quality controls.

REFERENCES

1. **Abraham, R., T. Chonmaitree, J. McCombs, B. Prabhakar, P. T. Lo Verde, and P. L. Ogra.** 1993. Rapid detection of poliovirus by reverse transcription and polymerase chain amplification: application for differentiation between poliovirus and nonpoliovirus enteroviruses. *J. Clin. Microbiol.* **31:**395–399.
2. **Abzug M. J., M. Loeffelholz, and H. A. Rotbart.** Polymerase chain reaction diagnosis of neonatal enterovirus infection. *J Pediatr.*, in press.
3. **Alksnis, M., M. Lindberg, P. Stalhandske, and H. Hultberg.** 1989. Use of synthetic oligodeoxyribonucleotides for type specific identification of coxsackie B viruses. *Mol. Cell. Probes* **3:**103–108.
4. **Bell, E. J., R. A. McCartney, D. Basquill, and A. K. R. Chaudhuri.** 1986. μ-Antibody capture ELISA for the rapid diagnosis of enterovirus infections in patients with aseptic meningitis. *J. Med. Virol.* **19:**213–217.
5. **Bruce, C., W. Al-Nakib, M. Forsyth, G. Stanway, and J. W. Almond.** 1989. Detection of enteroviruses using cDNA and synthetic oligonucleotide probes. *J. Virol. Methods* **25:**233–240.
6. **Chang, K. H., P. Auvienen, T. Hyypiä, and G. Stanway.** 1989. The nucleotide sequence of coxsackievirus A9; implications for receptor binding and enterovirus classification. *J. Gen. Virol.* **70:**3269–3280.
7. **Chapman, N. M., S. Tracy, C. J. Gauntt, and U. Fortmueller.** 1990. Molecular detection and identification of enteroviruses using enzymatic amplification and nucleic acid hybridization. *J. Clin. Microbiol.* **28:**843–850.
8. **Chatterjee, N. K., M. Kaehler, and R. Deibel.** 1988. Detection of enteroviruses using subgenomic probes of coxsackie virus B4 by hybridization. *Diagn. Microbiol. Infect. Dis.* **11:**129–136.
9. **Cherry, J. D.** 1987. Enteroviruses: polioviruses (poliomyelitis), coxsackieviruses, echoviruses, and enteroviruses, p. 1729–1841. *In* R. D. Feigin and J. D. Cherry (ed.), *Textbook of Pediatric Infectious Diseases*, 2nd ed. The W. B. Saunders Co., Philadelphia.
10. **Chonmaitree, T., C. Ford, C. Sanders, and H. L. Lucia.** 1988. Comparison of cell cultures for rapid isolation of enteroviruses. *J. Clin. Microbiol.* **26:**2576–2580.
11. **Chonmaitree, T., M. A. Menegus, and K. R. Powell.** 1982. The clinical relevance of CSF viral culture. A two-year experience with aseptic meningitis in Rochester, New York. *JAMA* **247:**1843–1847.
12. **Cova, L., H. Kopecka, M. Aymard, and M. Girard.** 1988. Use of cRNA probes for the detection of enteroviruses by molecular hybridization. *J. Med. Virol.* **24:**11–18.
13. **Dagan, R., and M. A. Menegus.** 1986. A combination of four cell types for rapid detection of enteroviruses in clinical specimens. *J. Med. Virol.* **19:**219–228.
14. **Dorries, R., and V. Ter Meulen.** 1983. Specificity of IgM antibodies in acute human coxsackievirus B infections, analyzed by indirect solid phase enzyme immunoassay and

immunoblot technique. *J. Gen. Virol.* **64:**159–167.
15. **Easton, A. J., and R. P. Eglin.** 1988. The detection of coxsackievirus RNA in cardiac tissue by *in situ* hybridization. *J. Gen. Virol.* **69:**285–291.
16. **Enders, J. F., T. H. Weller, and F. C. Robbins.** 1949. Cultivation of the Lansing strain of poliomyelitis virus in culture of various human embryonic tissues. *Science* **109:**85–99.
17. **Gow, J. W., W. M. H. Behan, G. B. Clements, C. Woodall, M. Riding, and P. O. Behan.** 1991. Enteroviral RNA sequences detected by polymerase chain reaction in muscle of patients with postviral fatigue syndrome. *Br. Med. J.* **302:**692–696.
18. **Grist, N. R., and E. J. Bell.** 1984. Paralytic poliomyelitis and nonpolio enteroviruses: studies in Scotland. *Rev. Infect. Dis.* **6:**S385–S386.
19. **Gutierrez, K. M., and M. J. Abzug.** 1990. Vaccine-associated poliovirus meningitis in children with ventriculo peritoneal shunts. *J. Pediatr.* **117:**424–427.
20. **Herrmann, E. C., Jr., D. A. Person, and T. F. Smith.** 1972. Experience in laboratory diagnosis of enterovirus infections in routine medical practice. *Mayo Clin. Proc.* **47:**577–586.
21. **Herrmann, J. E., R. M. Hendry, and M. F. Collins.** 1979. Factors involved in enzyme-linked immunoassay of viruses and evaluation of the method for identification of enteroviruses. *J. Clin. Microbiol.* **10:**210–217.
22. **Hogle, J. M., M. Chow, and D. J. Filman.** 1985. Three-dimensional structure of poliovirus at 2.9 Å resolution. *Science* **229:**1358–1365.
23. **Hsiung, G. D.** 1973. Enteroviruses, p. 54–67. In G. D. Hsiung (ed.), *Diagnostic Virology*. Yale University Press, New Haven, Conn.
24. **Hughes, P. J., C. North, P. D. Minor, and G. Stanway.** 1989. The complete nucleotide sequence of coxsackievirus A21. *J. Gen. Virol.* **70:**2843–2952.
25. **Hyypiä, T., P. Auvinen, and M. Maaronen.** 1989. Polymerase chain reaction for human picornaviruses. *J. Gen. Virol.* **70:**3261–3268.
26. **Hyypiä, T., C. Horsnell, M. Maaronen, M. Khan, N. Kalkkinen, P. Auvinen, L. Kinnunen, and G. Stanway.** 1992. A distinct picornavirus group identified by sequence analysis. *Proc. Natl. Acad. Sci. USA* **89:**8847–8851.
27. **Hyypiä, T., M. Maaronen, P. Auvinen, P. Stålhandske, U. Pettersson, G. Stanway, P. Hughes, M. Ryan, J. Almond, M. Stenvik, and T. Hovi.** 1987. Nucleic acid sequence relationships between enterovirus serotypes. *Mol. Cell. Probes* **1:**169–176.
28. **Hyypiä, T., P. Stalhandske, R. Vainionpaa, and U. Pettersson.** 1984. Detection of enteroviruses by spot hybridization. *J. Clin. Microbiol.* **19:**436–438.
29. **Iizuka, N., S. Kuge, and A. Nomoto.** 1987. Complete nucleotide sequence of the genome of coxsackievirus B1. *Virology* **156:**64–73.
30. **Jarvis, W. R., and G. Tucker.** 1981. Echovirus type 7 meningitis in young children. *Am. J. Dis. Child.* **135:**1009–1012.
31. **Jenkins, O., J. D. Booth, P. D. Minor, and J. W. Almond.** 1987. The complete nucleotide sequence of coxsackie B4 and its comparison to other members of the picornaviridae. *J. Gen. Virol.* **68:**1835–1848.
32. **Jin, O., M. J. Sole, J. W. Butany, W.-R. Chia, P. R. McLaughlin, P. Liu, and C.-C. Liew.** 1990. Detection of enterovirus RNA in myocardial biopsies from patients with myocarditis and cardiomyopathy using gene amplification by polymerase chain reaction. *Circulation* **82:**8–16.
33. **Johnston, S. L. G., and C. S. Siegel.** 1990. Presumptive identification of enteroviruses with RD, HEp-2, and RMK cell lines. *J. Clin. Microbiol.* **28:**1049–1050.
34. **Kandolf, R., D. Ameis, P. Kirschner, A. Canu, and P. H. Hofschneider.** 1987. *In situ* detection of enteroviral genomes in myocardial cells by nucleic acid hybridization: an approach to the diagnosis of viral heart disease. *Proc. Natl. Acad. Sci. USA* **84:**6272–6276.
35. **Kao, S.-Y., T. M. Coughran, M. J. Loeffelholz, B. Dale, and H. A. Rotbart.** 1994. Direct and uninterrupted RNA amplification of enteroviruses with colorimetric microwell detection. *Clin. Diagn. Virol.*, in press.
36. **Kapsenberg, J. G.** 1988. Picornaviridae: the enteroviruses (polioviruses, coxsackieviruses, echoviruses), p. 692–722. In E. H. Lennette, P. Halonen, and F. A. Murphy (ed.), *Laboratory Diagnosis of Infectious Diseases: Principles and Practice*. Springer-Verlag, New York.
37. **Klump, W. M., I. Bergmann, B. C. Muller, D. Ameis, and R. Kandolf.** 1990. Complete nucleotide sequence of infectious coxsackievirus B3 cDNA: two initial 5' uridine residues are regained during plus-strand RNA synthesis. *J. Virol.* **64:**1573–1583.
38. **Koch, F., and G. Koch.** 1985. *The Molecular Biology of Poliovirus*, p. 150–161. Springer-Verlag, New York.
39. **Kwok, S., and R. Higuchi.** 1989. Avoiding false positives with PCR. *Nature* (London) **339:**237–238.
40. **Linberg, A. M., P. O. K. Stalhandske, and**

U. Pettersson. 1987. Genome of coxsackievirus B3. *Virology* **156**:50–63.
41. **Lipson, S. M., R. Walderman, P. Costello, and K. Szabo.** 1988. Sensitivity of rhabdomyosarcoma and guinea pig embryo cell cultures to field isolates of difficult-to-cultivate group A coxsackieviruses. *J. Clin. Microbiol.* **26**:1298–1303.
41a. **Loeffelholz, M.** Unpublished observations.
42. **Loeffelholz, M., S. Fast, C. Lewinski, G. H. McCracken, M. Sawyer, and S. Young.** 1994. Detection of enteroviruses in cerebrospinal fluid using PCR. *Abstr. 4th Annu. Prog. Clin. Virol. Symp.*
43. **Loeffelholz, M. J., C. A. Lewinski, S. S. R. Silver, A. P. Purohit, S. A. Herman, D. A. Buonagurio, and E. A. Dragon.** 1992. Detection of *Chlamydia trachomatis* in endocervical specimens by polymerase chain reaction. *J. Clin. Microbiol.* **30**:2847–2851.
44. **Longo, M. C., M. S. Berninger, and J. L. Hartley.** 1990. Use of uracil DNA glycosylase to control carry-over contamination in polymerase chain reactions. *Gene* **93**:125–128.
45. **Martino, T. A., M. J. Sole, L. Z. Penn, C.-C. Liew, and P. Liu.** 1993. Quantitation of enteroviral RNA by competitive polymerase chain reaction. *J. Clin. Microbiol.* **31**:2634–2640.
46. **Melnick, J. L.** 1990. Enteroviruses: polioviruses, coxsackieviruses, echoviruses, and newer enteroviruses, p. 549–605. *In* B. N. Fields and D. M. Knipe (ed.), *Virology*. Raven Press, New York.
47. **Melnick, J. L., R. O. Proctor, A. R. Ocampo, A. R. Diwan, and E. Ben-Porath.** 1966. Free and bound virus in serum after administration of oral poliovirus vaccine. *Am. J. Epidemiol.* **84**:329–342.
48. **Melnick, J. L., V. Rennick, B. Hampil, N. J. Schmidt, and H. H. Ho.** 1973. Lyophilized combination pools of enterovirus equine antisera: preparation and test procedures for the identification of field strains of 42 enteroviruses. *Bull. W.H.O.* **48**:263–268.
49. **Melnick, J. L., N. J. Schmidt, B. Hampil, and H. H. Ho.** 1977. Lyophilized combination pools of enterovirus equine antisera: preparation and test procedures for the identification of field strains of 19 group A coxsackievirus serotypes. *Intervirology* **8**:172–181.
50. **Melnick, J. L., I. Tagaya, and H. Von Magnus.** 1974. Enteroviruses 69, 70, and 71. *Intervirology* **4**:369–370.
51. **Melnick, J. L., H. A. Wenner, and C. A. Phillips.** 1979. Enteroviruses, p. 471–534. *In* E. H. Lennette and N. J. Schmidt (ed.), *Diagnostic Procedures for Viral, Rickettsial and Chlamydial Infections*, 5th ed. American Public Health Association, Washington, D.C.
52. **Melnick, J. L., H. A. Wenner, and L. Rosen.** 1964. The enteroviruses, p. 194–242. *In* E. H. Lennette and N. J. Schmidt (ed.), *Diagnostic Procedures for Viral and Rickettsial Diseases*, 3rd ed. American Public Health Association, Inc., Washington, D.C.
53. **Menegus, M. A.** Enteroviruses, p. 943–947. *In* A. Balows, W. J. Hausler, Jr., K. L. Herrmann, H. D. Isenberg, and H. J. Shadomy (ed.), *Manual of Clinical Microbiology*, 5th ed. American Society for Microbiology, Washington, D.C.
54. **Miller, M. J.** 1993. Viral taxonomy. *Clin. Infect. Dis.* **16**:612–613.
55. **Minnich, L., E. Brown, R. Ashley, C. Andreou, D. Hirsch, E. Yanek, S. Oliver, W. Giles, and S. Maxwell.** 1993. *Abstr. 9th Annu. Clin. Virol. Symp.*, p. 50.
56. **Mintz, L., and W. L. Drew.** 1980. Relation of culture site to the recovery of nonpolio enteroviruses. *Am. J. Clin. Pathol.* **74**:324–326.
57. **Muir, P., F. Nicholson, M. Jhetam, S. Neogi, and J. E. Banatvala.** 1993. Rapid diagnosis of enterovirus infection by magnetic bead extraction and polymerase chain reaction detection of enterovirus RNA in clinical specimens. *J. Clin. Microbiol.* **31**:31–38.
58. **Newman, C. L., J. Modlin, R. H. Yolken, and R. P. Viscidi.** 1989. Solution hybridization and enzyme immunoassay for biotinylated DNA-RNA hybrids to detect enteroviral RNA in cell culture. *Mol. Cell. Probes* **3**:375–382.
59. **Olive, D. M., S. Al-Mufti, W. Al-Mulla, M. A. Khan, A. Pasca, G. Stanway, and W. Al-Nakib.** 1990. Detection and differentiation of picornaviruses in clinical samples following genomic amplification. *J. Gen. Virol.* **71**:2141–2147.
60. **Petitjean, J., M. Quibriac, F. Freymuth, F. Fuchs, N. Laconche, M. Aymard, and H. Kopecka.** 1990. Specific detection of enteroviruses in clinical samples by molecular hybridization using poliovirus subgenomic riboprobes. *J. Clin. Microbiol.* **28**:307–311.
61. **Phillips, C. A.** 1980. Enteroviruses and reoviruses, p. 823–828. *In* E. H. Lennette, A. Balows, W. J. Hausler, Jr., and J. P. Truant (ed.), *Manual of Clinical Microbiology*, 3rd ed. American Society for Microbiology, Washington, D.C.
62. **Pozzetto, B., O. G. Gaudin, M. Aouni, and A. Ros.** 1989. Comparative evaluation of immunoglobulin M neutralizing antibody response in acute-phase sera and virus isolation for the routine diagnosis of enterovirus infection. *J. Clin. Microbiol.* **27**:705–708.
63. **Reigel, F., F. Burkhardt, and U. Schilt.**

1985. Cross-reactions of immunoglobulin M and G antibodies with enterovirus-specific viral structural proteins. *J. Hyg.* **95**:469–481.
64. **Romero, J., J. R. Putnak, and E. Wimmer.** 1986. Abstr. 967. *Pediatr. Res.* **20**:319.
65. **Romero, J. R., and H. A. Rotbart.** 1993. PCR detection of the human enteroviruses, p. 401–406. *In* D. H. Persing, T. F. Smith, F. C. Tenover, and T. J. White (ed.), *Diagnostic Molecular Microbiology: Principles and Applications.* American Society for Microbiology, Washington, D.C.
66. **Romero, J. R., and H. A. Rotbart.** 1994. PCR-based strategies for the detection of human enteroviruses, p. 341–374. *In* G. D. Ehrlich and S. J. Greenberg (ed.), *PCR-Based Diagnostics in Infectious Disease.* Blackwell Scientific Publications, Boston.
66a. **Rotbart, H. A.** Unpublished observations.
67. **Rotbart, H. A.** 1990. Enzymatic RNA amplification of the enteroviruses. *J. Clin. Microbiol.* **28**:438–442.
68. **Rotbart, H. A.** 1990. Diagnosis of enteroviral meningitis with the polymerase chain reaction. *J. Pediatr.* **117**:85–89.
69. **Rotbart, H. A., M. J. Abzug, and M. J. Levin.** 1988. Development and application of RNA probes for the study of picornaviruses. *Mol. Cell. Probes* **2**:65–73.
70. **Rotbart, H. A., P. S. Eastman, J. L. Ruth, K. K. Hirata, and M. J. Levin.** 1988. Nonisotopic oligomeric probes for the human enteroviruses. *J. Clin. Microbiol.* **26**:2669–2671.
71. **Rotbart H. A., J. P. Kinsella, and R. L. Wasserman.** 1990. Persistent enterovirus infection in culture-negative meningoencephalitis—demonstration by enzymatic RNA amplification. *J. Infect. Dis.* **161**:787–791.
72. **Rotbart, H. A., M. J. Levin, and L. P. Villarreal.** 1984. Use of subgenomic poliovirus DNA hybridization probes to detect the major subgroups of enteroviruses. *J. Clin. Microbiol.* **20**:1105–1108.
73. **Rotbart, H. A., M. J. Levin, L. P. Villarreal, S. Tracy, B. L. Semler, and E. Wimmer.** 1985. Factors affecting the detection of enteroviruses in cerebrospinal fluid with coxsackievirus B3 and poliovirus type 1 cDNA probes. *J. Clin. Microbiol.* **22**:220–224.
74. **Rotbart, H. A., M. H. Sawyer, S. Fast, C. Lewinski, N. Murphy, E. F. Keyser, J. Spadoro, S.-Y. Kao, and M. Loeffelholz.** 1994. Diagnosis of enteroviral meningitis by using PCR with a colorimetric microwell detection assay. *J. Clin. Microbiol.* **32**:2590–2592.
75. **Ryan, M. D., O. Jenkins, P. J. Hughes, A. Brown, N. J. Knowles, D. Booth, P. D.**

Minor, and J. W. Almond. 1990. The complete nucleotide sequence of enterovirus type 70: relationships with other members of the picornaviridae. *J. Gen. Virol.* **71**:2291–2299.
76. **Sawyer, M. H., D. Holland, N. Aintablian, J. D. Connor, E. F. Keyser, and N. J. Waecker, Jr.** 1994. Diagnosis of enteroviral central nervous system infection by polymerase chain reaction during a large community outbreak. *J. Pediatr. Infect. Dis.* **13**:177–182.
76a. **Schlesinger, Y., M. H. Sawyer, and G. A. Storch.** 1994. Enteroviral meningitis in infancy: potential role for polymerase chain reaction in patient management. *Pediatrics* **94**:157–162.
77. **Schnurr, D., S. Yagi, and V. Devlin.** 1993. *Abstr. 9th Annu. Clin. Virol. Symp.*, p. 66.
78. **Strikas, R. A., L. J. Anderson, and R. A. Parker.** 1986. Temporal and geographic patterns of isolates of nonpolio enterovirus in the United States, 1970–1983. *J. Infect. Dis.* **153**:346–351.
79. **Takeda, N.** 1989. Complete nucleotide and amino acid sequences of enterovirus 70, p. 419–424. *In* K. Ishii, Y. Uchida, K. Miyamara, and S. Yamazaki (ed.), *Acute Hemorrhagic Conjunctivitis Etiology, Epidemiology, and Clinical Manifestations.* University of Tokyo Press, Tokyo.
79a. **Toyoda, H., M. Kohara, Y. Kataoka, T. Suganuma, T. Omata, N. Imura, and A. Nomoto.** 1984. Complete nucleotide sequences of all three poliovirus serotype genomes: implication for genetic relationship, gene function, and antigenic determinants. *J. Mol. Biol.* **174**:561–585.
80. **Tracy, S.** 1984. A comparison of the genomic homologies among the coxsackievirus B group: use of fragments of the cloned coxsackievirus B3 genome as probes. *J. Gen. Virol.* **65**:2167–2172.
81. **Tracy, S.** 1985. Comparison of genomic homologies in the coxsackievirus B group by use of cDNA:RNA dot-blot hybridization. *J. Clin. Microbiol.* **21**:371–374.
82. **Tracy, S., and R. A. Smith.** 1981. A comparison of the genomes of polioviruses by cDNA:RNA hybridization. *J. Gen. Virol.* **55**:193–199.
83. **Wadia, N. H., S. M. Katrak, V. P. Misra, P. N. Wadia, K. Miyamura, K. Hashimoto, T. Ogino, T. Hikiju, and R. Kono.** 1983. Polio-like motor paralysis associated with acute hemorrhagic conjunctivitis in an outbreak in 1981 Bombay, India: clinical and serologic studies. *J. Infect. Dis.* **147**:660–668.
84. **Webster, A. D. B., H. A. Rotbart, T. Warner, P. Rudge, and N. Hyman.** 1993.

Diagnosis of enteroviral brain disease in hypogammaglobulinemia by PCR. *Clin. Infect. Dis.* **17:**657–661.
85. **Wenner, H. A., and M. F. Lenahan.** 1961. Propagation of group A coxsackie viruses in tissue cultures. *Yale J. Biol. Med.* **34:**421–438.
86. **Wilfert, C. M., and J. Zeller.** 1985. Enterovirus diagnosis, p. 85–107. *In* L. M. de la Maza and E. M. Peterson (ed.), *Medical Virology IV*. Lawrence Erlbaum Associates, Publishers, Hillsdale, N. J.
87. **Wright, H. T., R. M. McAllister, and R. Ward.** 1962. "Mixed" meningitis: reports of a case with isolation of Haemophilus influenzae type b and echovirus type 9 from the cerebrospinal fluid. *N. Engl. J. Med.* **267:**142–144.
88. **Yagi, S., D. Schnurr, and J. Lin.** 1992. Spectrum of monoclonal antibodies to coxsackievirus B-3 includes type- and group-specific antibodies. *J. Clin. Microbiol.* **30:**2498–2501.
89. **Yolken, R. H., and V. M. Torsch.** 1980. Enzyme-linked immunosorbent assay for detection and identification of coxsackie B antigen in tissue cultures and clinical specimens. *J. Med. Virol.* **6:**45–52.
90. **Young, S., A. B. Strong, and R. Radloff.** 1993. *Abstr. 9th Annu. Clin. Virol. Symp.*, p. 67.
91. **Yousef, G. E., I. N. Brown, and J. F. Mowbray.** 1987. Derivation and biochemical characterization of an enterovirus group-specific monoclonal antibody. *Intervirology* **28:**163–170.
92. **Zhang, G., G. Wilsden, N. J. Knowles, and J. W. McCauley.** 1993. Complete nucleotide sequence of a coxsackie B5 virus and its relationship to swine vesicular disease virus. *J. Gen. Virol.* **74:**845–853.
93. **Zhang, H. Y., G. E. Yousef, N. E. Bowles, L. C. Archard, G. F. Mann, and J. F. Mowbray.** 1988. Detection of enterovirus RNA in experimentally infected mice by molecular hybridisation: specificity of subgenomic probes in quantitative slot blot and in situ hybridisation. *J. Med. Virol.* **26:**375–386.
94. **Zoll, G. J., W. J. G. Melchers, H. Kopecka, G. Jambroes, H. J. A. Van Der Poel, and J. M. D. Galama.** 1992. General primer-mediated polymerase chain reaction for detection of enteroviruses: application for diagnostic routine and persistent infections. *J. Clin. Microbiol.* **30:**160–165.

DEVELOPMENT OF ANTIVIRAL AGENTS FOR PICORNAVIRUS INFECTIONS

John O'Connell, Randi Albin, Deborah Blum, Paul Grint, and Jerome Schwartz

18

The discovery and development of antiviral agents for the treatment of picornavirus infections have been the focus of extensive research for more than 50 years. Since the advent of poliovirus replication in vitro (26) and the consequent production of poliovirus vaccine, picornaviruses have been extensively researched. Several major scientific breakthroughs have enhanced the possibility of developing successful chemotherapy for picornavirus infections: (i) the complete genomic sequences of several picornaviruses are known; (ii) the functions of the major gene products and elements in the 5' nontranslated region have been assigned; (iii) the three-dimensional structure of the viral capsid has been elucidated; (iv) complexes of inhibitors with the viral capsid have been described; (v) the cellular receptors for poliovirus, other enteroviruses, and the major group rhinoviruses have been identified; and (vi) systems for the replication of picornaviruses in culture and enteroviral infections in animal models have been established.

While many molecules have been shown to inhibit picornavirus, the identification of specific, selective inhibitors with potential as drug candidates has been slow. At present, no antiviral drugs are marketed for the treatment of rhinovirus or enterovirus infections. This chapter discusses the pharmaceutical advantages of newer molecules with respect to drug development. In reviewing the historical progression toward potent picornavirus antiviral agents, two classes of inhibitors (interferon and capsid-binding molecules) stand out as having demonstrated efficacy in clinical trials of picornavirus infections. A review of the activities of these agents and their corresponding clinical data is presented here. Finally, a discussion of problems in the further development of antipicornavirus agents is presented.

BACKGROUND

Experimental approaches to modulation of enteroviral infections have included research on chemotherapy, monoclonal antibodies, vaccines, interferons, and capsid-binding agents. In folk medicine, there are reports of attempts at treatment of epidemic enteroviral conjunctivitis with topical urine, ice, and plant juices, among other things (97). None of these attempts were successful. Scientific development of therapies began with the discovery that guanidine-HCl is a potent viral inhibitor in tissue culture (25). Guanidine interferes with

John O'Connell, Randi Albin, Deborah Blum, Paul Grint, and Jerome Schwartz, Departments of Antiviral Chemotherapy and Clinical Research, Schering-Plough Research Institute, 2015 Galloping Hill Road, Kenilworth, New Jersey 07033.

RNA synthesis and is believed to have a site of action on the viral protein 2C, a replicase complex protein, as determined by mutational analysis (88). Attempts at treatment were unsuccessful owing to the rapid development of viral resistance (68) and only marginal in vivo activity (9).

Ribavirin inhibits mouse encephalomyocarditis virus in tissue culture and in a myocarditis model (63). Ribavirin is a nucleoside analog that inhibits a wide spectrum of viruses, possibly by decreasing or interfering with intracellular guanine pools. Its clinical utility has not been definitely determined.

Enviroxime, a compound that acts after virus uncoating and inhibits replication, was used in clinical trials against rhinoviruses. The results of treatment were variable, and at times, no benefit was observed (59).

Monoclonal antibodies have demonstrated activity in Theiler's virus infection, with the VP1 epitope of the viral capsid being the neutralization target (30). In animal models, encephalomyocarditis was reduced by administration of neutralizing monoclonal antibodies raised against two distinct viral epitopes (101). Again, these promising results have not been extended to the clinic.

No vaccines for the nonpolio enteroviruses have been successfully developed. Because of the large number of enterovirus and rhinovirus immunotypes, such vaccines would have to be highly multivalent. Vaccines are in development for a related picornavirus, hepatitis A virus, and indications are that they cause a high rate of seroconversion (21).

INTERFERON

Interferons are potent, selective mediators of resistance to enteroviral infection (12, 31, 50, 53, 55, 57, 61, 77, 87). They act directly on cells and through cell receptor-mediated events. Interferon-induced resistance to viruses is not universal, and generally, cells become more resistant to infection with RNA viruses than to infection with DNA viruses, with retroviruses being intermediate with respect to resistance. Interferons are endogenously produced in response to certain stimuli such as virus infection, exposure to double-stranded RNA, or bacteria and are a major defense in limiting the spread of experimental enteroviral disease in animal models (12, 31, 80). In children with acute enteroviral meningitis, significant elevations in interferon levels in cerebrospinal fluid occur (16, 47), which is probably clinically important, but these levels cannot be of diagnostic value, as elevations are also seen in other meningeal infections (16). The genes for human interferons have been cloned and expressed, and both natural and recombinant interferons are being used clinically for several diseases, including hepatitis B and C. Although hepatitis A virus is sensitive to interferon in tissue culture, in hepatoma cells, and also clinically (60, 92), the virus itself is not a potent inducer of interferon (100). The potential overall utility of interferon in this indication is still unclear (94, 105).

Despite significant strain-to-strain variability (49), cells exposed to interferon become particularly resistant to infection with enteroviruses, and it is in these infections that interferon's mechanism of action has been most thoroughly studied. During enteroviral infection, generation of double stranded RNA intermediates (see chapter 4) causes induction of 2',5'-adenylate synthetase and synthesis of interferon (71, 74; Fig. 1). Interferon then activates adjacent cells to produce 2',5'-adenylate synthetase, generating 2',5'-poly(A), which in turn induces RNase L, and the RNase L can then degrade incoming viral enteroviral RNA, probably at the poly(A) 3' terminus (34, 39, 62). This cascade is believed to account for the observed viral resistance seen in vitro and in vivo. In addition, other interferon-induced cellular proteins, such as p68 and the eIF2 kinase (22), probably play important roles, but their mechanisms are not fully understood.

Although alpha interferon is itself a very potent inhibitor of enteroviral infection, additive or synergistic protective effects are seen when it is studied in conjunction with capsid-binding molecules like arildone (56), nucleoside analogs such as ribavirin (77), or gamma

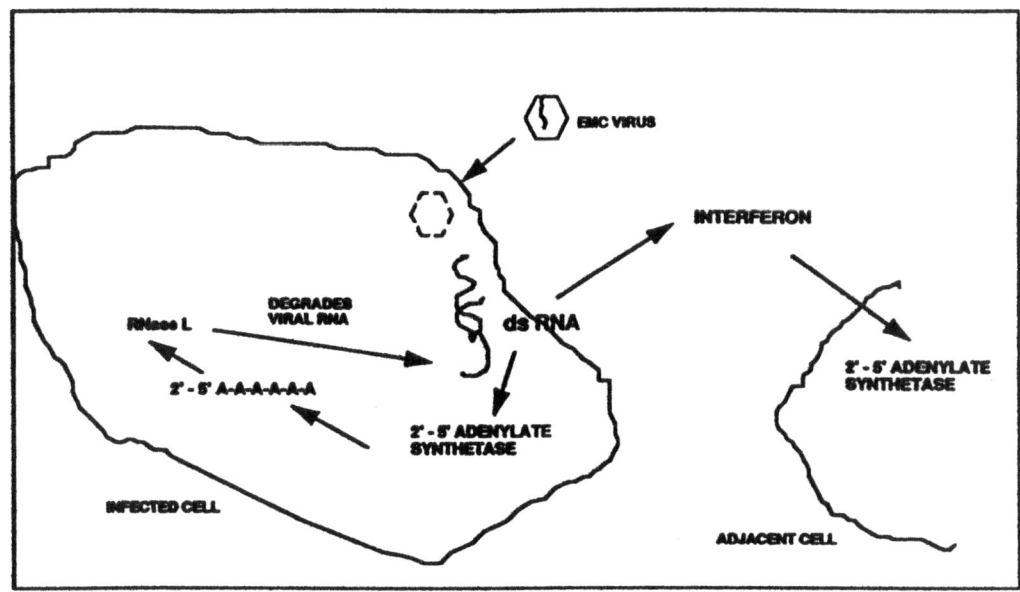

FIGURE 1 Induction of 2',5'-adenylate synthetase system by viral infection. Infection of HeLa cells with encephalomyocarditis (EMC) virus results in formation of double-stranded RNA (dsRNA), which has a dual activity: it activates 2',5'-adenylate synthetase and results in the production of interferon. The appearance of 2',5'(A)n induces RNase L, which degrades incoming viral RNA, probably at the poly(A) 3' terminus. Interferon induces 2',5'-adenylate synthetase in adjacent cells, inducing the cascade, which then prevents incoming EMC virus from replicating in the adjacent cell. The figure is based on studies by Hearl and Johnston (39) and Gribaudo et al. (34).

interferon (80). Interferons may also work in conjunction with humoral antibodies and cell-mediated immunity mechanisms, especially macrophages, to eliminate enteroviral infections (31).

CLINICAL STUDIES WITH INTERFERON

The clinical efficacy of interferon as prophylaxis for rhinovirus colds has been demonstrated in several treatment protocols (32, 35, 36, 70, 86). Using alpha-2 interferon in single or multiple doses for 4 to 5 days before infection, Hayden and Gwaltney (37) demonstrated a reduction of both infection and virus shedding in experimentally induced colds. Earlier studies by Merigan et al. (70) demonstrated protection against human rhinovirus type 4 (HRV4) infection and reduction of clinical symptoms when 14×10^6 IU alpha interferon were given prophylactically for 4 days. Prophylactic efficacy, as indicated by improvement in symptoms, was also observed by Samo et al. (86) and Greenberg et al. (32). An antihistamine was used in this last study to reduce mucous clearance and enhance exposure to human alpha-2 interferon (32). Additional studies demonstrated significant efficacy against naturally acquired rhinovirus infections (20) over a 6-month period and against contact spread of rhinoviruses within family groups after induction of an experimental cold (35). Interferon in high doses was associated with side effects that included nasal irritation, mucosal ulceration, and nasal stuffiness, especially after several weeks of treatment (35, 86).

When administered therapeutically beginning 28 h after experimental infection with HRV39, interferon in nasal spray or drops did not prevent infection or cold development (37). However, there were moderate reductions in virus shedding and lower symptom scores in the groups treated with interferon drops.

CAPSID-BINDING COMPOUNDS

Capsid-binding molecules take advantage of the unique structural organization of picornaviruses as delineated by crystallization and resolution of the three-dimensional structure of HRV14 and poliovirus by X-ray diffraction (44, 82, 85). The capsid, which houses the viral RNA, is composed of 60 protomers, each of which contains one copy of each viral protein, VP1, VP2, VP3, and VP4 (see chapters 3 and 7). Among the features on the viral capsid is the canyon formed by the junctions of VP1 and VP3. For HRV14, the canyon serves as the site for binding to the virus cellular receptor. For the major group rhinoviruses, the cellular receptor is ICAM-1 (33, 95, 98). The cellular receptors for poliovirus (69), echovirus type 1 (11), and coxsackievirus (17, 46) have also been described (see chapter 3). Underneath the canyon lies a hydrophobic cavity, the drug-binding pocket, that is accessible through a pore in the canyon floor. The structure of the canyon with its underlying hydrophobic pocket occurs 60 times per viral capsid, once at each fivefold axis of symmetry. The structure of the canyon and the cavity appears to be similar among all examined picornaviruses, with some differences in cavity length and the nature of the specific hydrophobic residues on amino acids lining the cavity.

A variety of diverse structures bind to the viral capsid in the drug-binding pocket. These include rhodamine (23, 24), flavonoids (48), chalcones (76), a series of aralkylamino-pyridines (51, 52), a series of oxazolinyl isoxazole compounds from Sterling-Winthrop (for example, arildone, WIN 51711, and WIN 54954; 19, 54, 66, 78, 102), a pyridazinamine series of molecules from Janssen Research Foundation (R61837 and R77975; 4, 6), and a (phenoxyl) imidazole series from the Schering-Plough Research Institute (SCH 38057; 84). Representative structures are shown in Fig. 2. Data from X-ray crystallographic studies and analysis of mutant viruses that demonstrate cross-resistance to several of the above-named compounds confirm that these molecules have similar binding sites. X-ray diffraction analyses of crystals of HRV14 infused with WIN molecules (8, 82, 93), with R61837 (15), or with SCH 38057 (107, 108) have shown that these capsid-binding molecules bind specifically within the hydrophobic pocket of VP1, the drug-binding pocket. A representation of SCH 38057 in HRV14 is shown in Fig. 3. Although the compounds bind to virus via a number of noncovalent, hydrophobic-type interactions, the binding affinity is high. Affinity constants determined by competition binding or Scatchard analysis for binding of WIN compounds to HRV14 range from 2.0×10^{-8} to 2.90×10^{-7} M (28).

Several factors appear to correlate with the abilities of a compound to bind to the drug-binding pocket and to manifest antiviral activity. These factors include (i) the number of molecules of compound bound to virus, (ii) the location of compound binding in the drug-binding pocket, (iii) the length and space-filling properties of the molecule, and (iv) the types of interactions with amino acids. Examples of the potential influence of these parameters on compound binding and antiviral activity are discussed below.

The average number of WIN molecules bound per HRV14 particle is 40 to 60, a result consistent with the maximum of 60 potential binding sites per virus (28). SCH 38057, a compound with less potent anti-HRV14 activity, has an average of 19 molecules bound per viral capsid (107). The minimum number of bound molecules necessary to inhibit virus infection is unknown.

Studies with HRV14 indicate that the more potent WIN 51711 binds near the opening of the pocket and, being a relatively long molecule, fills a greater region in the pocket, extending from the entrance to the innermost region. In contrast, SCH 38057, a less potent molecule (107), fits much deeper into the confines of the inner pocket (Fig. 4). R61837, which is also less potent than WIN 51711 against HRV14, binds closer to the entrance

4',6-dichloroflavan

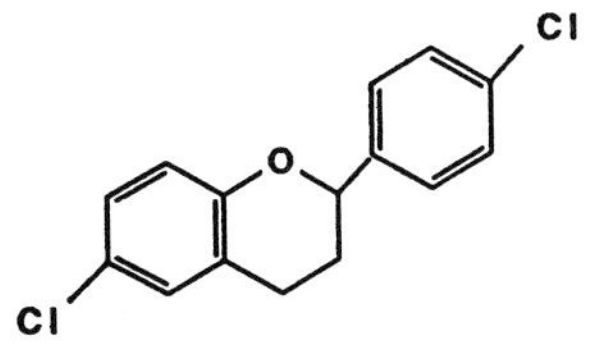

chalcone, Ro09-0410

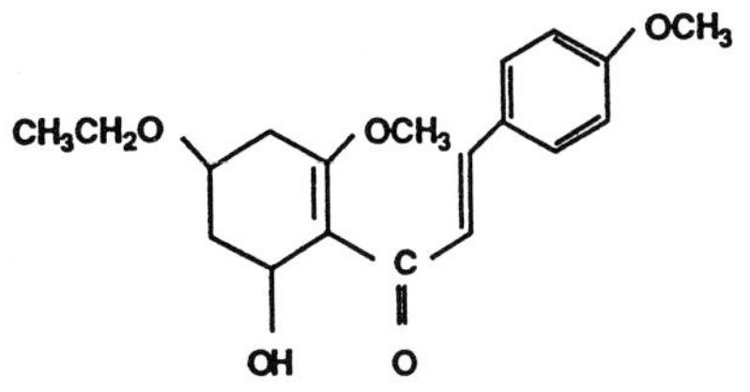

WIN 51711

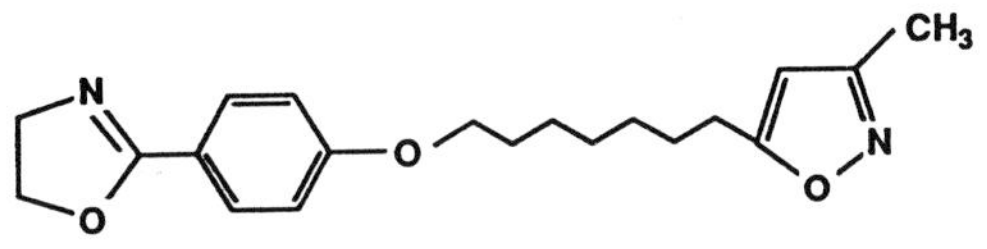

WIN 54954

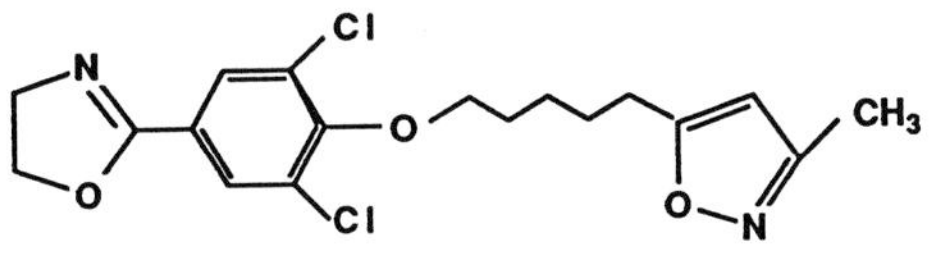

Janssen R61837

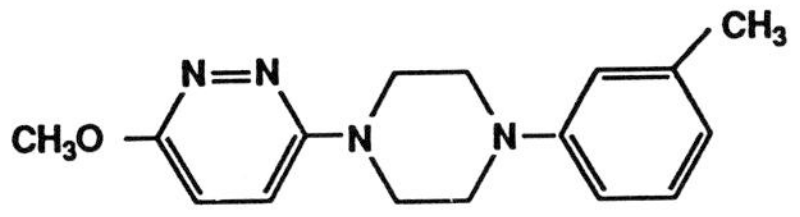

Janssen R77975

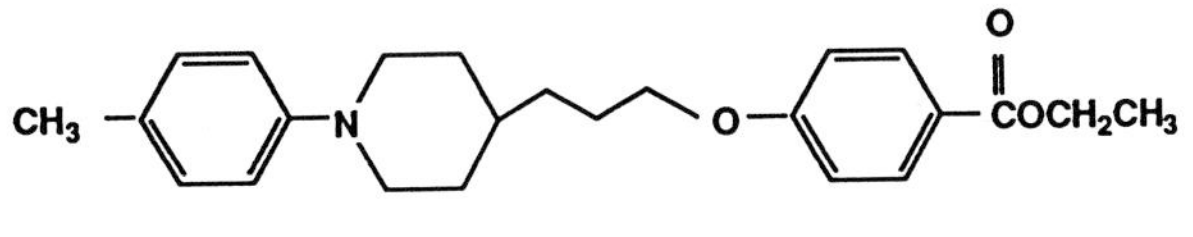

SCH 38057

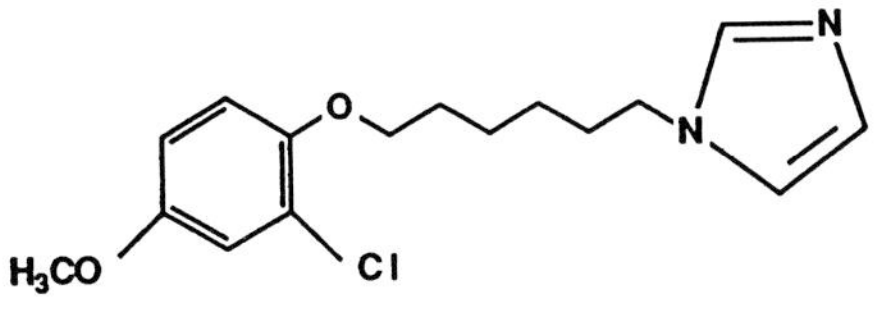

FIGURE 2 Chemical structures of representative picornavirus capsid binding inhibitors.

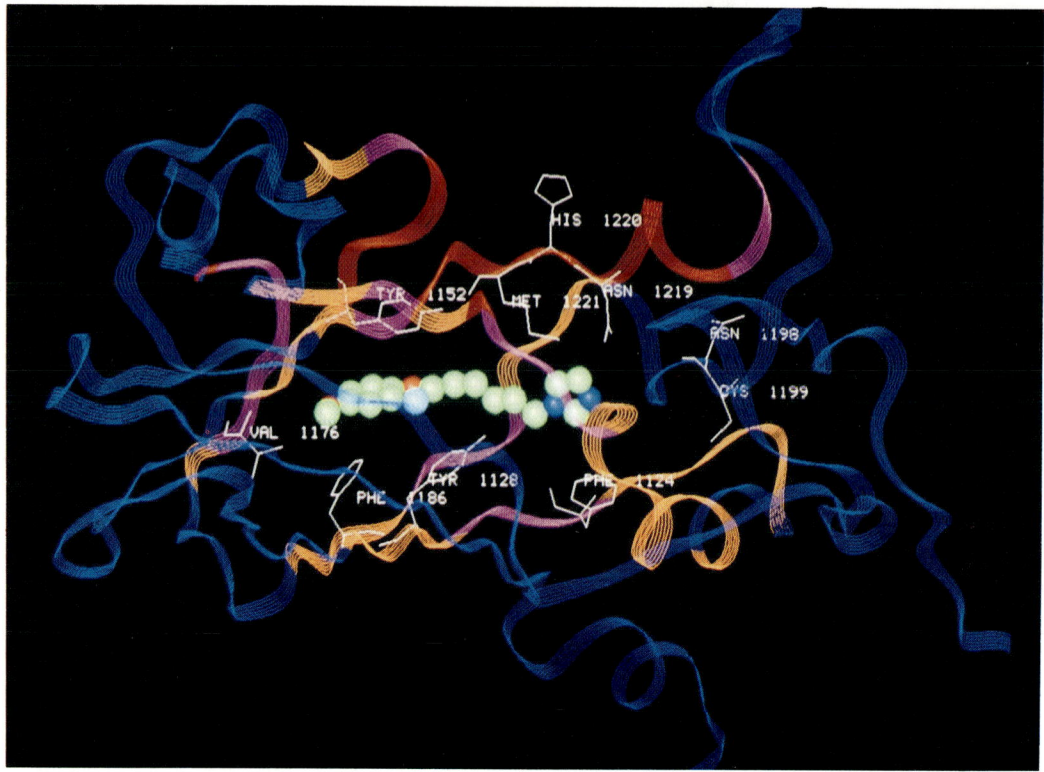

FIGURE 3 Binding of SCH 38057 to HRV14. Atoms of SCH 38057 are indicated by colored spheres. The main chain of VP1 is indicated by ribbons. Conformational changes induced by SCH 38057 are indicated as follows: blue, no significant conformational shifts in these residues; yellow, main chain shifts less than 0.5 Å (0.05 nm); pink, main chain shifts less than 1.0 Å (0.1 nm); red, main chain shifts more than 1.0 Å (0.1 nm). Selected pocket residues are indicated in white. (From Zhang et al., [108].)

of the pocket, but being a shorter molecule, it fills less of the pocket's internal space than WIN 51711 (28, 107, 108).

Hydrogen binding between inhibitor molecules and specific amino acids in the binding pocket has been noted. An examination of amino acids in close proximity to specific compounds suggests that interactions with some amino acids are shared among inhibitors (Table 1). However, many potential interactions with amino acids appear to be inhibitor specific. One consequence of amino acid changes in the pocket is that the interior space of the pocket fills, thereby restricting the binding of molecules. Mutations that replace amino acids with bulkier components result in a virus with a relatively high degree of resistance to the WIN molecules (40, 41, 79). It is suggested that these bulkier substitutions block the full entrance of a compound into the drug-binding pocket.

A comparison of the drug-binding pockets of rhinoviruses and enteroviruses indicates structural differences. Compared to the more elongated, narrower cavity of HRV14, that of HRV1A is open and broader. Similar to HRV1A, poliovirus has a broader pocket, which may be further expanded by the insertion of a naturally occurring lipid molecule. The prediction is that HRV1A and poliovirus can accommodate the binding of more space-filling antiviral compounds than HRV14. Knowledge of this geometry can guide chemists in the synthesis of more potent antiviral agents.

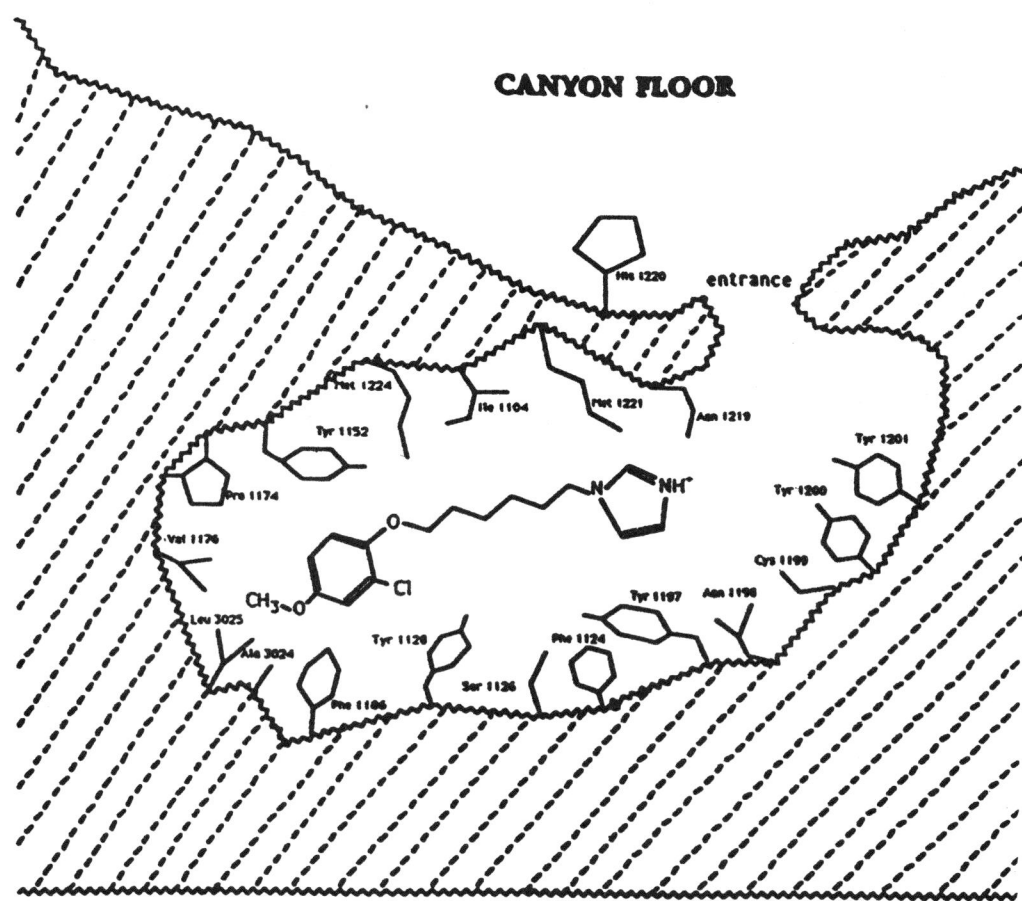

FIGURE 4 Schematic diagram of SCH 38057 in the hydrophobic pocket of HRV14 VP1. SCH 38057 is located in the innermost end of the pocket and leaves a large open space near the entrance of the pocket. This is in contrast to WIN compounds (93) and Janssen R61837 (15), which occupy the space nearest the entrance and leave open space in the innermost portion of the pocket. (Derived from Zhang et al.[107].)

While crystallography can provide valuable information regarding the fit of a given compound into the drug-binding pocket of a specific virus and the resulting conformational changes (see below), our ability to apply the information to predict broad-acting, anti-picornavirus activity is still somewhat limited. Optimizing activity against one serotype can select against activity for other serotypes. From a practical standpoint, selecting a compound as a candidate for clinical development often means choosing not the most active molecule against a particular serotype but the molecule with the broadest spectrum of activity. Whether there is an underlying structural organization shared among viral serotypes is not known. If a prototype viral structure could be determined, the modeling of compounds could incorporate an element of diversity, resulting in a wide antiviral spectrum and a potentially useful drug.

MECHANISM OF VIRAL INHIBITION BY CAPSID-BINDING MOLECULES

Capsid-binding molecules inhibit viral replication by blocking capsid attachment and/or uncoating (1, 6, 28, 54, 66, 76, 79, 106). While the exact mechanism of inhibition by capsid

TABLE 1 Comparison of amino acids in the drug-binding pockets of different picornaviruses[a]

Residue	Amino acid in:						
	HRV14	HRV1A	HRV39	HRV89	PV1M	CVA21	CVB1
1104	Ile	Ile	Ile	Val	Ile	Ile	Ile
1105	Asn	Thr	Thr	Ser	Thr	Thr	Asn
1106	Leu	Leu	Leu	Leu	Tyr	Tyr	Tyr
1124	Phe	Phe	Phe	Phe	Phe	Phe	Phe
1126	Ser	Ser	Ser	Ser	Met	Leu	Leu
1128	Try	Ile	Ile	Ile	Leu	Met	Leu
1150	Ala	Try	Try	Phe	Ile	Ile	Ile
1152	Try	Try	Try	Try	Try	Ile	Try
1174	Pro	Met	Ala	Ala	Pro	Pro	Pro
1176	Val	Ile	Val	Val	Ile	Ile	Val
1186	Phe	Phe	Phe	Phe	Ile	Met	Met
1188	Val	Ile	Leu	Ile	Val	Ile	Ile
1191	Val	Leu	Leu	Met	Val	Val	Ile
1197	Try	Try	Try	Try	Try	Try	Try
1199	Cys	Met	Met	Met	His	His	Cys
1219	Asn	Asn	Asn	Asn	Asn	Asn	Asn
1221	Met	Met	Met	Met	Phe	Phe	Met
1224	Met	Ile	Leu	Ile	Leu	Leu	Leu
3024	Ala	Ala	Ala	Ala	Ala	Ala	Ala
3025	Leu	Leu	Leu	Phe	Leu	Leu	Met

[a] PV1M, poliovirus 1 Mahoney. Table is adapted from Zhang et al. (108).

inhibitors is not known, several hypotheses have been proposed. One proposal is that to uncoat and release their RNAs, picornaviruses require a degree of capsid flexibility. Binding of molecules into the drug-binding pocket reduces this necessary flexibility, inducing a more rigid structure.

The binding of molecules in the drug-binding pocket also exerts significant conformational perturbations in the canyon floor. The canyon is the proposed site of viral attachment to its cellular receptor (HRV14 to ICAM), and conformational changes may account for the decreased virus attachment observed in the presence of inhibitors. However, the overall degree of conformational perturbations does not absolutely correlate with antiviral potency (Table 2 and Fig. 5). For example, SCH 38057, a compound less potent than WIN 51711 against HRV14, exerts a higher level of conformational changes than does the WIN molecule (107, 108). A more detailed analysis of the types of perturbational changes induced by compound binding may lead to a better understanding of the role of inhibitors in preventing attachment.

Since viral uncoating is a pH-dependent event that occurs in cellular endosomes (see chapter 3), it is proposed that the canyon and the cavity together serve as a channel for ion flow to the interior of the virus. According to this hypothesis, inhibitors function as physical blocks to ion flow, thereby blocking pH dependent uncoating.

An additional effect of compound binding is that the virus becomes resistant to thermal inactivation (81). It becomes possible to use a rapid screen, which measures thermal stability in order to identify molecules within certain structural series that possess capsid-binding activity. To date, the majority of molecules with potent antiviral activity also cause thermal stabilization. This correlation between thermal stability and antiviral activity is not absolute for all structural series. When a number of molecules in the Janssen series of capsid inhibitors were studied, no correlation between thermal stability and potency was observed (5).

TABLE 2 Conformational changes induced in main chains of HVR14 by capsid-binding antiviral compounds

Location of change	Conformational change in[a]:		
	SCH 38057	WIN 51711	R61837
βC	+	+	+
βD	+	−	+
βE	+	+	+
βF	+	−	−
βG	+	−	+
FMDV loop	+	+	+

[a] +, modeled conformational changes are present; −, modeled conformational changes are not present. Table is derived from Zhang et al. (108).

PRECLINICAL BIOLOGY OF CAPSID-BINDING MOLECULES

To be clinically useful, a drug exhibiting activity against picornaviruses must have broad activity against members of the *Enterovirus* and/or *Rhinovirus* genus, since a wide number of serotypes cause disease (83) (see Section II of this volume). Although about 70 types of enteroviruses are known (67), surveillance data from the Centers for Disease Control and Prevention from 1970 to 1983 show that 15 serotypes account for 65 to 89% of the enteroviral isolates for a given year in the United States. These are echoviruses 3, 4, 5, 6, 7, 9, 11, 24, and 30; coxsackievirus A9 (CVA9); and CVB1, CVB2, CVB3, CVB4, and CVB5 (13, 14, 96). Andries et al. (7) classified the rhinoviruses into groups A and B on the basis of susceptibility to known capsid-binding antirhinovirus agents. Isolation data from symptomatic individuals during the cold season indicate that rhinoviruses from the B group account for 84.5% of those recovered (27, 73), suggesting that rhinoviruses belonging to the B group are responsible for most colds.

Of the molecules studied to date, many possess broad-acting antiviral activity against both enteroviruses and rhinoviruses. For example, R77975 inhibits 80% of 100 rhinoviruses in vitro at a 50% inhibition level of 0.064 μg/ml (6). WIN 54954 inhibits both enteroviruses and rhinoviruses (102). The broad-spectrum activity is related to the conserved nature of the viral capsid and, more specifically, to the VP1 canyon-cavity structure. Cytotoxicity analyses of capsid-binding molecules support the notion that their antiviral activities act via a unique viral mechanism, as numerous molecules that do not have significant cytotoxicity in cell culture and thus have favorable therapeutic indices have now been identified.

The transition from in vitro antiviral activity to animal models of enteroviral disease has been accomplished by using a battery of in vivo tests. WIN 51711 and WIN 54954 are efficacious in adult mice infected with poliovirus type 2 (64, 102). Additional efficacy was observed in neonatal mice infected systemically with CVA9 or echovirus 9 (102). Efficacy in the neonatal and poliovirus models is demonstrated by the ability of the capsid-binding molecule to reduce viral titers, mortality, and paralysis. A reduction in viral titers and histopathology is observed after WIN 54954 treatment in a myocarditis model with CVA9 (91) and a pancreatitis model with CVB4 (90). While none of the models exactly reproduce the disease observed with human enteroviral infections, the models support the concept that capsid-binding molecules can have a significant impact on enterovirus replication in tissues such as heart, brain, spinal cord, and pancreas. HRVs do not replicate in nonprimate species; similar efficacy studies in animal models have therefore not been performed.

CLINICAL STUDIES WITH CAPSID-BINDING MOLECULES

Several capsid-binding molecules, including chalcones (2), Janssen's R61837 (10), Pirodavir (R77975) (38), and Sterling-Winthrop's WIN 54954 (88, 99), have been used in clinical trials. R61837 and Pirodavir were efficacious in experimentally induced rhinovirus colds when these drugs were administered intranasally before or after infection but prior to onset of symptoms (10, 38). For example, R77975 administered intranasally (2 mg per dose for a total of 25 doses per day) reduced the number of individuals shedding virus and the number of individuals experiencing a cold.

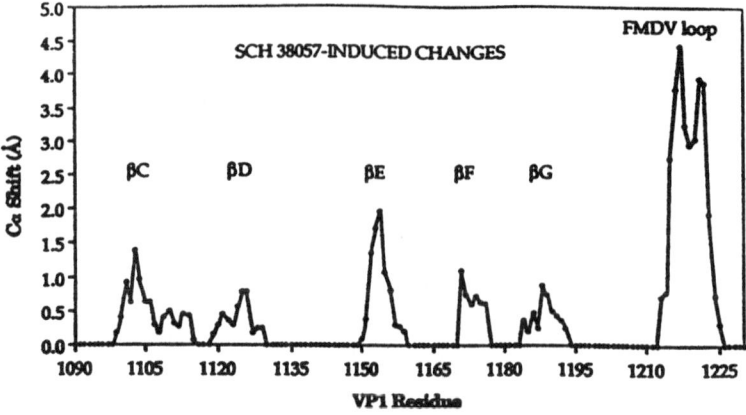

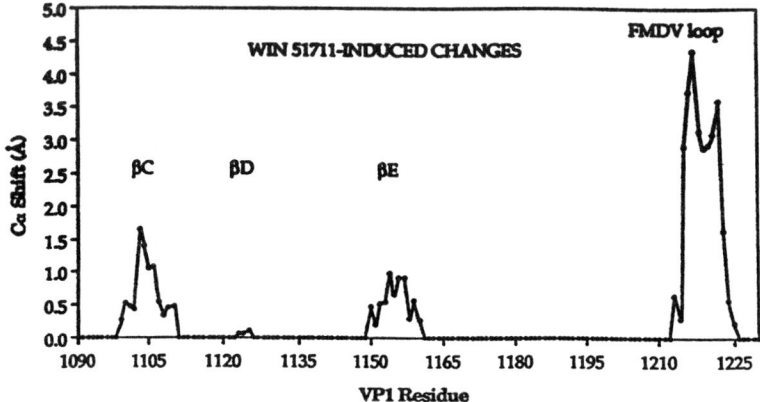

FIGURE 5 Comparison of conformational shifts in the HRV14 VP1 region upon binding of SCH 38057 and WIN 51711. Displacements of C-alpha atoms relative to the native HRV14 coordinates are shown as dots. Changes in the βC and βD strands are similar in the two compounds. However, changes in the βD, βF, and βG strands in the SCH 38057 complex are not reported in the WIN 51711 studies with HRV14. (Derived from Zhang et al. [107].)

WIN 54954 has been clinically tested in volunteers challenged with CVA21, an enterovirus capable of producing both respiratory and systemic symptoms (89). Starting 1 day before infection with CVA21, WIN 54954 was administered orally 3 times a day at 600 mg per dose (1,800 mg/day) to volunteers. WIN 54954 proved efficacious in reducing the number of individuals experiencing a cold, decreasing the severity of respiratory symptoms, decreasing the severity of systemic symptoms, and decreasing titers of virus in nasal secretions. This study was the first to demonstrate the efficacy of an antienterovirus compound in a human challenge trial. A similar set of volunteer trials was performed with a rhinovirus challenge, but efficacy of WIN 54954 was not observed (99).

Failure of compounds to demonstrate therapeutic efficacy in respiratory picornaviral infections could be due to (i) poor bioavailability in nasal secretions, (ii) high viral load during colds, or (iii) the complex biology of respiratory illness. The potential inability to adequately deliver high concentrations of compound to the nasal mucosa was noted in the chalcone and Janssen trials. In these trials, oral and nasal administrations may have been inadequate to provide high concentrations in nasal mucosa. Both the natural washing of drug by nasal mucosal flow and the fact that the compound must reach the nasal cells under the mucosa lining complicate drug delivery to the site of viral replication. The nature of the drug-binding pocket requires highly hydrophobic molecules to produce significant binding to the canyon. The majority of molecules studied have limited solubility in aqueous environments. In an attempt to circumvent this problem, Janssen used hydroxypropyl-β-cyclodextrin to facilitate administration of R61837 for distribution to the nasal mucosa.

The possibility that the lack of efficacy is related to higher virus concentrations requires more study. Viral load increases during the first few days of cold symptoms, and shedding can continue for as long as 2 weeks. In animals, compounds such as the WIN series are efficacious despite high-titer replication of enterovirus in mouse tissues (64, 90, 91, 102).

A dramatic result from both the interferon and the capsid-binding clinical studies is the lack of clinical efficacy when agents are administered therapeutically after viral infection or when symptoms appear. It does not appear that simply increasing the potency of compounds will address the shortcomings of current molecules. Rhinovirus colds induce inflammation and immune responses, and these nonviral factors may cause the symptoms of respiratory disease associated with colds. Potential mediators of respiratory illness include the production of interleukin-2 and interferon, an increased number of natural killer cells in nasal epithelium, and increased production of bradykinin and lysylbradykinins (45, 58, 75). A bradykinin inhibitor, NPC 567, did not reduce symptoms in a rhinovirus cold clinical trial (42). The role of immune mediators in rhinovirus or enterovirus colds remains to be investigated.

STUDIES OF VIRAL RESISTANCE

Consistent with the generation of other RNA viruses, that of picornaviruses resistant to capsid-binding molecules is relatively rapid. One or two passages in culture in the presence of drug generates a spectrum of viruses with reduced sensitivities. Detailed studies with the WIN series have indicated that low-level-resistant isolates were the result of a mutation that mapped to the canyon floor (40, 41, 79). However, high-level-resistant isolates had mutations mapping to the drug-binding pocket, resulting in amino acid residues containing bulkier groups in the interior of the pocket. Biological studies of resistant virus have demonstrated that the majority of these viruses have compromised growth in vitro. However, some viruses that are resistant to capsid-binding molecules replicate as well as wild-type strains (40).

Studies of resistance in clinical trials include the recovery of rhinoviruses from patients during a volunteer trial with the Janssen compound R61837. While the compound demonstrated efficacy in the trial, resistant virus was recovered from some patients. These viruses were compromised in their growth in vitro (6). Earlier studies with the chalcone Ro 09–0410 demonstrated that drug-resistant HRV2 could infect and produce disease in human volunteers, but infectivity was less than that of wild-type HRV2 (103).

An increased understanding of the potential role resistance will have in the use of capsid-binding inhibitors must await further clinical studies. The virulence profiles of drug-resistant viruses in the more serious enteroviral infections such as aseptic meningitis, are entirely unknown.

DISCUSSION

Significant progress has been made in the discovery and development of chemotherapeutic agents for picornaviruses. Molecules with improvements in potency, selectivity, and spectrum have been identified. Several molecules have been tested in clinical trials, and some (interferon and capsid-binding inhibitors) have demonstrated clinical efficacy when administered prophylactically during enterovirus- and/or rhinovirus-induced respiratory illness.

There are several significant remaining pharmaceutical hurdles to future drug development. These include (i) establishing drug delivery systems that maintain MICs within target tissues, (ii) determining the propensity of the virus to develop resistance and the significance of such resistance, and (iii) understanding the complex viral and nonviral pathogenesis of picornavirus disease. While respiratory illness has thus far been the focus of clinical efforts toward developing antipicornavirus molecules, a number of more serious illnesses, including encephalitis and aseptic meningitis (72) (see chapter 13), nonspecific febrile illness (18) (see chapter 11), neonatal sepsis (chapter 10), persistent infections in agammaglobulinemic patients (65) (see chapter 13), and acute hemorrhagic conjunctivitis (43, 104) (see chapter 1), are potential targets for therapy. The potential of antiviral agents for reducing morbidity and mortality in these diseases has yet to be determined but is an important and exciting area for future study.

ACKNOWLEDGMENTS

We thank our co-workers Stuart Cox, Peter Buontempo, Jacquelyn Wright-Minogue, Angela Skelton, and Jason DeMartino for their insights and hard work. We gratefully acknowledge Edward Arnold for providing the colored image of SCH 38057 in HRV-14.

REFERENCES

1. **Alacron, B., A. Zerial, C. Dupiol, and L. Carrasco.** 1986. Antirhinovirus compound 44 081 R.P. inhibits virus uncoating. *Antimicrob. Agents Chemother.* **30:**31–34.
2. **Al-Nakib, W., P. G. Higgins, G. I. Barrow, D. A. J. Tyrrell, K. Andries, G. Vanden Bussche, N. Taylor, and P. A. J. Janssen.** 1989. Suppression of colds in human volunteers challenged with rhinovirus by a new synthetic drug (R61837). *Antimicrob. Agents Chemother.* **33:**522–525.
3. **Andrei, G. M., O. I. Pieroni, H. S. Gatica, and C. E. Coto.** 1985. Substituted benzaldehyde thiosemicarbazone with antiviral activity against picornavirus. *Drugs Exp. Clin. Res.* **12:**869–873.
4. **Andries, K., B. Dewindt, M. De Brabander, R. Stokbroekx, and P. A. J. Janssen.** 1988. In vitro activity of R61837, a new rhinovirus compound. *Arch. Virol.* **101:**155–167.
5. **Andries, K., B. Dewindt, J. Snoeks, and R. Willebrords.** 1989. Lack of quantitative correlation between inhibition of replication of rhinoviruses by an antiviral drug and their stabilization. *Virology* **106:**51–61.
6. **Andries, K., B. Dewindt, J. Snoeks, R. Willebrords, K. Van Eemeren, R. Stokbroekx, and P. A. J. Janssen.** 1992. In vitro activity of pirodavir (R 77975), a substituted phenoxy-pyridazinamine with broad-spectrum antipicornaviral activity. *Antimicrob. Agents Chemother.* **36:**100–107.
7. **Andries, K., B. Dewindt, J. Snoeks, L. Wouters, H. Moereels, P. J. Lewi, and P. A. J. Janssen.** 1990. Two groups of rhinoviruses revealed by a panel of antiviral compounds present sequence divergence and differential pathogenicity. *J. Virol.* **64:**1117–1123.
8. **Badger, J., I. Minor, M. J. Kremer, M. A. Oliveira, T. J. Smith, J. P. Griffith, D. M. A. Guerin, S. Krishnaswamy, M. Luo, M. G. Rossmann, M. A. McKinlay, G. D. Diana, F. J. Dutko, M. Fancher, R. R. Rueckert, and B. A. Heinz.** 1988. Structural analysis of a series of antiviral agents complexed with human rhinovirus 14. *Proc. Natl. Acad. Sci. USA* **85:**3304–3308.
9. **Barrera-Oro, J. G., and J. L. Melnick.** 1961. The effect of guanidine. I. On the experimental poliomyelitis induced by oral administration of virus to cynomolgus monkeys. II. On naturally occurring enterovirus of cynomolgous monkeys. *Tex. Rep. Biol. Med.* **19:**529–536.
10. **Barrow, G. I., P. G. Higgins, D. A. J. Tyrrell, and K. Andries.** 1990. An appraisal of the efficacy of the antiviral R 61837 in rhinovirus infections in human volunteers. *Antiviral Chem. Chemother.* **5:**279–283.
11. **Bergelson, J. M., M. P. Shepley, B. M. C. Chan, M. E. Hemler, and R. W. Finberg.** 1992. Identification of the integrin VLA-2 as a receptor for echovirus 1. *Science* **255:**1718–1720.
12. **Capobianchi, M. R., D. Matteucci, A. Giovannetti, E. Soldaini, M. Bendinelli, J. G. Stanton, and F. Dianzani.** 1991. Role of interferon in lethality and lymphoid atrophy induced by coxsackievirus B3 infection in mice. *Virol. Immunol.* **5:**103–110.
13. **Centers for Disease Control.** 1989. Enterovirus surveillance—United States 1989. *Morbid.*

Mortal. Weekly Rep. **38**:563.
14. **Centers for Disease Control.** 1991. Aseptic meningitis—New York State and United States, weeks 1–36, *Morbid. Mortal. Weekly Rep.* **40**:773–775.
15. **Chapman, M. S., I. Minor, M. G. Rossmann, G. D. Diana, and K. Andries.** 1991. Human rhinovirus 14 complexed with antiviral compound R 61837. *J. Mol. Biol.* **217**:455–463.
16. **Chonmaitree, T., and S. Baron.** 1991. Bacteria and viruses induce production of interferon in the cerebrospinal fluid of children with acute meningitis: a study of 57 cases and review. *Rev. Infect. Dis.* **13**:1061–1065.
17. **Crowell, R. L., D. L. Krah, J. Mapoles, and B. J. Landau.** 1983. Methods of assay of cellular receptors for picornaviruses. *Methods Enzymol.* **96**:443–452.
18. **Dagan, R., C. B. Hall, K. R. Powell, and M. A. Menegus.** 1989. Epidemiology and laboratory diagnosis of infection with viral and bacterial pathogens in infants hospitalized for suspected sepsis. *J. Pediatr.* **115**:351–356.
19. **Diana, G. D., M. A. McKinlay, C. J. Brisson, E. S. Zalay, J. V. Miralles, and U. J. Salvador.** 1985. Isoxazoles with antipicornavirus activity. *J. Med. Chem.* **28**:748–752.
20. **Douglas, R. M., B. W. Moore, H. B. Miles, L. M. Davies, N. Graham, P. Ryan, D. Worswick, and J. Albricht.** 1986. Prophylactic efficacy of intranasal alpha A2–interferon against rhinovirus infections in the family setting. *N. Engl. J. Med.* **314**:65–70.
21. **Drugs and Market Development.** 1992. Hepatitis A vaccine development. *Drugs Market Dev.* **3**:86–90.
22. **Dubois, M. F., and A. G. Hovanessian.** 1990. Modified subcellular localization of interferon induced p68 kinase during encephalomyocarditis virus infection. *Virology* **179**:591–598.
23. **Eggers, H. J.** 1985. Antiviral agents against picornaviruses. *Antiviral Res. Suppl.* **1**:57–65.
24. **Eggers, H. J., M. A. Koch, A. Furst, G. D. Daves, Jr., J. J. Wilczynski, and K. Folkers.** 1970. Rhodanine: a selective inhibitor of the multiplication of echovirus 12. *Science* **167**:294–297.
25. **Eggers, H. J., and I. Tamm.** 1966. Antiviral chemotherapy. *Annu. Rev. Pharmacol.* **6**:231–250.
26. **Enders, J. F., T. H. Weller, and F. C. Robbins.** 1949. Cultivation of the Lansing strain of poliomyelitis virus in cultures of various human embryonic tissues. *Science* **109**:85–87.
27. **Fox, J. P., M. K. Cooney, C. E. Hall, and H. M. Foy.** 1985. Rhinoviruses in Seattle families, 1975–1979. *Am. J. Epidemiol.* **122**:830–846.
28. **Fox, M. P., M. A. McKinlay, G. D. Diana, and F. J. Dutko.** 1991. Binding affinities of structurally related human rhinovirus capsid-binding compounds are related to their activities against human rhinovirus type 14. *Antimicrob. Agents Chemother.* **35**:1040–1047.
29. **Fox, P. M., M. J. Otto, and M. A. McKinlay.** 1986. Prevention of rhinovirus and poliovirus uncoating by WIN 51711, a new antiviral drug. *Antimicrob. Agents Chemother.* **30**:110–116.
30. **Fuyinami, R. S., A. Rosenthal, P. W. Lampert, A. Zurhriggen, and M. Yamada.** 1989. Survival of athymic (*nu/nu*) mice after Theiler's murine encephalomyelitis virus infection by passive administration of neutralizing monoclonal antibody. *J. Virol.* **63**:2081–2087.
31. **Geniteau-Legendre, M., F. Forestier, A. M. Quero, and A. German.** 1987. Role of interferon, antibodies and macrophages in the protective effect of Corynebacterium parvum on encephalomyocarditis virus-induced disease in mice. *Antiviral Res.* **7**:161–167.
32. **Greenberg, S. B., M. W. Harmon, R. B. Couch, P. E. Johnson, S. Z. Wilson, C. C. Dacso, K. Bloom, and J. Quarles.** 1982. Prophylactic effect of low doses of human leukocyte interferon against infection with rhinovirus. *J. Infect. Dis.* **145**:542–546.
33. **Greve, J. M., G. Davis, A. M. Meyer, C. P. Forte, S. C. Yost, C. W. Marlor, M. E. Kamarck, and A. McClelland.** 1989. The major human rhinovirus receptor is ICAM-1. *Cell* **56**:839–847.
34. **Gribaudo, G., D. Lembo, G. Cavallo, S. Landolfo, and P. Lengyl.** 1991. Interferon action: binding of viral RNA to the 40 kilodalton 2',5'-oligoadenylate synthetase in interferon-treated HeLa cells infected with the encephalomyocarditis virus. *J. Virol.* **65**:1748–1757.
35. **Hayden, F., J. K. Albrecht, D. L. Kaiser, and J. M. Gwaltney.** 1986. Prevention of natural colds by contact prophylaxis with intranasal alpha2–interferon. *N. Engl. J. Med.* **314**:71–75.
36. **Hayden, F., and J. M. Gwaltney.** 1983. Intranasal interferon alpha2 for prevention of rhinovirus infection and illness. *J. Infect. Dis.* **148**:543–550.
37. **Hayden, F., and J. M. Gwaltney.** 1984. Intranasal interferon-a2 treatment of experimental rhinoviral colds. *J. Infect. Dis.* **150**:174–180.
38. **Hayden, F. G., A. Andries, and P. A. J. Janssen.** 1992. Safety and efficacy of intranasal pirodavir (R77975) in experimental rhinovirus infection. *Antimicrob. Agents Chemother.* **36**:727–732.

39. **Hearl, W. G., and M. I. Johnston.** 1987. Accumulation of 2',5'-oligoadenylates in encephalomyocarditis virus-infected mice. *J. Virol.* **61**:1586–1592.

40. **Heinz, B. A.** 1990. Escape mutant analysis of a drug-binding site can be used to map functions in the rhinovirus capsid, p. 173–186. *In* W. G. Laver and G. M. Air (ed.), *Use of X-Ray Crystallography in the Design of Antiviral Agents.* Academic Press, Inc., San Diego, Calif.

41. **Heinz, B. A., R. R. Rueckert, D. A. Shepard, F. J. Dutko, M. A. McKinlay, M. Fancher, M. G. Rossmann, J. Badger, and T. J. Smith.** 1989. Genetic and molecular analysis of spontaneous mutants of human rhinovirus 14 that are resistant to an antiviral compound. *J. Virol.* **63**:2476–2485.

42. **Higgins, P. G., G. I. Barrow, and D. A. Tyrrell.** 1990. A study of the efficacy of the bradykinin antagonist, NPC 567, in rhinovirus infections in human volunteers. *Antiviral Res.* **14**:339–344.

43. **Higgins, P. G., P. J. Scott, P. M. Daniels, and D. R. Gamble.** 1974. A comparative study of viruses associated with acute hemorrhagic conjunctivitis. *J. Clin. Pathol.* **27**:292–296.

44. **Hogle, J. M., M. Chow, and D. J. Filman.** 1985. Three-dimensional structure of poliovirus at 2.9 Å resolution. *Science* **229**:1358–1365.

45. **Hsia, J., A. Goldstein, G. Simon, M. Sztein, and F. Hayden.** 1990. Peripheral blood mononuclear cell interleukin-2 and interferon production, cytotoxicity, and antigen-stimulated blastogenesis during experimental rhinovirus infection. *J. Infect. Dis.* **162**:591–597.

46. **Hsu, K.-H. L., K. Lonberg-Holm, B. Alstein, and R. L. Crowell.** 1988. A monoclonal antibody specific for the cellular receptor for the group B coxsackieviruses. *J. Virol.* **62**:1647–1652.

47. **Ichimura, H., K. Shimase, I. Tamura, E. Kaneto, O. Kurimura, Y. Aramitsu, and T. Kurimura.** 1985. Neutralizing antibody and interferon-alpha in cerebrospinal fluids and sera of acute aseptic meningitis. *J. Med. Virol.* **15**:231–237.

48. **Ishitsuka, H., C. Ohsawa, T. Ohiwa, I. Umeda, and Y. Suhara.** 1982. Antipicornavirus flavone Ro 09–0179. *Antimicrob. Agents Chemother.* **22**:611–616.

49. **Jordan, G. W. and V. Bolton.** 1985. Interferon-sensitive Coxsackie virus variants in nature. *J. Interferon Res.* **5**:289–296.

50. **Kandolf, R., A. Canu, and P. H. Hofschneider.** 1985. Coxsackie B3 virus can replicate in cultured human foetal heart cells and is inhibited by interferon. *J. Mol. Cell. Cardiol.* **17**:167–181.

51. **Kenny, M. T., J. K. Dulworth, T. M. Bargar, and J. K. Daniel.** 1987. Antipicornavirus activity of some diaryl methanes and aralkylaminopyridines. *Antiviral Res.* **7**:87–97.

52. **Kenny, M. T., J. K. Dulworth, and H. L. Torney.** 1985. *In vitro* and *in vivo* antipicornavirus activity of some phenoxypyridinecarbonitriles. *Antimicrob. Agents Chemother.* **28**:745–750.

53. **Kishimoto, C., C. S. Crumpacker, and W. H. Abelmann.** 1988. Prevention of murine coxsackie B3 viral myocarditis and associated lymphoid organ atrophy with recombinant human leucocyte interferon alpha A/D. *Cardiovasc. Res.* **22**:732–738.

54. **Kuhrt, M. F., M. J. Fancher, V. Jasty, F. Pancic, and P. E. Came.** 1979. Preliminary studies of the mode of action of arildone, a novel antiviral agent. *Antimicrob. Agents Chemother.* **15**:813–819.

55. **Langford, M. P., J. C. Barber, V. E. Sklar, S. W. Clark III, P. A. Patriarca, I. M. Onarato, M. Yin-Murphy, and G. J. Stanton.** 1985. Virus-specific, early appearing neutralizing activity and interferon production in patients with acute hemorrhagic conjunctivitis. *Curr. Eye Res.* **4**:233–239.

56. **Langford, M. P., D. J. Carr, and M. Yin-Murphy.** 1985. Activity of arildone with or without interferon against acute hemorrhagic conjunctivitis viruses in cell culture. *Antimicrob. Agents Chemother.* **28**:578–580.

57. **Langford, M. P., R. M. Kadi, J. P. Ganley, and M. Yin-Murphy.** 1988. Inhibition of epidemic isolates of coxsackie virus type A24 by recombinant and natural interferon alpha and interferon beta. *Intervirology* **29**:320–327.

58. **Levandowski, R., and D. Horohov.** 1991. Rhinovirus induces natural killer-like cytotoxic cells and interferon alpha in mononuclear leukocytes. *J. Med. Virol.* **35**:116–120.

59. **Levandowski, R., C. T. Pachucki, M. Rubenis, and G. G. Jackson.** 1982. Topical enviroxime against rhinovirus infection. *Antimicrob. Agents Chemother.* **22**:1004–1007.

60. **Levin, S., E. Leibowitz, J. Torten, and T. Hahn.** 1989. Interferon treatment in acute progressive and fulminant hepatitis. *Isr. J. Med. Sci.* **25**:364–372.

61. **Lopez-Guerrero, J. A., F. X. Pimentel-Muinos, M. Fresno, and M. A. Alonso.** 1990. Role of soluble cytokines on the restricted replication of poliovirus in the monocytic U937 cell line. *Virus Res.* **16**:225–230.

62. **Matsumori, A., N. Tomika, and C. Kawai.** 1988. Protective effect of recombinant alpha

interferon on coxsackievirus B3 myocarditis in mice. *Am. Heart J.* **115**:1229–1232.
63. **Matsumori, A., H. Wang, W. H. Abelmann, and C. S. Crumpacker.** 1985. Treatment of viral myocarditis with ribavirin in an animal preparation. *Circulation* **71**:834–839.
64. **McKinlay, M. A., and B. A. Steinberg.** 1986. Oral efficacy of WIN 51711 in mice infected with human poliovirus. *Antimicrob. Agents Chemother.* **29**:30–32.
65. **McKinney, R. I., S. L. Katz, and C. M. Wilfert.** 1987. Chronic enteroviral meningoencephalitis in agammaglobulin patients. *Rev. Infect. Dis.* **9**:334–356.
66. **McSharry, J. J., L. A. Caliguiri, and H. J. Eggers.** 1979. Inhibition of uncoating of poliovirus by arildone, a new antiviral drug. *Virology* **97**:307–315.
67. **Melnick, J. L.** 1990. Enteroviruses: polioviruses, coxsackieviruses, echoviruses, and newer enteroviruses, p. 549–605. *In* B. N. Fields and D. M. Knipe (ed.), *Virology*. Raven Press Ltd., New York.
68. **Melnick, J. L., D. Cronither, and J. Barrera-Oro.** 1961. Rapid development of drug resistant mutants of poliovirus. *Science* **134**:551–552.
69. **Mendelsohn, C., E. Wimmer, and V. R. Racaniello.** 1989. Cellular receptor for poliovirus: molecular cloning, nucleotide sequence and expression of a new member of the immunoglobulin superfamily. *Cell* **56**:855–865.
70. **Merigan, T., S. Reed, T. Hall, and D. Tyrrell.** 1973. Inhibition of respiratory virus infection by locally applied interferon. *Lancet* **i**:536–567.
71. **Meurs, E., D. Krause, N. Robert, R. H. Silverman, and A. G. Hovanessian.** 1985. The 2–5A system in control and interferon-treated K/BALB cells infected with encephalomyocarditis virus. *Prog. Clin. Biol. Res.* **202**:307–315.
72. **Modlin, J. F.** 1990. Coxsackievirus, echovirus and newer enteroviruses, p. 1367–1383. *In* G. L. Mandell, R. G. Douglas, Jr., and J. E. Bennet (ed.), *Principles and Practice of Infectious Disease*. Churchill Livingstone, Inc., New York.
73. **Monto, A. S., E. R. Bryan, and S. Ohmit.** 1987. Rhinovirus infections in Tecumseh, Michigan: frequency of illness and number of serotypes. *J. Infect. Dis.* **156**:43–49.
74. **Morrissey, L. M., and K. Kirkegaard.** 1991. Regulation of a double-stranded RNA modification activity in human cells. *Mol. Cell. Biol.* **11**:3719–3725.
75. **Naclerio, R. M., D. Proud, L. M. Lichtenstein, A. Kagey-Sobotka, J. Hendley, J. Sorrentino, and J. M. Gwaltney.** 1988. Kinins are generated during experimental colds. *J. Infect. Dis.* **157**:133–142.
76. **Ninomiya, Y., M. Aoyama, I. Umeda, Y. Suhara, and H. Ishitsuka.** 1985. Comparative studies on the modes of action of the antirhinovirus agents Ro 09-0410, Ro 09-0179, RMI-15,731, 4',6-dichloroflavan, and enviroxime. *Antimicrob. Agents Chemother.* **27**:595–599.
77. **Okada, I., A. Matsumori, Y. Matoba, M. Tominaga, T. Yamada, and C. Kowai.** 1992. Combination treatment with ribavirin and interferon for coxsackievirus B3 replication. *J. Lab. Clin. Med.* **120**:569–573.
78. **Otto, M. J., M. P. Fox, M. J. Fancher, M. F. Kuhrt, G. D. Diana, and M. A. McKinlay.** 1985. *In vitro* activity of WIN 51711, a new broad-spectrum antipicornavirus drug. *Antimicrob. Agents Chemother.* **27**:883–886.
79. **Pevear, D. C., M. J. Fancher, P. J. Felock, M. G. Rossmann, M. S. Miller, G. Diana, A. M. Treasurywala, M. A. McKinlay, and F. J. Dutko.** 1989. Conformational change in the floor of the human rhinovirus canyon blocks adsorption to HeLa cell receptors. *J. Virol.* **63**:2002–2007.
80. **Pitkaranta, A., K. Linnavouri, and T. Houi.** 1991. Virus-induced interferon production in human leukocytes: a low responder to one virus can be a high responder to another virus. *J. Interferon Res.* **11**:17–23.
81. **Rombaut, B., R. Vrijsen, and A. Boeye.** 1985. Comparison of arildone and 3-methylquercetin as stabilizers of poliovirus. *Antiviral Res. Suppl.* **1**:67–73.
82. **Rossmann, M. G.** 1989. The structure of antiviral agents that inhibit uncoating when complexed with viral capsids. *Antiviral Res.* **11**:3–14.
83. **Rotbart, H. A.** 1989. Human enterovirus infections: molecular approaches to diagnosis and pathogenesis, p. 243–264. *In* B. L. Semler and E. Ehrenfeld (ed.), *Molecular Aspects of Picornavirus Infection and Detection*. American Society for Microbiology, Washington, D.C.
84. **Rozhon, E., S. Cox, P. Buontempo, J. O'Connell, W. Slater, J. DeMartino, J. Schwartz, G. Miller, E. Arnold, A. Zhang, C. Morrow, S. Jablonski, P. Pinto, R. Verace, T. Duelfer, and V. Girijavallabhan.** 1993. SCH 38057: a picornavirus capsid-binding molecule with antiviral activity after the initial stage of viral uncoating. *Antiviral Res.* **21**:15–35.
85. **Rueckert, R. R.** 1990. Picornaviridae and their replication, p. 507–548. *In* B. N. Fields and D. M. Knipe (ed.), *Virology*. Raven Press Ltd., New York.

86. Samo, T. C., S. B. Greenberg, R. B. Couch, J. Quarles, P. E. Johnson, S. Hook, and M. W. Harmon. 1983. Efficacy and tolerance of intranasal applied recombinant leukocyte A interferon in normal volunteers. *J. Infect. Dis.* **148**:535–542.
87. Sasaki, O., T. Karaki, and J. Imanishi. 1986. Protective effect of interferon on infections with hand, foot and mouth disease virus in newborn mice. *J. Infect. Dis.* **153**:498–502.
88. Saunders, K, and A. M. Q. King. 1982. Guanidine-resistant mutants of aphthovirus induce the synthesis of an altered nonstructural polypeptide, P34. *J. Virol.* **42**:389–394.
89. Schiff, G. M., J. R. Sherwood, E. C. Young, and L. J. Mason. 1992. Prophylactic efficacy of WIN 54954 in prevention of experimental human coxsackievirus A21 infection and illness. *Antiviral Res.* **17** (Suppl. 1):92.
90. See, D., and J. Tilles. 1993. WIN 54954 treatment of mice infected with a diabetogenic strain of group B coxsackievirus. *Antimicrob. Agents Chemother.* **37**:1593–1598.
91. See, D. M., and J. G. Tilles. 1992. Treatment of coxsackievirus A9 myocarditis in mice with WIN 54954. *Antimicrob. Agents Chemother.* **36**:425–428.
92. Sim, I. S., and R. L. Cerruti. 1987. Recombinant interferons alpha and gamma: comparative antiviral activity and synergistic interaction in encephalomyocarditis virus infection of mice. *Antiviral Res.* **8**:209–221.
93. Smith, T. J., M. J. Kremer, M. Luo, G. Vriend, E. Arnold, G. Kamer, M. G. Rossmann, M. A. McKinlay, G. D. Diana, and M. J. Otto. 1986. The site of attachment in human rhinovirus 14 for antiviral agents that inhibit uncoating. *Science* **233**:1286–1293.
94. Smith, R. A., and F. H. Norris. 1987. Antiviral therapy. *Adv. Exp. Med. Biol.* **209**:297–304.
95. Staunton, D. E., V. J. Merluzzi, R. Rothlein, R. Barton, S. D. Marlin, and T. A. Springer. 1989. A cell adhesion molecule, ICAM-1, is the major surface receptor for rhinoviruses. *Cell* **56**:849–853.
96. Strikas, R. A., L. J. Anderson, and R. A. Parker. 1986. Temporal and geographic patterns of isolates of nonpolio enterovirus in the United States, 1970–1983. *J. Infect. Dis.* **153**:346–351.
97. Taylor, H. R., J. C. Cadet, and A. Sommer. 1982. Folk medicines and acute hemorrhagic conjunctivitis. *Am. J. Ophthalmol.* **94**:555–560.
98. Tomassini, J. E., D. Graham, C. M. DeWitt, D. W. Lineberger, J. A. Rodkey, and R. J. Colonno. 1989. cDNA cloning reveals that the major group rhinovirus receptor on HeLa cells is intercellular adhesion molecule 1. *Proc. Natl. Acad. Sci. USA* **86**:4907–4911.
99. Turner, R. B., F. J. Dutko, N. H. Golstein, G. Lockwood, and F. G. Hayden. 1993. Efficacy of oral WIN 54954 for prophylaxis of experimental rhinovirus infection. *Antimicrob. Agents Chemother.* **37**:297–300.
100. Vallbracht, A., P. Gabriel, J. Zahn, and B. Fleming. 1985. Hepatitis A virus infection and the interferon system. *J. Infect. Dis.* **152**:211–213.
101. Vlaspolder, F., C. A. Kraaijeveld, R. Van Buuren, M. Harmsen, B. J. Benaissa-Trouw, and H. Snippe. 1988. Prophylaxis and therapy of virulent encephalomyocarditis virus in mice by monoclonal antibodies. *Arch. Virol.* **98**:123–130.
102. Woods, M. G., G. D. Diana, M. C. Rogge, M. J. Otto, F. J. Dutko, and M. A. McKinlay. 1989. In vitro and in vivo activities of WIN 54954, a new broad-spectrum antipicornavirus drug. *Antimicrob. Agents Chemother.* **33**:2069–2074.
103. Yasin, S. R., W. al-Nakib, and D. A. Tyrrell. 1990. Pathogenesis for humans of human rhinovirus type 2 mutants resistant to or dependent on chalcone Ro 09–0410. *Antimicrob. Agents Chemother.* **34**:963–966.
104. Yin-Murphy, M. 1984. Acute hemorrhagic conjunctivitis. *Prog. Med. Virol.* **29**:43–44.
105. Zachoval, R., M. Kroener, M. Brommer, and F. Deinhardt. 1990. Serology and interferon production during the early phase of acute hepatitis A. *J. Infect. Dis.* **161**:353–354.
106. Zeichardt, H., M. J. Otto, M. A. McKinlay, P. Willingmann, and K.-O. Habermehl. 1987. Inhibition of poliovirus uncoating by disoxaril (WIN 51711). *Virology* **160**:281–285.
107. Zhang, A., R. G. Nanni, G. F. Arnold, D. A. Oren, T. Li, A. Jacobo-Molina, R. L. Williams, G. Kamer, D. A. Rubenstein, Y. Li, E. Rozhon, S. Cox, P. Buontempo, J. O'Connell, J. Schwartz, G. Miller, C. Nash, B. Bauer, R. Versace, A. Ganguly, V. Girijavallabhan, and E. Arnold. 1991. Structure of a complex of human rhinovirus 14 with a water soluble antiviral compound SCH 38057. *J. Mol. Biol.* **230**:857–867.
108. Zhang, A., R. G. Nanni, D. A. Oren, E. J. Rozhon, and E. Arnold. 1992. Three-dimensional structure—activity relationships for antiviral agents that interact with picornavirus capsids. *Semin. Virol.* **3**:453–471.

INDEX

A particle, 82–83
Abortion, spontaneous, 224, 226–227
Acquired immunity, 176
Acquisition, *see* Transmission
Active surveillance, 6
Acute hemorrhagic conjunctivitis (AHC), 9, 13–14, 17, 240
Adaptation of enterovirus, 4–5
2′,5′-Adenylate synthetase, 420–421
ADP-ATP carrier autoantigen, 312, 326
Adriamycin, 331
Agammaglobulinemia, 177, 280
   X-linked, muscle disease with, 392
Age of host, 7–8
   insulin-dependent diabetes mellitus, 353
   meningitis and encephalitis, 273–274
   myocarditis and dilated cardiomyopathy, 294
   poliomyelitis, 204
AHC, *see* Acute hemorrhagic conjunctivitis
AIDS, 8
Alpha$_1$-adrenergic antagonists, 327
ALS, *see* Amyotrophic lateral sclerosis
Amniotic fluid, 224
Amyotrophic lateral sclerosis (ALS), 388, 395
Angiotensin-converting enzyme inhibitor, 327
Animal model
   diabetes mellitus, 355–356
   immune response to enterovirus, 175–176, 184–185
   myocarditis, 295–296
   neuromuscular disease, 388
Anorexia, infant, 247–249
Antigenic drift, 5
Antigenic mimicry, *see* Molecular mimicry
Anti-Ids, pathogenesis of myocarditis and dilated cardiomyopathy, 311

Antilaminin antibody, 326
Antimyosin autoantibody, 311–312
Anti-T-cell antibody, 330
Antiviral agents, 419–434, *see also specific agents*
   myocarditis and dilated cardiomyopathy, 328–329
Apnea, 247, 256
Apoptosis, 149–150, 389
Arildone, 82, 422
Assembly of virus, 155–174
Asthma, infectious, 256, 260, 263
att phenotype, *see* Attenuated strains
Attachment to cells, 73–81
Attenuated strains, 49–52
   in vivo variation, 52–53
Autoimmune disease, 178
Autoimmune mechanisms
   insulin-dependent diabetes mellitus, 354, 357–361, 363–364
   myocarditis and dilated cardiomyopathy, 309–313, 326
   neuromuscular disease, 387–398
Autopsy reports, insulin-dependent diabetes mellitus, 362–363
Azathioprine, 331–332

β-Adrenoceptor, cardiac, 326
β-Blocker, 329
β-Cell autoimmunity, insulin-dependent diabetes mellitus, 354, 357–361, 363–364
B-cell epitopes, 182
BIOPLF-70, 330
Birth defects, 227–228
Blood-borne transmission, 12–14
Blood-brain barrier, 275
Bornholm disease, *see* Pleurodynia

Bottle feeding, 240
Brain edema, 283
Breast-feeding, 240
Brefeldin A, 100–101, 145–146
Bronchiolitis, 256, 260, 263
Bronchitis, 260, 262–263
Buoyant density, virion, 156, 402

Calcium channel blocker, 329
Cap-binding protein, *see* Translation initiation factor eIF-4F
Capsid
 empty, 161–162, 165
 poliovirus, 31–33
Capsid protein(s), 156–159, 402
 gene organization, 158–159
 lytic function, 148–149
 modification during assembly, 165
 molecular size, 156
 myristoylation, 31–33, 165
 polyprotein cleavage, 158–159
 proteolytic processing of precursors, 158–160
 sequences that control receptor interaction, 75–77
 structure, 163–164
 virus architecture, 162–164
Capsid protein 1B, 182
Capsid protein 1C, 182
Capsid protein 1D, 180–184
Capsid-binding compounds, 422–425
 clinical studies, 427–429
 mechanism of viral inhibition, 425–426
 preclinical biology, 427
 viral resistance, 429
Captopril, 327
Cardiac myosin autoantigen, 312–313
Cardiomyopathy
 dilated, *see* Dilated cardiomyopathy
 peripartum, 295, 318
Cardiotropism, 296
Cardiovascular anomalies, 227
Carteolol, 329
Case finding, 6, 12
Case-control studies, insulin-dependent diabetes mellitus
 antiviral antibodies, 367
 viral nucleic acids, 371
CD44, poliovirus infection, 75, 87
CD55, *see* Decay-accelerating factor
cDNA clones, 5, 35–36, 96–97
cDNA probes, 405–407
Cell biology of infection, 135–154
Cell culture, 249–251, 264, 282, 403–405
Cell death, 148–150, 389
Cell entry, 81–84
Cell extract, factors interacting with IRES, 120–124
Cell lines, 403–404

Cell lysis, 147–150
Cell receptor, *see specific receptors*
Cell-free system, de novo synthesis of poliovirus, 104–106
Cell-mediated cytotoxicity
 gender, effect of, 306
 sex hormones, effect of, 306–307
Cell-mediated immune response, 175–176, 179–185
Central nervous system
 infection, 271–289
 virus entry into, 275
Cerebellar ataxia, 271
Cerebrospinal fluid, enteroviruses in, 243–245, 281–283
CFS, *see* Chronic fatigue syndrome
Chalcone, 423, 427–429
Chromatin, virus-infected cells, 141
Chronic fatigue syndrome (CFS), 388, 392–393
Classification, 27
Climate, 9, 11
Clinical studies
 capsid-binding compounds, 427–429
 interferon therapy, 421–422
Cloverleaf, poliovirus genome, 28
Coated vesicle, 144–145
Coding region, 97–98
Common cold, 256, 259–260
Complement fixation test, 413
Complementation, *see* Genetic complementation
Complementation index, 39
Computerized tomography, focal encephalitis, 280
Congenital anomalies, 227–228
Congenital rubella syndrome, 359–360
Conjunctivitis
 acute hemorrhagic, *see* Acute hemorrhagic conjunctivitis
 infant, 247–249
Copy choice mechanism, 44
Corticosteroid therapy, 329–330
Cortisone, 329
Coxsackievirus
 febrile illness in infant, 239–254
 host range, 85
 neonatal infections, 231
 tissue tropisms, 87
Coxsackievirus receptor, 81
CPE, *see* Cytopathic effect
CRC system, positive-strand RNA synthesis, 102–104
Crops, contaminated, 10–11
Croup, 256, 260, 262
Crowding, 8–9, 14, 256–257
CTL, *see* Cytolytic T lymphocytes; Cytotoxic T lymphocytes
Cyclicity, 11

Cyclosporin A, 331–332
Cytokine, pathogenesis of myocarditis and dilated cardiomyopathy, 313–314
Cytolytic T lymphocytes (CTL)
  autoreactive, 309–310
  pathogenesis of myocarditis and dilated cardiomyopathy, 296–297, 304–305, 309–310
Cytopathic effect (CPE), 124–154, 264–265
Cytoplasmic membrane, virus-infected cells, 143–147
Cytoskeleton, virus-infected cells, 141–143
Cytotoxic T lymphocytes (CTL), 183–184, 303–307

DAF, see Decay-accelerating factor
DCM, see Dilated cardiomyopathy
Decay-accelerating factor (DAF), 80
Dermatomyositis (DM), 388–392
Developing world
  poliomyelitis, 209–210
  poliovirus vaccine, 210–212
Devil's grippe, see Pleurodynia
DI genome, 45, 47, 106
DI particle, 45, 47, 106
Diabetes mellitus, insulin-dependent (IDDM), 353–385
  β-cell autoimmunity, 354, 357–361, 363–364
  environmental factors, 371–373
  epidemiology, 353–354, 367–371
  gene-environment interactions, 371–372
  genetics, 354–355, 371–373
  HLA phenotype, 354–355, 357, 372–373
  human studies
    autopsy reports, 362–363
    disease following enteroviral infections, 363–364
    ecological studies, 364–367
    seroepidemiology, 367–371
  incubation period, 354
  outbreaks, 365–366
  pathophysiology, 355–362
    acute cytolytic infection, 355–356
    hit-and-run model, 357–359
    innocent bystander theory, 356–357
    persistent infection and autoimmunity, 359–361
    trigger for autoimmunity, 357–359
  polio model, 367
  prevention, 373
  protective effect of viral infection, 362
  vaccine, 373
  without β-cell lysis or autoimmunity, 361–362
Diagnosis, 401–418
  direct detection of viral components, 405–411
  electron microscopy, 405
  evaluation and interpretation of results, 413–414
  immunoassay, 405
  isolation of virus, see Isolation of virus
  meningitis and encephalitis, 281–283
  myocarditis and dilated cardiomyopathy, 318–324, 326
  nonpolio enterovirus in infant, 249–251
  nucleic acid hybridization, 405–407
  PCR methods, see PCR methods
  perinatal enterovirus infections, 231–232
  respiratory infections, 264–265
  serologic, 412–413
  serotype identification, 411–412
  specimen collection and storage, 402–403
Diaphragmatic spasm, see Pleurodynia
Diarrhea, infant, 247–249
4',6-Dichloroflavan, 423
Dicistronic virus, 37–38, 41, 167
Dilated cardiomyopathy (DCM), 291–351
  age and, 294
  clinical presentation, 325–327
  diagnosis, 326
  enterovirus detection, 318–322
  epidemiology, 292–295
  evidence linking myocarditis to, 325
  gender and, 295
  genetic factors, 326–327
  geography and, 295
  immunologic abnormalities, 326
  incidence as proportion of all heart disease, 293
  incidence from population surveys, 293
  pathogenesis, 295–318
    cell-mediated destruction of myofibers, 303–307
    coxsackievirus infection and cardiac dysfunction, 313–315
    host defense mechanisms, 299–303
    immune and autoimmune mechanisms, 309–313
    viral replication in heart, 296–299
    virus in chronic heart disease, 307–309
  pregnancy and, 295
  prevalence of associated enteroviral infection, 292–293
  prognosis, 327
  race and, 295
  serologic diagnosis, 318–319
  severity of disease
    environmental factors, 318
    physiologic factors, 316–317
    viral factors, 315–316
  treatment
    alpha$_1$-adrenergic antagonists, 327
    angiotensin-converting enzyme inhibitor, 327
    antiviral agents, 328–329
    β-blockers, 329
    calcium channel blocker, 329
    conventional, 327–332

corticosteroids, 329–330
immunization, 330
immunomodulating therapy, 330–331
immunosuppressive therapy, 331–332
nonsteroidal anti-inflammatory drugs, 332
thrombolytic agent, 332
virus detection
RNA detection, 320–322
virus isolation, 319–320
Disoxaril, 328
DM, see Dermatomyositis
DNA polymerase I, 138–139
inhibition, 140–141
DNA polymerase II, 138–139
inhibition, 139–140
DNA polymerase III, 138–139
inhibition, 141
DNA-binding proteins, 140–141
Doxazosin, 327
Drug-binding pocket, 422–425

Echovirus
febrile illness in infant, 239–254
host range, 85
neonatal infections, 231
Echovirus receptor, see Integrin VLA-2
Electron microscopy, 405
Elevation, 9
Empty capsid, 161–162, 165
Encapsidation of RNA, 100, 159, 165–167
Encephalitis, 6, 271–289
clinical manifestations, 277–281
diagnosis, 281–283
epidemiology, 271–275
focal, 279–280
neonatal, 229–231
pathogenesis and pathology, 275–277
prevention, 283–284
sequelae, 278–279
treatment, 283–284
Encephalomyelitis, 279
Encephalomyocarditis virus, 355–356
Enclave, virus-susceptible, 14–15
Endemic (sporadic) disease, 6, 11
Endomyocardial biopsy, 323–324
Endoplasmic reticulum, 143–147
Enterocolitis, necrotizing, 277
Enterovirus
characteristics, 401–402
definition of genus, 27
relationship among members of genus, 33–35
Enterovirus infection
cell biology, 135–154
cytoskeleton, 141–143
immune response, 175–191
inhibitors, 145–146
membrane rearrangements, 143–147

nuclear effect, 135–141
Entry into cells, 81–84
Environmental factors, insulin-dependent diabetes mellitus, 371–373
Environmental persistence, 5, 9–11
Enviroxime, 420
Epidemic cyclicity, 11
Epidemic disease, 6, 11
myocarditis, 294
poliomyelitis, 196–198
Epidemiology, 3–23, see also Incidence of disease; Prevalence of disease; Transmission
descriptive, 7–11
dilated cardiomyopathy, 292–295
encephalitis, 271–275
host factors, 294–295
insulin-dependent diabetes mellitus, 353–354, 367–371
meningitis, 271–275
molecular, 15–18
myocarditis, 292–295
nonpolio enterovirus infections in infants, 239–242
outbreaks and epidemics, 294
perinatal enterovirus infection, 221–223
person, 7–9, see also Host characteristics
place, 9–11
poliomyelitis, 6–10, 12, 15, 197–198
respiratory infections, 256–257
surveillance data, 5–7
time factors, 11–12
Epitope distribution, 15
Eradication, poliovirus, 18
Ethnic identity of host, 9
Evolution of virus, 4, 16
Exercise
meningitis and encephalitis and, 274
myocarditis and dilated cardiomyopathy and, 316–317
poliomyelitis and, 204
Exit of viruses, 147–150

Febrile illness, nonpolio enterovirus, 239–254
Fecal-oral transmission, 5, 12, 14, 256, 275
Fetal infection, 221, 317–318, see also Perinatal enterovirus infection
Fingerprinting studies, 16–18
FK-506, 330
Flaccid paralysis, acute, 240
Fomite transmission, 11, 13, 256–257
Food-borne transmission, 10, 12–13

GAD, see Glutamate decarboxylase
Gamma globulin, 283
Gastroenteritis, 4
Gender, 8
effect on cell-mediated cytotoxicity, 306

meningitis and encephalitis and, 274
myocarditis and dilated cardiomyopathy and, 294–295, 317
Genetic complementation, 39–41
  intergenic, 39
  intragenic, 39
  intragenomic, 41
  poliovirus replication, 39–41
Genetic conservation, 33–35
Genetic drift, 5
Genetic recombination, 25, 43–47
  homologous, 43–46
  nonhomologous, 45–47
Genetics/genetic factors, 25–72
  dilated cardiomyopathy, 326–327
  insulin-dependent diabetes mellitus, 354–355, 371–373
  pathogenesis, 47–53
  T-lymphocyte responses, 305–306
Genome, 25
  coding region, 97–98
  conservation and diversity, 33–35
  genetic dissection, 35–39
  noncoding region, see Noncoding region
  organization, 26, 95–96
  poliovirus, 27–33, 96–98
Genome sequencing, 15
Genomic masking, 40
Genotype conservation, 42–43
Geographic parameters, 9
  insulin-dependent diabetes mellitus, 353
  myocarditis and dilated cardiomyopathy, 295
Glutamate decarboxylase (GAD), 357–359
Golgi apparatus, 145–146
Groundwater, 10
Guanidine, 419–420
Guillain-Barré syndrome, 204, 271

Half-shell intermediates, 161–162
Hand-foot-mouth syndrome, 240, 277
Health status of host, 8
Heart, viral replication in, 296–299
Heart disease, see also Dilated cardiomyopathy; Myocarditis
  chronic, 307–309
  enterovirus-associated, general population, 292
Heart-reactive autoantibody (HRA), 310–311
Hemagglutination inhibition test, 413
Hemorrhagic conjunctivitis, acute, see Acute hemorrhagic conjunctivitis
Heparin, 332
Hepatic necrosis, 277
Hepatitis, neonatal, 229, 232
Herd immunity, 15
Herpangina, 258, 260–262
Histidyl-tRNA synthetase, see Jo-1 antigen
Hit-and-run model, 357–359

HLA phenotype
  insulin-dependent diabetes mellitus, 354–355, 357, 372–373
  myocarditis and dilated cardiomyopathy, 326–327
Homologous recombination, 43–46
Host cell shutoff, 124–128
Host characteristics
  age, 7–8, see also Age
  ethnic identity, 9
  gender, 8, 294–295, see also Gender
  health status, 8
  meningitis and encephalitis, 273–274
  myocarditis and dilated cardiomyopathy, 316–317
  race, 295
  socioeconomic status, 8–9, 240
  susceptibility status, 9
Host defense, myocarditis, 299–303
Host range, 48–49
  coxsackievirus, 85
  echovirus, 85
  poliovirus, 84–86
  receptors and, 84–86
Household secondary attack rates, 14
Household transmission, 14, 257
HRA, see Heart-reactive autoantibody
Humoral immunity, 175–179
  poliovirus, 202
  poliovirus vaccine, 205–208

Ibuprofen, 332
ICA, see Islet cell antibodies
ICAM-1, see Intercellular adhesion molecule 1
Icosahedral virus, 156
IDDM, see Diabetes mellitus, insulin-dependent
Ig, see Immunoglobulin
Immune response, 5, 175–191
  cell-mediated, 175–176, 179–185
  humoral, 175–179
  pathogenesis of myocarditis and dilated cardiomyopathy, 309–313, 326
Immunity
  acquired, 176
  respiratory infection, 258–259
Immunization, myocarditis and dilated cardiomyopathy, 330
Immunoassay, 405
Immunocompromised patient, 8
  meningitis and encephalitis, 274–275, 280–282
  poliomyelitis, 204
Immunoglobulin A (IgA), antienteroviral, 177, 258
Immunoglobulin G (IgG), antienteroviral, 177, 258, 412–413
Immunoglobulin M (IgM), antienteroviral, 177, 258, 318–319, 358, 367–371, 413
Immunoglobulin (Ig) therapy

meningitis, 280–281, 283
nonpolio enterovirus infections in infant, 252
perinatal enterovirus infections, 232
prevention of perinatal enterovirus infections, 233
Immunosuppressive therapy, myocarditis and dilated cardiomyopathy, 331–332
In situ hybridization, 321–322
Inactivated poliovirus vaccine (IPV), 202, 207–208
  efficacy, 208
  exclusive use, 209
  sequential IPV-OPV immunization, 209
  virus transmission by immunized children, 208
Incidence of disease, 6, 11–12
Inclusion body myositis, 391
Incubation period
  insulin-dependent diabetes mellitus, 354
  respiratory disease, 258
Indomethacin, 332
Infant, see also Neonate
  maternal antibodies, 240–241
  meningitis, 277–279
  nonpolio enterovirus infection, 239–254
    clinical presentation, 247–249
    diagnosis, 249–251
    epidemiology, 239–242
    historical background, 239
    pathogenesis, 242–246
    treatment, 252
  perinatal enterovirus infection, see Perinatal enterovirus infection
Inflammatory disease, 175, 183
Inflammatory myopathy, 389–392
Initiation factor, see Translation initiation factor
Injection, poliomyelitis risk, 204
Innocent bystander theory, 356–357
Inoculation, 5
Inoculation acquisition, 13
Insulin-dependent diabetes mellitus, see Diabetes mellitus, insulin-dependent
Integrin, coxsackievirus receptor, 81
Integrin VLA-2, 48, 79–81
Intercellular adhesion molecule 1 (ICAM-1), 48, 81, 357
Interferon, pathogenesis of myocarditis and dilated cardiomyopathy, 302–303
Interferon therapy, 420–421
  clinical studies, 421–422
  myocarditis, 328–329
Intergenic complementation, 39
Interleukin
  in insulin-dependent diabetes mellitus, 356–357
  in myocarditis and dilated cardiomyopathy, 313–314
Interleukin therapy, myocarditis and dilated cardiomyopathy, 330
Interleukin-2 receptor antagonist, 330

Intermediate filaments, 142
Internal ribosome entry site (IRES), 28–30, 115–120
  binding of cellular peptides, 123
  boundaries, 119–120
  cellular and viral factors interacting with, 120–124
  types, 118–119
Intestinal lining, 48, 275
Intrafamily transmission, 14, 257
Intragenic complementation, 39
Intragenomic complementation, 41
Intrauterine infection, 221, 224–226
IPV, see Inactivated poliovirus vaccine
IRES, see Internal ribosome entry site
Iron lung, 200
Irritability, infant, 247–249
Islet cell antibodies (ICA), 354–355
Isolation of virus, 403–405
  different components of blood, 251
  isolation rates from different sites, 251
  myocarditis and dilated cardiomyopathy, 319–320
  speed, 250
  tissue culture, 249–251

Janssen R61837, 423, 427–429
Janssen R77975, 423, 427–429
Jo-1 antigen, 387–390

L protein, 127
La protein, 121–122
Lameness survey, 12
Latitude, 353
Lck-deficient mice, 303–304
LEEKGI sequence, 180
Lethargy, infant, 247–249
Levamisole, 330
LS 2616, see Quinoline-3-carboxamide
Lymphocytic choriomeningitis virus, mice, 359–360
Lysosomal enzymes, 136

Macrophages, pathogenesis of myocarditis and dilated cardiomyopathy, 299–302
Major histocompatibility complex (MHC), see also HLA phenotype
  class I molecules, 176, 303, 326–327
  class II molecules, 176, 303, 326–327, 355
Membranous vesicle, see Vesicle
Meningitis, 6, 240, 271–289
  chronic, 280–281
  clinical course, 277–278
  clinical manifestations, 277–281
  diagnosis, 281–283
  epidemiology, 271–275
  infant, 239

neonatal, 223, 229–230, 277–279
pathogenesis and pathology, 275–277
prevention, 283–284
sequelae, 278
treatment, 283–284
Meningoencephalitis, 279–280
Metabolic T lymphocytes, 305
Metoprolol, 329
MHC, see Major histocompatibility complex
Microtubule-associated protein 4, 142
Microvascular damage, pathogenesis of myocarditis and dilated cardiomyopathy, 315
Microwell-based, colorimetric reverse transcription-PCR kit, 409–410
Molecular epidemiology, 15–18
Molecular mimicry, 311–312, 357, 387, 390
Mononuclear cells, interaction with enteroviruses, 243, 245–246, 276
Morphogenesis, 164–166
Motor neuron disease, 387–398
Mouse
  coxsackievirus infection, 175
  Lck-deficiency, 303–304
  lymphocytic choriomeningitis virus, 359–360
  myocarditis, 184–185, 388
  myositis, 388
Mucosal immunity
  poliovirus, 202–203
  poliovirus vaccine, 208
Muscle disease, 387–398
Mutagenesis, 36
Mutant
  characterization, 37–39
  reversion, 41–43
  selection and generation, 36
Mutation, 25
Mutation frequency, 42
Mutation rate, 28, 41–42
Myalgia, epidemic, see Pleurodynia
Myelitis
  paralytic, 271
  transverse, 271
Myocarditis, 4, 47, 175, 178–179, 184–185, 277, 291–351
  age and, 294
  animal model, 295–296
  clinical presentation, 322–325
  clinicopathologic classification, 325
  Dallas criteria, 292, 323–324
  diagnosis, 323–324
  enterovirus detection, 318–322
  epidemiology, 292–295
  evidence linking to dilated cardiomyopathy, 325
  fetal, 227
  gender and, 294–295
  geography and, 295
  histomorphic presentation, 323–324
  immunologic abnormalities, 326
  incidence from postmortem examination, 292
  mouse, 388
  neonatal, 229–230
  outbreaks and epidemics, 294
  pathogenesis, 295–318
    cell-mediated destruction of myofibers, 303–307
    coxsackievirus infection and cardiac dysfunction, 313–315
    host defense mechanisms, 299–303
    immune and autoimmune mechanisms, 309–313
    viral replication in heart, 296–299
    virus in chronic heart disease, 307–309
  pregnancy and, 295, 317–318
  prevalence of associated enteroviral infection, 292–293
  prognosis, 324–325
  race and, 295
  seasonality, 294
  serologic diagnosis, 318–319
  severity of disease
    environmental factors, 318
    physiologic factors, 316–317
    viral factors, 315–316
  treatment
    alpha$_1$-adrenergic antagonists, 327
    angiotensin-converting enzyme inhibitor, 327–328
    antiviral agents, 328–329
    β-blockers, 329
    calcium channel blocker, 329
    conventional, 327–332
    corticosteroids, 329–330
    immunization, 330
    immunomodulating therapy, 330–331
    immunosuppressive therapy, 331–332
    nonsteroidal anti-inflammatory drugs, 332
    thrombolytic agent, 332
  virus detection
    RNA detection, 320–322
    virus isolation, 319–320
Myocytolysis, 297–299
Myopathy, inflammatory, 389–392
Myosin
  antimyosin autoantibody, 311–312
  cardiac myosin autoantigen, 312–313
Myositis, 387–388
Myristoylation, 31, 165

Nasal specimen, 265
Natural killer (NK) cells, pathogenesis of myocarditis and dilated cardiomyopathy, 302, 326
NCR, see Noncoding region
Neonatal mortality, 224

Neonate, 13, 177, *see also* Infant; Perinatal enterovirus infection
  meningitis, 277–279
Neuromuscular disease, 387–398, *see also specific diseases*
  animal model, 388
  viral persistence in muscle or motor neurons, 388–389
  with X-linked agammaglobulinemia, 392
Neurotropism, 276
Neurovirulence, 123, 276
Neutralization test, 413
Neutralizing antibody, pathogenesis of myocarditis and dilated cardiomyopathy, 299
Neutralizing antigenic sites, 31, 177–179
Nitric oxide, pathogenesis of myocarditis and dilated cardiomyopathy, 314–315
NK cells, *see* Natural killer cells
3' Noncoding region (NCR), 97
5' Noncoding region (NCR), 97, 113–115, 276
  AUG codons, 114, 117–118
  binding of cellular peptides and proteins, 122–123
  model, 114–115
  sequence analysis, 114–115
Nonhomologous recombination, 45–47
Nonsteroidal anti-inflammatory drugs, 332
3' Nonterminal repeat (NTR), 30
5' Nonterminal repeat (NTR), 27
Nosocomial transmission, 14, 222–223
NPC 567, 429
NTR, *see* Nonterminal repeat
Nuchal rigidity, 277
Nucleoside triphosphatase, 166
Nucleotide sequence, 15, 25–26, 33–35
Nucleus, virus-infected cells, 135–141
Nutrition, susceptibility to myocarditis and dilated cardiomyopathy, 317

Oligomeric probes, 405–407
Oligonucleotide hybridization test, 16–18
OPV, *see* Oral poliovirus vaccine
Oral poliovirus vaccine (OPV), 201–202, 205–207
  developing world, 210–212
  efficacy, 206, 208
  exclusive use, 209
  OPV-associated poliomyelitis, 206–207
  sequential IPV-OPV immunization, 209
  transmission of OPV viruses, 206
Otitis media, 256, 259–261

Pancarditis, neonatal, 226
Paralytic disease, nonpolio enterovirus, 203–204
Pathogenesis
  genetics, 47–53
  variants with altered properties, 49
PCR methods, 15, 272, 407–411

  cerebrospinal fluid, 281–283
  colorimetric microwell plate assay, 409–410
  myocarditis and dilated cardiomyopathy, 320–321
  neuromuscular disease, 390–393
  universal primers, 407–409
Pentamer, 161–162, 165–166
Perinatal enterovirus infection, 221–238, 277
  clinical presentations, 226–231
  diagnosis, 231–232
  epidemiology, 221–223
  insulin-dependent diabetes mellitus and, 361
  nonpoliovirus, 228–231
  pathogenesis, 223–226
  prevention, 232–233
  sequelae, 230–231
  treatment, 232
Peripartum cardiomyopathy, 295, 318
Persistent infection, 148–149
  chronic heart disease, 308–309
  insulin-dependent diabetes mellitus, 360–361
  neuromuscular disease, 387–398
Pharyngitis, 260
Pharyngotonsillitis, 256, 260
Phenotypic mixing, 40
Physical properties of virion, 155–158
Picornaviridae, 25, 401
Pirodavir, *see* Janssen R77975
Placentitis, 223
Pleurisy, epidemic benign, *see* Pleurodynia
Pleurodynia, 4, 260, 264, 387
PM, *see* Polymyositis
Pneumonia, 256, 260, 263–264
  neonatal, 229
Pneumonitis, fetal, 259
Poliomyelitis, 4, 195–220
  acute, 203, 394
  bulbar, 203
  clinical features, 203–205
  complications, 203
  developing world, 209–210
  differential diagnosis, 203–204
  epidemics, 196–198
  epidemiology, 6–10, 12, 15, 197–198
  experimental infection, 198
  history, 195–201
  major illness, 203
  neonatal, 221–222, 226, 228
  paralytic, 203, 394
  pathogenesis, 198
  population immunity, 197–198
  in pregnancy, 221
  prevention, 200
  prognosis, 204–205
  risk factors, 204
  treatment, 199–200
  vaccine-associated, 206–207

worldwide control, 209–210
Poliovirus
   in amyotrophic lateral sclerosis, 395
   architecture, 162–164
   CD44 in infection, 75, 87
   cell entry, 81–84
   cell-free system for de novo synthesis, 104–106
   characterization, 199
   coding region, 97–98
   complementation map, 41
   cultivation, 199
   dicistronic, 37–38
   discovery, 197
   eradication, 18
   functions of viral proteins, 31–33
   genome structure and function, 27–33, 96–98
      cloverleaf, 28
      IRES, 28–30
   host cell shutoff, 124–128
   host range, 84–86
   humoral immunity, 202
   identification of vaccine strains, 16–17, 411–412
   mucosal immunity, 202–203
   3' noncoding region, 97
   5' noncoding region, 97
   3' nonterminal repeat, 30
   5' nonterminal repeat, 25
   pathogenesis, 201–202
   polyprotein, 30
   postpolio syndrome, 205, 388, 394
   protomer, 157
   replication, complementation in, 39–41
   secretory antibody response, 202–203
   3' terminal polyadenylic acid, 30–31
   tissue tropisms, 86–87
   transmission, 201
      IPV-immunized children, 208
Poliovirus receptor, 48, 73–81, 84–87, 394
   regions that interact with virus, 77–79
Poliovirus vaccine, 15–16, 52–53, 177, 195–220
   adverse vaccine events, 201
   attenuated strains, 49–52
   developing world, 210–212
   development, 195–201
   distinguishing vaccine strains from nonpolio enterovirus, 16–17, 411–412
   efficacy, 206, 210–212
   inactivated (Salk-type), 200, 202, 207–209
   live, attenuated, 201
   oral, 201–202, 205–207, 209
   sequential IPV-OPV immunization, 209
   vaccination strategy and public policy in U.S., 208–209
Polyadenylic acid, 3' terminal, 30–31
Polymyositis (PM), 387, 389–392
Polyprotein
   cleavage, 158–159

   poliovirus, 30
   processing, 158–160
Polypyrimidine tract-binding protein (PTB), 122
Population immunity, poliomyelitis, 197–198
Postpolio syndrome (PPS), 205, 388, 394
PPS, see Postpolio syndrome
Prednisolone, 329
Prednisone, 329–332
Pregnancy, see also Perinatal enterovirus infection
   myocarditis and dilated cardiomyopathy, 295, 317–318
   nonpoliovirus enterovirus infection, 222
   poliomyelitis, 204, 221
   poliomyelitis risk, 204
Prevalence of disease, 6, 11–12
Procapsid, 161–162, 166
Prospective studies, insulin-dependent diabetes mellitus, 371
Protein(s), see also Capsid protein(s)
   interacting with IRES, 120–124
   poliovirus, 31–33
   in RNA synthesis, 98–99
   RNA-protein interactions, 120–124
   secretion in virus-infected cells, 146
Protein 2A, 31–32, 123–128, 158, 161
Protein 2B, 31–32, 98, 143, 146
Protein 2BC, 143–146, 166
Protein 2C, 31–32, 98, 143–145, 166, 180
Protein 3A, 32–33, 143, 146, 149
Protein 3AB, 32–33, 98, 143
Protein 3B, 32–33
   priming model for positive-strand synthesis, 102–104
Protein 3C, 32–33, 99, 125, 127–128, 141, 158–159
Protein 3CD, 32–33, 159, 162
Protein 3D, 99, 159, 166
Protein p220, 124–128
Protein p50, 121
Protein p52, 121–122
Protein p56^{lck}, 303–304
Protein p57, 122
Proteinase, 32–33, 99, 124–126, 141, see also specific proteins
Protomer, 156
   poliovirus, 157
Provirion, 161–162
Prozosin, 327
Pseudotypes, 40, 167
PTB, see Polypyrimidine tract-binding protein
Public health, poliovirus vaccination policy, 208–209

"Quasispecies," 28, 36, 42–43, 47
Quinoline-3-carboxamide, 331

Race, myocarditis and dilated cardiomyopathy, 295

Rainfall, 9
Rash, 277
　　infant, 247–249
RC, see Replication complex
Receptor, 48, 73–93, 276, see also *specific receptors*
　　capsid sequences that control receptor interaction, 75–77
　　　　host range and, 84–86
　　　　regions that interact with virus, 77–79
　　　　tissue tropisms and, 86–87
Recombination, see Genetic recombination
Reinfection, viral heart disease, 316
Replication, see also RNA synthesis
　　poliovirus, complementation in, 39–41
Replication complex (RC), 96, 100–101, 166
　　in vivo specificity, 106
　　structural organization, 100
Replicative cycle, 95
Replicative intermediate (RI), 100, 102
Replicative-form (RF) RNA, 100, 102
Respiratory infection, 255–270
　　clinical presentations, 259–264
　　diagnosis, 264–265
　　epidemiology, 256–257
　　immunity, 258–259
　　infant, 247–249
　　pathogenesis and pathology, 257–259
　　treatment, 265
Respiratory transmission, 5, 12–14, 257
Retrograde transport, 144–145
Reverse transcription PCR, 407–410
Reversion, 37–39, 41–43
RF RNA, see Replicative-form RNA
RI, see Replicative intermediate
Ribavarin, 329, 420
Ribosome landing pad, see Internal ribosome entry site
RNA, 402
　　detection
　　　　insulin-dependent diabetes mellitus, 371
　　　　myocarditis and dilated cardiomyopathy, 320–322
　　encapsidation, 100, 159, 165–167
　　persistence in chronic heart disease, 307–308
　　single-stranded, 100
　　uncoating, 81–84
RNA polymerase
　　cellular, 127–128
　　RNA-dependent, 99, 106
　　viral, 46–47, 166
RNA probes, 405–407
RNA synthesis, 44–45, 95–112
　　biphasic, 101
　　cell-free system, 104–106
　　cellular, 127–128
　　coupling to encapsidation, 166–167
　　coupling to translation, 106–107
　　in vitro systems, 101
　　in vivo specificity of replication complex, 106
　　inhibitors, 145–146
　　initiation, 99
　　membrane-associated, 143–147
　　negative-strand, 99, 101–102
　　positive-strand, 99–100, 102–104
　　processive mechanism, 44–46
　　products, 100
　　proteins involved, 98–99
　　RNA sequences involved, 99
　　site of replication complex, 100–101, 142
　　two-step process, 101
RNA translocase, 166
RNA-binding protein, 99, 120–124
RNA-protein interactions, 120–124
RNase L, 420–421
Ro 09-0410, 423, 429
Rp-α protein, 81
Rubella, congenital, 359–360
Rural-urban occurrence, 9

Salicylates, 332
Salk vaccine, 200
Sanitation, 8, 12
SCH 38057, 423–428
Seasonality, 11, 256, 294, 353, 364
Secondary attack rates, household, 14
Secretory antibody response
　　poliovirus, 202–203
　　poliovirus vaccine, 206
Secretory pathways, 144–145
　　inhibitors, 145–146
　　virus-infected cells, 146
Secular trends, 11
Sedimentation coefficient, virion, 156
Sepsis, infant, 241–242
Seroepidemiology, insulin-dependent diabetes mellitus, 367–371
Serologic diagnosis, 412–413
　　myocarditis and dilated cardiomyopathy, 318–319
Serosurvey, 6, 412
Serotypes, 401–402
　　serotype identification, 411–412
Sewage, 10, 13, 197
Sex hormones, effect on cell-mediated cytotoxicity, 306–307
Shellfish, 10
Single-stranded RNA, 100
Site-directed mutagenesis, 36
Slot blot hybridization, 320–321
Snapback model, HF-dependent, 102
Socioeconomic status, 8–9, 240
Soil, contaminated, 10–11
Soluble-receptor-resistant mutants, 75–76, 83
Specimen

collection and storage, 402–403
processing
    for inoculation of cell culture, 404
    for PCR studies, 407
Sporadic (endemic) disease, 6, 11
Stillbirth, 224, 226–227
Strand switching, 43–44
Surface water, 10
Surveillance data, 5–7
Susceptibility status, 9
Swimming area, 10
Syndrome of inappropriate antidiuretic hormone, 278, 283

T cells, 176, 179–185
  cytolytic, see Cytolytic T lymphocytes
  epitopes, 176, 182–183
  host genetics and, 305–306
  metabolic, 305
  pathogenesis of myocarditis and dilated cardiomyopathy, 303–307
  splenic, reactive against virus-infected myofibers, 304
TATA-binding protein (TBP), 128
  cleavage, 140–141
Taxonomy, 401
TBP, see TATA-binding protein
Temporal trends, insulin-dependent diabetes mellitus, 364–365
3' Terminal polyadenylic acid, 30–31
Terminal uridylyl transferase (TUTase), 102
Throat specimen, 265
Thrombolytic agent, 332
Tissue culture, see Cell culture
Tissue tropism, 48–49, 276
  coxsackievirus, 87
  poliovirus, 86–87
  receptors and, 86–87
Tonsillectomy, during incubation period of poliomyelitis, 204
Tonsillitis, 260
Transcription, infectious viral RNA, 35–36
Transcription factor CREB/ATF, 128
Transcription factor IID, 140
Transcription factor IIIC, 128
trans-initiation model, positive-strand RNA synthesis, 104–105
Translation, 113–124
  coupling to RNA synthesis, 106–107
  initiation, 113–118
Translation initiation factor eIF-3, 125–126
Translation initiation factor eIF-4B, 125
Translation initiation factor eIF-4F, 124–125
Transmission, 5, 9, 12–15, 256–257, see also specific routes
  poliovirus, 201, 206–208
Transplacental transmission, 7, 223–224, 277
Transport vesicle, 144–145
Trauma, poliomyelitis risk, 204
Treatment
  antiviral agents, 419–434
  meningitis and encephalitis, 283–284
  nonpolio enterovirus in infant, 252
  respiratory infection, 265
Tumor necrosis factor, pathogenesis of myocarditis and dilated cardiomyopathy, 313–314
Tumor necrosis factor therapy, myocarditis and dilated cardiomyopathy, 331
TUTase, see Terminal uridylyl transferase

Uncoating of RNA, 81–84
Urban area, 9
Urogenital anomalies, 227–228

Vaccine
  poliovirus, see Poliovirus vaccine
  vaccine-associated disease, 177
Vascular injury, pathogenesis of myocarditis and dilated cardiomyopathy, 315
Venereal transmission, 13
Verapamil, 329
Vesicle, 100–101, 135, 143–147
  formation in uninfected and infected cells, 144–145
  inhibition of formation, 145–146
Viral exit, 147–150
Viremia, 242–244, 258, 275
Virion, physical properties, 155–158
Virus-encoded oligopeptide (VPg), 27, 32, 102–104, 113–114
Vomiting, infant, 247–249
VPg, see Virus-encoded oligopeptide

Waterborne transmission, 5, 10, 12–13
Wheezing, 256, 263
WIN 51711, 422–424, 426–428
WIN 54954, 329, 373, 422–423, 427–429
WIN compounds, 82–83, 422–429